Thieme

Lower Extremity Reconstruction

A Practical Guide

Joon Pio Hong, MD, PhD, MMM
Professor of Plastic Surgery
Asan Medical Center University of Ulsan
Seoul, Korea

Geoffrey G. Hallock, MD
Consultant
Division of Plastic Surgery
Sacred Heart Campus
St. Luke's Hospital
Allentown, Pennsylvania, USA

608 illustrations

Thieme
New York • Stuttgart • Delhi • Rio de Janeiro

Library of Congress Cataloging-in-Publication Data is available from the publisher.

Thieme Publishers New York
333 Seventh Avenue, New York, NY 10001 USA
+1 800 782 3488, customerservice@thieme.com

Georg Thieme Verlag KG
Rüdigerstrasse 14, 70469 Stuttgart, Germany
+49 [0]711 8931 421, customerservice@thieme.de

Thieme Publishers Delhi
A-12, Second Floor, Sector-2, Noida-201301
Uttar Pradesh, India
+91 120 45 566 00, customerservice@thieme.in

Thieme Publishers Rio de Janeiro
Thieme Publicações Ltda.
Edifício Rodolpho de Paoli, 25º andar
Av. Nilo Peçanha, 50 – Sala 2508
Rio de Janeiro 20020-906 Brasil
+55 21 3172 2297 / +55 21 3172 1896

Cover design: Thieme Publishing Group
Typesetting by DiTech Process Solutions, India

Printed in USA by King Printing Company, Inc. 5 4 3 2 1

ISBN 978-1-62623-808-4

Also available as an e-book:
eISBN 978-1-62623-809-1

Important note: Medicine is an ever-changing science undergoing continual development. Research and clinical experience are continually expanding our knowledge, in particular our knowledge of proper treatment and drug therapy. Insofar as this book mentions any dosage or application, readers may rest assured that the authors, editors, and publishers have made every effort to ensure that such references are in accordance with **the state of knowledge at the time of production of the book.**

Nevertheless, this does not involve, imply, or express any guarantee or responsibility on the part of the publishers in respect to any dosage instructions and forms of applications stated in the book. **Every user is requested to examine carefully** the manufacturers' leaflets accompanying each drug and to check, if necessary in consultation with a physician or specialist, whether the dosage schedules mentioned therein or the contraindications stated by the manufacturers differ from the statements made in the present book. Such examination is particularly important with drugs that are either rarely used or have been newly released on the market. Every dosage schedule or every form of application used is entirely at the user's own risk and responsibility. The authors and publishers request every user to report to the publishers any discrepancies or inaccuracies noticed. If errors in this work are found after publication, errata will be posted at www.thieme.com on the product description page.

Some of the product names, patents, and registered designs referred to in this book are in fact registered trademarks or proprietary names even though specific reference to this fact is not always made in the text. Therefore, the appearance of a name without designation as proprietary is not to be construed as a representation by the publisher that it is in the public domain.

FSC
www.fsc.org
100%
Paper from well-managed forests
FSC® C103101

Contents

Videos

Foreword

Time flies! It is hard to imagine that three decades ago, the concept of perforator flaps was at its infancy, and it was 16 years ago when I put together the first issue in *Clinics in Plastic Surgery* on perforator flaps.

The devoted and relentless effort put forth by numerous reconstructive microsurgeons since then has brought about marvelous advancements.

Indeed, the leap the field of reconstructive microsurgery has taken with the introduction of perforator flap surgery has revolutionized our approach.

The muscle or fascia is no longer considered an essential blood supply carrier to skin, and they can be left in place to serve their original function with none to minimal damage.

Donor site morbidity has been minimized. Reconstruction has evolved from simple wound coverage to functional restoration in a more refined manner, and to better benefit the patient.

The "Gent" consensus on perforator flap terminology in 2003 reminds us this is truly a field that has progressed through international collaboration.

One should not forget that the current state-of-the-art free tissue transfers is the result of unprecedented work by giants who contributed either directly or indirectly to perforator flaps.

Ian Taylor's angiosome studies laid down the anatomic foundation of our work today. Nakajima, Kroll, Allen, Koshima, Blondeel, and many others have not only pioneered this field but created a propelling force that carried us into the new century.

Hallock is one of the founding fathers and a pioneer of perforator flaps. For decades, he never ceased to inspire me with his profound contribution to this field and its nomenclature. And, while the definition of a true perforator remains a matter of debate, we all agree that Hallock has shaped much of our language on perforator flaps, not to mention all the beautiful and complex cases he has mastered.

JP is a star in reconstructive microsurgery and perforator flaps. His work, based on Koshima's earlier contribution, has taken perforator flaps to new frontiers such as the thin and ultra-thin flaps and supermicrosurgery. I like how he reminds us that there is always room to innovate and create.

Writing the foreword of this new book on lower extremity reconstruction with an emphasis on perforator flaps has been a pleasure to me. I loved witnessing two generations of surgeons working together to capture it all: origin, evolution and progress, state of the art, and future in one beautifully-crafted and exciting book. This is no doubt a must-read and must-have book.

Fu-Chan Wei, MD, FACS
Distinguished Chair Professor
Department of Plastic and Reconstructive Surgery
Chang Gung Memorial Hospital
Chang Gung University Medical College
Taoyuan, Taiwan

Preface

On the first day of my training as a resident in plastic surgery, I was led to a room where a patient with a near total degloving of the entire thigh and leg was lying on the table. I really thought that I had come into the wrong operating room as I did not comprehend the harsh reality of the reconstruction world. After this case of debridement and dressings, I realized what reconstruction can be. Plastic surgery is not a glamorous field, but a field where we hope to restore the subnormal to normal. And when I saw the patient walk again, I knew this was what I needed to do. But lower extremity reconstruction is one of the most difficult fields of reconstruction. I not only had to learn through tough training but also seek wisdom from publications from masters from all over the world. Dr Hallock in my opinion was the leading figure from whom I obtained the knowledge to provide better care for these patients. Every time I had a question and looked up papers to satisfy my curiosity, his paper would always be addressing those issues or be guiding me further to seek more evidence. Ultimately, I met my hero through a meeting in India, and I have been privileged since to become a close friend. Not surprisingly, we had very similar interests and questions.

As we discussed together over the years afterwards, we realized that plastic surgeons have a conception that lower extremity reconstruction is more difficult than other fields of our specialty. Although this may be true, we believe with the right understanding and approach, lower extremity care can be interesting and as worthwhile as any other reconstruction procedure. I am proud to see my fellows and residents, whom I was honored to train, also do lower extremity reconstruction as they do any other reconstruction procedure. Learning proper preoperative, intraoperative, and postoperative care led them to practice in lower extremity reconstruction with confidence and to accept new challenges.

As a co-editor of this book with Dr Hallock, I am now privileged to share what I have learned and experienced throughout my career. Our common idea was to make this book to be as practical as possible in the hope that it will help you to guide in your lower extremity practice with less anxiety. Sometimes as surgeons we are faced with cases where a new procedure is required or a new approach is necessary. This book will hopefully guide you through any clinical situations you might encounter.

I have written this book for any reconstructive surgeon who will be or is currently faced with demands for lower extremity reconstruction in the hope that you will not have to endure the problems of a trial & error approach as I have. My best example is the diabetic foot which is not just surgery treating wounds, but involving various other factors that require a multidisciplinary approach and collegiality with our other subspecialty colleagues. Since I have identified these factors and began working closely with these other professionals, my complication rate after reconstruction has been reduced significantly. Throughout the book, we will talk about these factors and how to address them or altogether avoid them accordingly. The accompanying videos will help you see how the other experts perform these surgeries as appropriate.

Finally, we will be very interested in your feedback. Your criticism and opinions are important to further extend our knowledge and improve our format to be more reader or learner friendly. It is our goal to bring together all reconstructive surgeons to share their work and passion in the field of lower extremity reconstruction which ultimately will lead to further evolution and progress within this discipline.

Joon Pio Hong, MD, PhD, MMM

Preface

Unlike today when training in microsurgical techniques is just another standard regimen that must be endured by all in every fellowship program, this was not always true. In my era, the so-called random flaps, length to width ratios, and delay maneuvers were skills that had to be mastered by every novice including this enthusiastic newcomer in plastic and reconstructive surgery. Lower extremity coverage was routinely achieved with distant flaps, like what we called "cross-leg flaps." These were usually safe yet cumbersome procedures, and very time consuming from the patients' perspective. Pedicle division prior to adequate neovascularization from the recipient site would be a disaster, as we would then have to start from the beginning again. Usually, we soon learned the tricks to know when and how to prevent this from occurring, but not always. Stress centered around the dictum that "no wound left the hospital unhealed," and rounds had to be done every day sometimes for weeks.

Change indeed is the only thing that is predictable. Becoming an attending was not the light at the end of the tunnel. Starting afresh in a trauma center, it was impossible to avoid the cornucopia of lower extremity defects that needed basic soft tissue coverage. Here there was a live animal vivarium and a microscope that the director used to teach tuboplasties for sterilization reversal by the obstetricians. It seemed reasonable to try to raise free flaps in the available rats, which, once mastered (if that were possible?), extended our reach to real patients to hopefully better solve the treatment of their complex wounds. By then muscle flaps had just become acceptable, and soon thereafter fasciocutaneous flaps. In a few laborious years, microsurgical tissue transfers became our standard preference; and after a few hundred flaps so routine that admittedly it became boring. Fortunately, the advent of perforator flaps just some two decades ago became not just a fascination, but an obsession, and quite frankly a career rejuvenation. Perforator flaps—never the same, always mindful for anomalies, always stimulating, always an intellectual challenge. The flap became the thing, as after all, the microsurgery was just "work."

Teaching became a privilege, and not just an excuse for not to have to "work." While trying to spread the gospel of the perforator flap at our annual international meeting in Coimbatore, India, one of the "free paper" presenters introduced himself to me during the afterwards social events. Networking—it was no other and none better than "jp" (as he is known) Hong! By the next year, he, too, was on the faculty! For that matter, thereafter at every meeting of every kind no matter where in the world, there too was "jp" Hong—and usually in my absence as I would be "working"! We repeatedly found that we had common interests besides just perforator flaps and their application to the lower extremity reconstruction. Several times we even teamed up to do live surgery, and it was amazingly fast and efficient. Probably because he was always challenging dogma and the status quo. But had I not endured just that when I introduced microsurgery in my own youth as a better way to treat the victims of trauma? We recognized that especially the reconstruction of the lower extremity will always require our love of both flaps and microsurgery. Even local perforator flaps, now more commonly used, still require the dexterity and cautiousness typical of microsurgical techniques. Microsurgery has become inescapable.

So who could really be surprised that we decided to compile together our thoughts and experiences, and those of our most esteemed colleagues, in a book, specifically on reconstruction of the lower extremity? We wanted to challenge the concept that all books must be encyclopedias. We sought a practical resource that includes all the basic flaps, which can be quickly reviewed via videos, as well as some more complex means to care for the lower extremity properly. Hopefully, our format will prove to be easily accessible and provide just the right smattering of esoteric knowledge, including a step-by-step demonstration of each technique with some pertinent case examples. If users say that they have not read a single written chapter, but have found the videos to be priceless, have we not achieved our goal without compromise? Indeed amazing, the "young and the restless" blended perfectly with the wisdom of this ancient historian.

Geoffrey Hallock, MD

Acknowledgment

First of all, I would like thank my co-author and friend, Dr Geoffrey Hallock. Every step of the way in the making of this book, never was there a dull moment. It was a huge treat working with my hero and sharing the hope that this book with bring more confidence in reconstructive surgeons in providing reconstruction for lower extremity cases.

I was privileged to have many wonderful mentors and there are few mentors that have really had a profound impact and shaped me the way I am today. My life as a reconstructive surgeon all started with professor Yoon Kyu Chung back at Wonju, Korea. He opened my eyes to reconstruction. He taught me that there is always something to learn from a good as well as a bad experience. I still consult with him on various cases and feel grateful that I have a "reconstruction family home" to go to when I am facing a challenge. Dr David Chang from University of Chicago has shown me the importance of sharing. Not only sharing knowledge with your peers but also serving in case of need. His guidance has made me realize what my calling is. To be a part of peoples' path and help them grow. Jason Yoon, the former Chairman to Daewoong Pharmaceutical and my confidant, has led me to understand the world of business. He taught me how to use constraint and to be consciously aware of decisions you make in your life. Finally, my father, Soon-Young Hong, who passed away few years ago. He has always taught me to follow the right path even though it meant taking the long road. I miss him dearly as I walk along this road of life today.

I am grateful that I have a wonderful team led by my friend and partner Dr Hyunsuk Peter Suh. Working with him, and with plastic surgery colleagues, anesthesiologists, fellows, residents, nurses, and other specialists at Asan Medical Center is an unbelievable experience. It is always a pleasure coming to work and engaging with this group of professionals, aiming to provide better solutions to help our patients. All the past fellows and residents, to be a part of your path was a privilege.

Finally, I want to thank God and my family. Without God's never-ending grace, mercy, and provision I would not have had this wonderful life to serve others. Without my family's support and love, I would not be where I am today.

Thank you.

Joon Pio Hong, MD, PhD, MMM

Acknowledgments

If anyone needs to be appreciated, I realize that none of this would have happened without the gentle persuasion and enthusiasm of my young co-editor, "jp" Hong. I also realize that no microsurgery would have ever been possible without all the nurses, orderlies, anesthesiologists, and consultants who have tolerated me for so long. My physician extender, David C. Rice, B.S., and I learned from rats not just how to do free flaps, but how to do them using the essential team approach format for decades.

My focused learning continues to be derived from my extraordinary fellow members of the International Perforator Flap Faculty—Bob Allen, Claudio Angrigiani, Mark Ashton, Isao Koshima, Koen van Landuyt, Jaume Masia, Nathalie Roche, Eric Santamaria, G. Ian Taylor, Fu chan Wei, as well as many others perhaps overlooked; and, of course, the other three from our "Gang of 4," Phillip Blondeel, Steve Morris, and Peter Neligan. Recently, even more extraordinary for this country doctor has been the numerous invitations to Asia, where my interest in perforator flaps in particular has been accelerated well beyond my dreams and abilities. I hope my meager educational forays there have been successful, and surely the ability for cross-communication bolstered by the efforts of my "leftover" Chinese translator, Wu yang Zhang, with whom I have been privileged to simultaneously explore many worlds not usually open to Americans.

Geoffrey Hallock, MD

Contributors

Mouchammed Agko, MD
Assistant Professor of Surgery
Department of Surgery
Section of Plastic Surgery
Medical College of Georgia
Augusta University
Augusta, Georgia, USA

Oskar C. Aszmann, MD
Professor
Division of Plastic and Reconstructive Surgery
Department of Surgery
Clinical Laboratory for Bionic Extremity Reconstruction
Medical University of Vienna
Vienna, Austria

Christopher Attinger, MD
Professor
Plastic and Orthopedic Surgery
Medstar Georgetown University Hospital
Washington, DC, USA

Karim Bakri, MD
Assistant Professor of Plastic Surgery and Orthopedics
Program Director, Plastic Surgery Residency
Division of Plastic Surgery
Department of Surgery
Mayo Clinic
Rochester, Minnesota, USA

Oded Ben-Amotz, MD
Attending Physician
Maccabi Health System
Tel Aviv, Israel

Pedro C. Cavadas, MD, PhD
Chief of Clínica Cavadas
Associate Professor of Microsurgery
Department of Surgery
CEU University School of Medicine
Valencia, Spain

Hung-Chi Chen, MD, PhD, FACS
Professor of Plastic Surgery
Chairman, Department of Plastic and Reconstructive Surgery
China Medical University
China Medical University Hospital International Medical Service Center
Taichung, Taiwan

Rachel M. Clancy, MBChB, MA, MRCS, Med
Plastic Surgery Fellow
University of Toronto
Toronto, Ontario, Canada

David L. Colen, MD
Assistant Professor of Surgery (Plastic and Reconstructive)
Yale School of Medicine
New Haven, Connecticut, USA

Lawrence B. Colen, MD, FACS
Professor of Surgery (Plastic and Reconstructive)
Eastern Virginia Medical School
Norfolk, Virginia, USA

Michael V. Defazio, MD
Plastic and Reconstructive Surgeon
Florida Plastic Surgery Group
Baptist MD Anderson Cancer Center
Jacksonville, Florida, USA

Karen K. Evans, MD
Professor
Department of Plastic and Reconstructive Surgery
MedStar Georgetown University Hospital
Washington, DC, USA

Waleed Gibreel, MBBS
Chief Resident
Division of Plastic Surgery
Department of Surgery
Mayo Clinic
Rochester, Minnesota, USA

Lawrence J. Gottlieb, MD, FACS
Professor of Surgery
The University of Chicago Medicine and Biological Sciences
Chicago, Illinois, USA

Clemens Gstoettner, MD, PhD
Resident
Clinical Laboratory for Bionic Extremity Reconstruction
Medical University of Vienna
Vienna, Austria

Geoffrey G. Hallock, MD
Consultant
Division of Plastic Surgery
Sacred Heart Campus
St. Luke's Hospital
Allentown, Pennsylvania, USA

Mitsunobu Harima, MD
Senior Resident
Plastic and Reconstructive Surgery
The University of Tokyo
Tokyo, Japan

Alexander de Heinrich, MD
Attending, Department of Plastic, Reconstructive, Hand and Burn Surgery
Muenchen Klinik Bogenhausen
Academic Teaching Hospital Technical University
Munich, Germany

Joon Pio Hong, MD, PhD, MMM
Professor of Plastic Surgery
Asan Medical Center University of Ulsan
Seoul, Korea

Hirofumi Imai, MD
Assistant Professor
International Center for Lymphedema
Hiroshima University Hospital
Hiroshima city, Japan

Marco Innocenti, MD
Professor of Plastic Surgery
University of Florence;
Director, Plastic Surgery Department
Careggi University Hospital
Florence, Italy

Matthew Iorio, MD
Associate Professor
Director, Plastic and Reconstructive Hand Surgery
Co-Director, Extremity Microsurgical Reconstruction
Co-Director, Wound Care Program
Division of Plastic Surgery
University of Colorado Hospital
Aurora, Colorado, USA

Jeffrey E. Janis, MD, FACS
Professor of Plastic Surgery, Neurosurgery, Neurology, and Surgery
Chief of Plastic Surgery, University Hospital
Ohio State University Wexner Medical Center
Columbus, Ohio, USA

Ibrahim Khansa, MD
Clinical Assistant Professor of Plastic and Reconstructive Surgery
The Ohio State University;
Craniofacial Surgeon
Director, Hemangioma and Vascular Malformations Program
Columbus, Ohio, USA

Isao Koshima, MD
Professor and Chief
International Center for Lymphedema
Hiroshima University Hospital
Hiroshima, Japan

Stephen J. Kovach, MD, FACS
Herndon B. Lehr Endowed Associate Professor of Surgery
Associate Professor, Division of Plastic Surgery
Associate Professor, Department of Orthopaedic Surgery
University of Pennsylvania Health System
Philadelphia, Pennsylvania, USA

Casey T. Kraft, MD
Resident
Ohio State University Wexner Medical Center
Columbus, Ohio, USA

L. Scott Levin, MD, FACS
Paul B. Magnuson Professor of Bone and Joint Surgery
Chairman, Department of Orthopaedic Surgery
Professor of Surgery, Division of Plastic Surgery
University of Pennsylvania Health System
Philadelphia, Pennsylvania, USA

Samir Mardini, MD
Professor of Surgery
Chair, Division of Plastic Surgery
Department of Surgery
Mayo Clinic
Rochester, Minnesota, USA

Shaun D. Mendenhall, MD
Assistant Professor of Surgery
Hand and Plastic Surgery
University of Utah Health
Salt Lake City, Utah, USA

Haruki Mizuta, MD,
Senior Resident
Plastic and Reconstructive Surgery
University of Tokyo
Tokyo, Japan

Steven L. Moran, MD
Professor of Plastic Surgery and Orthopedic Surgery
Mayo Clinic
Rochester, Minnesota, USA

Steven F. Morris, MD, MSc, FRCSC
Professor of Surgery and Medical Neurosciences
Dalhousie University
Halifax, Nova Scotia, Canada

Shogo Nagamatsu, MD
Lecturer
Plastic and Reconstructive Surgery
Hiroshima University Hospital
Hiroshima, Japan

Manas Nigam, MD
Academic Chief Resident
Department of Plastic and Reconstructive Surgery
MedStar Georgetown University Hospital
Washington, DC, USA

Marina Ninković, MD
Assistant Professor
Physical Medicine and Rehabilitation
Department of Visceral, Transplant and Thoracic Surgery
Center of Operative Medicine
Innsbruck Medical University
Innsbruck, Austria

Milomir Ninković, MD, PhD
Chairman, Department of Plastic, Reconstructive, Hand and Burn Surgery
Muenchen Klinik Bogenhausen
Academic Teaching Hospital Technical University
Munich, Germany

Changsik John Park, MD, PhD
Assistant professor of Plastic Surgery
Asan Medical Center University of Ulsan
Seoul, Korea

Madhu Periasamy, MBBS, MS, MRCS, DNB
Consultant
Plastic, Trauma, and Chronic Wound Reconstructive Surgery
Ganga Hospital
Coimbatore, India

Patrick L. Reavey, MD, MS
Assistant Professor of Surgery
Assistant Professor Orthopedic Surgery
University of Rochester Medical Center
Rochester, Minnesota, USA

S. Raja Sabapathy, MS, MS (Gen), MCh (Plastic), DNB (Plastic), FRCS (Edin.), Hon FRCS (Glas), FAMS, DSc (Hon)
Chairman
Department of Plastic, Hand, Reconstructive Microsurgery and Burns
Ganga Hospital
Coimbatore, India

Stefan Salminger, MD, PhD
Resident
Division of Plastic and Reconstructive Surgery
Department of Surgery
Clinical Laboratory for Bionic Extremity Reconstruction
Medical University of Vienna
Vienna, Austria

Eric Santamaria, MD
Professor Of Reconstructive Microsurgery
Universidad Nacional Autonoma De Mexico
Department Of Plastic And Reconstructive Surgery
Hospital General Dr. Manuel Gea Gonzalez
Mexico City, Mexico

Stephen Andrew Sems, MD
Assistant Professor of Orthopaedics
Division Chairman, Orthopaedic Trauma Surgery
Mayo Clinic
Rochester, Minnesota, USA

Agnes Sturma, MSc, BSc, PhD
Physiotherapist
Clinical Laboratory for Bionic Extremity Reconstruction
Medical University of Vienna
Vienna, Austria;
Department of Bioengineering
Imperial College London
London, UK

Hyunsuk Peter Suh, MD, PhD
Assistant Professor
Department of Plastic Surgery
Asan Medical Center University of Ulsan
Seoul, Korea

Young Chul Suh, MD
Clinical Assistant Professor of Plastic Surgery
Bucheon St. Mary Hospital
The Catholic University of Korea
Gyeonggi-do, South Korea

Hari Venkatramani, MS, MCh, DNB EDHS
Senior Consultant
Plastic and Trauma Reconstructive Surgery Department
Ganga Hospital
Coimbatore, India

Alison Wong, MD
Plastic Surgery Resident
Department of Surgery
Division of Plastic Surgery
Dalhousie University
Halifax, Nova Scotia, Canada

Karen W . Wong, MD, MSc, FRCSC
Assistant Professor
University of Toronto;
Staff Surgeon
Hospital for Sick Children
Toronto, Ontario, Canada

Shuji Yamashita, MD
Associate Professor
Plastic and Reconstructive Surgery
The University of Tokyo
Tokyo, Japan

Kazunori Yokota, MD
Professor
Plastic and Reconstructive Surgery
Hiroshima University Hospital
Hiroshima, Japan

Shuhei Yoshida, MD
Associate Professor
International Center for Lymphedema
Hiroshima University Hospital
Hiroshima, Japan

Nicole A. Zelenski, MD
Hand Fellow
Mayo Clinic
Rochester, Minnesota, USA

Ronald M. Zuker, MD, FRCSC, FACS, FAAP, FRCSEd (Hon)
Staff Surgeon
Division of Plastic and Reconstructive Surgery
The Hospital for Sick Children;
Professor of Surgery
The University of Toronto
Toronto, Ontario, Canada

1 Our Introduction to Lower Extremity Reconstruction

Joon Pio Hong and Geoffrey G. Hallock

Summary
For a myriad of reasons, the lower extremity may be considered the most challenging of all body regions to reconstruct. Do not forget that the goal will always be to restore ambulatory function as much as possible, while ensuring long-term retention of vital structures or prosthesis, and obtaining an appearance that is satisfactory to the patient. Our capabilities to achieve this are in a constant state of evolution, as new techniques and/or innovations must be carefully scrutinized as to their efficacy. Although in the past amputation may have been the only treatment option, many surgical and nonsurgical means are now available to allow success in limb salvage. It behooves everyone interested in the management of these lower limb dilemmas to be aware of the long history of dealing with these challenges and to be familiar with the cornucopia of choices that must be made to best accomplish the outcome expected by the patients and their families (▶ Fig. 1.1).

Keywords: lower extremity reconstruction, lower limb salvage, amputation, microsurgery, perforator flaps

1.1 Introduction

Lower extremity reconstruction, whether needed for a sequela of severe trauma, cancer ablation, diabetes and/or vascular disease, or chronic infections, remains the most challenging of all reconstructions of the human body. The involvement of multiple discrete structures including bone, muscle, tendon, vessel, and nerve, all contained within the skin itself, makes it difficult to achieve the goal of restoring function, having long-term coverage of vital structures, and obtaining a satisfactory appearance of the lower limb. The objective of our effort then is to provide a pragmatic guide for our readers to understand the preoperative, intraoperative, and postoperative processes that will ultimately help them to develop a logical approach to lower extremity reconstruction that will more likely lead to a successful outcome.

Everyone must also understand that the management of lower extremity defects, whether complex or the most simple, is in a constant state of evolution as we are inundated daily by numerous new techniques and/or innovations that must be carefully scrutinized as to their worthiness. This has allowed the salvage of extremities today, whereas in the past amputation may have been the only alternative. For example, significant bone gaps can now be overcome by the current availability of vascularized bone grafts, Ilizarov lengthening, bone matrices, and growth factors. This coupled with new insights derived from our enhanced knowledge of anatomy like negative pressure wound therapy, tissue expansion or creep, and perforator flaps including propeller flaps has permitted superior soft-tissue coverage. Advances in microsurgery now reliably allow the use of small arteries (even < 1 mm in caliber for donor or recipient site anastomoses), or similarly permit lymphatic vessel interventions that will provide better surgical solutions for lymphedema.

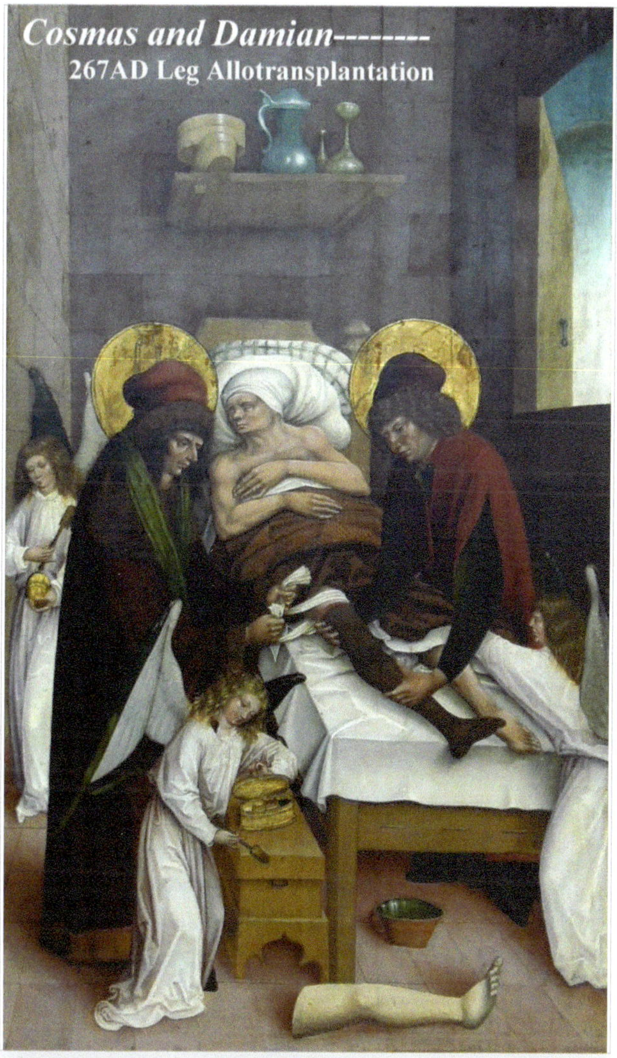

Fig. 1.1 Non-vascularized composite tissue allotransplantation.

Any attempt at lower extremity salvage must be recognized as a long and complex process for both the medical professional and the patients and their support systems. Therefore, as physicians it is important to ensure that all patients and family members are properly informed and included in any decision-making process,[1] while maintaining on their part an accurate awareness of the expected prognosis. This approach should impact positively on any patient's motivation and compliance while retaining the support of the family that will be critical not only during the necessary surgeries and hospitalization but also throughout the long phases of physical and psychological recovery.

1.2 History

Many say that the best use of the present is to rely on the past to make the future. What was the best solution may still be so, and at the least it has already had a definitive outcome that can

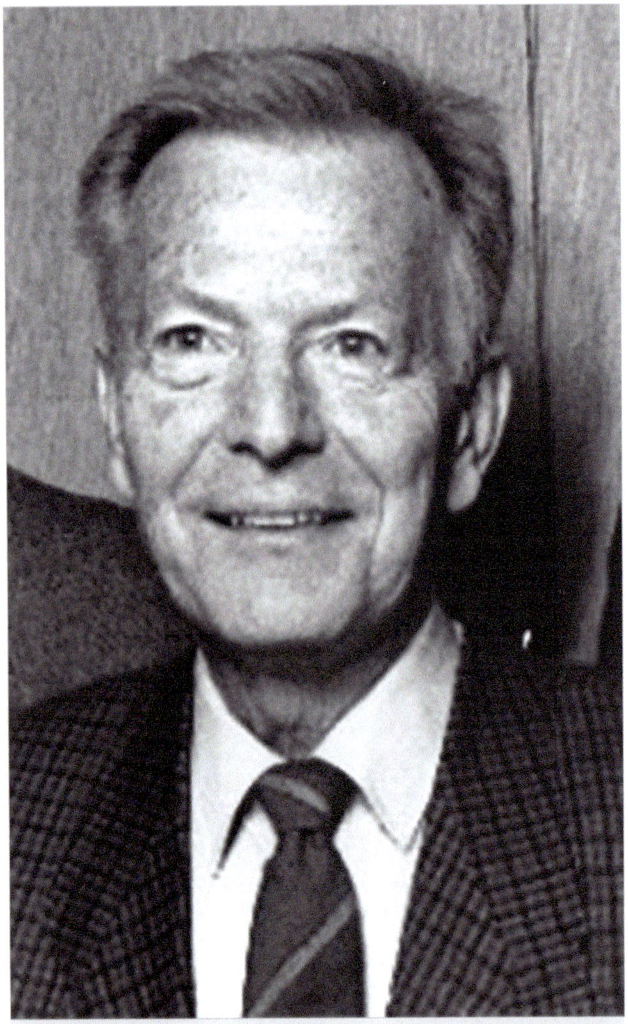

Fig. 1.2 Bengt Pontén: rediscovered fasciocutaneous flaps.

appear predictable. So, history *is* important, and this has been acknowledged by us in the introduction of every chapter, where that pertinent saga has been included.

The early history of lower extremity reconstruction dates back to Hippocrates (460–370 BC), when amputation was the norm, and procedures trying to improve the success of amputation and survival of life itself were the main practice up to World War I.[2] Although early amputation and rapid prosthetic fitting was believed to offer the potential of faster recovery at a lower cost, recent reports have differed from this traditional viewpoint. Undeniably, the choice of reconstruction will be a more challenging path to be taken; yet, the Lower Extremity Assessment Project (LEAP) study showed no significant difference in outcome when compared to amputation at 2 years.[3] Interestingly, a cost analysis derived from this study concluded that amputation was more expensive than limb salvage, and amputation yielded fewer quality-adjusted life-years than salvage.[4] Other reports have shown similar findings where projected lifetime health care costs for amputation may be as high as three times that spent on limb salvage.[5,6] Even if the entire lower extremity cannot be salvaged, the primary goal now should be to maintain maximal limb length with durable soft-tissue coverage of any stump that can then be fitted properly with a prosthesis that will allow a functional gait. Preservation of the knee joint as in a below-knee amputation requires far less energy consumption, and has the potential for two- to threefold greater mobility when compared to an above-knee amputation.[7,8]

Not until the First and Second World Wars were pedicled flaps of some form used extensively to repair lower extremity injuries (▸ Fig. 1.2). Many of these had a discrete vascular supply, which today would be called “axial pattern flaps.”[9] Stark[10] and later Ger[11] recognized that the leg muscles themselves were reliable flaps for leg coverage, having an abundant blood supply if outside the zone of injury (▸ Fig. 1.3).

With the advent of microsurgical capabilities, extensive and complex defects even after severe trauma and truly radical debridements could be solved (▸ Fig. 1.4).

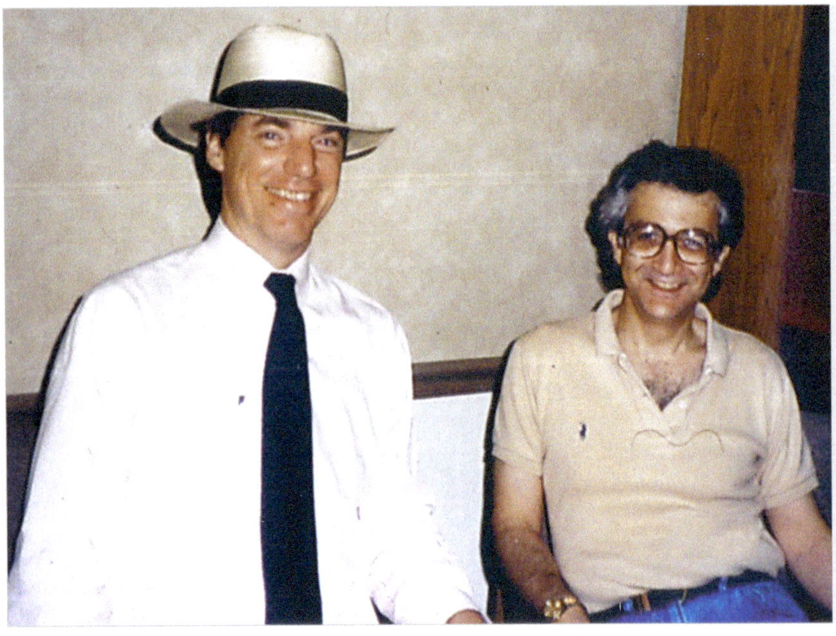

Fig. 1.3 Stephen Mathes and Foad Nahai: classification of muscle flaps.

In 1986, a landmark publication for reconstructive lower extremity microsurgery by Godina established the principles of early extensive debridement, immediate free tissue transfer, and aggressive rehabilitation that routinely salvaged functional limbs.[12] Radical debridement and coverage within 72 hours compared to more delayed treatment had superior outcomes, as only 0.75% of flaps failed, 1.5% of limbs became infected, and early bony union within 6.8 months was the norm.[12]

This dramatic deviation from established principles was followed by the development of functioning muscle transfers,[13] innervated flaps to regain protective sensation of the sole,[14,15,16] and tissue expansion to create a local flap option for large chronic defects[17,18] or to minimize donor site morbidity.[19] By the 1990s, Koshima (▶ Fig. 1.5) and Soeda[20] provided convincing evidence of the value of perforator flaps (▶ Fig. 1. 6), a cutaneous flap that best ensured preservation of muscle function. The anterolateral thigh flap—first introduced by Song et al,[21]

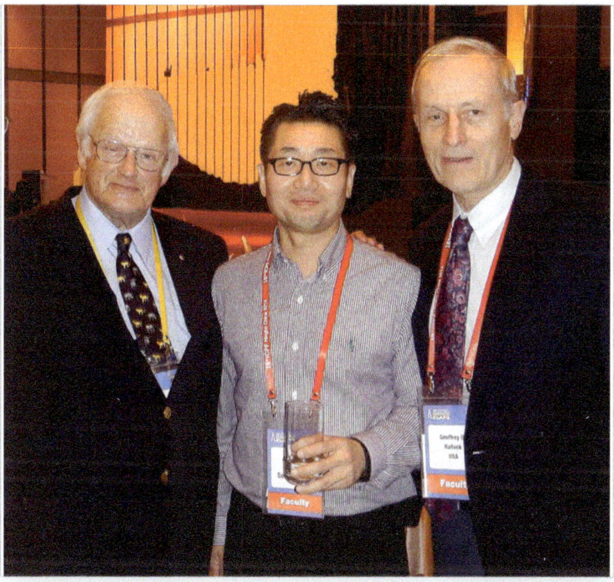

Fig. 1.4 G. Ian Taylor: anatomist and microsurgeon extraordinaire.

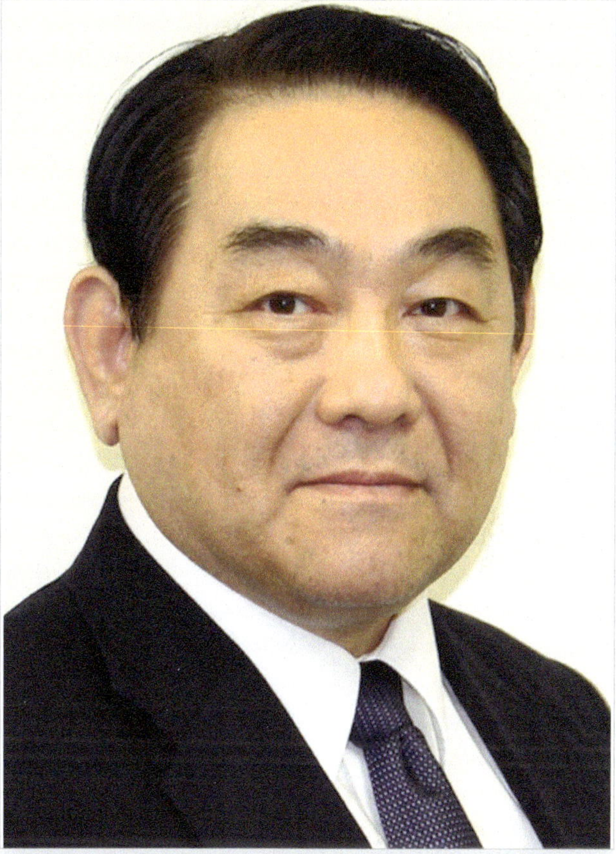

Fig. 1.5 Isao Koshima: father of Perforator Flaps.

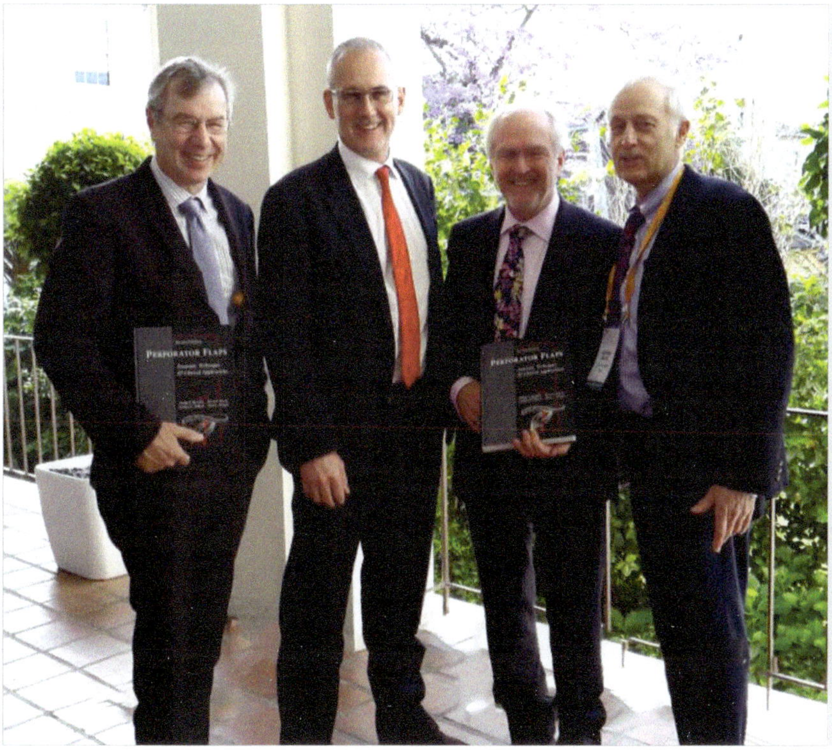

Fig. 1. 6 Steven Morris, Phillip Blondeel, Peter Neligan, Geoffrey Hallock: the perforator "gang of 4."

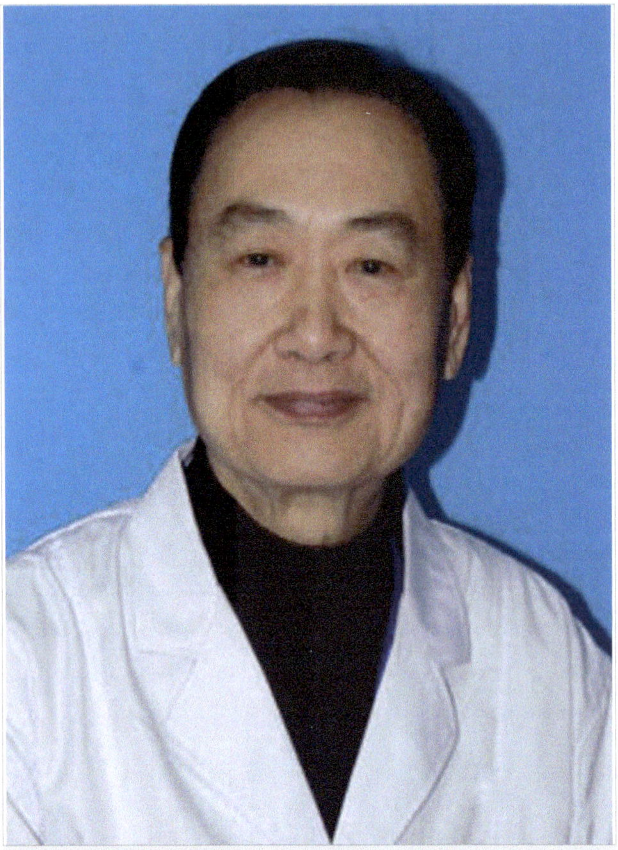

Fig. 1.7 Ye-guang Song: introduced the anterolateral thigh flap.

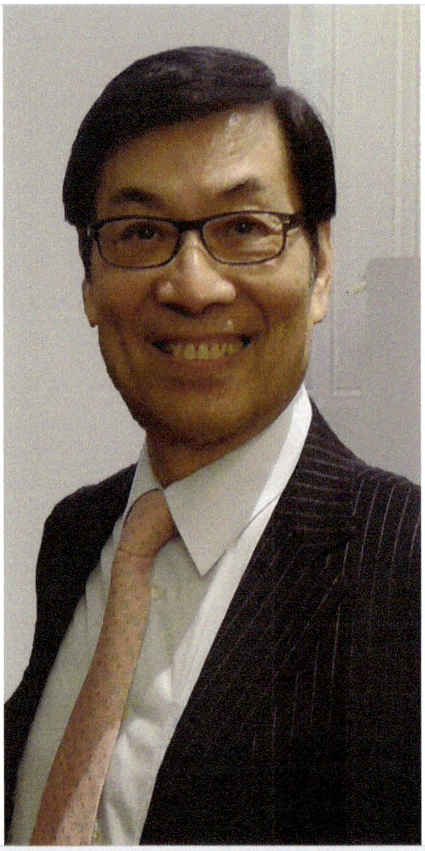

Fig. 1.8 Fu-Chan Wei: master of microsurgical reconstruction.

(▶ Fig. 1.7) just as Wei et al[22] (▶ Fig. 1.8) proposed as the ideal soft-tissue flap for all purposes—is widely used worldwide today. However, currently perforator flaps in general allow better choice of a donor site that best matches the tissue qualities needed at the recipient site.[23] Though originally utilized primarily as microvascular tissue transfers, increasingly they have become a local perforator flap option applicable to all zones of the lower extremity.[24]

Advances in nonsurgical alternatives should not be overlooked as well. Subatmospheric pressure devices provide a stable temporary dressing intended to promote a better environment for ultimately a skin graft or flap coverage,[25] although healing by secondary intention or wound contraction may instead be possible. What the future will bring will surely encompass the pioneering fields of tissue engineering, genetic engineering, lower limb replantation or allotransplantation, and supermicrosurgery.

1.3 Basic Principles

We abhor dogma, and we would be the first to challenge any if something better were available. On the other hand, classical dictums are of paramount importance if nothing more than a guideline to at least keep us near the beaten path. Always remember that the primary goal of surgical reconstruction of the lower extremity is to restore or maintain ambulatory function. That is better assured with a well-vascularized extremity, presence of a skeletal structure able to support both necessary weight bearing and gait, and optimally an innervated plantar surface to provide protective sensation. Without restoration of proper function, the value of any attempted reconstruction will be reduced significantly, increasing both the emotional and the financial burden on the patient.

An early evaluation of the patient as a whole will allow proper decisions to be made, considering not just their overall physical condition but also their socioeconomic status and rehabilitative potential. The lower extremity injury, thus, is best approached by a team of physicians and not just surgeons, with a knowledge base including skeletal, vascular, neurologic, and soft-tissue anatomy, not to forget psychology. According to a study by Lange[26] limited to open tibial fractures, absolute indications for an amputation were anatomically complete disruption of the posterior tibial nerve in adults or crush injuries with warm ischemia time greater than 6 hours. Relative indications listed were serious associated polytrauma, severe ipsilateral foot trauma, and anticipation of a protracted course to obtain soft-tissue coverage and tibial reconstruction.[26] Other means for initial assessments such as the Mangled Extremity Severity Score (MESS), the Predictive Salvage Index, and the Limb Salvage Index can assist the team in making a decision for amputation, but they must never be the sole criterion in making that decision and must always be individualized for each patient.[27,28,29,30]

The initial evaluation of a lower extremity wound requires a competent physical examination, both visual and manual, to document the location, size, depth, extent, and character of the

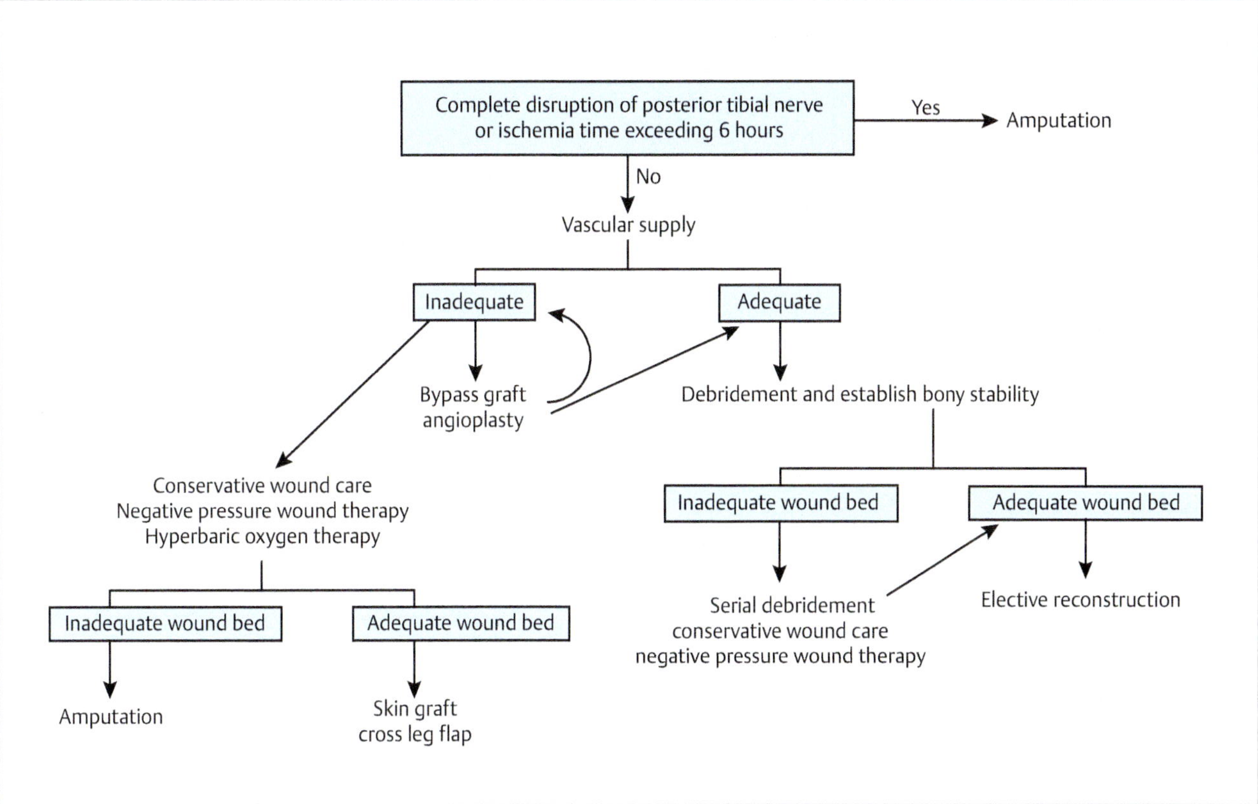

Fig. 1.9 A reconstruction algorithm as a useful guideline for a traumatic injury of the lower extremity.

wound. A neurological, vascular, and skeletal evaluation is essential to ascertain the extent of injuries, which helps the development of a solid plan for reconstruction (▶ Fig. 1.9). A thorough vascular profile using whatever clinical or diagnostic tools are available should be foremost in the examiner's mind. Inadequate perfusion that cannot be rectified may dictate consideration in favor of life over limb preservation. Yet amputated or avulsed tissues should never be thrown away until absolutely not needed, as these may be potential donor sites for skin grafts or even flaps.[31,32,33,34,35] Nothing currently available can mimic the superiority of autologous tissues, no matter how they are attained.

If the vascular supply is reasonable, then stability of skeletal structures would next be in order, followed by debridement until all nonviable tissues have been removed. Only then should soft-tissue coverage be considered. This may be achieved by following the traditional concept of the reconstructive ladder, or reconstructive elevator, or reconstructive paradigm (see also Chapter 11).[36,37] The simplest reconstructive option may not necessarily provide the most optimal result in the long term. Think not just about today, but also about tomorrow. Skin grafts or bioengineered acellular dermal matrices[38] may be totally appropriate. Similarly, so may be local muscle or perforator flaps, but if the intent is to avoid the vagaries of microvascular tissue transfers, beware of the substandard outcome. The selection process from this cornucopia of choices is elaborated in more detail in other pertinent chapters that follow, where attributes as well as detriments are listed.

Microsurgery always has and always will have a role in lower extremity reconstruction. Recognize that any perforator flap,

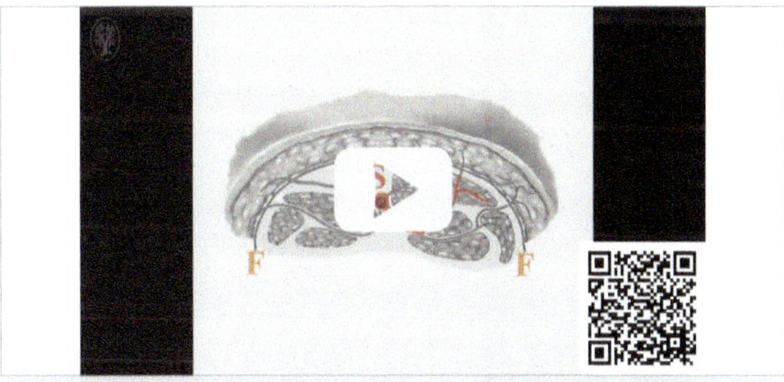

Video 1.1 How to Dissect a Musculocutaneous Perforator. https://www.thieme.de/de/q.htm?p=opn/cs/20/7/12265287-f398be45

whether as a local or free flap, when the perforator is dissected, requires meticulous microsurgical technique (▶ Video 1.1). Traditionally, recipient sites should be chosen outside the zone of injury.[39,40] End-to-side arterial anastomoses are always preferable to preserve distal flow as much as possible especially in those complex, mangled injuries seen so often in this region.[41] End-to-end venous adjacent to that of the arterial microanastomosis are logistically the most convenient, but do not hesitate to seek out the superficial venous system if the deep venae comitantes are unusable.[42]

Note the confusion if obeying all of these points caused by the successful anastomosis of perforators to perforators found adjacent to or within the zone of injury, and usually anastomosed in an end-to-end fashion.[43] Postoperative monitoring of all flaps is imperative, but it is mandatory for free flaps. There is no shortcut that can replace meticulous surgical technique and early diagnosis of flap compromise so that take-back, if needed, will more likely be successful.[44] If the free flap fails, unless infected, do not hastily remove it, as it will have an excellent role as a biologic dressing. More often than expected, healthy granulation tissue during this period may have developed, so that some other treatment modality might be possible.

1.4 Conclusion

Proper management of the multitude of tissue deficits encountered in the mangled lower extremity, exposure after oncologic ablations, or from the ravages of systemic diseases requires a thorough examination and contemplative approach before embarking on what may be the most difficult challenge in attempting limb salvage, not just for the reconstructive surgeon but also for the patient who has not volunteered for this predicament. Today we can better diagnose, better support, and better intervene to assist these unfortunate souls in our common goal to restore ambulatory function. Whether surgical capabilities or nonsurgical devices may be apropos, how we get there is not as important as is getting there. Although complete lower limb restoration is rarely possible, do not forget that the most reasonable endpoint should also be that which minimizes scars and preserves appearance as well as possible using whatever aesthetic plastic surgery techniques are available. All these things are our patient's expectation, and should also be ours.

References

[1] Hughes CD, Tran BNN, Rinkinen J, Lee BT, Iorio ML. Readability, suitability, and complexity of online resources for lower extremity reconstruction. Ann Plast Surg. 2019; 82(1):2–6

[2] Aldea PA, Shaw WW. The evolution of the surgical management of severe lower extremity trauma. Clin Plast Surg. 1986; 13(4):549–569

[3] Higgins TF, Klatt JB, Beals TC. Lower Extremity Assessment Project (LEAP): the best available evidence on limb-threatening lower extremity trauma. Orthop Clin North Am. 2010; 41(2):233–239

[4] Chung KC, Saddawi-Konefka D, Haase SC, Kaul G. A cost-utility analysis of amputation versus salvage for Gustilo type IIIB and IIIC open tibial fractures. Plast Reconstr Surg. 2009; 124(6):1965–1973

[5] Williams MO. Long-term cost comparison of major limb salvage using the Ilizarov method versus amputation. Clin Orthop Relat Res. 1994(301):156–158

[6] MacKenzie EJ, Jones AS, Bosse MJ, et al. Health-care costs associated with amputation or reconstruction of a limb-threatening injury. J Bone Joint Surg Am. 2007; 89(8):1685–1692

[7] Dormandy J, Heeck L, Vig S. Major amputations: clinical patterns and predictors. Semin Vasc Surg. 1999; 12(2):154–161

[8] Gonzalez EG, Corcoran PJ, Reyes RL. Energy expenditure in below-knee amputees: correlation with stump length. Arch Phys Med Rehabil. 1974; 55 (3):111–119

[9] McGregor IA, Morgan G. Axial and random pattern flaps. Br J Plast Surg. 1973; 26(3):202–213

[10] Stark WJ. The use of pedicled muscle flaps in the surgical treatment of chronic osteomyelitis resulting from compound fractures. J Bone Joint Surg Am. 1946; 28:343–350

[11] Ger R. The technique of muscle transposition in the operative treatment of traumatic and ulcerative lesions of the leg. J Trauma. 1971; 11(6):502–510

[12] Godina M. Early microsurgical reconstruction of complex trauma of the extremities. Plast Reconstr Surg. 1986; 78(3):285–292

[13] Lin CH, Lin YT, Yeh JT, Chen CT. Free functioning muscle transfer for lower extremity posttraumatic composite structure and functional defect. Plast Reconstr Surg. 2007; 119(7):2118–2126

[14] Irwin MS, Jain A, Anand P, Nanchahal J. Free innervated sole of foot transfer for contralateral lower limb salvage. Plast Reconstr Surg. 2006; 118(4):93e–97e

[15] Hong JP, Kim EK. Sole reconstruction using anterolateral thigh perforator free flaps. Plast Reconstr Surg. 2007; 119(1):186–193

[16] Santanelli F, Tenna S, Pace A, Scuderi N. Free flap reconstruction of the sole of the foot with or without sensory nerve coaptation. Plast Reconstr Surg. 2002; 109(7):2314–2322, discussion 2323–2324

[17] Ong YS, Levin LS. Lower limb salvage in trauma. Plast Reconstr Surg. 2010; 125(2):582–588

[18] Borges Filho PT, Neves RI, Gemperli R, et al. Soft-tissue expansion in lower extremity reconstruction. Clin Plast Surg. 1991; 18(3):593–599

[19] Hallock GG. Tissue expansion techniques to minimize morbidity of the anterolateral thigh perforator flap donor site. J Reconstr Microsurg. 2013; 29 (9):565–570

[20] Koshima I, Soeda S. Inferior epigastric artery skin flaps without rectus abdominis muscle. Br J Plast Surg. 1989; 42(6):645–648

[21] Song YG, Chen GZ, Song YL. The free thigh flap: a new free flap concept based on the septocutaneous artery. Br J Plast Surg. 1984; 37(2):149–159

[22] Wei FC, Jain V, Celik N, Chen HC, Chuang DCC, Lin CH. Have we found an ideal soft-tissue flap? An experience with 672 anterolateral thigh flaps. Plast Reconstr Surg. 2002; 109(7):2219–2226, discussion 2227–2230

[23] Saint-Cyr M, Schaverien MV, Rohrich RJ. Perforator flaps: history, controversies, physiology, anatomy, and use in reconstruction. Plast Reconstr Surg. 2009; 123(4):132e–145e

[24] Koh K, Goh TLH, Song CT, et al. Free versus pedicled perforator flaps for lower extremity reconstruction: a multicenter comparison of institutional practices and outcomes. J Reconstr Microsurg. 2018; 34(8):572–580

[25] Stannard JP, Volgas DA, McGwin G, III, et al. Incisional negative pressure wound therapy after high-risk lower extremity fractures. J Orthop Trauma. 2012; 26(1):37–42

[26] Lange RH. Limb reconstruction versus amputation decision making in massive lower extremity trauma. Clin Orthop Relat Res. 1989(243):92–99

[27] Helfet DL, Howey T, Sanders R, Johansen K. Limb salvage versus amputation. Preliminary results of the Mangled Extremity Severity Score. Clin Orthop Relat Res. 1990(256):80–86

[28] Johansen K, Daines M, Howey T, Helfet D, Hansen ST, Jr. Objective criteria accurately predict amputation following lower extremity trauma. J Trauma. 1990; 30(5):568–572, discussion 572–573

[29] Howe HR, Jr, Poole GV, Jr, Hansen KJ, et al. Salvage of lower extremities following combined orthopedic and vascular trauma. A predictive salvage index. Am Surg. 1987; 53(4):205–208

[30] Russell WL, Sailors DM, Whittle TB, Fisher DF, Jr, Burns RP. Limb salvage versus traumatic amputation. A decision based on a seven-part predictive index. Ann Surg. 1991; 213(5):473–480, discussion 480–481

[31] Anderson WD, Stewart KJ, Wilson Y, Quaba AA. Skin grafts for the salvage of degloved below-knee amputation stumps. Br J Plast Surg. 2002; 55(4):320–323

[32] Ghali S, Harris PA, Khan U, Pearse M, Nanchahal J. Leg length preservation with pedicled fillet of foot flaps after traumatic amputations. Plast Reconstr Surg. 2005; 115(2):498–505

[33] Akyurek M, Fudem G, Leclair W, Babbitt R, Dunn RM. Salvage of a lower extremity by microsurgical transfer of tibial bone from the contralateral extremity traumatically amputated at the ankle level. Ann Plast Surg. 2009; 63(4):389–392

[34] Weinberg A, Mosheiff R, Liebergall M, Berlatzky Y, Aner H, Neuman RA. Amputated lower limbs as a bank of organs for other organ salvage. Injury. 1999; 30 Suppl 2:B34–B38

[35] Hallock GG. Isle of palm and sole fillet flaps. Ann Plast Surg. 1991; 26(6):514–519

[36] Gottlieb LJ, Krieger LM. From the reconstructive ladder to the reconstructive elevator. Plast Reconstr Surg. 1994; 93(7):1503–1504

[37] Erba P, Ogawa R, Vyas R, Orgill DP. The reconstructive matrix: a new paradigm in reconstructive plastic surgery. Plast Reconstr Surg. 2010; 126 (2):492–498

[38] Burke JF, Yannas IV, Quinby WC, Jr, Bondoc CC, Jung WK. Successful use of a physiologically acceptable artificial skin in the treatment of extensive burn injury. Ann Surg. 1981; 194(4):413–428
[39] Arnez ZM. Immediate reconstruction of the lower extremity: an update. Clin Plast Surg. 1991; 18(3):449–457
[40] Isenberg JS, Sherman R. Zone of injury: a valid concept in microvascular reconstruction of the traumatized lower limb? Ann Plast Surg. 1996; 36 (3):270–272
[41] Hallock GG. The mangled foot and ankle: soft tissue salvage techniques. Clin Podiatr Med Surg. 2014; 31(4):565–576
[42] Hallock GG. Both superficial and deep extremity veins can be used successfully as the recipient site for free flaps. Ann Plast Surg. 2000; 44(6):633–636
[43] Hong JP. The use of supermicrosurgery in lower extremity reconstruction: the next step in evolution. Plast Reconstr Surg. 2009; 123(1):230–235
[44] Chen KT, Mardini S, Chuang DC, et al. Timing of presentation of the first signs of vascular compromise dictates the salvage outcome of free flap transfers. Plast Reconstr Surg. 2007; 120(1):187–195

2 Assessment of the Normal and Impaired Lower Extremity

Rachel M. Clancy and Ronald M. Zuker

Summary

Before embarking on any lower extremity treatment intervention, not only must an accurate hands-on physical examination be performed but an in-depth history should first be obtained, as often the patient may be the best source of factual information. A complete knowledge of the normal lower limb anatomy and physiology is imperative before attempting to evaluate the impaired lower extremity. Often bone and soft-tissue compromise occurs simultaneously, and thus an orthoplastic approach is preferable to solve not just limb but also life-threatening issues like crush or degloving injuries, as well as the risk of a compartment syndrome. The omnipresent risk of osteomyelitis and the high frequency of diabetic foot wounds today, as with all impaired lower extremities, require a multidisciplinary treatment plan.

Keywords: Gustilo–Anderson classification, orthoplastic approach, compartment syndrome, degloving injury, crush syndrome, Cierny osteomyelitis classification

2.1 Introduction

A comprehensive history as well as a hands-on physical examination is always necessary for the proper assessment of what may be the normal, and definitely for an impaired, lower extremity. Each unit needs to develop a systematic process to achieve this evaluation that is routinely followed to facilitate efficiency and completeness. The impaired lower extremity will, in addition, need to be observed for any acute and chronic complications that may have arisen, whatever the etiology. The complications may include lower extremity fractures, identification of surgical emergencies such as compartment syndromes, the possibility of a crush syndrome, and degloving injuries. A description of the pathology expected with chronic diseases, and in particular osteomyelitis and the diabetic foot, will complete this introduction.

2.2 Assessment of the Normal Lower Extremity

Physicians should have at the least a personal routine for the assessment of the lower extremity to ensure a thorough and focused examination is performed in a timely manner. This should be guided by the history, if available, and requires a complete understanding of lower extremity anatomy, biomechanics, and neurovascular supply as is apropos. In this context, the examination should include assessment of the skin; soft tissues; and the vascular, neurological, and musculoskeletal systems. Selection of appropriate bedside tests as well as more involved investigations to aid with this assessment and an exact diagnosis will be important. An understanding of when and why different imaging modalities should be used such as plain radiographs, computed tomography (CT), magnetic resonance imaging (MRI), ultrasound, and the audible Doppler is imperative. The choices should be made efficiently and timely without redundancy, as extraneous studies in the presence of a critical or life- or limb-threatening injury may lead to a delay in transfer to the operating room which could compromise not only the immediate management of the patient but also ultimate outcome.

2.2.1 Lower Extremity Anatomy

Humans are bipedal; so in the erect position, full weight bearing will be on the lower extremity.[1] The fibula and tibia are the bony support of the leg with the latter sustaining 85% of the weight-bearing forces necessary to maintain ambulation.[1] This is an important consideration when examining the lower extremity and then selecting potential reconstructive options. The tibia articulates with the femur at the knee joint and joins with the fibula to articulate with the talus to form the ankle joint. The fibula, as does the tibia, serves as a bony surface for multiple muscle and fascial attachments important for integrated locomotion.[1]

The leg itself is divided into four muscle compartments: anterior, lateral, and posterior—which is again subdivided into a superficial and deep compartment. Knowledge of the location of these compartments and anatomical markers to facilitate their decompression when indicated is essential (▶ Fig. 2.1). The anterior compartment contains the tibialis anterior, extensor hallucis longus, extensor digitorum longus, and peroneus tertius muscles. All four of these muscles are supplied by branches of the anterior tibial artery and innervated by the deep peroneal nerve. The peroneus longus and brevis are found in the lateral compartment of the leg. The peroneus longus receives blood supply from branches of the anterior tibial and peroneal arteries, whereas the peroneus brevis is supplied by only the peroneal artery. Both the peroneus longus and brevis are innervated by the superficial peroneal nerve. The posterior compartment is divided into superficial and deep compartments. The superficial compartment includes both heads of the gastrocnemius, soleus, plantaris, and popliteus muscles. Circulation to the gastrocnemius is supplied by the sural branches of the popliteal artery. The soleus is supplied by the posterior tibial, peroneal, and branches of the popliteal artery. The plantaris muscle is supplied by the sural branches of the popliteal artery. The popliteus is supplied by the genicular branches of the popliteal artery. All muscles of the superficial compartment of the leg are innervated by the tibial nerve. The flexor hallucis longus, flexor digitorum longus, and tibialis posterior muscles are found in the deep compartment. The flexor hallucis longus is supplied by the peroneal artery. The flexor digitorum longus and tibialis posterior are supplied by branches of the posterior tibial artery. All muscles of the deep posterior compartment are innervated by the tibial nerve.

The common vascular anatomy as stated earlier, however, has numerous anomalies thought to be the result of a generalized defect in the mesoderm.[2] The venous anatomy of the lower limb

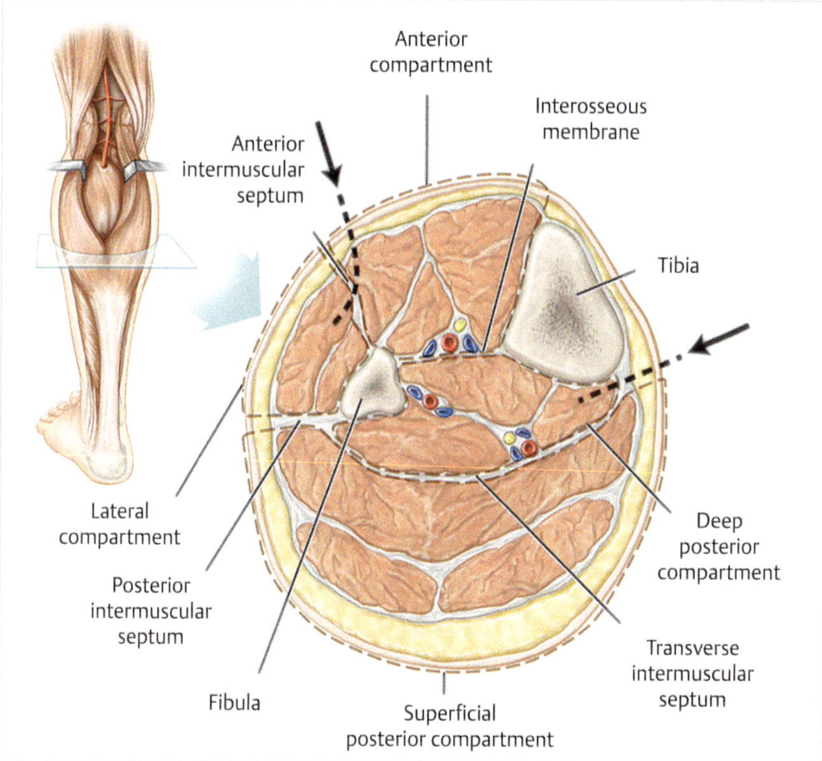

Fig. 2.1 Left mid-leg cross-section showing the four muscle compartments of the leg and the relative location of their investing fascia. The dotted lines emphasized by the arrows should be the direction followed by the anterolateral and posteromedial incisions needed for four-compartment decompression if a compartment syndrome is suspected.

can be highly variable as a result of venous malformations occurring during embryonic development in the final phase of embryogenesis.[2,3] Park et al[4] described four distinct anatomical variations of the femoral and popliteal veins: agenesis, multiplications, variation in anatomical course, and a high union of the tibial veins. Variations in arterial anatomy have also been reported, such as an anterior tibial artery with a high origin; a trifurcation of the anterior tibial artery, peroneal artery, or posterior tibial artery; and a hypoplastic or aplastic posterior tibial artery.[5]

There are also unique factors of the lower limb that can lead to predictable compromise. For example, there is minimal soft tissue overlying the tibia anteriorly. Therefore, even the most minor trauma can lead to exposure of the tibia, and the lack of adjacent soft tissue limits the use of local flaps for its coverage. Adequacy of distal lower extremity blood supply can be complicated by the ubiquitous presence of atherosclerosis. Dependency of the leg and consequently enhanced hydrostatic pressures can contribute to an increased incidence of deep vein thrombosis and venous disease, making reconstruction with any form of soft-tissue flap more susceptible to venous congestion. In addition, following even the slightest insult, patients can be susceptible to venous stasis ulcers which are most difficult to treat.[1,6] Finally, unlike other areas of the body, normal sensation to the foot best allows proper ambulation and rehabilitation.

2.3 Assessment of the Impaired Lower Extremity

Treatment of the impaired lower extremity must begin just as for the normal lower extremity with a comprehensive evaluation of not just the defect of the ipsilateral limb but the whole patient. The etiology of these defects may be multifactorial and secondary to trauma, neoplasia, infection, poorly controlled systemic disease, and/or arterial and venous compromise. Regardless of the origin of the defect, the patient should be treated by a multidisciplinary team, and always with a respect for the patient's autonomy. The patient's comorbidities, premorbid state, American Society of Anesthesiologists (ASA) grade, smoking status, rehabilitative potential, as well as expectations and motivation should always be taken into consideration before embarking on any treatment course. Following the preservation of life and then limb, the goal of reconstruction will be to restore function. In this context, an acceptable reconstruction will require a stable skeleton capable of supporting the patient's weight, a robust tissue envelope with satisfactory proprioception and plantar sensibility, as well as having a reasonable appearance.[6]

2.3.1 Lower Extremity Trauma

Lower extremity trauma should be considered as a potential life-threatening injury due to the risk of high-volume blood loss and the sequelae of inadequate resuscitation, such as hypothermia, hypovolemia or shock, coagulopathy, and adult respiratory distress syndrome.[6] Lower extremity injuries should also be considered potentially limb threatening: so obvious after a traumatic amputation, less obvious with a serious vascular injury causing ischemia or a compartment syndrome, but even possible with any open fracture or fracture dislocations resulting in nerve injury.[7] Universally, the most common mechanisms of lower extremity trauma still remain motor vehicle accidents, falls, and interpersonal violence.[8]

2.3.2 History

Open lower extremity fractures are usually a result of high-energy trauma. Treatment can be difficult, as these injuries are usually not solitary but involve multiple-organ systems and each must be assessed and treated simultaneously.[9] As well as the mechanism of injury, a thorough history including any past medical or surgical history, allergies, known medications, social history, and premorbid condition must be known. A primary and secondary survey should be performed to look for specific signs indicative of high-energy trauma that would include the presence of other injuries, a large soft-tissue defect, a degloving injury, or a transverse or segmental fracture pattern with comminution.[9] Complex bony and soft-tissue injuries may be a clue also of the presence of associated neurovascular compromise.

2.3.3 Examination

Open tibial fracture is one of the most common lower extremity injuries that requires an orthoplastic approach. The Gustilo–Anderson classification schema (▶ Table 2.1) remains the most widely used system for the classification of open lower extremity fractures (▶ Fig. 2.2).[10] The classification is relatively straightforward and offers orthoplastic surgeons a prognostic framework that guides management.

The BOA/BAPRAS guidelines are a robust set of evidenced-based principles also devised to aid in the assessment and management of open tibial fractures.[9] They have revolutionized the management of many aspects of lower limb trauma in the United Kingdom and are being increasingly implemented in other European countries. The relevant areas following these guidelines will be summarized as follows.

ATLS principles are employed with airway and spinal management as well as with breathing and circulation support even prior to the arrival of the patient in the emergency department. This should include intravenous access and analgesia. External hemorrhage is stopped via direct pressure or as a last resort by application of a tourniquet. The neurovascular status should be ascertained and documented. Neurovascular examination should include assessment of the capillary refill of the skin, palpation of pedal pulses, as well as the presence or absence of sensation of the medial plantar surface (tibial nerve) and first web space of the foot (deep peroneal nerve).

Repeated neurovascular examinations must be performed particularly for evolving injuries and following any intervention.[9] Gross contamination should be removed, and the limb realigned as long as no iatrogenic injury would occur. Photographs ideally need to be taken before the wound is covered with a sterile moist dressing, and this dressing should then not be interfered with until the patient is taken to the operating room. The fracture must be temporarily splinted and radiographs taken (two orthogonal views, as well as the joint above and below). A more thorough examination of the injury should follow in the operating room jointly by a senior plastic and orthopaedic surgeon. This scenario ensures that sterility, illumination, anesthesia, and an expert opinion will be optimal. On-table femoral angiography most simply can also be performed in the operating room if indicated. This initial surgery should be performed at least within 24 hours of the injury. In some cases, however, more immediate surgery without delay should be strongly considered, including the presence of gross contamination, a suspected compartment syndrome, vascular compromise, or other life-threatening injuries.

Table 2.1 The Gustilo–Anderson classification of open fractures[10]

Gustilo grade definition
I: Low-energy trauma wound < 1 cm
II: Wound > 1 cm without extensive soft-tissue damage or avulsions
III: Extensive soft-tissue damage/loss including any segmental comminuted fractures or fracture open more than 8 h before treatment
• IIIA: Type III fracture with periosteal coverage of the fracture; extensive soft-tissue laceration or damage
• IIIB: Type III fracture with periosteal stripping, extensive soft-tissue loss, and bone damage; usually associated with massive contamination
• IIIC: Type III fracture associated with a vascular injury requiring repair

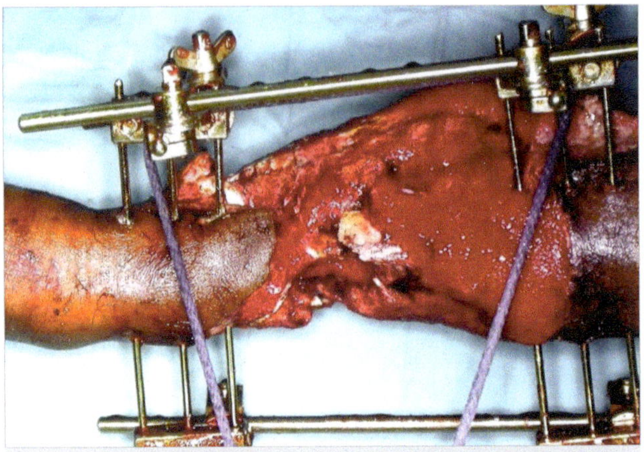

Fig. 2.2 Typical high-energy trauma injury with open left tibia and fibula fracture, with extensive soft-tissue loss. This would be considered a Gustilo grade IIIB fracture and invariably will require a flap for reconstruction.

2.4 Compartment Syndrome

A compartment syndrome is defined as the elevation of the interstitial pressure in a closed osseofascial compartment resulting in microvascular compromise.[8] A missed diagnosis will result in irreversible neuromuscular ischemia (▶ Fig. 2.3). Any form of tissue injury can disrupt normal tissue hemostasis leading to increased tissue pressure. Capillary blood flow will decrease when the tissue pressure exceeds the capillary pressure. This causes hypoxia which exacerbates the existing tissue injury, ultimately leading to tissue necrosis.[8] Muscle necrosis will occur after 3 to 4 hours of warm ischemia.[9]

Compartment syndrome can be caused by both closed and open fractures. The incidence of a compartment syndrome with tibial shaft fractures is 9.1%.[11] This is anything but negligible. It should never be assumed that an open fracture has allowed adequate compartment decompression, as it may have actually increased the risk. A compartment syndrome can also be caused by soft-tissue trauma alone, an arterial injury, severe burns, and prolonged compression due to immobility as often occurring in an obtunded patient.[8]

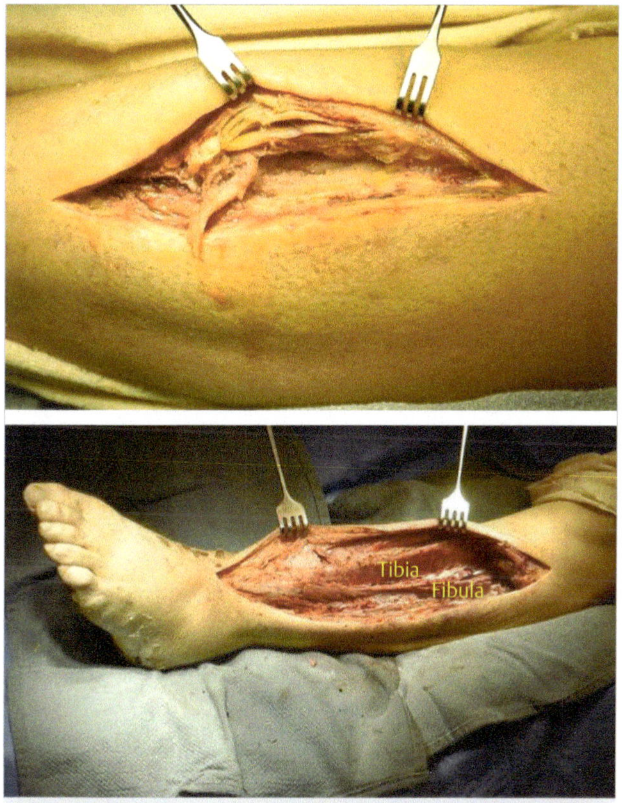

Fig. 2.3 Inadequate anterior compartment decompression of a compartment syndrome through this short mid-tibial incision eventually required debridement of all necrotic muscle, exposing the tibia and fibula sidewalls virtually in their entirety.

The presence of a compartment syndrome can be difficult to diagnose during the initial assessment. Surgeons must have a high index of suspicion, and should always be considered in any patient with a severe lower extremity injury. Remember that the classic signs of onset of an acute compartment syndrome can be easily missed in patients with severe hypovolemia or in the unconscious patient.[7] Otherwise, the signs and symptoms that should raise clinical suspicion are the following:

1. **Pain** with passive stretch of the limb out of proportion with the injury. The tibial nerve and the common peroneal nerve should be assessed by plantar flexion and dorsiflexion of the foot, respectively. In practice, however, this evaluation of pain is difficult as patients are often in a splint or traction device, which by itself is painful as well as limits any such testing. The pain often is described as a burning pain. The possibility of a more proximal injury to the sciatic nerve, nerve roots, or the spinal cord itself should also be considered.[9]
2. **Pressure** and tightness from tense and palpably swollen compartments will be obvious with gentle palpation. While compartment syndrome remains a clinical diagnosis, devices enabling direct measurement of the pressure in certain groups of patients is helpful, that is, those who are unresponsive or uncooperative (children, intoxicated), and those with premorbid lower limb injuries or compromise.
3. **Paresthesias** in the involved compartment. Perception of touch will be diminished. This can be elicited for the tibial and deep peroneal nerve by touch of the medial sole of the foot and the first dorsal web space, respectively.
4. **Paralysis** of muscle occurs following prolonged ischemia after arterial injury, and can be a sign of a prolonged compartment syndrome. The degree of paralysis is again difficult to assess if patients are in pain, splinted, or have a bony injury.
5. **Pallor** of the skin alone is not a reliable sign. A pale limb with slow capillary refill should immediately arouse suspicion of a major arterial injury, which if present will require immediate intervention.
6. **Pulselessness** must be explained. The posterior tibial and dorsalis pedis pulses, should be palpated. However, distal pulses may or may not be palpable, and absent pulses is considered a late finding. On the other hand, the presence of a pulse does not exclude the risk of a compartment syndrome. Absent pulses are more suggestive of arterial injury, or preexisting conditions such as atherosclerosis.

If a compartment syndrome is suspected, the encompassing fascia of all compartments of the leg can be released by an anterolateral and posteromedial 15- to 20-cm-long longitudinal incisions. The anterolateral incision is made between the tibial crest and the fibular shaft extending from about 3 cm distal to the tibial crest to the lateral malleolus, passing from the anterior compartment through the anterior intermuscular septum to reach the lateral compartment (▶ Fig. 2.1). The posteromedial incision is made approximately 2 cm posterior to the posteromedial border of the tibia to extend from the tibial tuberosity to the medial malleolus, through which the posterior intermuscular septum that separates the superficial and deep posterior compartments is released.

2.5 Degloving Injuries

Degloving soft-tissue injuries, albeit somewhat of a misnomer, describe the avulsion or tearing of a large portion of skin and subcutaneous tissues that will usually be detached from the underlying fascia and muscle.[12] Degloving injuries can be open with obvious skin lacerations (▶ Fig. 2.4) or closed, making the diagnosis not so obvious. These can occur as a consequence of torsion, crush, and avulsion or shear forces. Degloving injuries are very often associated with other severe injuries. They are also often underestimated in severity due to a lack of diagnostic indicators and established treatment guidelines, which makes it difficult to set standard management protocols and to predict outcomes (▶ Fig. 2.5).[13] After a degloving, it is often impossible to distinguish between viable and nonviable tissues, as extensive ecchymosis and any underlying hematoma can frequently mask what is actually viable tissue. In the immediate phase postinjury, this makes it difficult to decide on which tissue can be salvaged and which needs to be debrided, the latter being potentially life or limb threatening as this could progress to a fulminant infection or necrotizing fasciitis.[12]

Newly available tools such as laser-assisted indocyanine green dye angiography,[14] or dynamic infrared thermography now inexpensive using a Smartphone[15] app, may make any surgical decisions safer.

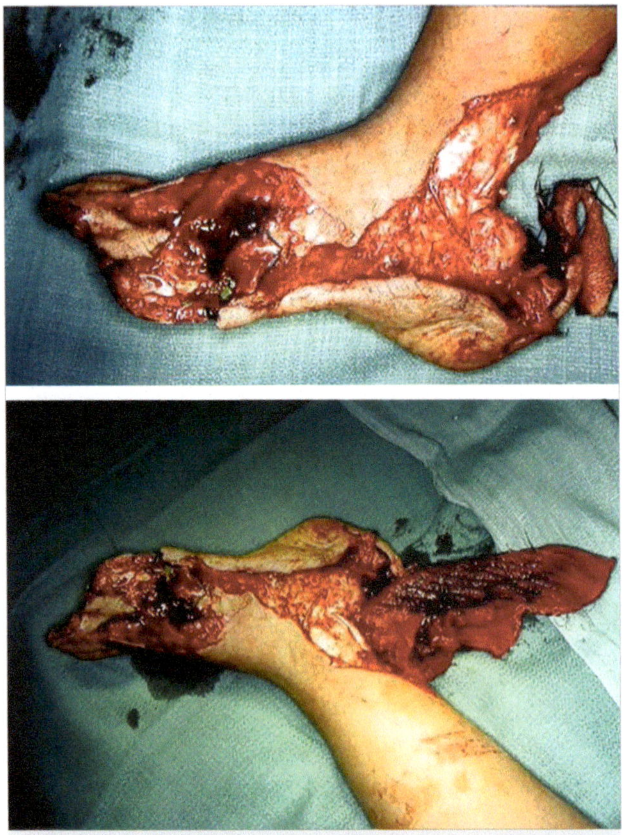

Fig. 2.4 Near circumferential multiplanar open degloving injury of the foot.

Four patterns of degloving have been described by Tyler and coworkers to aid in the assessment and management of these potentially complex situations.[9,16]

1. Localized degloving such as an abrasion/avulsion.
2. Noncircumferential single-plane degloving.
3. Circumferential single-plane degloving.
4. Circumferential and multiplanar degloving.

Remember that any degloved skin may still be valuable as a split-thickness skin graft, perhaps not so much so for the traumatized recipient site, but as a method if onlayed to hasten reepithelialization of the graft donor site.[17,18]

2.6 Crush Syndrome

Crush syndrome, traumatic rhabdomyolysis, or Bywaters syndrome is a severe life-threatening condition resulting from prolonged external pressure on muscle, and, if left untreated, may result in acute renal failure.[7] The physiological insult is due to direct muscle injury, muscle ischemia, muscle cell death, and release of myoglobin. Muscular trauma can progress to rhabdomyolysis and acute renal failure resulting in hypovolemia, hypocalcemia, hyperkalemia, metabolic acidosis, and disseminated intravascular coagulation. As part of the initial assessment and patient monitoring, the urine should be routinely examined. Note that myoglobin produces dark urine, and mandates further investigation.[7]

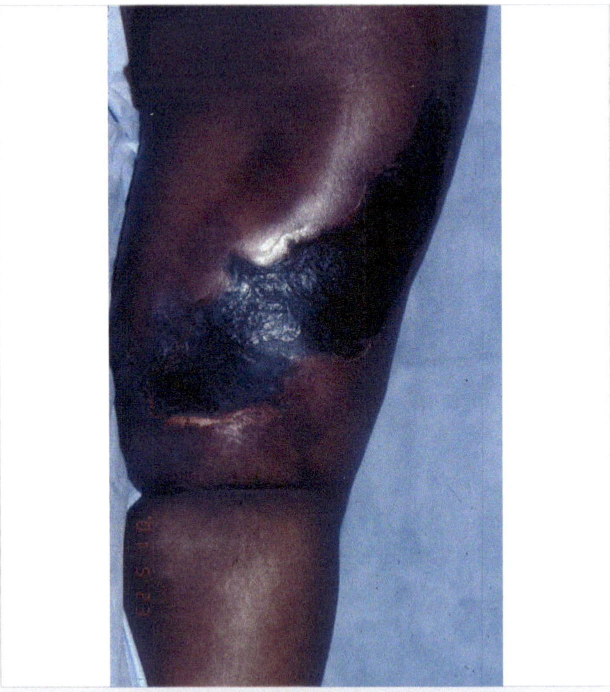

Fig. 2.5 Unsuspected closed degloving injury of the thigh demarcated with extensive eschar requiring debridement prior to skin grafting.

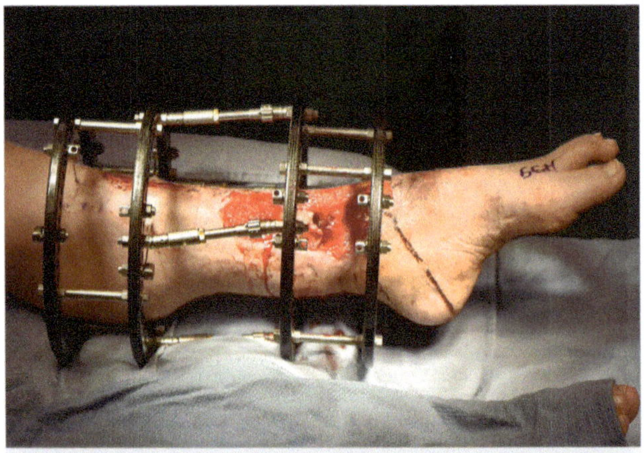

Fig. 2.6 Following a fall causing open Gustilo grade IIIB tibial fracture, inadequate soft-tissue cover resulted in an infection that becomes an obvious chronic osteomyelitis surrounded by extensive granulation tissues.

2.7 Osteomyelitis

Osteomyelitis is an acute or chronic inflammation of bone secondary to infection (▶ Fig. 2.6). The duration and mechanism of onset define osteomyelitis.[6] The term "acute osteomyelitis" is generally used to describe the first 6 weeks of a bone infection, whereas chronic osteomyelitis is a more prolonged infection where patients have developed long-term radiologic changes and fistulas.[6] Osteomyelitis is considered an ischemic disease of bone as well as an infection of bone.[6] This infection can be exogenous in origin (following open fractures, iatrogenic, or contiguous spread from an adjacent local infection) or hematogenous as if caused by a bacteremia. Hematogenous spread of infection is more common in children and adolescents. Osteomyelitis by definition is resistant to nonoperative management. According to the Cierny classification, adult chronic osteomyelitis can be divided into four categories[6]:

1. **Medullary osteomyelitis**, an endosteal disease.
2. **Superficial osteomyelitis**, which is a periosteal disease secondary commonly to trauma and associated with inadequate soft-tissue coverage. In this case, the disease is focal and cortical bone is not breached.
3. **Localized osteomyelitis**, where there is a full-thickness defect in cortical bone. The mechanical integrity of the bone is maintained. It may represent a progression from a medullary or superficial osteomyelitis.
4. **Diffuse osteomyelitis** is defined as a full-thickness defect with a cortical breach of the bone. Thus, the mechanical integrity of bone is no longer maintained.

Although some patients with osteomyelitis do not report any symptoms and examination does not elucidate any signs, some may describe severe bone pain or have fevers and chills of undetermined etiology. Lethargy or generalized irritability may be the only manifestation in young children. Clinical signs of osteomyelitis include swelling, erythema, and warmth over the affected area. Early radiological changes of osteomyelitis are often subtle and may not be observed for 5 to 7 days in children and double this period in adults. Generally, osteomyelitis must extend at least 1 cm and compromise 30 to 50% of bone mineral content before producing visible changes in radiographs. However, early changes that should arouse suspicion are adjacent soft-tissue swelling, loss of normal fat planes, and in some cases joint effusion.[19] A number of late changes such as regional osteopenia, periosteal reaction, cortical loss, endosteal scalloping, loss of trabecular architecture, new bone apposition, and peripheral sclerosis may be noted.[19] MRI is more sensitive and specific than CT and so a superior diagnostic tool, whereas ultrasound is not recommended.[19] A definitive diagnosis can only be confirmed by tissue samples in the form of bone biopsy, which will also facilitate obtaining proper antibiotic sensitivities.

2.8 Diabetic Foot

The number of individuals worldwide living with diabetes mellitus continues to expand. It is estimated that by 2030 the number will be over 552 million or 9.9% of the adult population.[20] Diabetes is the leading cause of foot ulcers and their subsequent infections and amputations in Europe and the United States.[21] The lifetime incidence of a diabetic patient developing a foot ulcer is estimated to be 25%.[22] Every 20 seconds a lower limb is lost as a consequence of diabetes somewhere in the world.[20] This can be the result of a combination of neuropathy, peripheral arterial disease, foot and skeletal deformities, and infection.[23] Infections in the diabetic foot can range from a superficial cellulitis to chronic osteomyelitis, and not so infrequently in the worst-case scenario a gangrenous extremity that requires amputation. The most common findings are overviewed but discussed more completely in Chapters 7 and 18.

2.8.1 Neuropathy

Neuropathy is the most important risk factor for development of a diabetic foot ulcer and the need for an amputation.[21,24] The neuropathic changes observed in the diabetic foot are the direct result of abnormalities in the sensory, motor, and autonomic nervous systems. Sensory changes include loss of protective sensation and poor proprioception, which leads to impaired balance. Reduced or impaired sensation over bony prominences or between toes can lead to a delay in the detection of skin breaks. Loss of motor function leads to atrophy of the intrinsic muscles of the foot. This may result in foot deformities such as a claw foot that is a result of overpowering of long flexors over the extensors.[21] Autonomic neuropathy will cause dryness of the foot, with onset of cracks and fissures secondary to anhidrosis and hyperkeratosis. All these problems may disrupt the skin integrity and then become a portal of entry for infection.

2.8.2 Charcot Arthropathy or Neuropathy

Charcot arthropathy or neuropathy is characterized by abnormal sensory and motor function with a normal vascular examination. This is manifest clinically by loss of protective sensation, diminished or even absent vibration sensation, and absent deep tendon reflexes in the presence of bounding peripheral pedal pulses.[21] Fractures and dislocation of the foot and ankle, and most commonly bones of the midfoot, leads to Charcot arthropathy.[21] It is widely accepted that the observed joint collapse is a result of accumulated damage as a result of insensitivity to pain. These destructive changes alter the biomechanics of gait and cause strain on ligaments binding the small bones that form the arch of the foot. This leads to further alteration in gait, resulting in abnormal weight-bearing stress and ultimately collapse of the foot. Charcot deformities occur in a small but high-risk proportion of the diabetic population. When present, the tarsometatarsal joints are involved in 30% of cases, the metatarsophalangeal joints also in 30%, the intertarsal joints in 24%, and the interphalangeal joints in 4%.[25,26]

Other common structural deformities in the diabetic include ankle equinus, hallus valgus, hammertoe, claw toe, and dislocation of the metatarsophalangeal joints. Careful physical examination will reveal loss of footpads, joint stiffness, and decreased range of motion. Ulcers seen are caused by a number of these factors usually related to pressure and repetitive trauma.[21] Note that in some cases, radiographic findings in Charcot arthropathy can mimic osteomyelitis. As such, the constant risk of infection requires a daily surveillance of their feet by the patients themselves. The physician must also be wary of any complaints of pain and signs of erythema, emphysema, or abscess.

2.9 Conclusion

Any physician dealing with the impaired lower extremity must be thoroughly familiar with the examination of the normal. Any abnormalities must be assessed along with evaluation of the patient's history and a complete whole body physical exam, before embarking on what should be a multidisciplinary treatment plan. Nonviable tissue always requires debridement, then debridement, and finally more debridement until eliminated. Exposed bone, fixation devices, or other vital structures need selection of an appropriate method of reconstruction in a timely fashion. Maximum form and function of the lower extremity should be preserved whenever reasonable by restoring vascularity, stability, and musculoskeletal structure in that order. Contour and any donor-site morbidity are always important considerations, but these must always be secondary to salvage of a functioning limb whenever that is feasible.

References

[1] Kasabian AK, Karp NS. Lower extremity reconstruction. In: Aston SJ, Beasley RW, Thorne CHM, eds. Grabb And Smith's Plastic Surgery. 5th ed. Philadelphia, PA: Lippincott-Raven; 1997:1031

[2] Silva MAM, Mesquita HFP, Carneiro IG, Krupa AE, Silva SGJ, Cardoso RS. Variação anatômica venosa rara em membros inferiores. J Vasc Bras. 2016; 15(4): 334–338

[3] Uhl JF, Gillot C, Chahim M. Anatomical variations of the femoral vein. J Vasc Surg. 2010; 52(3):714–719

[4] Park EA, Chung JW, Lee W, et al. Three-dimensional evaluation of the anatomic variations of the femoral vein and popliteal vein in relation to the accompanying artery by using CT venography. Korean J Radiol. 2011; 12(3): 327–340

[5] Kropman RH, Kiela G, Moll FL, de Vries JP. Variations in anatomy of the popliteal artery and its side branches. Vasc Endovascular Surg. 2011; 45(6):536–540

[6] Mackenzie D, Seyfer A. Reconstructive surgery: lower extremity coverage. In: Mathes S, Hentz V, eds. Plastic Surgery Volume 6 Trunk And Lower Extremity. 2nd ed. Philadelphia: Saunders Elsevier; 2006

[7] American College of Surgeons Committee on Trauma. Advanced Trauma Life Support. 8th ed. Chicago: American College of Surgeons Committee on Trauma; 2008:187–203

[8] Richards A, Dafydd H. Key Notes on Plastic Surgery. 2nd ed. Hoboken: Wiley; 2014

[9] Standards for the Management of Open Fractures of the Lower Limb. London: Royal Society of Medicine Press; 2009. Available at: http://www.bapras.org.uk/docs/default-source/commissioning-and-policy/standards-for-lower-limb.pdf?sfvrsn=0. Accessed October 20, 2017

[10] Gustilo RB, Merkow RL, Templeman D. The management of open fractures. J Bone Joint Surg Am. 1990; 72(2):299–304

[11] Janis J, O'Reilly E. Lower extremity reconstruction. In: Janis J, ed. Essentials of Plastic Surgery. 2nd ed. Boca Raton, FL: Taylor and Francis; 2014:651–665

[12] Latifi R, El-Hennawy H, El-Menyar A, et al. The therapeutic challenges of degloving soft-tissue injuries. J Emerg Trauma Shock. 2014; 7(3):228–232

[13] Hakim S, Ahmed K, El-Menyar A, et al. Patterns and management of degloving injuries: a single national level 1 trauma center experience. World J Emerg Surg. 2016; 11(1):35

[14] Phillips BT, Munabi NCO, Roeder RA, Ascherman JA, Guo L, Zenn MR. The role of intraoperative perfusion assessment: what is the current state and how can i use it in my practice? Plast Reconstr Surg. 2016; 137(2):731–741

[15] Hardwicke JT, Osmani O, Skillman JM. Detection of perforators using smartphone thermal imaging. Plast Reconstr Surg. 2016; 137(1):39–41

[16] Arnez ZM, Khan U, Tyler MP. Classification of soft-tissue degloving in limb trauma. J Plast Reconstr Aesthet Surg. 2010; 63(11):1865–1869

[17] Khan U, Ho K, Deva A. Exchanging split-skin grafts to reduce donor morbidity in limited pretibial degloving injuries. Plast Reconstr Surg. 2004; 113(5): 1523–1525

[18] Bradow BP, Hallock GG, Wilcock SP. Immediate regrafting of the split thickness skin graft donor site assists healing. Plast Reconstr Surg Glob Open. 2017; 5(5):e1339

[19] Gaillard F. Osteomyelitis | Radiology Reference Article | Radiopaedia.org. Radiopaediaorg. 2017. Available at: https://radiopaedia.org/articles/osteomyelitis. Accessed October 20, 2017

[20] IWGDF | The International Working Group on the Diabetic Foot. Iwgdforg. 2017. Available at: http://iwgdf.org/. Accessed October 21, 2017

[21] Reddy G. Foot ulcers. In: Janis J, ed. Essentials of Plastic Surgery. 2nd ed. Boca Raton, FL: Taylor and Francis; 2014:667–680

[22] Singh N, Armstrong DG, Lipsky BA. Preventing foot ulcers in patients with diabetes. JAMA. 2005; 293(2):217–228

[23] Noor S, Khan RU, Ahmad J. Understanding diabetic foot infection and its management. Diabetes Metab Syndr. 2017; 11(2):149–156

[24] Lavery LA, Armstrong DG, Vela SA, Quebedeaux TL, Fleischli JG. Practical criteria for screening patients at high risk for diabetic foot ulceration. Arch Intern Med. 1998; 158(2):157–162

[25] Colen L, Uroskie T. Foot reconstruction: lower extremity coverage. In: Mathes S, Hentz V, eds. Plastic Surgery: Volume 6, Trunk and Lower Extremity. 2nd ed. Philadelphia, PA: Saunders Elsevier; 2006

[26] Conrad MC. Large and small artery occlusion in diabetics and nondiabetics with severe vascular disease. Circulation. 1967; 36(1):83–91

3 Indications for Vascular Intervention in Lower Extremity Reconstruction

David L. Colen and Lawrence B. Colen

Summary

Proper initial assessment of the peripheral vascular status of the impaired lower limb should never be overlooked, as a balance between the arterial and venous systems is essential for equilibrium of the homeostatic mechanisms responsible for tissue regeneration and wound healing. Vascular laboratory evaluations that include basic ankle-brachial indices and pulse volume recordings, as well as standard imaging technologies, may be required for staging and characterizing the extent of any disease processes. These will aid in determining if a vascular surgery consultation would be essential, often mandatory before any reconstructive endeavor.

Keywords: peripheral vascular disease, ankle-brachial index, pulse volume recordings

3.1 Introduction

Uncomplicated lower extremity wound healing relies on adequate tissue perfusion. Satisfactory arterial inflow allows access for immune cells and provides metabolic factors for the inflammatory process and the subsequent anabolic stages of healing. Likewise, venous outflow will provide for the elimination of undesirable metabolites and byproducts. This important balance underlies the homeostatic mechanisms of wound healing and tissue remodeling; likewise, disturbances in this perfusion–drainage equilibrium will contribute to pathologic changes in the healing process and may cause *de novo* wounds to develop from ischemia, venous stasis, or a combination of the two.

The lower extremity is at increased risk for peripheral vascular disease (PVD) and often presents a significant challenge for the reconstructive surgeon. Patients with known peripheral arterial disease (PAD) or the stigmata thereof (i.e., claudication, ulceration) and those with risk factors for atherosclerotic disease (smoking, obesity, diabetes) must be carefully evaluated and screened. Failure to first appreciate vascular disease is the cardinal sin of lower extremity reconstruction as it will lead to catastrophic outcomes.

The progress realized in reconstructive surgery over the past three decades has been paralleled by our vascular surgery colleagues. In the 1970s, aortofemoral bypass and/or profundaplasty were the only vascular surgical options to improve the blood supply to a chronically ischemic limb. Today, bypass grafting and endovascular procedures below the popliteal artery, and all the way into the foot are commonplace.

3.2 Principles of Limb Salvage

Successful limb salvage or reconstruction depends on proper patient selection, judicious preoperative preparation, and meticulous postoperative care. Anyone embarking upon a career in the management of lower extremity wounds must understand the relationship between the reconstructive options conferred by the phasic nature of blood flow into the limb and the amount of tissue required for the reconstructive effort. It is critically important that the reconstructive surgeon is well versed in the lexicon and arsenal of his vascular surgery counterpart. An appropriate understanding of the tools of the vascular laboratory and the interventional options available will both improve collaboration and optimize outcomes in lower extremity reconstruction.

Proper management of dysvascular lower extremity wounds requires a multidisciplinary approach including, but not limited to, plastic surgery, vascular surgery, podiatry, endocrinology, neurology, infectious disease, and physical/occupational therapy. Institution of a "limb salvage team" dedicated to the comprehensive management of lower extremity wounds is becoming increasingly common and has many benefits. This team typically consists of a vascular surgeon, plastic surgeon, and a podiatrist with additional members added as necessary via consultation. This team should be able to perform several important tasks to optimize limb salvage including assessing wounds; recognizing signs of infection and ischemia; performing a thorough vascular evaluation; performing wound debridements at the bedside or, when necessary, in the operating room; and initiating and modifying culture-specific antibiotic therapy.[1]

Prior to intervention, patients should be in optimal medical condition (e.g., smoking cessation, glycemic control) and evaluated for potential barriers to successful rehabilitation as well as risk factors for wound recurrence. Diabetic patients present a challenge, as these lower extremity ulcerations occur because of both ischemic and neuropathic changes in most patients. These same factors can predispose diabetic patients to either a reconstructive failure or wound recurrence. A full neurologic evaluation is vital for both treatment planning and patient selection. In addition, the closure of foot wounds in the presence of diabetic neuropathy with Charcot deformity should include proper biomechanical manipulation of the limb to prevent recurrent ulceration.[2]

3.3 Anatomy

It is well understood that sufficient blood supply is crucial for wound healing. To properly address lower extremity limb salvage, one must understand both the longitudinal courses and branches of the lower extremity vessels as well as the musculoskeletal and integumentary domains supplied by that vasculature. This latter part, known as the angiosome theory, becomes crucially important when planning a reconstruction. Understanding which vessels are responsible for the perfusion to the different anatomical locations in the lower extremity can be the difference between success and failure in the dysvascular patient.

All arterial inflow to the lower extremity below the inguinal ligament is derived from the external iliac artery, which becomes the common femoral artery (CFA) upon entering the thigh. It then bifurcates into the superficial femoral artery (SFA) and profunda femoris artery (PFA). Although much of the medial, lateral, and posterior thigh are supplied by the terminal branches of the PFA, the SFA gives segmental branches to the sartorius and rectus femoris muscles as it spirals inferomedially and distally enters the Hunter canal. In the popliteal fossa, the SFA becomes the popliteal artery and gives off superior medial and lateral genicular branches (important contributors to the genicular anastomosis supplying the knee joint) and the medial and lateral sural arteries that nourish the gastrocnemius muscle bellies. At the level of the tibial and fibular metaphyses, the popliteal artery branches into the anterior tibial artery, which pierces the interosseous membrane to supply the anterior and lateral compartment soft tissues, and the tibioperoneal trunk. The latter in turn branches into the posterior tibial and peroneal arteries, the last two of the three "runoff" arteries in the lower leg and foot. Although the peroneal artery terminates as calcaneal branches after descending in the lateral compartment of the leg, the posterior tibial artery provides flow directly to the foot as does the anterior tibial that terminates as the dorsalis pedis artery. Within the tarsal tunnel, the posterior tibial artery divides into the medial and lateral plantar arteries.

In 1987, Taylor and Palmer introduced the concept that discrete arterial segments reliably perfuse tissues within well-defined three-dimensional territories, or angiosomes.[3] This concept provided an anatomical understanding of flap perfusion as well as ischemic wound etiology and now provides the basis for safe planning of surgical incisions to maximize healing capacity. Since then, these authors have clarified the angiosome anatomy specifically of the lower extremity,[3,4] improving our understanding of soft-tissue perfusion and the etiology of ischemic wounds of the lower extremity.[4,5]

As a result, many advocate an angiosome-directed intervention to maximize the likelihood of success and a recent meta-analysis showed improved healing of foot wounds treated with an angiosome-directed intervention.[6] However, critics of this method suggest that chronically ischemic extremities develop compensatory collateral circulation which makes the angiosome anatomy irrelevant in those situations.[7]

3.4 Vascular Evaluation

Prior to any lower extremity reconstructive intervention, the vascular status of the leg must be completely evaluated. This begins with a pertinent history and physical examination (▶ Table 3.1).

Table 3.1 History and physical examination of vascular disease

Clinical history
• Rest pain, claudication
• Weakness
• Changes in sensation (numbness, hypersensitivity)
• Discoloration (pallor, ecchymosis)
• Swelling
• Ulceration, tissue loss
• Varicosities
• Comorbidity: obesity, smoking, diabetes, autoimmune disease, trauma, hypercoagulability, deep vein thrombosis, hyperhomocysteinemia, chronic renal insufficiency
Physical examination
• Edema (pitting, nonpitting, lymphedema stage)
• Varicosities
• Atrophy
• Cyanosis
• Mottling
• Pallor
• Rubor
• Temperature
• Hair distribution
• Abnormal nail growth
• Ulceration, tissue loss
• Pulses, signals
• Motor function

3.4.1 History Assessment

A thorough clinical history describes symptoms based on the timing and circumstances of their initial onset (acute vs. chronic), progression over time, location, contribution to disability, and their association with aggravating or mitigating factors, such as activity, dependency, or temperature. Peripheral arterial and venous disease follow a common pattern of progression, and deviations from this pattern should raise suspicion for other disease processes (e.g., autoimmune, oncologic) that may be contributing to wound physiology. Comorbid conditions must also be thoroughly documented and managed. In patients without lower extremity vascular symptoms, important historical concerns include any cerebrovascular events (transient ischemic attack, stroke), cardiovascular events (myocardial infarction, arrhythmia), or thrombotic episodes.

3.4.2 Physical Examination

Physical examination is an important source of information that builds from the clinical history and gives the surgeon insight into the severity and chronicity of the patient's disease. In the reconstructive setting, vascular disease is a formidable opponent to wound healing and clues to its presence are crucial for proper patient selection and a successful outcome. PAD symptoms vary based on the severity and chronicity of the process, from mild/intermittent claudication to ischemic rest pain and limb-threatening trophic changes/wounds (▶ Table 3.1).

3.4.3 Vascular Laboratory Evaluation

Any suspicion of vascular disease on the physical exam (▶ Table 3.1) prompts the need for further evaluation in the vascular laboratory. Determining ankle-brachial index (ABI) and pulse volume recordings (PVRs) is important in staging and characterizing the extent of PVD. Obtaining directional Doppler flow studies and vascular imaging is helpful in planning reconstruction.

Ankle-Brachial Indices

The ABI is a simple measurement that can be done with a sphygmomanometer and continuous wave Doppler probe. Brachial arterial systolic pressure serves as a reference for the determination of the ABI, giving an indication of the relative degree of ischemia. In addition, the absolute pressure measured at the ankle seems to correlate well with the prognosis of healing of skin wounds. Most surgeons would agree that absolute pressures less than 50 mm Hg signify rather severe PVD with a poor prognosis for healing.[8,9] However, the ankle pressure measurement is not always accurate. Rigid arteries because of medial sclerosis, as most frequently seen in patients with diabetes, yield erroneously high-pressure measurements in the leg, giving falsely elevated ankle-brachial pressure indices. It is quite important, then, to obtain additional information with other noninvasive techniques, to assess the distal circulation more accurately. Patients with calcified arteries about the ankle should have measurements obtained from the great toe rather than the ankle vessels, as the toe digital arteries are less likely to have become calcified and can give a more reliable indication of pedal perfusion[10] (▶ Fig. 3.1). Normal reference values for the ABI are shown in ▶ Table 3.2.

Pulse Volume Recordings

Pulse volume recordings provide a functional assessment of arterial perfusion of the lower extremity. PVRs use air plethysmography to determine changes in volume in the extremity during systole. Cuffs are placed at each segment of the extremity and inflated to a known pressure and volume. Pulse volume changes are measured as a change in pressure within the cuff and converted to an analog pressure pulse curve. Normal PVR waveforms have a systolic upstroke and a sharp systolic peak followed by a diastolic down stroke with a distinct dicrotic notch (▶ Fig. 3.1). Alterations in the pulse volume curve and amplitude suggest aberrant arterial flow with loss of the dicrotic notch and a widening of the complex, in mild to moderate disease, and eventual loss of amplitude in severe disease. PVRs are paired with segmental pressures and particularly helpful when extensive arterial calcinosis renders vessels noncompressible and gives falsely elevated ABIs. Waveforms are recorded from high in the thigh, the distal thigh, the calf, the ankle, and the great toe to detect and localize the region of the vascular disease.

Analog Doppler Waveforms

Though similar in many respects to a PVR, some patients, especially those with known PVD, benefit from the evaluation of Doppler velocity recordings. These are recorded from peripheral arteries and are important for the diagnosis and localization of occlusive PAD. The normal Doppler blood flow velocity waveform is triphasic, consisting of forward flow, reverse flow, and a second forward flow component (▶ Fig. 3.2a). Distal to an arterial stenosis or occlusion, the waveform is dampened, the amplitude of the velocity wave is decreased, the peak is delayed, and the reverse flow component is attenuated or absent (▶ Fig. 3.2b). In the usual vascular laboratory study, waveforms are recorded from the femoral, popliteal, dorsalis pedis, and posterior tibial arteries to detect and localize the region of the vascular disease. Although these studies provide only qualitative flow profiles, they assist both the vascular surgeon and plastic surgeon in planning their reconstructive approaches.

3.4.4 Imaging

Vascular imaging plays a crucial role in planning lower extremity reconstruction and provides important information about the patency of vessels, location of vascular lesions or obstructions, and the character of blood flow into the foot. Lower extremity angiography is the gold standard for diagnosing and characterizing the quality of arterial flow of the lower extremity. Angiography is an invasive procedure that must be done in a specialized room often with hybrid technology, making it expensive and cumbersome. Therefore, CT angiography (CTA), when available, has now supplanted conventional angiography in many cases. Atherosclerotic occlusive disease occurs and progresses in recognizable patterns. Lesions typically originate at the ostia of branch vessels or at main arterial

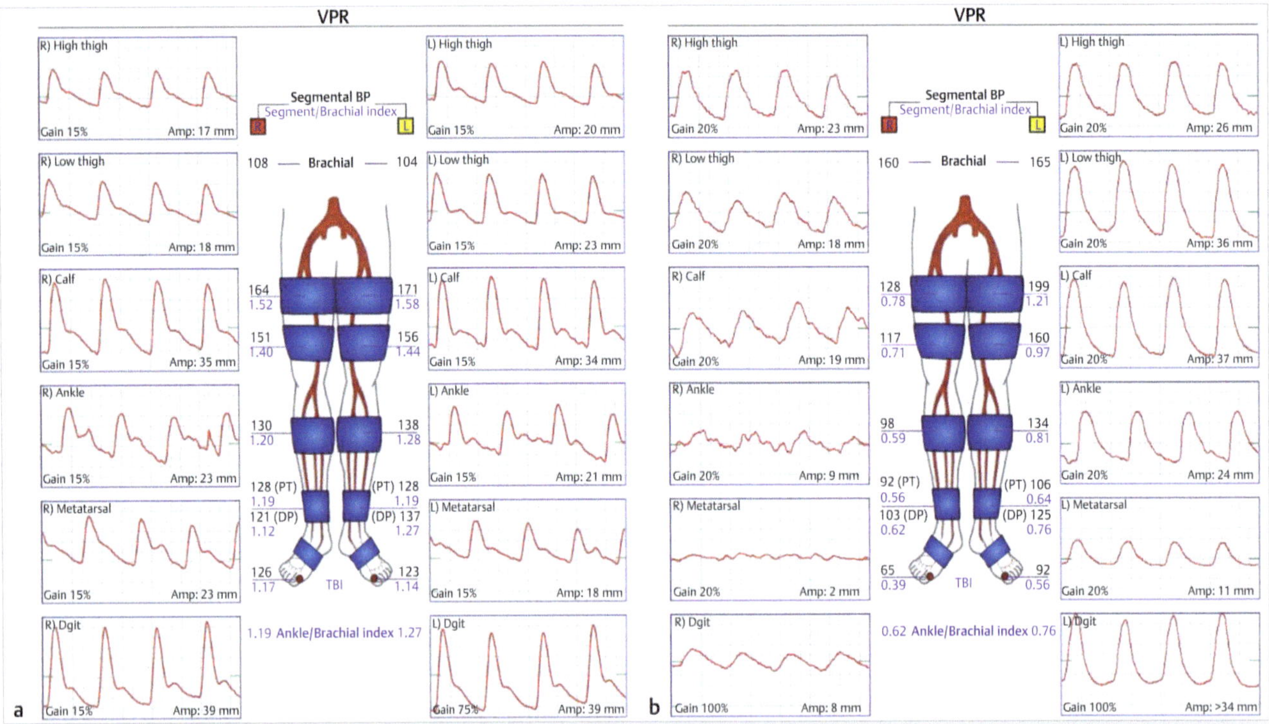

Fig. 3.1 Ankle-brachial index (ABI) and pulse volume recording (PVR). **(a)** Normal ABI and PVR morphology distally. This patient has a clean systolic upstroke, a sharp systolic peak, and a diastolic down stroke with a dicrotic notch indicating healthy and elastic arteries. **(b)** It is important to obtain toe-brachial indices in patients with calcified or noncompressible vessels around the ankle, as the digital vessels are less prone to calcification. For example, this patient has poor waveforms around the right ankle and foot, but a better PVR waveform in the right great toe.

Table 3.2 Reference values for ABI

ABI value (ankle SBP/brachial SBP)	Interpretation	Recommendation
> 1.4	Calcified, noncompressible vessels	Consider referral to vascular surgery
1.0–1.4	Normal	Proceed with reconstruction
0.9–1.0	Satisfactory	
0.8–0.9	Mild arterial disease	Treat modifiable risk factors, proceed with reconstruction
0.5–0.8	Moderate arterial disease	Refer to vascular surgeon for possible revascularization • If able to obtain "good" monophasic flow, can proceed with free tissue transfer • If able to improve ABI to > 0.5, can attempt local tissue reconstruction

Abbreviations: ABI, ankle-brachial indices; SBP, systolic blood pressure.

bifurcations, and progress over time to affect multiple levels of the arterial tree. As a rule, younger patients will have isolated aortoiliac and focal superficial femoral arterial disease, whereas older patients may have occlusive disease that is more diffusely distributed. Patients with diabetes, however, are prone to isolated tibial and peroneal lesions rather than more proximal disease.[11]

Magnetic resonance angiography (MRA) offers an alternative, albeit costlier, method for vascular imaging. MRA may be required in patients who cannot tolerate intravenous radiopaque contrast either due to allergy or nephropathy. It has an important advantage over conventional angiography, as the visualization of vessels on MRA is solely dependent on the presence of blood flow, not contrast, making MRA more sensitive than conventional angiography when assessing the distal circulation.[12]

Duplex imaging has been very helpful in the preoperative planning for lower extremity microsurgery, both in the post-traumatic and dysvascular patient. It provides meaningful information about both the arterial and venous circulation of the foot and ankle when free tissue transfer is contemplated. A combination of anatomic, geometric, and velocity data, as well as blood flow measurements from most desired locations within the vascular system can be obtained. It is possible to scan the arteries about the leg and foot and precisely locate sites of disease as well as measure quantitatively the velocity patterns and changes across such segments. Duplex imaging combines a real-time B-mode imaging system with a pulsed

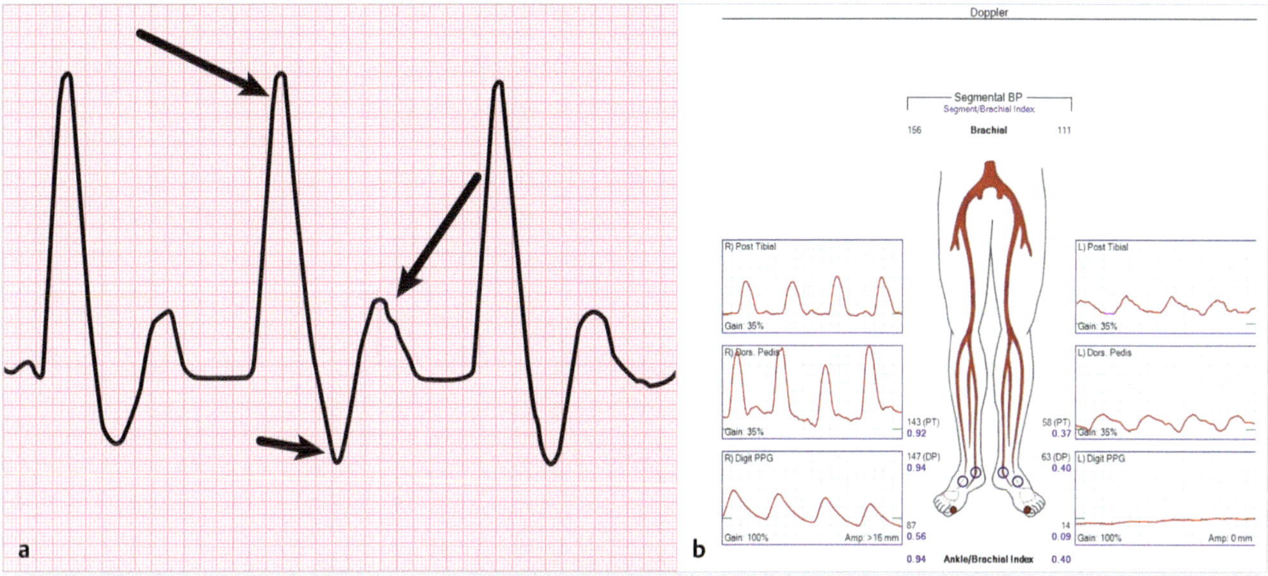

Fig. 3.2 Analog Doppler assessment. **(a)** Normal study from a posterior tibial artery showing two forward flow components (*long arrows*) and a reverse flow component (*short arrow*). **(b)** Abnormal study (left leg) distal to an arterial stenosis/occlusion. There is loss of the normal waveform with very poor monophasic flow in the dorsalis pedis and posterior tibial vessels and aphasic flow in the left great toe.

Doppler unit. Images of the vessel being scanned are stored electronically on the monitor so that accurate measurements of vessel diameter, luminal irregularities, and blood flow velocity may be obtained. We have found Duplex imaging to be invaluable in the assessment of the venous circulation as well. The presence or absence of deep venous pathology can determine the most effective management of venous outflow from free tissue transfer surgery. Assessment of the zone of injury in the posttraumatic patient will help determine the most appropriate location for arterial and venous anastomosis (either proximal or distal to the zone of injury).[13] Identification of perforators that can be used as recipient vessels even in the presence of otherwise severe occlusive disease can allow free tissue transfers using supermicrosurgery.[14,15]

Recently, fluorescence angiography, using indocyanine green (ICG), has been incorporated into the vascular evaluation of lower extremity wounds.[16] This method uses intravascular ICG injection and quantitative tissue fluorescence to characterize skin perfusion which can provide very meaningful information regarding the ability of the wound to heal either with or without flap or skin graft surgery. In many patients, it can provide the needed information to guide the need for vascular surgical intervention or level of amputation if limb salvage is not feasible.

3.5 Plastic Surgery Indications for Vascular Surgical Intervention

Abnormalities in vascular testing are to be expected in patients with known PVD and may necessitate vascular intervention prior to performing soft-tissue reconstruction. Every effort should be made to maximize blood flow to the lower extremity prior to performing wound closure surgery. If pedal pulses are not palpable, vascular laboratory evaluation is mandatory. If any abnormalities of flow are found, vascular surgery consultation is requested. It is quite common that a relatively simple endovascular intervention will set the stage for uncomplicated healing either with or without plastic surgery assistance.

In our experience, the need for vascular intervention is determined by two important variables: how much tissue is required for wound repair and the phasic nature of the blood flow recorded via Doppler waveform assessment (PVR). For smaller wounds on the foot, that can be closed with local tissue using either advancement or rotation techniques, we have found that an ABI of 0.5 or greater is satisfactory to allow for uncomplicated wound healing. This, generally, would be manifested as a "good" monophasic waveform on PVRs. Larger tissue requirements will often necessitate free tissue transfer techniques which will demand blood flow in the recipient artery to be, at least, "good" monophasic flow.[17] When free tissue transfer is deemed necessary for reconstruction, either due to size and complexity of the wound or because of a lack of local tissue options, we have found that the nature of the arterial waveform becomes an important variable to consider. Both clinically and in our laboratory, we have found that, at least, a "good" monophasic" signal is necessary to maintain patency of a microvascular anastomosis.[17]

Patients with total occlusion of the SFA present a unique challenge when contemplating the use of an ipsilateral anterolateral thigh free flap for soft-tissue repair. Upon review of CT angiograms from 673 diabetic patients, Suh et al[18] found that most limbs (96%) rely on collaterals from both the profunda femoral *and* descending branch of the lateral circumflex femoral arteries (compared to profunda femoral artery alone [3%] or descending branch of the lateral circumflex femoral artery alone [1%]). Thus, when SFA occlusion is suspected, choosing a flap based on the lateral circumflex femoral artery (the vastus lateralis muscle flap or the anterolateral thigh flap) could deprive the distal extremity of more than half of its inflow and compromise the foot. Vascular surgery consultation in this patient population is crucial prior to selecting this flap.[18]

3.6 Special Considerations for the "Vascular/Diabetic" Patient

For relatively small wounds on the plantar surface of the foot, local flap options are usually the best reconstructive alternative. These options generally require antegrade blood flow in the posterior tibial artery and its medial and lateral plantar branches. Many diabetic patients with plantar wounds who have single vessel runoff to the foot via the dorsalis pedis artery or who have had a vascular bypass procedure to the distal anterior tibial or dorsalis pedis arteries will be found to have retrograde flow through the plantar vessels making use of intrinsic muscle flaps or medial plantar flaps unsafe. As such, these wounds generally require the use of a free tissue transfer (▶ Fig. 3.3). It is important when evaluating the blood supply to the foot that the surgeon listen to the blood flow in the dorsalis pedis and posterior tibial arteries with the handheld Doppler. The surgeon should listen over the posterior tibial artery at the ankle and while occluding the dorsalis pedis blood flow by digital compression. If flow through the posterior tibial artery is retrograde, the Doppler signal will disappear.

Successful microvascular anastomosis is best performed on noncalcified recipient vessels. It is common for diabetic patients and particularly those who are on dialysis to have significant arterial calcifications. Though preoperative Duplex imaging may help the reconstructive surgeon find an area of vessel wall that is relatively free of calcium (▶ Fig. 3.4), if no suitable noncalcified segment of the recipient vessels can be identified within a reasonable distance from the wound, then vascular surgery can help by performing a saphenous vein bypass graft, which can then be used as the recipient site artery to ensure flap perfusion.

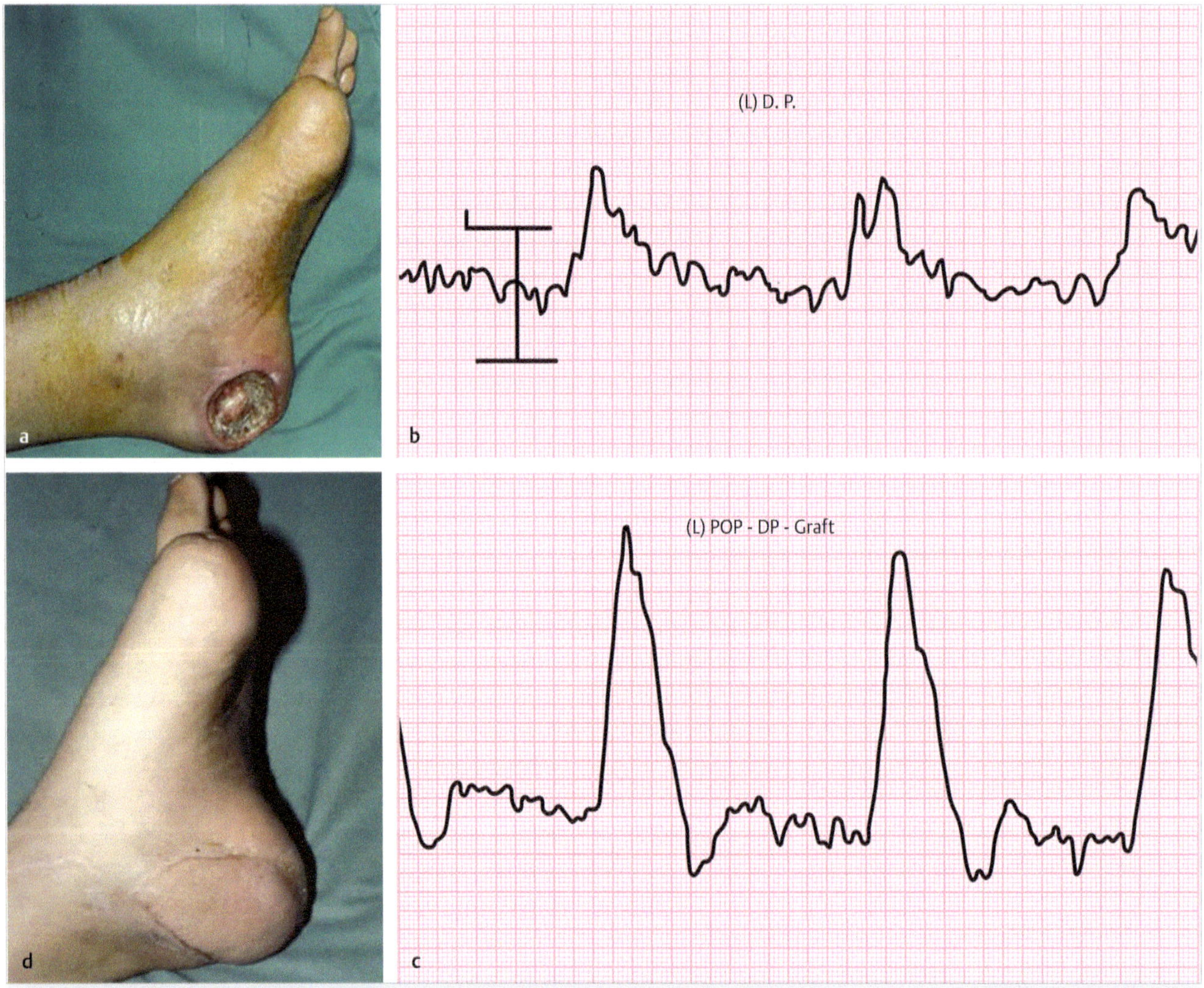

Fig. 3.3 **(a)** Left heel wound. **(b)** Preoperative dorsalis pedis (DP) waveform. **(c)** Improved DP waveform following bypass grafting to the dorsalis pedis artery that restored flow to the foot. The medial and lateral plantar vessel blood flow was retrograde as expected so that a local plantar flap was inadvisable. **(d)** Successful serratus anterior muscle flap and skin graft using the now adequate dorsalis pedis vessels as the recipient site.

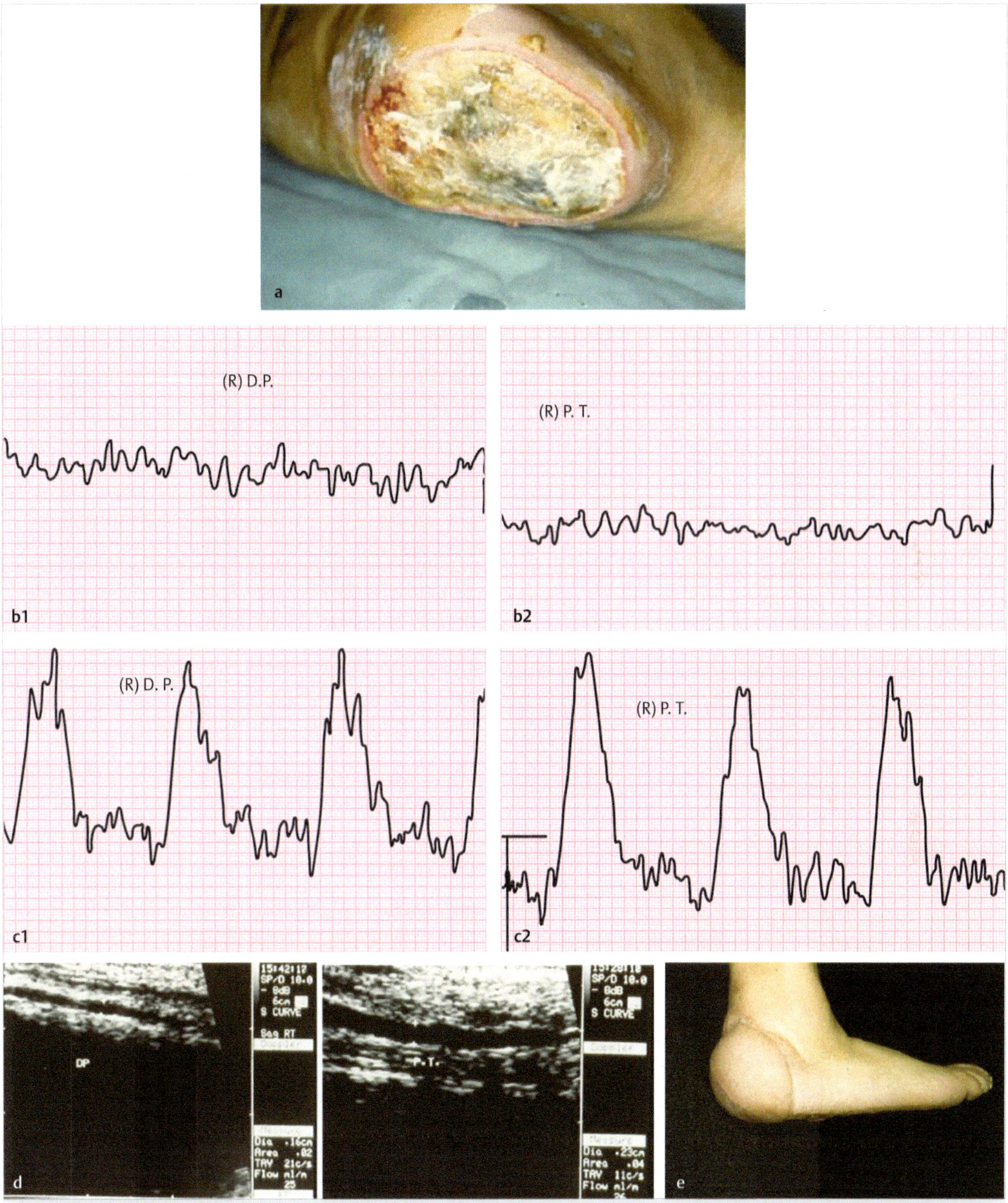

Fig. 3.4 **(a)** Large necrotic right heel wound in this diabetic patient on long-term dialysis. **(b)** Initial Doppler waveforms of the dorsalis pedis and posterior tibial vessels show aphasic blood flow. **(c)** Following femoral-popliteal bypass grafting, the ankle waveforms are improved without evidence of one vessel being "dominant." **(d)** Duplex scans show the posterior tibial artery to be larger than the dorsalis pedis artery and relatively free of intraluminal irregularities even though blood flow velocity was similar. **(e)** Well-healed scapular free flap reconstruction using the deemed preferable posterior tibial vessels.

References

[1] Fitzgerald RH, Mills JL, Joseph W, Armstrong DG. The diabetic rapid response acute foot team: 7 essential skills for targeted limb salvage. Eplasty. 2009; 9:e15

[2] Colen LB, Kim CJ, Grant WP, Yeh JT, Hind B. Achilles tendon lengthening: friend or foe in the diabetic foot? Plast Reconstr Surg. 2013; 131(1):37e–43e

[3] Taylor GI, Palmer JH. The vascular territories (angiosomes) of the body: experimental study and clinical applications. Br J Plast Surg. 1987; 40(2): 113–141

[4] Taylor GI, Pan WR. Angiosomes of the leg: anatomic study and clinical implications. Plast Reconstr Surg. 1998; 102(3):599–616, discussion 617–618

[5] Attinger CE, Evans KK, Bulan E, Blume P, Cooper P. Angiosomes of the foot and ankle and clinical implications for limb salvage: reconstruction, incisions, and revascularization. Plast Reconstr Surg. 2006; 117(7) Suppl:261S–293S

[6] Biancari F, Juvonen T. Angiosome-targeted lower limb revascularization for ischemic foot wounds: systematic review and meta-analysis. Eur J Vasc Endovasc Surg. 2014; 47(5):517–522

[7] McCallum JC, Lane JS, III. Angiosome-directed revascularization for critical limb ischemia. Semin Vasc Surg. 2014; 27(1):32–37

[8] Holstein P, Lassen NA. Healing of ulcers on the feet correlated with distal blood pressure measurements in occlusive arterial disease. Acta Orthop Scand. 1980; 51(6):995–1006

[9] Lassen NA, Tönnesen KH, Holstein P. Distal blood pressure. Scand J Clin Lab Invest. 1976; 36(8):705–709

[10] Collins KA, Sumpio BE. Vascular assessment. Clin Podiatr Med Surg. 2000; 17(2):171–191

[11] Sumpio BE, Lee T, Blume PA. Vascular evaluation and arterial reconstruction of the diabetic foot. Clin Podiatr Med Surg. 2003; 20(4):689–708

[12] Owen RS, Carpenter JP, Baum RA, Perloff LJ, Cope C. Magnetic resonance imaging of angiographically occult runoff vessels in peripheral arterial occlusive disease. N Engl J Med. 1992; 326(24):1577–1581

[13] Colen LB. Limb salvage in the patient with severe peripheral vascular disease: the role of microsurgical free-tissue transfer. Plast Reconstr Surg. 1987; 79(3): 389–395

[14] Hallock GG. Evaluation of fasciocutaneous perforators using color duplex imaging. Plast Reconstr Surg. 1994; 94(5):644–651

[15] Hong JP. The use of supermicrosurgery in lower extremity reconstruction: the next step in evolution. Plast Reconstr Surg. 2009; 123(1):230–235

[16] Samies JH, Gehling M, Serena TE, Yaakov RA. Use of a fluorescence angiography system in assessment of lower extremity ulcers in patients with peripheral arterial disease: a review and a look forward. Semin Vasc Surg. 2015; 28(3-4):190–194

[17] Colen LB, Hamdy E, Totan S, Potparic Z, Badran H. Effect of monophasic blood flow on the patency of microvascular anastomoses. J Reconstr Microsurg. 1999; 15(8):609–613

[18] Suh HP, Kim Y, Suh Y, Hong J. Multidetector computed tomography (CT) analysis of 168 cases in diabetic patients with total superficial femoral artery occlusion: is it safe to use an anterolateral thigh flap without CT angiography in diabetic patients? J Reconstr Microsurg. 2018; 34(1):65–70

4 Orthopaedic Evaluation of the Lower Extremity and the Concept of the Orthoplastic Approach

Shaun D. Mendenhall, Nicole A. Zelenski, Oded Ben-Amotz, Stephen J. Kovach, and L. Scott Levin

Summary

If salvage of a lower extremity is the chosen path, any reconstruction will require stable skeletal support as well as adequate and durable soft-tissue coverage. The former is within the realm of the orthopaedic surgeon, whereas the latter typically is in the domain of the plastic surgeon or sometimes the orthopaedic soft-tissue expert. Most often, these are complementary roles best performed by a mutual cooperation in using the principles of both specialties to obtain the optimum functional result, and that is the *orthoplastic approach.* If focusing on the traumatic wound, treatment should be initiated as soon as reasonable, and always after a complete evaluation of the patient for concomitant medical issues. Radical debridement is then essential. If necessary, serial debridement may be required before contemplating closure, and that will be more likely the higher the Gustilo grade of injury. Fracture fixation should be performed so as not to be an obstacle to later soft-tissue management or even vascularized bone transfer. The choice, instead of amputation, must always be individualized, as injury severity scoring systems have been found not to be reliably predictable.

Keywords: orthoplastic approach, Gustilo classification, medial femoral condyle flap, debridement.

4.1 Introduction

Just as in the craft of carpentry, a stable foundation and framework is absolutely essential to uphold the final function of a building, but no more important than the sheetrock, trim, and paint that make the building functional, durable, and livable. Reconstruction of the lower extremity is similar, where the orthopaedic surgeon must obtain stable fixation of the damaged bone while the plastic or orthopaedic soft-tissue surgeon must provide vascularized, stable coverage over that damaged bone. These two components are complementary, not adversarial, and both contribute to the success or failure of functional limb restoration. The quality of bone repair and healing will predict the ultimate weight-bearing status, while the vascularized envelope will bring nourishment, immune system elements, antibiotics, and protection to the repaired bone. When both aspects are properly attended to, the result is often a functional limb with an acceptable appearance. While a single surgeon need not perform both of these tasks (although some may choose to do so), the orthopaedic and plastic surgeons involved in this care must have a clear understanding of the other's role and the importance of each other for a good outcome. This is what we call the *orthoplastic approach* to reconstructive surgery of the extremities, that is, *the application of the principles of both the specialties of orthopaedic and plastic surgery simultaneously to optimize the outcomes in limb reconstruction.*[1,2,3,4] We plan to discuss the pertinent history and key elements of orthoplastic surgery along with the factors that lead to good outcomes in lower extremity reconstruction. These will always include a thorough orthopaedic evaluation of the extremity; the role and timing of debridement and then flap coverage; the key elements of bone fixation, limb salvage versus amputation; and other applications of orthoplastic surgery.

4.2 The Orthoplastic Approach

Since the days of Hippocrates, surgeons have treated traumatized extremities by providing fracture stabilization using splints or external fixators, and soft-tissue injuries have been treated with various potions and salves. The need for proper limb alignment and healing of soft tissue and bone has been the subject of medicine throughout both the ancient and modern eras. It is the history of medicine that allows us to introduce the concept of orthoplastic surgery. Individuals such as Ambroise Pare, Gaspar Tagliacozzi, Dupuytren, Velpau, and Malgaigne had careers as master surgeons ranging from the 16th century to the middle of the 19th century. If we read the history of orthopaedic surgery or the history of plastic surgery, each of these individuals is mentioned as founding fathers of these respected specialties.

The evolution of distinct surgical specialties really developed at the conclusion of the 19th century. Modern plastic surgery has its roots in the trenches of World War I and is approximately 100 years old. Probably the first modern orthopaedic plastic collaboration was between W. Arbuthnot Lane and Sir Harold Gilles. In 1919, Lane, an orthopaedic surgeon, wrote the preface for Major Gilles' textbook, and so began the modern era of "orthoplastic surgery."[4]

The development of reconstructive microsurgery allowed modern orthoplastic surgery to develop. In 1960, Jacobsen and Suarez introduced the operating microscope for the suture of small vessels.[5,6] In 1968, Tamai reported the first successful digital replantation.[7,8] Other microsurgical successes evolved in the later part of the 1960s.[5,9] Composite transfer of vascularized tissues became commonplace in the 1980s, with an explosion of techniques, flaps, and the popularization of microvascular surgery not just for the traumatic injury of the extremities and replantation but also for elective reconstructive surgery. Refinements such as flap expansion, prefabrication, and modification of tissue transfers continued to take place in the 1990s.[7] During this era, innovations have continued including a better understanding of the angiosome concept and the microvasculature territories of skin, leading to a wide array of new free tissue transfer options for complex defects, for example, by utilizing perforator-based flaps.[10] The modern reconstructive microsurgeon today has an armamentarium of flap options: skin, fascia, adipofascial, fasciocutaneous, muscle, or vascularized bone flaps, as well as combined tissue flaps or chimeric flaps. Over the last two decades, vascularized composite allotransplantation has also developed to become the highest rung on the reconstructive ladder.[11,12] This explosion of microsurgical advancements has become one of the pillars of orthoplastic surgery.

A better understanding of orthoplastic surgery can be obtained by analyzing the two specialties involved. Plastic surgery specialization over the last 50 years has come to include:

- Microsurgery.
- Hand surgery.
- Burn care.
- Aesthetic surgery.
- Breast reconstruction.
- Craniofacial surgery.

Plastic surgeons tend to place emphasis on:

- Careful soft-tissue handling and reconstruction.
- Detailed suture and layered closure techniques.
- Aesthetics and improving appearance.

Similarly, orthopaedic specialization has occurred with development of separate societies concentrating on:

- Pediatric orthopaedics.
- Trauma.
- Musculoskeletal oncology.
- Joint reconstruction.
- Hand surgery.
- Sports medicine.

Orthopaedic surgeons tend to focus on:

- Functional outcomes.
- Biomechanics.
- Stable bone and joint reconstruction.
- Rehabilitation.

Therefore, the blending of all these strengths of the two specialties constitutes the definition of orthoplastic surgery:

"The principles and practices of both specialties applied to clinical problems simultaneously, either by a single provider or team of providers working in concert for the benefit of the patient."[1,6]

This combined "orthoplastic" approach to patients with severe injuries to the lower extremities will lead to not only better outcomes such as quicker time to bone union, more durable soft-tissue coverage, less pain, and better function, but also fewer complications, shorter hospital stays, and higher patient satisfaction, which are all important in the current health care climate of bundled payments and outcomes-based reimbursement, a landmine more easily traversed by always obtaining optimal results.

4.3 Orthopaedic Evaluation of the Injured Extremity

Combined bone and soft-tissue injuries to the lower extremity come in many different shapes, locations, and sizes. The Gustilo classification has become the most widely accepted and simple way to classify open fractures of the lower extremity.[13,14] This classification consists of three main categories of open fractures with three subtypes (▶ Table 4.1).

The group from New York University Langone Medical Center has further substratified the Gustilo grade 3B category with a 3–2-1 modification with the numbers stating the total of uninjured source vessels intact in the limb at the initial evaluation.[15,16] This better reflects the difficulties to be expected by the reconstructive surgeon, as unplanned returns to the operating room and flap failure rates were found to be significantly greater the fewer the vessels that remained.[15] A grade 3B-3 limb with all vessels intact intuitively would appear to have been less injured than a grade 3B-1 limb with only one vessel intact, and therefore the former would be expected to have a superior outcome.

Other key elements of the orthopaedic evaluation of the traumatized lower extremity include[1]:

- Timing and environment of injury.
- Mechanism and amount of energy absorption.
- Fracture configuration and amount of bone loss.
- Systemic conditions, medical status, other associated injuries.

Table 4.1 The Gustilo-Anderson Classification of Open Fractures

Gustilo grade[13,14]	Description	Treatment
I	Open fracture, clean wound < 1 cm in length	Irrigation, debridement, ORIF/EF, primary closure
II	Open fracture, wound > 1 cm but < 10 cm in length without extensive soft-tissue damage, flaps, avulsions	Irrigation, debridement, ORIF/EF, primary closure
III	Open fracture with extensive soft-tissue laceration (> 10 cm), damage, or loss or an open segmental fracture. This type also includes open fractures caused by gunshot injuries, farm injuries, fractures requiring vascular repair, or fractures that have been open for 8 h prior to treatment	Variable, see below
IIIA	Adequate soft-tissue coverage of the fractured bone despite the extensive soft-tissue laceration or flaps, or high-energy trauma irrespective of wound size	Irrigation, debridement, ORIF/EF, primary closure, or sometimes requires STSG or local soft-tissue flap coverage
IIIB	Extensive soft-tissue injury with periosteal stripping and bone exposure. Usually associated with massive contamination	Irrigation, debridement, ORIF/EF, often requires free tissue transfer or local muscle flaps or perforator-based flaps
IIIC	Open fracture associated with an arterial injury requiring repair, irrespective of degree of soft-tissue injury	Irrigation, debridement, ORIF/EF, vascular repair, often requires free tissue transfer or local muscle flaps or perforator-based flaps

Abbreviations: ORIF/EF, open reduction internal fixation or external fixation; STSG, split-thickness skin graft.

- Extent of surrounding soft-tissue injury, shearing, tissue loss (including integument, muscle, fascia, and periosteum).
- Vascularity, sensibility, and motor function of the limb.
- Possibility of compartment syndrome.

Location of soft-tissue injuries along the axis of the leg is also an important factor to analyze. Traditionally, the traumatized lower extremity has been divided into thirds in an algorithmic manner to help guide treatment:

- Upper one-third: gastrocnemius pedicled flaps.
- Middle one-third: hemisoleus pedicled flaps.
- Lower one-third: free tissue transfer.

However, with modern-day microsurgical techniques including perforator-based local flaps such as propeller flaps and reverse flow flaps, and improvement in free tissue transfers, many options now exist for each region of the extremity. A more modern approach to analyzing a lower extremity defect is to focus on the nature of the defect, what is missing and therefore what needs to be replaced, and what local or distant options exist for the achievement of a well-vascularized sealed wound regardless of specific location. However, vital to the success of any reconstruction is the process of preparing the wound by thorough debridement.

4.4 The Role and Timing of Debridement

4.4.1 Timing of Debridement of Open Fractures of the Lower Extremity

Urgent administration of antibiotics is well established in preventing infection of open fractures[17] with delays in greater than 3 hours resulting in 1.63 times greater odds of infection.[18] However, timing of operative debridement remains controversial. Historically, open fractures were taken emergently to the operating room within 6 hours of injury.[19,20,21] However, this practice was extrapolated from data prior to administration of intravenous antibiotics and has been challenged in recent literature. Although most clinical studies challenging the "6-hour rule" have been small retrospective series with fewer than 200 patients,[22,23] several prospective studies exist. One such study of 237 patients demonstrated no significant difference in infection rates for operative management earlier or beyond 6 hours.[24] In a prospective study of 736 patients, Weber et al demonstrated increasing Gustilo grade and tibia fractures to be associated with a higher risk of infection, but not time to surgery.[25] Additionally, several meta-analyses demonstrate no difference in rate of infection with the delay of initial debridement beyond 6 hours.[26,27] However, several recent studies still advocate for debridement within 6 hours. One prospective study of 404 patients demonstrated that delayed irrigation of lower extremity fractures beyond 8 hours, higher Gustilo grade, and higher Injury Severity Score increased the risk of infection, but not of the upper extremity.[28] In 2009, the British Association of Plastic, Reconstructive and Aesthetic Surgeons revised their guidelines in favor of debridement within 24 hours of injury.

4.4.2 Type of Irrigation Fluid

There is much variation in the manner and content of irrigation solution used in open fractures.[17] High as well as low pressure irrigation has been recommended. High-pressure irrigation is thought to be more effective at debriding contaminants from wounds,[29,30] whereas those in favor of low pressure have shown high pressure causes potential damage to fractured bone[31] as well as bacterial propagation into the soft tissue or femoral canal.[32] Yet in 2016, a large prospective multicenter study demonstrated no difference in clinical outcomes with varying pressures of the irrigation solution. They did demonstrate a detrimental effect of using castile soap in the irrigation solution when compared with normal saline.[33]

4.4.3 Timing of Wound Closure

There are currently no objective clinical guidelines to determine the timing of wound closure.[34] Multiple debridements may be required in the case of gross wound contamination or tenuous soft-tissue envelope.[17] In these scenarios, delayed wound closure allows for repeated reassessment of the wound, more precise operative planning, and thorough cleansing of the tissue bed.[17] Lenarz et al[34] instituted a protocol wherein an open fracture underwent serial debridement until cultures were negative before definitive wound culture. Mean number of days to closure ranged from 0.76 for Gustilo grade I to 18.5 for IIIC injuries, indicating that several debridements are often necessary with the increasing complexity of the wound. Using this approach, they obtained an impressively low infection rate of 4.3%.[34] Russell et al in an early study found wounds closed primarily after the first debridement had significantly greater risk of infection compared with those closed in delayed fashion (20 vs. 3%).[35] However, more recent studies have challenged this approach and have consistently shown that delays in reconstructive wound coverage are associated with increased infection and flap failure rates.[36] Godina's classic work demonstrated that delayed reconstruction beyond 72 hours resulted in an increase in infection rate from 1.5 to 17.5% and a higher free-flap failure rate.[37] Fischer et al showed that soft-tissue coverage beyond 10 days of injury was associated with a higher infection rate (18 and 69%).[38] Nevertheless, it must be recognized that the magnitude of the soft-tissue damage may affect outcomes. For example, Hohmann et al compared low-grade open tibia fractures and found no difference in the infection rate between primary closure and delayed closure, with a significant cost reduction in the primary closure group.[39]

In our practice, the following principles of irrigation, debridement, and coverage have proven successful:

- Get the patient to the operating room as soon as reasonably possible (considering vascular status, level of contamination, concomitant injuries, availability of qualified personnel, etc.).
- Perform a "radical necrectomy," treating the wound as a "pseudotumor" by removing all devitalized soft tissue, bone, and surface contaminated tissue.
- If unhappy with the wound's appearance (continued bacterial colonization, purulent appearance, or ongoing necrotic or fibrinous debris), take the patient back for a second or third look.
- Irrigation with normal saline at low pressure.
- Use a Versajet for surface decontamination or minor debridements.

- Keep wound moist at all times.
- Negative pressure wound therapy can keep the wound clean and buy more time.
- Early coverage desirable.
- Manage edema.
- Prevent equinus contracture.

▶ Fig. 4.1 demonstrates a representative case of an 8-year-old child with a Gustilo 3C injury to the lower extremity where these principles were applied. This orthoplastic approach led to successful limb salvage and a good outcome.

4.5 Basic Principles of Bone Fixation

Open fractures with soft-tissue defects necessitate coordinated care to achieve bony union, guard against infection, and maximize

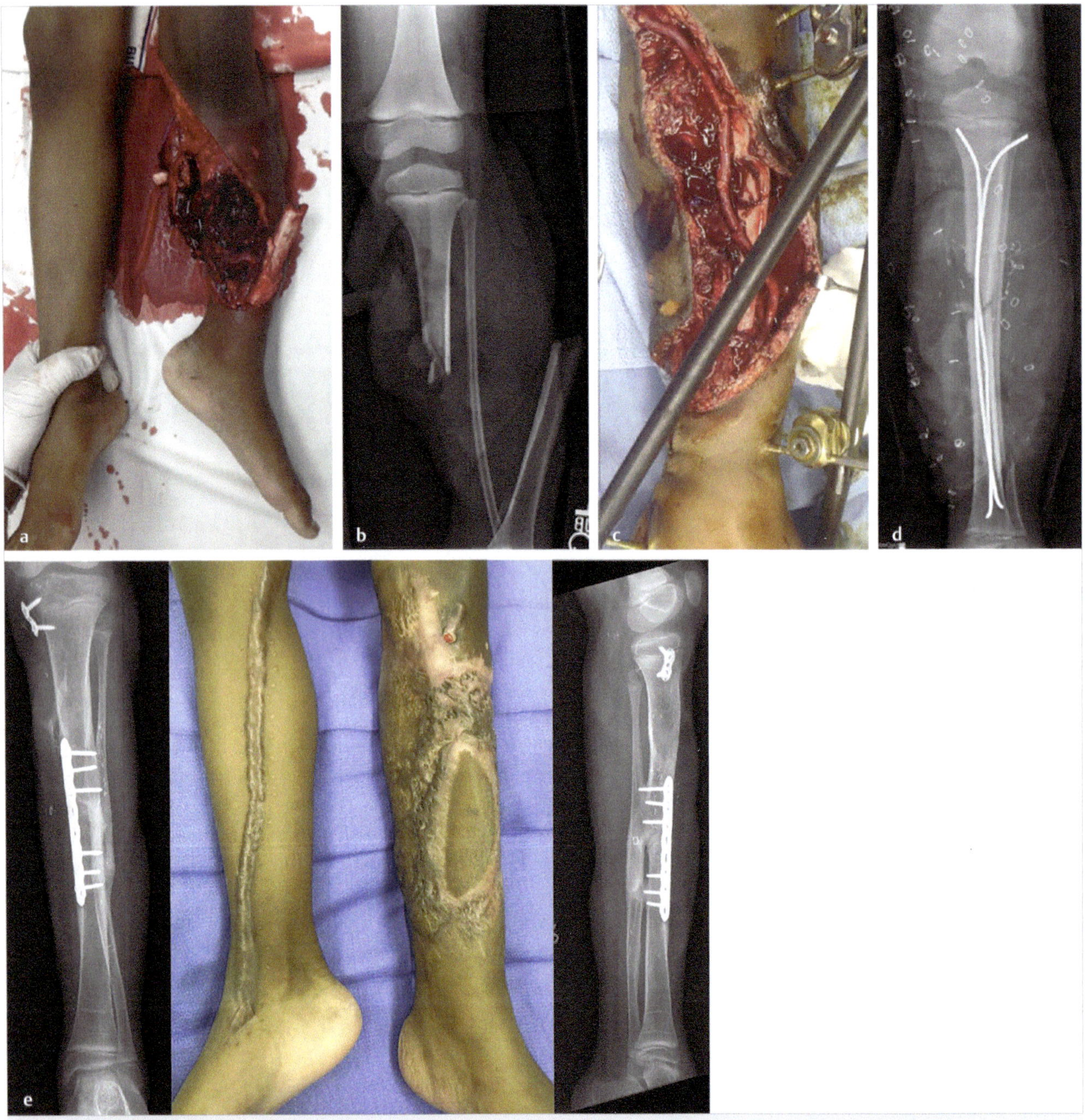

Fig. 4.1 Orthoplastic approach to Gustilo 3C injury in an 8-year-old child with a severe limb-threatening injury after being struck by a car **(a, b)**. This required immediate stabilization with an external fixator and revascularization with a reversed saphenous vein graft **(c)**. After multiple debridements, conversion to internal fixation and free latissimus myocutaneous flap reconstruction was performed **(d)**. Although the patient developed hypertrophic scaring and required revision open reduction internal fixation with bone grafting, he went on to union with an acceptable outcome **(e)**.

functional outcome. In the late 1950s, the Arbeitsgemeinschaft für Osteosynthesefragen (AO) group developed four basic principles for the surgical treatment of fractures. These include:

1. Fracture reduction and fixation to restore anatomical relationships.
2. Fracture fixation providing absolute or relative stability as the fracture, patient, or injury requires.
3. Preservation of blood supply to soft tissues and bone by gentle reduction techniques and careful handling.
4. Early mobilization and rehabilitation of the injured part and patient as a whole.

The development of these principles emphasized the importance of soft tissue, and has led to the awareness that successful management of major orthopaedic trauma is inseparable from successful management of the soft-tissue envelope.

Mutilating extremity injuries often involve significant bony comminution and contamination which require temporary external fixation and repeated irrigation and debridements. If the bone contamination is significant or there is concern for ongoing infection, these fractures require external fixation as the definitive treatment until bone healing. Important soft-tissue reconstruction principles must be considered with placement of external fixation pins and bars as follows:

- Pins should be as far from the wound as possible while maintaining fracture stability.
- Bars should not obstruct the soft-tissue window around the zone of injury.
- In the leg, mid anterior pins are better than medial or lateral pins to allow for vascular access for free flaps and rotational muscle and perforator flaps.
- The frame must be easily loosened for adjustments needed during reconstruction.

Conversion from external fixation to plates or intramedullary nails in open fractures that have been thoroughly debrided in combination with immediate soft-tissue coverage has proven effective in the treatment of severe extremity trauma (▶ Fig. 4.1).[40,41] This approach is ideal when possible and allows for reconstruction to proceed without interference of external fixator devices.

It is imperative that both the orthopaedic surgeon and the reconstructive plastic surgeon be familiar with the needs and approaches of the other to optimize a functional outcome for the patient. This orthoplastic approach to limb salvage will maximize outcomes, although at times amputation must be considered before embarking on the often lengthy limb salvage journey.[4]

4.6 Limb Salvage versus Amputation

A number of studies have been performed in an attempt to determine factors predicting success of limb salvage. The largest of these was a subset of the Lower Extremity Assessment Project (LEAP) study which evaluated 556 patients by using five different injury severity scoring systems. None of the indicators were useful for determining limbs that require amputation or those likely to be successfully salvaged. They did find that low scores could be used to predict limb-salvage potential; however, the converse was not true. They concluded that the low sensitivity of their indices failed to support the validity of the scores as predictors of amputation.[42] A separate study examined seven lower extremity injury severity indices and found none were predictive of ultimate functional outcome at 2 years.[43] The LEAP study group investigated the outcome of limb salvage versus reconstruction, and found that patients who underwent limb salvage versus primary amputation had no difference in long-term outcomes and both were found to have less than ideal outcomes.[44] Importantly, the LEAP studies demonstrated that overall function was affected by patients' economic, social, and emotional recourses more so than by treatment course. Factors associated with poor outcomes included poverty, lack of health insurance, poor social network, involvement in litigation, nonwhite race, and smoking.[44]

Given this information and the lack of accurate prediction of outcomes with scoring systems, the decision to reconstruct or amputate must often be made based on the judgment of the multidisciplinary orthoplastic team with input from the patient. In our practice, factors that encourage amputation include a mangled lower extremity and the following:

- Prolonged warm ischemia time (> 3 hours).
- Severe muscle damage.
- Multilevel injury including ipsilateral tibia and foot crush injury.
- Proximal or severe tibial nerve injury that would preclude plantar sensation even with repair.
- Poor psychosocial support and coping mechanisms.
- Concomitant medical conditions or injuries that make patient a significant surgical risk.

If amputation is to be performed, the orthoplastic surgeon should attempt to preserve sufficient length and sensibility for effective prosthetic use, and utilize the principles of spare-part surgery, fillet flaps, island pedicle flaps, and free flaps as needed.[4]

4.7 Other Applications of Orthoplastic Surgery

Orthoplastic principles can be applied with a variety of reconstructive options. One of the most exciting aspects of orthoplastic surgery is the combination of bone healing principles and microvascular surgery to fill large bone defects after trauma, avascular osteonecrosis, tumor extirpation, or osteomyelitis. Microsurgery has revolutionized the treatment of large segmental bone defects through the use of vascularized bone transfer. Since its description by Taylor et al in 1975, the vascularized fibula has been used extensively due to its size, acceptable donor-site morbidity, and predictable dissection.[45] Free fibular vascularized grafts have been utilized for segmental defects of the upper and lower extremity and have a pivotal role in traumatic reconstruction.[46] A unique orthoplastic application of the free vascularized fibula flap is in the setting of

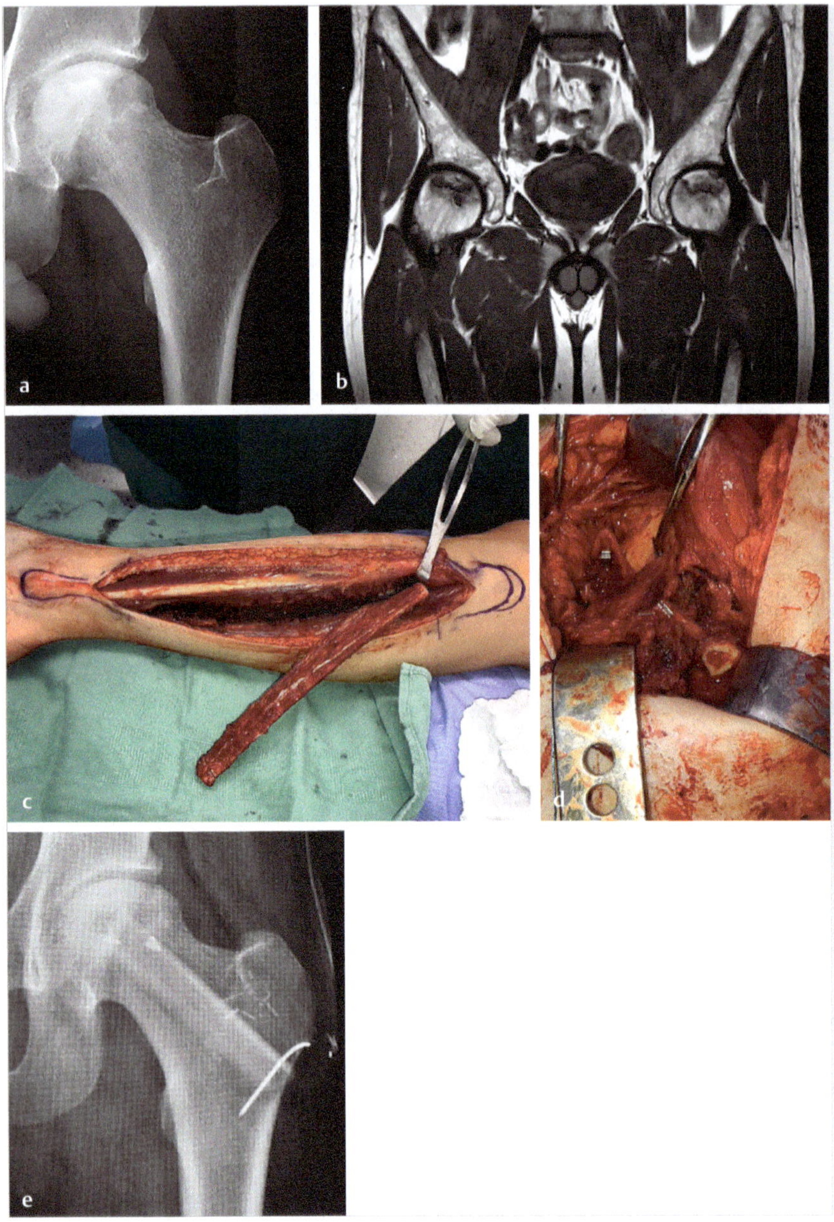

Fig. 4.2 Free vascularized fibula for hip avascular necrosis. A 27-year-old male with bilateral idiopathic avascular necrosis of the femoral heads as demonstrated on plain radiograph **(a)** and T1-weighted MRI **(b)**. To avoid total hip arthroplasty in this young patient, a free vascularized fibula bone flap in situ **(c)** was placed in the femoral head and neck to revitalize the bone with the peroneal pedicle anastomosed to the ascending branch of the lateral femoral circumflex vessels **(d)**. Plain radiograph of the bone flap in place in the femoral neck and head **(e)**.

osteonecrosis of the femoral head in the young patient (▶ Fig. 4.2). Long-term follow-up of this technique has demonstrated it to be the most effective method of joint preservation with a low conversion rate to total hip arthroplasty.[47]

Free vascularized bone grafts from the medial femoral condyle are increasing in versatility and popularity. The medial femoral condyle flap or medial genicular artery flap as a source of vascularized bone transfer has had a surge in use in a variety of bony reconstructions. It has been utilized with increased frequency for larger bone grafting procedures, and has become a reliable alternative to free fibular grafts for intermediate to large osseous defects.[48,49,50] The flap has more recently been described as a method of supplying well-vascularized cortico-periosteum as a method of treating recalcitrant nonunions all over the body including the foot/ankle, tibia, femur, scaphoid, radius, ulna, humerus, and clavicle.[51] We have found this to be a versatile flap with reliable anatomy, with a wide array of orthoplastic applications (▶ Fig. 4.3).

4.8 Conclusion

The concept of the orthoplastic approach brings together the strengths of orthopaedic surgery of stable bone reconstruction and rehabilitation with the microvascular soft tissue and aesthetic principles of plastic surgery simultaneously to maximize outcomes in extremity reconstruction. When both perspectives are clearly understood and applied, outcomes in reconstruction and salvage are maximized. Key aspects of orthoplastic include building a foundation of effective debridement and stable fracture fixation followed by well-vascularized bone grafts or soft-tissue coverage as needed that together bring success in treating composite injuries of the lower extremity.

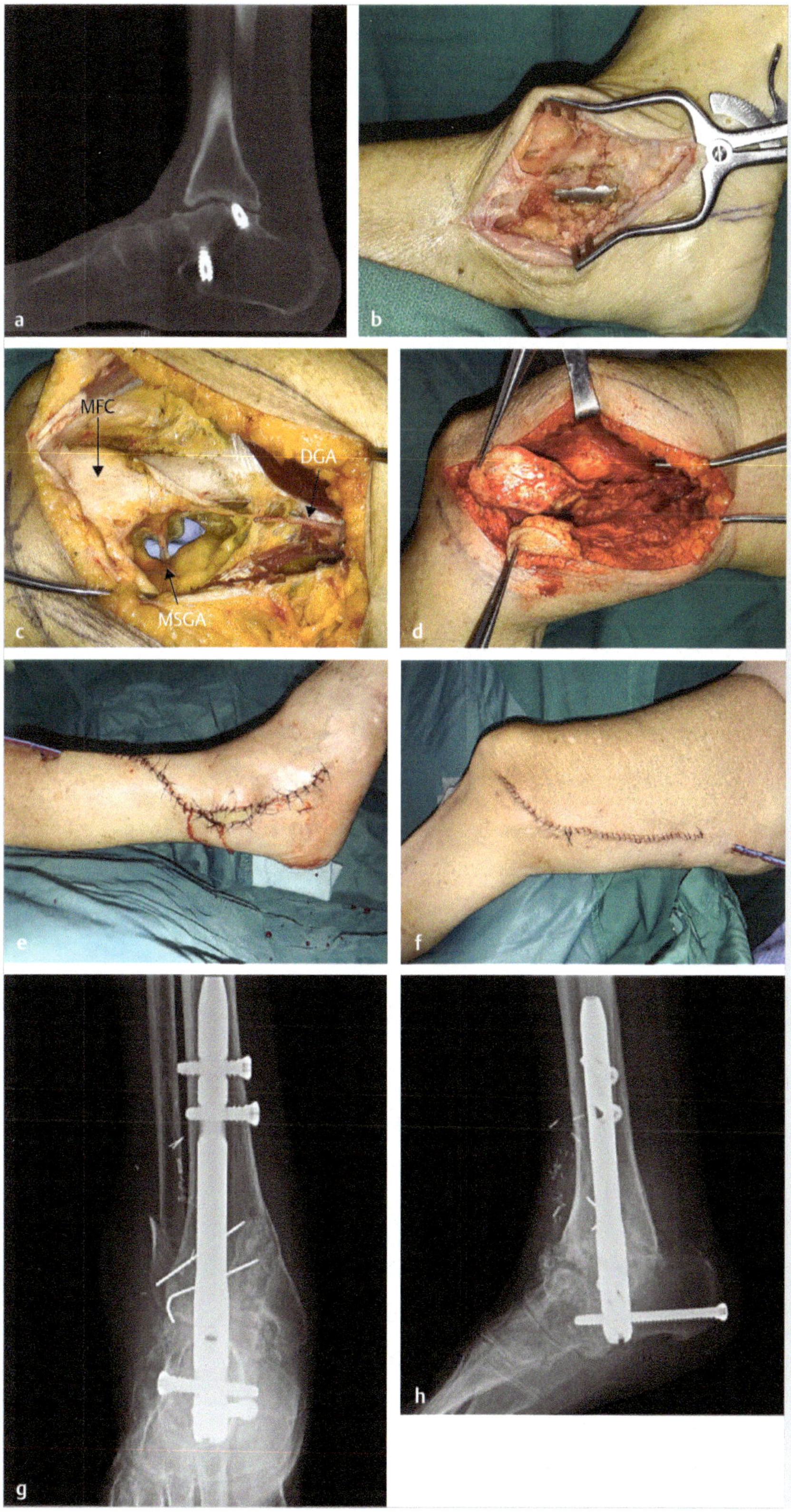

Fig. 4.3 Medial geniculate artery osteocutaneous flap for a tibiotalar fusion nonunion. A 75-year-old female with a persistent nonunion 1 year after attempt at ankle fusion as demonstrated on CT scan **(a)**. Revision fusion was performed by debriding the nonunion site and placing an intramedullary ankle fusion nail **(b)**. A medial femoral condyle (MFC) osteocutaneous flap was performed to augment bone healing. In this particular case, the descending genicular artery (DGA) was quite diminutive; therefore, the medial superior genicular artery (MSGA) was used as the main pedicle **(c)**. In situ as chimeric island flap combined with skin paddle **(d)**, the latter was inset in the ankle and used as a sentinel monitoring flap **(e)**. Knee donor-site closure **(f)**. Plain radiographs of the bone flap in place at the fusion site **(g, h)**.

References

[1] Levin LS. The reconstructive ladder. An orthoplastic approach. Orthop Clin North Am. 1993; 24(3):393–409

[2] Levin SL. Orthoplastic reconstruction of the hand. Curr Opin Orthop. 1993; 4(4):10–13

[3] Heitmann C, Levin LS. The orthoplastic approach for management of the severely traumatized foot and ankle. J Trauma. 2003; 54(2):379–390

[4] Lerman OZ, Kovach SJ, Levin LS. The respective roles of plastic and orthopedic surgery in limb salvage. Plast Reconstr Surg. 2011; 127 Suppl 1:215S–227S

[5] Tsai TM, Breyer JM, Panattoni JB. History of microsurgery: curiosities from the sixties and seventies. Microsurgery. 2013; 33(2):85–89

[6] Tintle SM, Levin LS. The reconstructive microsurgery ladder in orthopaedics. Injury. 2013; 44(3):376–385

[7] Tamai S. History of microsurgery. Plast Reconstr Surg. 2009; 124(6) Suppl: e282–e294

[8] Tamai S. History of microsurgery–from the beginning until the end of the 1970s. Microsurgery. 1993; 14(1):6–13

[9] Buncke HJ, Buncke GM, Kind GM. The early history of microsurgery. Plast Reconstr Surg. 1996; 98(6):1122–1123

[10] Taylor GI. The angiosomes of the body and their supply to perforator flaps. Clin Plast Surg. 2003; 30(3):331–342, v

[11] Shores JT, Malek V, Lee WPA, Brandacher G. Outcomes after hand and upper extremity transplantation. J Mater Sci Mater Med. 2017; 28(5):72

[12] Sosin M, Rodriguez ED. The face transplantation update: 2016. Plast Reconstr Surg. 2016; 137(6):1841–1850

[13] Gustilo RB, Mendoza RM, Williams DN. Problems in the management of type III (severe) open fractures: a new classification of type III open fractures. J Trauma. 1984; 24(8):742–746

[14] Gustilo RB, Anderson JT. Prevention of infection in the treatment of one thousand and twenty-five open fractures of long bones: retrospective and prospective analyses. J Bone Joint Surg Am. 1976; 58(4):453–458

[15] Ricci JA, Stranix JT, Lee ZH, et al. Comparing reconstructive outcomes in patients with Gustilo Type IIIB fractures and concomitant arterial injuries. Plast Reconstr Surg. 2019; 143(5):1522–1529

[16] Levin LS. Discussion: comparing reconstructive outcomes in patients with Gustilo Type IIIB fractures and concomitant arterial injuries. Plast Reconstr Surg. 2019; 143(5):1530

[17] Rozell JC, Connolly KP, Mehta S. Timing of operative debridement in open fractures. Orthop Clin North Am. 2017; 48(1):25–34

[18] Patzakis MJ, Wilkins J. Factors influencing infection rate in open fracture wounds. Clin Orthop Relat Res. 1989(243):36–40

[19] Crowley DJ, Kanakaris NK, Giannoudis PV. Debridement and wound closure of open fractures: the impact of the time factor on infection rates. Injury. 2007; 38(8):879–889

[20] Sungaran J, Harris I, Mourad M. The effect of time to theatre on infection rate for open tibia fractures. ANZ J Surg. 2007; 77(10):886–888

[21] Srour M, Inaba K, Okoye O, et al. Prospective evaluation of treatment of open fractures: effect of time to irrigation and debridement. JAMA Surg. 2015; 150(4):332–336

[22] Khatod M, Botte MJ, Hoyt DB, Meyer RS, Smith JM, Akeson WH. Outcomes in open tibia fractures: relationship between delay in treatment and infection. J Trauma. 2003; 55(5):949–954

[23] Tripuraneni K, Ganga S, Quinn R, Gehlert R. The effect of time delay to surgical debridement of open tibia shaft fractures on infection rate. Orthopedics. 2008; 31(12). DOI: 10.3928/01477447-20081201-27

[24] Al-Arabi YB, Nader M, Hamidian-Jahromi AR, Woods DA. The effect of the timing of antibiotics and surgical treatment on infection rates in open long-bone fractures: a 9-year prospective study from a district general hospital. Injury. 2007; 38(8):900–905

[25] Weber D, Dulai SK, Bergman J, Buckley R, Beaupre LA. Time to initial operative treatment following open fracture does not impact development of deep infection: a prospective cohort study of 736 subjects. J Orthop Trauma. 2014; 28(11):613–619

[26] Schenker ML, Yannascoli S, Baldwin KD, Ahn J, Mehta S. Does timing to operative debridement affect infectious complications in open long-bone fractures? A systematic review. J Bone Joint Surg Am. 2012; 94(12):1057–1064

[27] Prodromidis AD, Charalambous CP. The 6-hour rule for surgical debridement of open tibial fractures: a systematic review and meta-analysis of infection and nonunion rates. J Orthop Trauma. 2016; 30(7):397–402

[28] Malhotra AK, Goldberg S, Graham J, et al. Open extremity fractures: impact of delay in operative debridement and irrigation. J Trauma Acute Care Surg. 2014; 76(5):1201–1207

[29] Longmire AW, Broom LA, Burch J. Wound infection following high-pressure syringe and needle irrigation. Am J Emerg Med. 1987; 5(2):179–181

[30] Barnes S, Spencer M, Graham D, Johnson HB. Surgical wound irrigation: a call for evidence-based standardization of practice. Am J Infect Control. 2014; 42(5):525–529

[31] Bhandari M, Adili A, Lachowski RJ. High pressure pulsatile lavage of contaminated human tibiae: an in vitro study. J Orthop Trauma. 1998; 12(7):479–484

[32] Hassinger SM, Harding G, Wongworawat MD. High-pressure pulsatile lavage propagates bacteria into soft tissue. Clin Orthop Relat Res. 2005; 439(439): 27–31

[33] Bhandari M, Jeray KJ, Petrisor BA, et al. FLOW Investigators. A trial of wound irrigation in the initial management of open fracture wounds. N Engl J Med. 2015; 373(27):2629–2641

[34] Lenarz CJ, Watson JT, Moed BR, Israel H, Mullen JD, Macdonald JB. Timing of wound closure in open fractures based on cultures obtained after debridement. J Bone Joint Surg Am. 2010; 92(10):1921–1926

[35] Russell GG, Henderson R, Arnett G. Primary or delayed closure for open tibial fractures. J Bone Joint Surg Br. 1990; 72(1):125–128

[36] Melvin JS, Dombroski DG, Torbert JT, Kovach SJ, Esterhai JL, Mehta S. Open tibial shaft fractures: II. Definitive management and limb salvage. J Am Acad Orthop Surg. 2010; 18(2):108–117

[37] Godina M. Early microsurgical reconstruction of complex trauma of the extremities. Plast Reconstr Surg. 1986; 78(3):285–292

[38] Fischer MD, Gustilo RB, Varecka TF. The timing of flap coverage, bone-grafting, and intramedullary nailing in patients who have a fracture of the tibial shaft with extensive soft-tissue injury. J Bone Joint Surg Am. 1991; 73(9):1316–1322

[39] Hohmann E, Tetsworth K, Radziejowski MJ, Wiesniewski TF. Comparison of delayed and primary wound closure in the treatment of open tibial fractures. Arch Orthop Trauma Surg. 2007; 127(2):131–136

[40] Gopal S, Majumder S, Batchelor AG, Knight SL, De Boer P, Smith RM. Fix and flap: the radical orthopaedic and plastic treatment of severe open fractures of the tibia. J Bone Joint Surg Br. 2000; 82(7):959–966

[41] Bhandari M, Guyatt GH, Swiontkowski MF, Schemitsch EH. Treatment of open fractures of the shaft of the tibia. J Bone Joint Surg Br. 2001; 83(1):62–68

[42] Bosse MJ, MacKenzie EJ, Kellam JF, et al. A prospective evaluation of the clinical utility of the lower-extremity injury-severity scores. J Bone Joint Surg Am. 2001; 83(1):3–14

[43] Ly TV, Travison TG, Castillo RC, Bosse MJ, MacKenzie EJ, LEAP Study Group. Ability of lower-extremity injury severity scores to predict functional outcome after limb salvage. J Bone Joint Surg Am. 2008; 90(8):1738–1743

[44] MacKenzie EJ, Bosse MJ. Factors influencing outcome following limb-threatening lower limb trauma: lessons learned from the Lower Extremity Assessment Project (LEAP). J Am Acad Orthop Surg. 2006; 14(10 Spec No): S:205–210

[45] Taylor GI, Miller GD, Ham FJ. The free vascularized bone graft. A clinical extension of microvascular techniques. Plast Reconstr Surg. 1975; 55(5):533–544

[46] Jupiter JB, Gerhard HJ, Guerrero J, Nunley JA, Levin LS. Treatment of segmental defects of the radius with use of the vascularized osteoseptocutaneous fibular autogenous graft. J Bone Joint Surg Am. 1997; 79(4):542–550

[47] Korompilias AV, Lykissas MG, Beris AE, Urbaniak JR, Soucacos PN. Vascularised fibular graft in the management of femoral head osteonecrosis: twenty years later. J Bone Joint Surg Br. 2009; 91(3):287–293

[48] Hayashi A, Maruyama Y. The medial genicular artery flap. Ann Plast Surg. 1990; 25(3):174–180

[49] Sakai K, Doi K, Kawai S. Free vascularized thin corticoperiosteal graft. Plast Reconstr Surg. 1991; 87(2):290–298

[50] Kazmers NH, Thibaudeau S, Steinberger Z, Levin LS. Upper and lower extremity reconstructive applications utilizing free flaps from the medial genicular arterial system: A systematic review. Microsurgery. 2018; 38(3):328–343

[51] Deng AD, Innocenti M, Arora R, Gabl M, Tang JB. Vascularized small-bone transfers for fracture nonunion and bony defects. Clin Plast Surg. 2017; 44(2): 267–285

5 Surgical Approach to Pediatric Bone and Soft-Tissue Tumors of the Lower Extremity

Rachel M. Clancy, Karen W. Wong, and Ronald M. Zuker

Summary
Sarcomas are a diverse class of malignant tumors originating from mesenchymal tissues such as bone, cartilage, muscle, blood vessels, or lymphoid tissue. Dramatic improvements in chemotherapy have resulted in increased survival rates so that limb salvage has become the standard of care rather than amputation, as had been the norm in the past. Diagnosis and staging should precede surgical management. This will require a biopsy in a location that will not impede the definitive surgical intervention. Adequate resection margins are routinely required, realizing that the child will then need a durable reconstruction of bone, tendon, nerve, and/or soft tissues that will meet their expected high functional demands as well as the likelihood of limb length inequality as they grow and reach maturity. In the lower extremity, this could be an intercalary resection with preservation of the epiphyses and concomitant vascularized bone reconstruction, joint resection with replacement with an endoprosthesis or rotationplasty, or amputation. All these variations will also often require standard local or free flap soft-tissue coverage.

Keywords: pediatric sarcomas, osteosarcoma, Ewing sarcoma, Rhabdomyosarcoma, synovial sarcoma, intercalary resection, rotationplasty

5.1 Introduction

Sarcomas are a heterogeneous group of malignant tumors derived from mesenchymal origin: bone, cartilage, muscle, blood vessels, or lymphoid tissue. Osteosarcoma, Ewing sarcoma, and rhabdomyosarcoma are the most common pediatric sarcomas.[1]

Long-term survival of pediatric sarcoma patients has dramatically improved with advances in chemotherapy regimens. With increased survival rates, considerable effort has gone into limb salvage, which is now the standard of care for primary bone tumors, rather than amputation.[2,3] The overriding goal in surgical management is always oncological safety. To prevent tumor recurrence, wide resection of bone and soft tissue is usually required. Secondary considerations include function, durability, and appearance. Given the extensive resection required, the immature skeleton of a child will usually need a durable reconstruction with bone, tendon, nerve, and soft tissues to address their high functional demands and the likelihood of limb length inequality as they continue to grow and mature.[2,3] To achieve this, a multidisciplinary approach is essential, which encompasses patient and family preference as well as a wide range of surgical expertise, oncology, radiology, pathology, nursing, physiotherapy, and psychosocial support. As advances in treatment have prolonged survival, quality of life has become a more pertinent consideration. The aims of this chapter are to provide an overview of the surgical approach to pediatric bone and soft-tissue tumors and to describe reconstructive options for lower extremity defects.

5.2 Types of Sarcoma

5.2.1 Osteosarcoma

Osteosarcoma is an aggressive primary bone tumor that most commonly presents in the long bones (▶ Fig. 5.1). Most cases occur in the absence of radiation exposure or inherited syndromes. The peak incidence is at 16 years or during puberty, suggesting a potential association with rapid bone growth.[4] Approximately 20% of patients present with metastases, which are most commonly found in the lung.[5] Osteosarcoma is generally resistant to radiotherapy; however, chemotherapy in combination with surgery for presumed micrometastases has increased survival rates.

5.2.2 Ewing Sarcoma

Ewing sarcoma tumors are defined under the umbrella of "Ewing sarcoma family of tumors (ESFT). ESFT also includes Askin tumors and peripheral primitive neuroectodermal tumors. Ewing sarcoma is usually classified as a bone tumor and is most commonly found in the diaphysis and metaphyses of long bones as well the pelvis (▶ Fig. 5.2). Soft tissue tumors

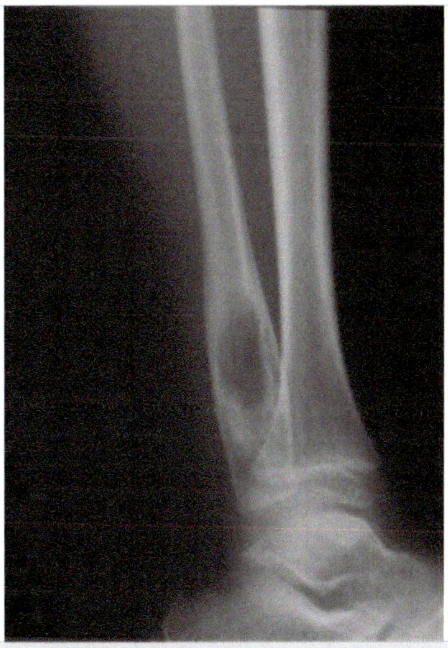

Fig. 5.1 Osteosarcoma: this is an aggressive primary bone tumor. On X-ray, characteristically will be found a lytic lesion with bone destruction, surrounded by an aggressive periosteal reaction.

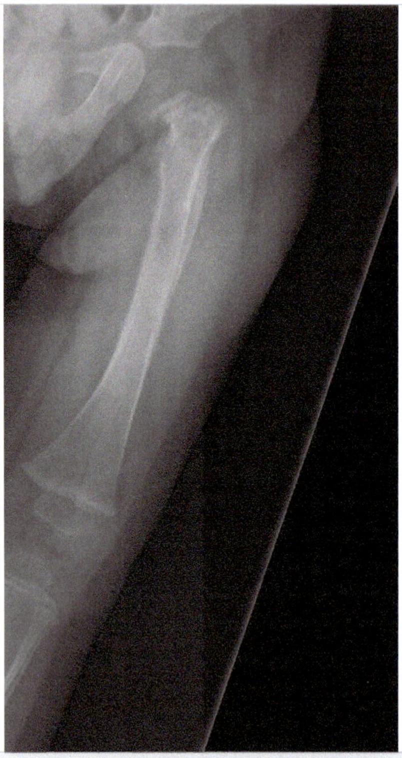

Fig. 5.2 Ewing sarcoma: as seen here in the proximal femur, there is extensive bone destruction with a moth-eaten appearance. Poor margination is observed with an aggressive periosteal reaction that is often laminated and described as "onion skin."

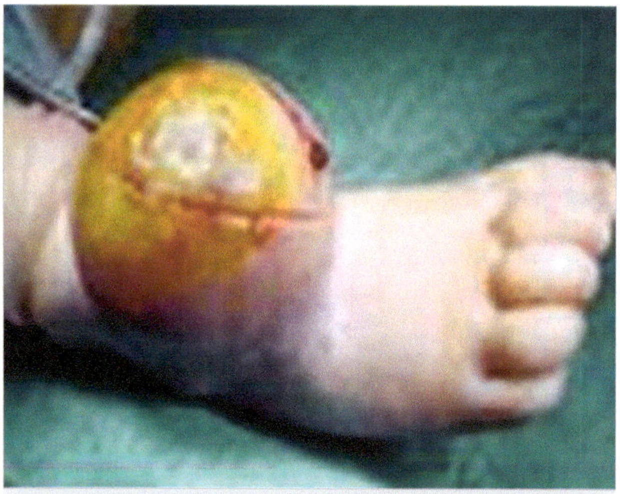

Fig. 5.3 Rhabdomyosarcoma: this is the most common soft tissue sarcoma and can be found throughout the body. There will be an expanding and distorting soft tissue mass, with possibly bony erosion adjacent to the tumor. Source: Prof. Dr. med. Günter German, Ethianum, Heidelberg, Germany.

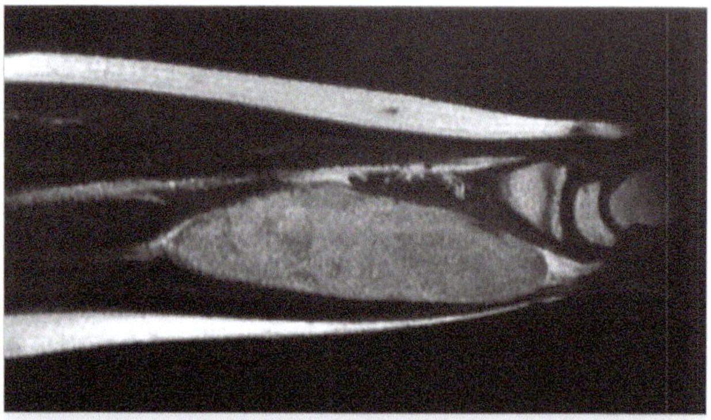

Fig. 5.4 Synovial sarcoma: albeit rare, this is the most common of the nonrhabdomyosarcoma soft-tissue sarcomas. This is typically a slow-growing, deep-seated mass, as seen here on an upper extremity MRI that was used to assess the involvement of adjacent tissues and extent of damage.

with similar characteristics of mesodermal and ectodermal origin have also been described, making it difficult to classify.[4,6] Approximately 25% of patients present with metastases of the lung, bone marrow, or bone.[7] Ewing sarcoma occurs over a wide age range from infants to adults with a peak incidence in the second decade.[8] Intensive multimodal treatment with combination chemotherapy, radiotherapy, and surgery is used in those with Ewing sarcoma and has increased survival rate from less than 10% to approximately 50%.[8]

5.2.3 Rhabdomyosarcoma

Rhabdomyosarcoma is the most common soft-tissue sarcoma in children. Rhabdomyosarcoma can develop in any soft tissue (▶ Fig. 5.3) and is grouped according to anatomical site, the extremities and genitourinary tract being the most common.[4] The peak incidence is bimodal occurring in children aged 2 to 6 and 15 to 19 years[1]; 15 to 20% of patients present with metastases which can be widespread.[7] Chemotherapy, radiotherapy, and surgery are all useful treatment modalities in the management of rhabdomyosarcoma.

5.2.4 Nonrhabdomyosarcomas

The term "nonrhabdomyosarcomas" is used to describe all other soft-tissue sarcomas, of which synovial sarcoma, a relatively rare tumor (▶ Fig. 5.4), is the most common. These tumors are usually managed by surgical excision. The use of radiotherapy and chemotherapy is inconsistent.

5.3 Staging

There are two staging systems used to classify sarcomas: the Musculoskeletal Tumor Society, also referred to as the Enneking System, and the American Joint Committee on Cancer (AJCC). The Enneking System classifies sarcomas on the basis of grade, whether the tumor is intra- or extracompartmental, and the presence of metastasis.[9] As anatomical features are included, this system is useful for guiding surgical resection. The AJCC uses the tumor, node, metastases, grade (TNMG) to stage sarcomas.[9,10] Within this system, information relating to the latter can be grouped into four stages for a more simplistic classification. The Intergroup Rhabdomyosarcoma Study Group uses a modified AJCC TNM for the classification of soft-tissue tumors.

5.4 Diagnosis

The clinical presentation of sarcomas is variable depending on the tissue of origin. Soft-tissue sarcomas typically present with gradual swelling and a firm, painless, enlarging palpable mass. They may also present with symptoms of compression. Bone tumors can present with a pathological fracture or more commonly swelling and pain. When evaluating a patient with a potentially malignant mass, the physician should clarify the duration of symptoms; any recent change in size or consistency of the mass; the constellation of symptoms including fever, pyrexia, and paraesthesia; as well as history of trauma, and any other relevant environmental factors.[11]

The type of imaging will often depend on the size and location of tumor. Regional and whole-body imaging is essential through various modalities. Radiography, computed tomography (CT), and magnetic resonance imaging (MRI) are a key component of diagnosis and should be done prior to biopsy. Ultrasound can be used for soft-tissue tumors. Following local imaging, systemic imaging should be performed, specifically an MRI to assess lymph node basins, a CT of the chest and abdomen, positron emission tomographic (PET) scans, as well as whole-body bone scans to assess for the presence of metastases.

Blood work should include full blood count, erythrocyte sedimentation ratio, C-reactive protein, electrolytes (including calcium, magnesium, and phosphate), serum alkaline phosphatase, and serum lactate dehydrogenase.

A biopsy should be obtained and careful consideration should be given to the location with regard to the definitive surgical excision. For extremity tumors, biopsies should be positioned longitudinal with an extensible incision where possible. The biopsy tract should be excised during tumor resection.

5.5 Surgical Management

Oncologic safety is the primary guiding principle in the surgical management of pediatric sarcoma. To reiterate, secondary principles include function, durability, appearance, and minimization of complications.[4] The type of resection required is determined by tumor characteristics. There are four types of excision used in the treatment of sarcomas: intralesional excision, marginal excision (margins of excision are at margin of tumor), wide excision (margins include a cuff of normal tissue surrounding the tumor), and radical excision (excision of entire compartment containing the tumor).[9] Neoadjuvant chemotherapy is commonly used because of the theoretical increase in safety, the ease of obtaining a negative surgical margin, and its ability to target systemic disease directly.[4]

5.5.1 Surgical Approach

There are several key factors which should be taken into consideration, and a number of key questions that surgeons will need to ask when planning sarcoma excision. The most important of these are to ensure adequate margins, and to determine which structures can be preserved. Then ask if the joint is involved? If the joint cannot be preserved, can supporting structures be preserved? If the joint is preserved, will there be significant joint stiffness? Will the function of the limb following surgery be adequate or better than that offered by a prosthesis? Is the aesthetic appearance acceptable? What are the patient's and family's wishes?

5.5.2 Our Approaches for Surgical Reconstruction after Tumor Excision of the Extremities

Defect size, location, tissue composition, and question of joint involvement determine the type of reconstruction needed to achieve adequate coverage and restoration of form and function. See ▶ Table 5.1.

5.5.3 Soft-Tissue Reconstruction Only

There are numerous reconstructive options available for soft-tissue reconstruction following sarcoma excision (▶ Table 5.1). Closure can range from the direct approximation of skin to free flap coverage of critical structures and bone. Zenn and Jones[12] provided helpful guidance in relation to lower limb reconstruction, as will be found in the rest of this book.

Reconstruction of the Thigh

When reconstructing the thigh, the need for free flap coverage is rare and the use of local muscles is often more superior. The most common local muscles used are sartorius, gracilis, and tensor fascia lata. If a free flap is required, the surgical approach at the recipient sites should always be to use an end-to-side arterial anastomoses to allow preservation of distal blood flow.[12]

Reconstruction of the Knee

One of the most important considerations surgeons need to take into account when reconstructing the knee is the range of

Table 5.1 A pragmatic guide for approaches to extremity reconstruction following sarcoma excision

Soft-tissue reconstruction

Intercalary bony reconstruction
• Bone only
  ○ Allograft (cadaver bone)
  ○ Autograft (fibula)
  ○ Allograft and autograft combination
• Bone and soft tissue
  ○ Allograft and vascularized coverage
  ○ Autograft and vascularized coverage

Joint resection and reconstruction
• Reconstruction with bone
  ○ Allograft (cadaver joint)
  ○ Autograft (vascularized head of fibula)
• Reconstruction with an endoprosthesis

Rotationplasty • New knee powered by calf muscles (distal femoral tumors) • New knee powered by thigh muscles (proximal tibial tumors)
Amputation

motion associated with the joint. The knee has an extensive surface area, and some surgeons advocate creating a template with the knee in the flexed position prior to the definitive surgery. The medial head of the gastrocnemius is an ideal local muscle for reconstruction of the knee due to its larger size (in comparison to the lateral head), minimal donor-site morbidity, and ease of transposition. Disadvantages include a long scar and lasting contour defect. The distal-based anterolateral thigh perforator flap or vastus lateralis muscle, sometimes may also be an alternative, but perhaps not quite as reliable.[12]

Reconstruction of the Leg

Reconstructive options vary depending on the location of the tumor and resulting defect in the leg. Often it is feasible to use local muscle flaps for reconstruction of defects of the upper two-thirds of the leg. Although there are some local options available for reconstruction of the lower third of the leg, depending on the size of the defect more often this area is better served by a free flap. If possible, two venous anastomoses (using both the deep and superficial system) should be performed to accompany the arterial anastomosis. Again in this situation, end-to-side anastomoses are preferable to preserve venous outflow that may have been jeopardized by the tumor resection.

Reconstruction of the Foot

The foot is a challenging area to reconstruct due to increased venous pressure, the distant nature of the blood supply, and the extensive postoperative swelling that invariably occurs. The planter surface requires a durable option to allow for weight bearing. Wound healing, postoperative complications, and the patients' ability to ambulate are similar with muscle free flaps covered by a skin graft as would be a free skin flap. Patients generally need an external fixator at the time of surgery to maintain foot position even in the absence of bony injury or resection.[12]

5.5.4 Intercalary Excision and Free Flap Reconstruction

An intercalary excision is indicated when the adjacent epiphysis is considered free of tumor and edema. Most pediatric high-grade periosteal tumors arise in the metadiaphysis and eventually extend to the epiphysis. If MRI following neoadjuvant chemotherapy shows no evidence of epiphyseal edema, surgeons can be reassured no microscopic tumor is present.[4,13]

Reconstruction of intercalary defects has previously included the use of allograft bone. However, the development of microsurgical techniques using primarily a vascularized free fibula flap (FFF) has revolutionized this reconstruction with improved outcomes. The fibula provides a long segment of bone and can include a skin paddle if required. The fibula can be used as a single strut or a double-barreled construct. The FFF represents the ideal bone graft as it heals by primary union rather than by creeping substitution, and it can replace the loss of a large segment of bone.[14] The FFF provides autogenous bone that actively participates in the healing process, unites quickly, remains reliably organized, and has shown decreased infection rates, increased ambulation potential without aid, and excellent functional outcomes. The bone is alive and generally avoids resorption. In the skeletally immature pediatric population, incorporation of the proximal fibular epiphysis in a reconstruction can result in continued growth of the autograft. In addition, vascularized autografts can undergo hypertrophy resulting in increased strength. However, strength may be insufficient until hypertrophy occurs, and bone fractures have been reported.[14]

5.5.5 Joint Resection and Reconstruction

If the epiphysis is involved, intracapsular resection is indicated. If extracapsular structures can be preserved, a joint reconstruction with bone is a sensible option. The fibula, including the fibula head, can be transferred as living bone and joint. Circulation will be based on the peroneal vessel and/or anterior tibial vessels.[15,16] With time, the fibula head will remodel to mimic the joint surface of the joint reconstructed. However, to again reiterate, oncologic safety is always the priority; and, if a joint is devascularized as a result of the tumor resection, limb salvage is not an option. Instead, future growth and limb length discrepancies should be considered when planning the reconstruction. In children, the anticipated discrepancy can be functionally limiting especially in the lower limb, and they may require further surgical intervention. Surgical options include contralateral epiphyseodesis, acute contralateral shortening, and ipsilateral leg lengthening.

The most common reconstructive option after joint resection in children is endoprosthesis or rotationplasty. For patients with large tumors, the latter may be the only option as limb salvage may not be indicated or oncologically safe. In these cases, the family and patient with the clinician's support will have to make a decision based on how they value appearance versus durability, with oncological safety being the overriding guiding principle.

Endoprosthetic reconstruction is a reasonable option for patients who require joint resection. It is most appropriate in those who are content not to engage in high-impact activities and favor limb salvage. These patients need to be prepared for the likelihood of multiple surgeries and revisions due to anticipated septic loosening and unanticipated complications such as infection and implant failure.[4]

Endoprosthesis

The use of a prosthesis can result in rapid mobilization. However, the prosthesis requires adequate coverage with well-vascularized tissue. Hemiarthroplasty for the hinge-type knee joint is relatively straightforward unlike using a prosthesis at the hip or proximal femur. Pediatric patients are likely to require revision due to device failure and lack of longevity of devices.[17] To account for limb growth, expandable endoprostheses are available. These devices are lengthened in a closed manner, limiting the number of open surgeries required. However, such devices are mechanically weaker than solid implants. Custom sized solid implants are an alternative option but require management of limb length. Endoprostheses require coverage with well-vascularized tissue to minimize infection.

Soft-tissue coverage is best undertaken during the initial surgery.[16] The proximal femur is deep and has enough endogenous soft-tissue coverage even for those requiring wide tumor resection. The knee may require additional coverage and the medial gastrocnemius muscle can be used. If local tissues have been resected, free tissue transfer is needed to ensure adequate coverage of the endoprosthesis.

Rotationplasty

Rotationplasty is an acceptable alternative to endoprosthetic reconstruction following joint resection. Rotationplasty is usually performed at the level of the knee for resections of the proximal tibial and distal femur. Rotationplasty involves resecting a segment of the limb including the entire knee joint and rotating the leg and ankle 180 degrees before reconnecting the tibia to the proximal femur.[18,19,20,21] Knee prosthesis is no longer required as the ankle becomes the new knee joint.[22] The tibial nerve powers the knee into extension. Involvement of the tibial nerve with tumor is a contraindication to rotationplasty.[4]

Future leg length discrepancy must be taken into consideration for endoprosthetic reconstruction and rotationplasty. For patients having rotationplasty, the reconstructed femur is usually left longer than the contralateral limb to accommodate for future growth and skeletal maturity. Procedures to address limb-length discrepancy include lengthening using distraction osteogenesis, epiphysiodesis of the long limb to limit growth, and limb shortening of the contralateral limb.

If surgeons need to resect long bones such as the tibia or femur, the corresponding segment of major vessels will also need to be resected. However, one can generally resect vessels and proceed with arterial and venous repair, as there is almost always enough vessel that can be preserved and so no graft is necessary.

5.5.6 Amputation

For large tumors at any site in the lower limb, if resection necessitates the sacrifice of multiple critical structures, salvage is not appropriate. In these cases, amputation, a last resort, is the most appropriate option. Where amputation is necessary, creating a durable stump to enable future mobility and the prevention of painful neuroma formation are critical.

5.6 Conclusion

Lower limb reconstruction following tumor resection in pediatric patients requires careful application of the principles of oncologic safety, as well as optimizing function and quality of life. The most common types of resection of extremity tumors include intercalary resection with vascularized bony reconstruction, joint resection with an endoprosthesis or rotationplasty, and amputation. Consideration for skeletal maturity is important in pediatrics. The goal of the reconstructive surgeon with the multidisciplinary team is to provide the best functional outcome possible with the lowest treatment burden.

References

[1] HaDuong JH, Martin AA, Skapek SX, Mascarenhas L. Sarcomas. Pediatr Clin North Am. 2015; 62(1):179–200

[2] Piper M, Irwin C, Sbitany H. Pediatric lower extremity sarcoma reconstruction: a review of limb salvage procedures and outcomes. J Plast Reconstr Aesthet Surg. 2016; 69(1):91–96

[3] Ver Halen JP, Soto-Miranda MA, Hammond S, Konofaos P, Neel M, Rao B. Lower extremity reconstruction after limb-sparing sarcoma resection of the proximal tibia in the pediatric population: case series, with algorithm. J Plast Surg Hand Surg. 2014; 48(4):238–243

[4] Wong KY, Hopyan S, Borschel GH, Zuker RM. Pediatric soft tissue and bony sarcomata of the extremities: considerations and reconstruction. In: Bentz M, Bauer B, Zuker R, eds. Principles and Practice of Paediatric Plastic Surgery. 2nd ed. Boca Raton, FL: CRC Press; 2016:1683–1706

[5] Meyer WH, Spunt SL. Soft tissue sarcomas of childhood. Cancer Treat Rev. 2004; 30(3):269–280

[6] Longtin R. Ewing's sarcoma: a miracle drug waiting to happen? J Natl Cancer Inst. 2003; 95(21):1574–1576

[7] Hawkins DS, Spunt SL, Skapek SX, COG Soft Tissue Sarcoma Committee. Children's Oncology Group's 2013 blueprint for research: soft tissue sarcomas. Pediatr Blood Cancer. 2013; 60(6):1001–1008

[8] Rivera-Valentin RK, Zhu L, Hughes DP. Bone sarcomas in paediatrics: progress in our understanding of tumour biology and implications for therapy. Paediatr Drugs. 2015; 17(4):257–271

[9] Enneking WF, Spanier SS, Goodman MA. A system for the surgical staging of musculoskeletal sarcoma. Clin Orthop Relat Res. 1980(153):106–120

[10] Jawad MU, Scully SP. In brief: classifications in brief: Enneking classification: benign and malignant tumors of the musculoskeletal system. Clin Orthop Relat Res. 2010; 468(7):2000–2002

[11] Morrison BA. Soft tissue sarcomas of the extremities. Proc Bayl Univ Med Cent. 2003; 16(3):285–290

[12] Zenn MR, Jones G. Guide to flap selection. In: Zenn MR, Jones G, eds. Reconstructive Surgery; Anatomy, Technique and Clinical Applications. St. Louis, MO: Quality Medical Publishing; 2012:81–151

[13] San-Julian M, Aquerreta JD, Benito A, Cañadell J. Indications for epiphyseal preservation in metaphyseal malignant bone tumors of children: relationship between image methods and histological findings. J Pediatr Orthop. 1999; 19(4):543–548

[14] Belt PJ, Dickinson IC, Theile DR. Vascularised free fibular flap in bone resection and reconstruction. Br J Plast Surg. 2005; 58(4):425–430

[15] Taylor GI, Wilson KR, Rees MD, Corlett RJ, Cole WG. The anterior tibial vessels and their role in epiphyseal and diaphyseal transfer of the fibula: experimental study and clinical applications. Br J Plast Surg. 1988; 41(5):451–469

[16] Mastorakos DP, Disa JJ, Athanasian E, Boland P, Healey JH, Cordeiro PG. Soft-tissue flap coverage maximizes limb salvage after allograft bone extremity reconstruction. Plast Reconstr Surg. 2002; 109(5):1567–1573

[17] Longhi A, Errani C, De Paolis M, Mercuri M, Bacci G. Primary bone osteosarcoma in the pediatric age: state of the art. Cancer Treat Rev. 2006; 32(6):423–436

[18] Kotz R, Salzer M. Rotation-plasty for childhood osteosarcoma of the distal part of the femur. J Bone Joint Surg Am. 1982; 64(7):959–969

[19] Borggreve J. Kneiegelenksersatz durch das in der Beinlängsachse um 180° gedrehte Fußgelenk. Arch. Orthop. Trauma Surg. 1930; 28:175–178

[20] van NES CP. [Some cases of reparative and reconstructive surgery]. Brux Med. 1950; 30(41):2093–2115

[21] Salzer M, Knahr K, Kotz R, Kristen H. Treatment of osteosarcomata of the distal femur by rotation-plasty. Arch Orthop Trauma Surg. 1981; 99(2):131–136

[22] Krajbich JI. Modified Van Nes rotationplasty in the treatment of malignant neoplasms in the lower extremities of children. Clin Orthop Relat Res. 1991 (262):74–77

6 Spare-Part Surgery

Marco Innocenti, Eric Santamaria, and Young Chul Suh

Summary

The use of discarded tissue for reconstruction is referred to as "spare-part surgery." It is an important strategy to utilize tissue otherwise wasted. Although there are no core principles or techniques, successful application can be made by understanding the basic concepts of flaps and grafts.

Keywords: spare-part surgery, reconstruction, trauma, microsurgery

6.1 Introduction

Limb-mutilating injuries or oncologic radical amputations are a challenge for the surgeon to restore effective function and appearance of the upper or lower extremities. When tissue needs to be harvested from donor sites for reconstruction, this may be in the form of single tissue grafts such as skin, bone, nerve, or veins, or vascularized composite flaps. These procedures invariably require violation of various sites in the body with additional donor site morbidity. The surgeon needs to weigh cost-effectiveness between the gain of function from reconstruction of the injured limb and the morbidity of harvesting from an uninjured donor site. An alternative strategy is to scavenge tissue for reconstruction from parts that are nonsalvageable amputated sites.[1]

The "spare parts" concept involves using parts of amputated or otherwise nonsalvageable limbs, allowing the harvest of flaps for reconstruction without additional donor-site morbidity. These undamaged and potentially usable elements include skin, bone, nerves, tendons, vessels, or portions of composite functional units. Fillet flaps, a component of the spare parts concept, can be used as pedicled or free flaps. In severe traumatic injury, pedicled fillet flap is a good option for reconstruction. But in the case of cancer reconstruction, tumor involvement of the proximal limb and trunk often precludes the use of the limb fillet flap as a pedicled flap. Thus, free fillet flap coverage is required.[2]

Spare parts represent those components that may be overlooked in a pile of presumed unusable and mutilated tissues. Every traumatic injury of the extremity is different; the surgeon must weigh the value of the remains of a mutilated extremity to carefully distinguish the viable from the nonviable. Of what is available, one must then determine the prospective use and contribution of the remaining constituents to the overall function and form of the limb.

The unique aspect of spare-part surgery in trauma is that the surgeon has to assess and create a strategy on the spot to maximize the use of tissues that otherwise would be discarded. This requires surgical expertise, experience, and planning at the time of primary surgery. Certain factors should be taken into consideration in the decision-making, the first being prerequisites that must be satisfied when the surgeon contemplates spare-part surgery.

6.2 Debridement

Debridement is the first step in any limb amputation and it is the only way to reduce bacterial burden for early reconstructive procedure. Debridement aims to convert a dirty contaminated wound into a clean surgical wound by removing all tissue that is devitalized, including the zone of injury, that is of marginal viability, or that is contused and likely to be nonfunctional. The approach is similar in concept to tumor surgery. Especially, there is little role of staged debridement for spare-part surgery. There is only one chance of debridement before doing spare-part surgery for urgent reconstruction. According to Büchler, a conservative approach with preservation of contused and partially devascularized structures can result in fibrosis and scarring, which compromise the ultimate functional result.[3]

After all life-threatening emergencies are addressed and the patient is medically stabilized, operative surgical debridement and irrigation can be initiated. Thorough removal of all nonviable skin, soft tissue, muscle, bone, and foreign bodies is crucial in obtaining a clean wound bed, reducing bacterial contamination, and preventing subsequent infection.

In the amputated part, however, consistency, color, contractility, and circulation are uncheckable to determine muscle viability. It is also difficult to assess the amount of excision in skin because there is no fresh-bleeding skin edge. Spare-part surgery is usually performed in severely crushed limb, not in clearly cut amputation, so debridement amount can be only dependent on surgeon's experience.

At the end of the procedure, the wound should be washed with copious quantities of saline, preferably as pulsed lavage or Versajet. The Versajet hydrosurgery system (Smith & Nephew, Key Largo, FL) offers a unique way of performing debridement: a high-pressure fluid jet running parallel to the surface draws devitalized soft tissues into a cutting chamber for excision and evacuation.

6.3 Extracorporeal Membrane Oxygenation Circuit

Spare-part surgery can be a "hot potato," in the case of marginally crushed amputated limbs in which it is difficult to make a clear decision on whether urgent replantation, spare-part surgery, or stump revision would be the best choice for the patient. Even in the cases of clear-cut amputation with marginal ischemic time, decision-making between urgent replantation and spare-part surgery is still difficult because there is only one chance of utilizing an amputated part. Even in a clear-cut, and not crushed, amputated part with short ischemic time, it requires a couple of days for the patient's condition to be stabilized after having undergone prolonged general anesthesia.

Greaney et al reported that utilization of the extracorporeal membrane oxygenation (ECMO) circuit allows for preservation of the extremity for several days, thus allowing an extended period of time for patient stabilization.[4] The abilities to optimize oxygenation, induce cooling, and titrate the concentration of hemoglobin in the circuit are the additional benefits of isolating the limb on an ECMO circuit. Due to the complex nature of ECMO and the many variables that must be taken into account when implementing this technology, an in-depth discussion of this technology is warranted herein. Among the factors that were carefully evaluated in conjunction with the cardiac perfusion team to optimize tissue perfusion in this patient's extremity were circuit size, oxygen delivery, anticoagulation, perfusion temperature, and the ECMO's laminar blood flow.

The concept of isolating the circulation of the limb to prevent harm to the body is not new. However, it is more commonly applied in the setting of isolated limb perfusion for oncologic purposes. Isolated limb perfusion is primarily utilized in the setting of treatment of melanomas and sarcomas that cannot be surgically excised.[5] It can also be used to deliver thrombolytic medications in the setting of extensive arterial or venous thrombosis.[6]

When ECMO is used after cleansing the amputation part, during the couple of days while waiting for stabilization of the patient, debridement can be done to remove all devitalized tissue, as described earlier.

Even though the ultimate limit of viable limb preservation is not defined, it may help extend perfusion time, slow down metabolism, and/or help regenerate damaged tissue during the time of perfusion.[7] These also help enhance the survival of each tissue graft such as arterial or vein graft, nerve graft, or bone graft if availability of fillet flap or replantation is decreased.

6.4 Tissue Graft

Tissue graft is the most common form of spare-part surgery. Amputated or nonsalvageable components can be used as sources of tissue grafts. These include skin grafts, nerve grafts, arterial or vein grafts, and bone grafts for reconstruction of the remaining limb. These components fall within the zone of injury and a careful assessment is necessary, especially for vascular and nerve grafts where there is a high chance of surgical failure if injured segments are used.

Skin graft from an amputated part can be stored at most for 14 days from the time of injury. This graft can be used not only in emergency operation setting, but also in elective setting after amputation stump is stabilized (▶ Fig. 6.1a–c). Bone is also resistant to ischemia for up to 48 hours.[8] Short segment of the bone chip can be useful as a nonvascularized bone graft. However, nerve graft should be carefully chosen because it has limited threshold of ischemia (only 6 hours) and can easily be damaged by traction injury more than any other type of tissue graft.

Arterial or vein graft is also suitable for reconstruction of amputation stumps with flaps. They can contribute to preventing shortening of stump because of vascular crushing injury. Based on the length of ischemia, vigorous irrigation with heparin or urokinase is necessary to ensure washing out of all thrombosis along the graft. Although there are no certain data that demonstrate the time of ischemic threshold of vessels, thrombosis inside of the graft lumen is a major limiting factor of availability of the graft.

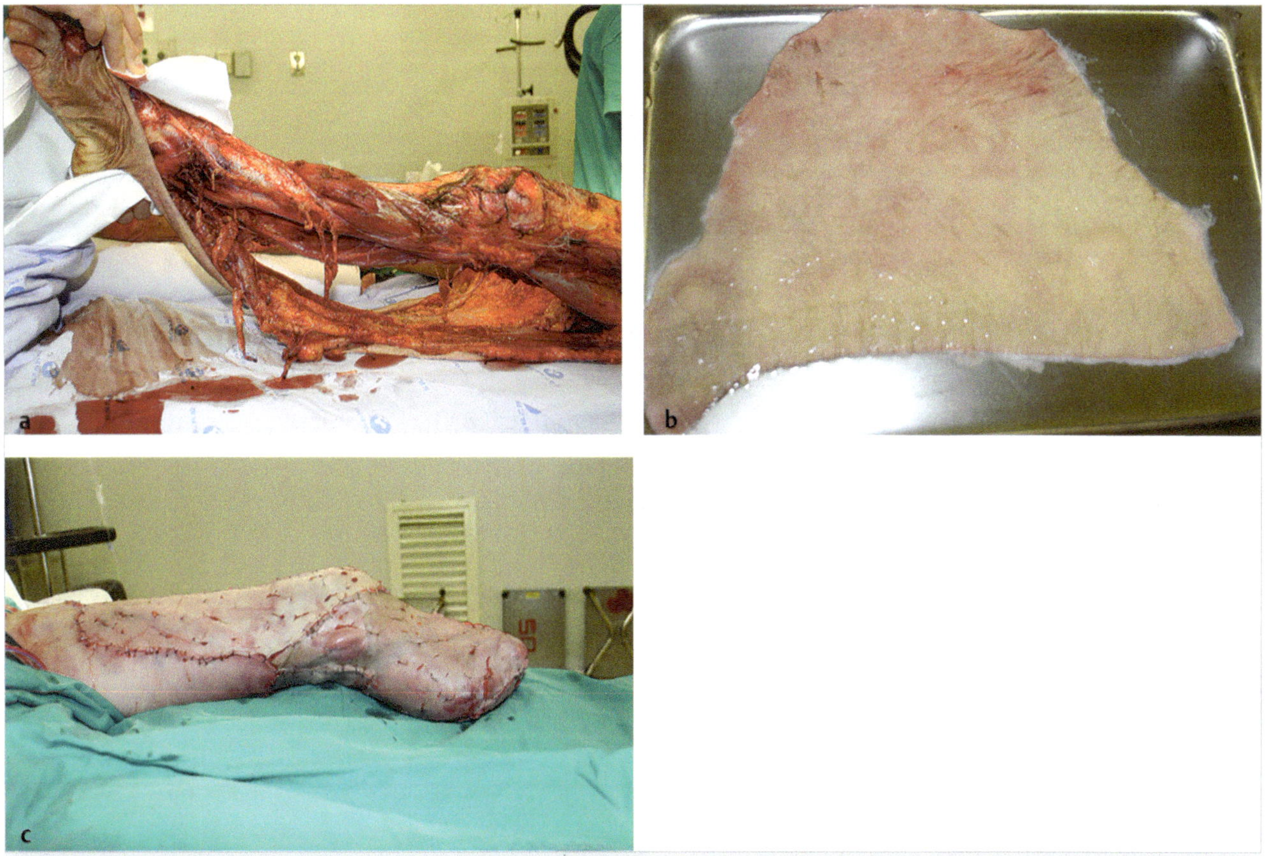

Fig. 6.1 **(a)** A 51-year-old man is shown to have a mangled lower extremity without the chance for limb salvage. **(b)** In the case of below-knee amputation, there will not be adequate skin coverage. Thus, all the skin was harvested from the amputated part to be used as a graft. **(c)** After below-knee amputation, the skin was used as a graft.

6.5 Fillet Flaps

By definition, fillet flaps are axial-pattern flaps that can function as composite-tissue transfers. They can be used as pedicled or free flaps and are a beneficial reconstruction strategy for major defects, provided there is tissue available adjacent to these defects.[9] The use of fillet flaps can be extended to the reconstruction of major defects caused by tumor resection or to the treatment of recurrent pressure sores.[2,10]

Fillets of the lower limb have been used to salvage amputation stumps in lower-leg amputations. Length of preservation is of the utmost importance in lower-leg amputations because the performance and quality of life of the patient correlate significantly with the level of amputation.[11,12,13,14,15] Amputation level has a significant impact on patient rehabilitation with below-knee amputation (BKA) well recognized as being functionally and aesthetically superior to above-knee amputation (AKA). Functionally, unilateral amputation, distal amputation level, and younger age have been shown to be predictive of better walking ability.[16] Comparison of metabolic requirements of walking within a prosthesis also demonstrates energy expenditure of transtibial amputees to be the lowest and that of transfemoral amputees to be the highest.[17] Hence, when possible, BKA remains the amputation level of choice. This requires a functional knee articulation, sufficient tibial length, and adequate soft-tissue coverage to provide a well-padded, robust, and ideally sensate stump able to withstand the rigors of ambulating within a prosthesis. If the soft-tissue requirements cannot be met, then further tibial shortening, through knee amputation, AKA, or free tissue transfer, becomes the only remaining option.

6.5.1 Pedicled Fillet Flap

The fillet plantar flap can be easily raised on the posterior tibial neurovascular pedicle and provides adequate size, soft-tissue bulk, stability, and strength to withstand the shear forces associated with walking. Use of the "spare part" provides a single-stage reconstruction, relative ease of flap dissection, and no further donor site morbidity in a patient already undergoing major surgery. With a two-team approach, operative time can be further shortened with harvesting of the flap performed on a side table after amputation of the limb.[18]

While this flap could be raised as a pedicled flap, preserving continuity of the tibial nerve, this would introduce the difficulties of length dissection within an inflamed field, pedicle redundancy, and risk of kinking during flap inset. Sensory recovery facilitates early weight bearing, better proprioceptive feedback during gait training, and reduction of prosthesis-related complications such as ulcers, neuroma, and pain.

These flaps are reliable. Technical difficulties include placement of the redundant neurovascular bundle in the distal thigh or under the flaps.

Case Example

A 64-year-old man had recurrent rhabdomyosarcoma on his right hand. The tumor extended to both the second and third metacarpal heads (▶ Fig. 6.2a). Radical resection of the metacarpal joints was performed including skin, margins free of disease. Pedicled fillet flap based on radial neurovascular bundle was performed including skin and proximal interphalangeal joint of the second ray, which transferred to the metacarpal bone of the

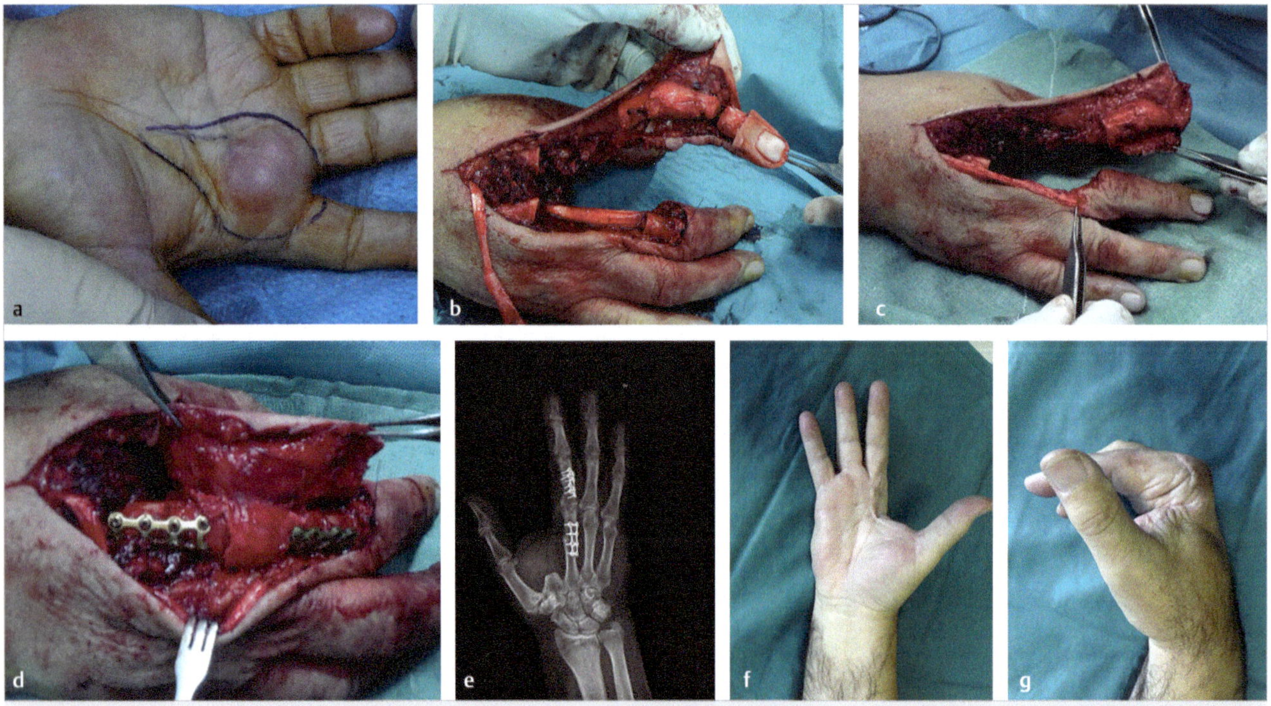

Fig. 6.2 **(a)** A patient with a malignant cancer on the hand involving the second and third metacarpal bones is noted with threat of amputation of both digits. **(b)** After wide resection of the involved bones, the distal digital structures were saved for both digits. **(c–e)** The phalangeal bone from the second digit was transposed to reconstruct the missing parts of the third digit. **(f, g)** Note the functional recovery after using these spare parts from the hand.

third ray (▶ Fig. 6.2b, c). Bony fixation was performed with metallic plate and screw (▶ Fig. 6.2d, e). The reconstructed hand achieved a range of motion of 0 to 80 degrees at 6 months postoperative (▶ Fig. 6.2f, g).

6.5.2 Free Fillet Flap

Indications and Contraindications

The amputated part and recipient site must be both available and in satisfactory condition for the free fillet flap. Lower extremity and upper arm fillet free flap may also be indicated in a child. The child possesses improved nerve regeneration that may allow improved function for amputations at these levels. Patients who have lost multiple digits also deserve an extra consideration in replantation. In upper extremity trauma, where a single digit loss may be well tolerated, patients who have lost multiple digits have a significantly greater disability. Salvaging one or two fingers in a mutilated hand may preserve essential function of the hand. In multiple-digit amputations, consideration should also be made for "spare-parts surgery." If an amputation is through the metacarpophalangeal joint of the long finger and more proximal on the index finger, replantation of the index finger to the long finger ray, preserving the joint, may increase the patient's overall function.

The absolute contraindication to performing fillet free flap is preserving life over limb. A patient with life-threatening injuries or multiple medical problems who cannot withstand prolonged surgery should not undergo free flap surgery. Also, tumor extension into the fillet flap should also be contraindicated. An uncooperative patient is also a contraindication for microsurgery. In a patient with acute major life-threatening injuries, an amputated hand or leg may be kept in cold storage and the patient reassessed in 24 hours. If the patient is stable enough to undergo surgery, delayed replantation may be considered.

Contraindications for free fillet flap include the following:

- Concomitant life-threatening injury.
- Tumor extension into the fillet flap.
- Systemic illness (e.g., small-vessel disease).
- Poor anesthesia risk.
- Mentally unstable patients.
- Multiple segmental injuries in the amputated part.
- Severe crushing or avulsion of the tissues.
- Extreme contamination.
- Prior surgery or trauma to the amputated part.
- Prolonged warm ischemia time.
- Ribbon sign and red-line sign.
- Limb necrosis.

Operative Technique

It should proceed in an organized and deliberate fashion. When fillet free flap is considered feasible, the amputated part is brought to the operating room and explored to identify the neurovascular structures. This may even be performed while the patient is still in the emergency room being evaluated and stabilized.

If two surgical teams are available (at least for a short time during this surgery), both the amputated part and the patient can undergo simultaneous surgery. If there is any delay in getting the patient to the operating room, the amputated part is brought to the operating room first. Using loupe magnification, all structures are examined. The blood vessels and nerves are usually examined at high magnification with the operating microscope before committing to perform free fillet flap. Under the operating microscope, the part is examined for suitability of fillet flap. Tissue loss is evaluated, along with the level of amputation. The neurovascular structures should be evaluated for evidence of avulsion injuries. A string sign or ribbon sign means the digit is not suitable for microanastomosis.[19] These signs are indicated by a red streaking of blood along the path of the artery, usually implying an avulsion injury.

Fillet flaps are classically elevated based on perforators. Similar to debridement, it is not easy to determine the best perforator to supply the angiosome because there is no pulsation, so capturing as many perforators as possible in one fillet flap is beneficial to supply enough vascularity. The artery and nerves should be identified and tagged with a 7–0 polypropylene suture or microclips.

Once the patient is under anesthesia, the proximal level of the injury is explored. Free fillet flap surgery is usually performed under general anesthesia. Foley catheter is inserted and proper body warming is assured by utilizing a warming blanket and warming the operating room. All pressure points should be well padded to avoid pressure injuries; this includes the occiput to avoid scalp alopecia.

Arteries should be debrided to beyond the zone of injury. The lumen of the artery should be explored to make certain there are no intimal flaps that can cause thrombosis. The arteries should be examined and cut back, as necessary, prior to inflation of the tourniquet. The vessel is flushed with a dilute heparin solution at a concentration of 100 units/mL.

If after proper debridement the gap precludes primary repair, a vein graft should be used. Theoretically, an increased potential of thrombosis exists when vein grafts are used since there are two microvascular anastomoses. However, clinical studies do not support an increased incidence of thrombosis. When vein grafts are utilized, venous discrepancies may be managed by a variety of techniques, including fish mouth incisions, sleeve anastomosis, or end-to-side coupling or step-down vein grafts.[20]

Repair of the veins is one of the most crucial steps in fillet free flap. In a complete amputation, the vein repair is critical. The veins are usually repaired after repair of one artery. Veins grafts to bridge segments of venous loss are used as required. At least one vein should be repaired prior to release of the arterial clamp. If a vein could not be identified on the initial exploration of the amputated part, release of the arterial clamp will allow visualization of the dorsal veins as they fill with blood, but the resulting bleeding may obscure the clean microvascular field.

Sensory restoration of the extremities with innervated free tissue transfer has been mentioned by several authors.[21,22,23] Sensibility in the replanted finger is an important factor in final functional outcome. Sensibility is even more important than range of motion. Superior results may be achieved if neural continuity is preserved.[24] The concept of reinnervation should be considered whenever practical, if donor and recipient nerves are present. Primary repair of the nerve can be performed in most clean guillotine-type injuries.

Nerve grafts or conduits can be used for small nerve defects. Conduits may be constructed utilizing a variety of materials,

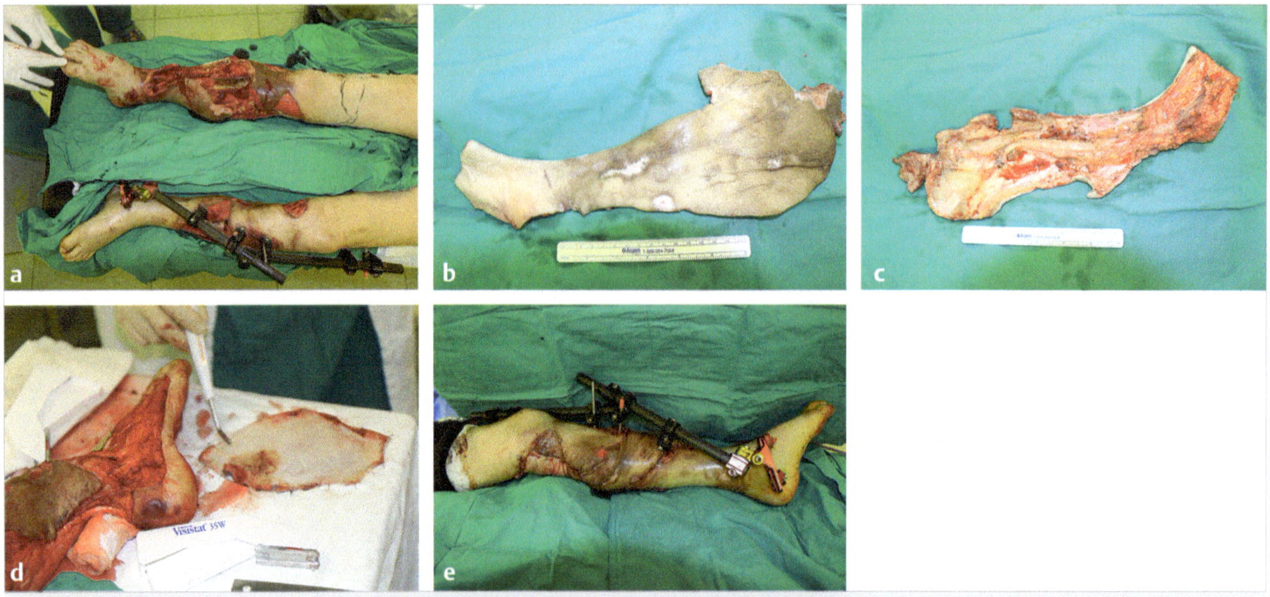

Fig. 6.3 **(a)** Note the patient with open tibiofibular fractures of both legs after trauma. **(b)** The right leg was determined impossible to salvage; thus, a skin flap was elevated from the right leg prior to amputation. **(c)** The flap was used to reconstruct the left leg. **(d)** Part of the skin was also used for graft after removal of fat. **(e)** The immediate postoperative photograph of the reconstructed leg.

including segments of vein, collagen, silicone, Gore-Tex, polyester, and polyglycolide.[25] Conduits are best limited to defects of less than 2 cm in length.[25] Some conduits are extremely rigid and may impede motion if placed over a joint or are at risk for erosion of overlying skin. Conduits are best used for sensory nerve defects; for motor nerves, standard nerve grafts are preferred. Nerve grafts can be harvested from a variety of donor sites. In the upper extremity, these include the posterior interosseous or median antebrachial cutaneous nerves. Sural nerve is the standard donor graft in the lower extremity. The fascicles of the sural nerve match the digital nerve topology well.

Case Example

A 51-year-old man sustained severe crushing injury of both legs. The right leg was severely ischemic due to popliteal artery dissection and had multiple fractures on both tibia and fibula (▶ Fig. 6.3a). AKA of the right leg was decided. Fillet flap was harvested from the right side of the posterior tibial angiosome (▶ Fig. 6.3b, c). Microanastomosis was performed in an end-to-side manner between the donor site posterior tibial artery and left posterior tibial artery. The accompanying vein was connected to the posterior tibial vein. Flap inset was done and skin was harvested from the amputated part and coverage of the residual defect was also performed (▶ Fig. 6.3d, e).

6.6 Postoperative Care

Pharmacological management of replantation and revascularization remains a controversial topic. Platelet aggregation is the most prevalent underlying cause of arterial thrombosis. Venous thrombosis is generally caused by fibrin clotting. The risk of thrombosis is highest in the first 2 postoperative days, with 80% of thromboses being seen in this time period. Various schemes of pharmacological management have been utilized. No consensus exists on the use of anticoagulation therapy after microsurgery. The most commonly utilized agents are heparin, low-molecular-weight dextran, and aspirin, but little evidence is available on the efficacy of any of these regimens. A survey of microsurgeons showed that 90% used anticoagulation in free flap and microvascular surgery.[26]

6.7 Complications

The most significant complication after replantation and revascularization is anastomotic failure. Close observation of the patient postoperatively for signs of thrombosis and urgent re-exploration of the vessel is the essential first step in successful re-exploration. In the patient's room, the dressing should be removed and if skin sutures appear to be constricting venous outflow, they should also be removed. The patient is given a bolus of intravenous heparin and the operating room is readied. The anastomosis is opened, and clots are atraumatically evacuated. The use of a Fogarty catheter is considered; however, a catheter can cause significant intimal damage. If white thrombus or intimal injury is present, a vein graft should be utilized. Intravascular tissue plasminogen activator is considered; however, there are very limited clinical data and outcome of its effectiveness. After establishing flow, prophylactic therapy with aspirin or heparin should be strongly considered.

References

[1] Peng YP, Lahiri A. Spare-part surgery. Semin Plast Surg. 2013; 27(4):190–197

[2] Ver Halen JP, Yu P, Skoracki RJ, Chang DW. Reconstruction of massive oncologic defects using free fillet flaps. Plast Reconstr Surg. 2010; 125(3):913–922

[3] Büchler U. Traumatic soft-tissue defects of the extremities. Implications and treatment guidelines. Arch Orthop Trauma Surg. 1990; 109(6):321–329

[4] Greaney PJ, Jr, Cordisco M, Rodriguez D, Newberger J, Legatt AD, Garfein ES. Use of an extracorporeal membrane oxygenation circuit as a bridge to salvage

a major upper-extremity replant in a critically ill patient. J Reconstr Microsurg. 2010; 26(8):517–522
[5] Brady MS, Brown K, Patel A, Fisher C, Marx W. Isolated limb infusion with melphalan and dactinomycin for regional melanoma and soft-tissue sarcoma of the extremity: final report of a phase II clinical trial. Melanoma Res. 2009; 19(2):106–111
[6] Quiñones-Baldrich WJ, Colburn MD, Gelabert HA, Barcliff LT, Moore WS. Isolated limb thrombolysis with extracorporeal pump and urokinase. J Surg Res. 1994; 57(3):344–351
[7] Kueckelhaus M, Dermietzel A, Alhefzi M, et al. acellular hypothermic extracorporeal perfusion extends allowable ischemia time in a porcine whole limb replantation model. Plast Reconstr Surg. 2017; 139(4):922e–932e
[8] Berggren A, Weiland AJ, Dorfman H. The effect of prolonged ischemia time on osteocyte and osteoblast survival in composite bone grafts revascularized by microvascular anastomoses. Plast Reconstr Surg. 1982; 69(2):290–298
[9] Küntscher MV, Erdmann D, Homann HH, Steinau HU, Levin SL, Germann G. The concept of fillet flaps: classification, indications, and analysis of their clinical value. Plast Reconstr Surg. 2001; 108(4):885–896
[10] Niazi ZB, Salzberg CA. Operative repair of pressure ulcers. Clin Geriatr Med. 1997; 13(3):587–597
[11] Foster RJ, Barry RJ, Holloway A, Burney DW, III. A 50-cm fillet flap for preservation of maximal lower extremity residual limb length. Clin Orthop Relat Res. 1983(178):216–219
[12] Frieden RA. Amputation after tibial fracture: preservation of length by use of a neurovascular island (fillet) flap of the foot. J Bone Joint Surg Am. 1989; 71(7):1109–1110
[13] Katsaros J, Proudman TW. The very long posterior tibial artery island flap. Br J Plast Surg. 1991; 44(8):599–601
[14] Holden D, Shayan R, Edwards E, Bruscino-Raiola F. Elective spare parts free flap-calcaneal fillet of foot flap. Eur J Trauma Emerg Surg. 2013; 39(4):415–419
[15] Erdmann D, Sundin BM, Yasui K, Wong MS, Levin LS. Microsurgical free flap transfer to amputation sites: indications and results. Ann Plast Surg. 2002; 48(2):167–172
[16] Chung KC, Saddawi-Konefka D, Haase SC, Kaul G. A cost-utility analysis of amputation versus salvage for Gustilo type IIIB and IIIC open tibial fractures. Plast Reconstr Surg. 2009; 124(6):1965–1973
[17] Göktepe AS, Cakir B, Yilmaz B, Yazicioglu K. Energy expenditure of walking with prostheses: comparison of three amputation levels. Prosthet Orthot Int. 2010; 34(1):31–36
[18] Tancharoen C, Ek E, Ramakrishnan A.. Spare parts surgery: salvage of a below knee amputation stump. Modern Plastic Surgery. 2012; 2:28–30
[19] Waikakul S, Sakkarnkosol S, Vanadurongwan V, Un-nanuntana A. Results of 1018 digital replantations in 552 patients. Injury. 2000; 31(1):33–40
[20] Suri MP, Ahmad QG, Yadav PS. Managing venous discrepancy: simple method. J Reconstr Microsurg. 2009; 25(8):497–499
[21] Goldberg JA, Trabulsy P, Lineaweaver WC, Buncke HJ. Sensory reinnervation of muscle free flaps for foot reconstruction. J Reconstr Microsurg. 1994; 10(1): 7–9
[22] Potparić Z, Rajacić N. Long-term results of weight-bearing foot reconstruction with non-innervated and reinnervated free flaps. Br J Plast Surg. 1997; 50(3): 176–181
[23] Yamauchi T, Yajima H, Kizaki K, Kobata Y, Fukui A, Tamai S. Sensory reconstruction in sensate radial forearm flap transfer. J Reconstr Microsurg. 2000; 16(8):593–595
[24] Arnez ZM, Valdatta L, Sassoon E, Planinsek F, Ahcan U. Salvage of a below knee amputation stump with a free sensate total sole flap preserving continuity of the posterior tibial nerve. Br J Plast Surg. 1998; 51(6):470–472
[25] Houschyar KS, Momeni A, Pyles MN, et al. The role of current techniques and concepts in peripheral nerve repair. Plast Surg Int. 2016; 2016:4175293
[26] Askari M, Fisher C, Weniger FG, Bidic S, Lee WP. Anticoagulation therapy in microsurgery: a review. J Hand Surg Am. 2006; 31(5):836–846

7 Using the Flap and Angiosome Concepts to Optimize Functional Lower Leg and Foot Amputations

Christopher Attinger

Summary

The key factor when considering salvage or amputation of the lower leg or foot is to optimize the functional result appropriate for the age and activity level of the patient. In either case, first, assurance of an adequate blood flow to allow healing and eradication of any residual infection is imperative. This next may require serial radical debridement with removal of any biofilm while retaining any critical interconnections between source vessel angiosomes. Retention of all available viable tissues, especially in the foot, should be routine at the initial debridement, as this may be a source of healthy soft tissue for later wound closure. Once these conditions have been satisfied, and a level of amputation determined, the actual techniques are outlined in necessary detail to allow a toe, transmetatarsal, Lisfranc, Chopart, Syme, or below-knee amputation.

Keywords: toe amputation, transmetatarsal amputation, Lisfranc amputation, Chopart amputation, Syme amputation, below-knee amputation, Ertl modification

7.1 Introduction

When salvaging a limb, it is critical to assess the type of function the reconstructed limb can potentially achieve. The physician has to accurately determine the activities that the patient desires and will be physically capable of eventually. This then determines what best meets those goals: the planned reconstructed limb versus an amputation. Salvaging a limb just to salvage the limb is no longer an acceptable goal. One has to salvage a **functiona**l limb that meets the patient's realistic goals whether it is a reconstructed or an amputated limb. The younger the patients, the more they will demand of their reconstructed leg. As such, the reconstructed limb may not be able to meet the patient's desired expectations, and the decision to go to an amputation may be more appropriate. However, the older the patient, the less will be demanded of the reconstructed leg as long as it allows them to accomplish their activities of daily living so that they can maintain their independence.

The intent here will not be to discuss the basic amputation techniques of the foot and lower leg. Instead, this discussion will be from a plastic surgery perspective using flaps and myodesis to optimize function. Because plastic surgeons have mastered the art of shaping soft tissue and are comfortable with handling both bone and tendon, they are fully qualified to perform the most functional of amputations. As such, the key factors to consider with every amputation to optimize those functional results will be reviewed. This will be critical if one is to be capable of planning whether to salvage or amputate part of the foot or the lower leg.

7.1.1 Preoperative Preparation

The need for a decision to potentially perform an amputation occurs because of inadequate available soft tissue or bone for reconstruction of a functional limb, uncorrectable blood flow, or presence of overwhelming infection. To assess the leg for possible reconstruction, one has to accomplish three things: ensure adequate blood flow for healing, eradicate any residual infection, and have a functional result in mind.

When presented with a diabetic or irradiated patient, it is often difficult to clinically assess blood flow. The angiosome concept must be kept in mind at all times to be sure that the area in question will be well perfused. Ankle-brachial indices are unreliable in diabetics and renal failure patients because of their calcified vessels. Doppler signals can be misleading, but doppler waveforms are more reliable. The most trustworthy is an angiogram with magnified views of the foot. This actually allows the surgeon to visualize the rate of flow in each artery. This can be done with very little dye (< 10 mL of dye) especially in patients with kidney function at risk. This will demonstrate the contributions of each of the three source arteries to the foot, and the arterial–arterial interconnections between each other.[1] The planned amputation may lead to the sacrifice of some of those arterial–arterial connections on which part of the foot may depend as collaterals and could lead to poor outcomes, so that a revision of that plan might be in order.

To ensure the best vascular supply to the impaired limb, it is essential to have a good vascular team to rely upon. They must excel in angioplasty, bypass surgery, and venous surgery. Review of the angiogram with the respective vascular interventionist is critical so that he or she understands exactly what type of blood flow is needed in order for the surgery to be successful. This is especially true if microsurgery is one of the possible reconstructive options. Angioplasties tend to have a shorter half-life when compared to that of a bypass, and that must be considered within the time frame of the required reconstruction. The optimal flow to the downstream foot [as measured by total carbon dioxide (TCO_2)] with bypass surgery is 5 to 8 days versus as long as 30 days with angioplasty. Any microsurgical anastomosis to a major artery should always be in an end-to-side fashion so as not to sacrifice distal flow that already may be compromised. The exception is when the recipient site will be a small perforator, where an end-to-end anastomosis using supermicrosurgery is preferable. When doing microvascular surgery, the venous flow also has to be evaluated to make sure that the venous return from the flap travels via the venous system (superficial or deep) that has the least amount of resistance.[2]

Dealing with an infection can be difficult because the exact diagnosis will be affected by the way the specimen is collected, the way the laboratory handles it, the presence of biofilm, and assessing the PCR (polymerase chain reaction) data. In addition, one has to consider host factors, as the more medically compromised the patient, the more vulnerable they will be for harboring a residual infection.

The quality of debridement can often vary. We recommend removing all exposed tissue after painting the wound with blue dye to accurately demarcate the wound surface.[3] Only by excisional debridement to normal red, yellow, and white tissue can one be certain that all the surface bacteria has been removed. The thicker the excision, the more likely will be removed any underlying biofilm, which can be as deep as 4 mm under the surface. The resection of any indurated tissue at the edges of the wound also helps remove all potentially inflamed tissue. Pre- and postdebridement tissue cultures (vs. culture swabs) are essential to assess the quality of that debridement. Once the postdebridement results are available, the surgeon can then make the decision as to whether to close the wound or not. Meanwhile, a close working arrangement with the infectious disease service ensures that the initial broad-spectrum antibiotics and subsequent culture-specific antibiotic coverage are appropriate to minimize the potential toxicity of any antibiotics. If the bone infection has been resected, note that antibiotics are needed for only 1 week as per the guidelines of the Infectious Diseases Society of America (IDSA)[4] and the International Society of Infectious Diseases (ISID).

After completion of the preoperative preparation, finally a decision has to be made as to what will be the best type of reconstruction. Remember that if an ulcer does heal in a diabetic foot, the chances of ulcer recurrence at 2 years can be as high as 80%.[5] The final result therefore has to be a functional foot that will also minimize the risk of recidivism. If the surgeon believes that the function of a salvaged limb will not meet the physical capacity and expectations of the patient, then amputation has to be considered. That can be either a foot amputation or a below-knee amputation (BKA). The proposed procedure and possible options must be fully discussed with not only the patient but also their entire family or other caregivers. A peer amputee discussion with the patient can be very helpful, as the patient is more likely then to understand the implications of an amputation. Also important is that a prosthetist and orthotist talk to the patient about the consequences of shorter foot amputations versus a BKA. All these factors will permit the patient and their family to make the most intelligent decision as to which option should be chosen.

7.1.2 Toe Amputation

The amputation of toes distal to the metatarsophalangeal (MTP) head should be done either with vertical or horizontal clamshell flaps. The key is to design them so that direct blood flow to the skin is retained, and the closure does not lead to a bulbous toe tip. The diameter of the closure should be the same as that of the more proximal intact toe. One should try to keep part of the proximal phalanx intact to help prevent medial or lateral deviation of the adjacent toes. When only the distal toe is to be amputated, the germinal matrix of the nail bed must be removed to avoid new nail growth in unexpected parts of the line of closure.

When doing a hallux amputation, first determine whether hallux rigidus is present. If it is, it is preferable to amputate the hallux at the MTP joint rather than preserving part of the proximal phalanx. Recurrent ulceration at the distal toe is three or four times higher with partial hallux amputations in patients who have hallux rigidus.[6] Otherwise, preserving as much of the hallux as possible works well.

If the metatarsal head is exposed and the neighboring toe is intact, one can consider fillet of the existing or neighboring toe to cover the defect rather than cutting the metatarsal head shorter to close the defect. A filleted toe never creates as much of a flap as one thinks. The key to filleting a toe is to remove bone without damaging the underlying existing blood supply. The incision can be medial or lateral along a line that separates the top one-third of the toe from the bottom third (▶ Fig. 7.1a). A cut is then made around the distal phalanx staying proximal to the germinal matrix to expose the interphalangeal (IP; hallux) or distal IP (DIP) joint (lesser toes; ▶ Fig. 7.1b). A towel clamp used to grasp the distal phalanx allows retraction to flip it from proximal to distal a complete 180 degrees while the soft tissue is dissected off (▶ Fig. 7.1c, d). The same is done for the proximal phalanx (▶ Fig. 7.1e, f). The volar plates under the IP joints are cut by placing a scissor in the flexor tendon sheath (▶ Fig. 7.1g) and splitting it in two. Each hemivolar plate is carefully removed to avoid damaging the plantar digital vessels that pass just lateral and inferior to it. The flexor tendons are then removed (▶ Fig. 7.1h). The filleted toe is ready to be transferred (▶ Fig. 7.1i, j). Using a fillet of toe can be very useful for preservation of the proximal phalanx (▶ Fig. 7.1k) or filling in large forefoot defects that can occur as when doing transmetatarsal amputations (TMAs; ▶ Fig. 7.2).

7.1.3 Transmetatarsal Amputation

When planning a TMA, the surgeon has to establish whether there is arterial inflow in both the dorsal and plantar surfaces. The direction of the flow and its source artery must be known. Any critical arterial interconnections between the dorsal and plantar foot occur just distal to Lisfranc joint. The main one is from the dorsalis pedis artery that dives between the first and second proximal metatarsals to join the lateral plantar artery. If there is good independent inflow from both the dorsalis pedis and the lateral plantar artery, the dorsal and plantar flaps can be designed with impunity as there will be direct inline flow to each. However, if only one of the two arteries is supplying blood flow to the entire foot, then it is imperative to keep the arch between the dorsalis pedis and lateral plantar arteries intact. This is of particular concern when a proximal TMA or Lisfranc amputation is required. Under those circumstances, to avoid damaging this arch, the first metatarsal is removed medially without visualizing the tissue between the proximal first and second metatarsals to avoid damaging it. The second through fifth metatarsals are removed laterally, again without visualizing the connection between the dorsal and plantar circulation.

When initially debriding any foot that is going to later undergo potential amputation, any soft tissue that is viable should be preserved (▶ Fig. 7.2a–d). This means only removing what is necrotic and saving everything else that can then be a possible option for any subsequent reconstructive surgery needed to preserve length. Salvaged toes or even portions thereof can be extremely valuable for closure of forefoot amputations (▶ Fig. 7.2, ▶ Fig. 7.3). At the time of skin closure, the metatarsals are cut to recreate the normal arch of the metatarsal heads (▶ Fig. 7.2e, f). The residual toes are filleted and used

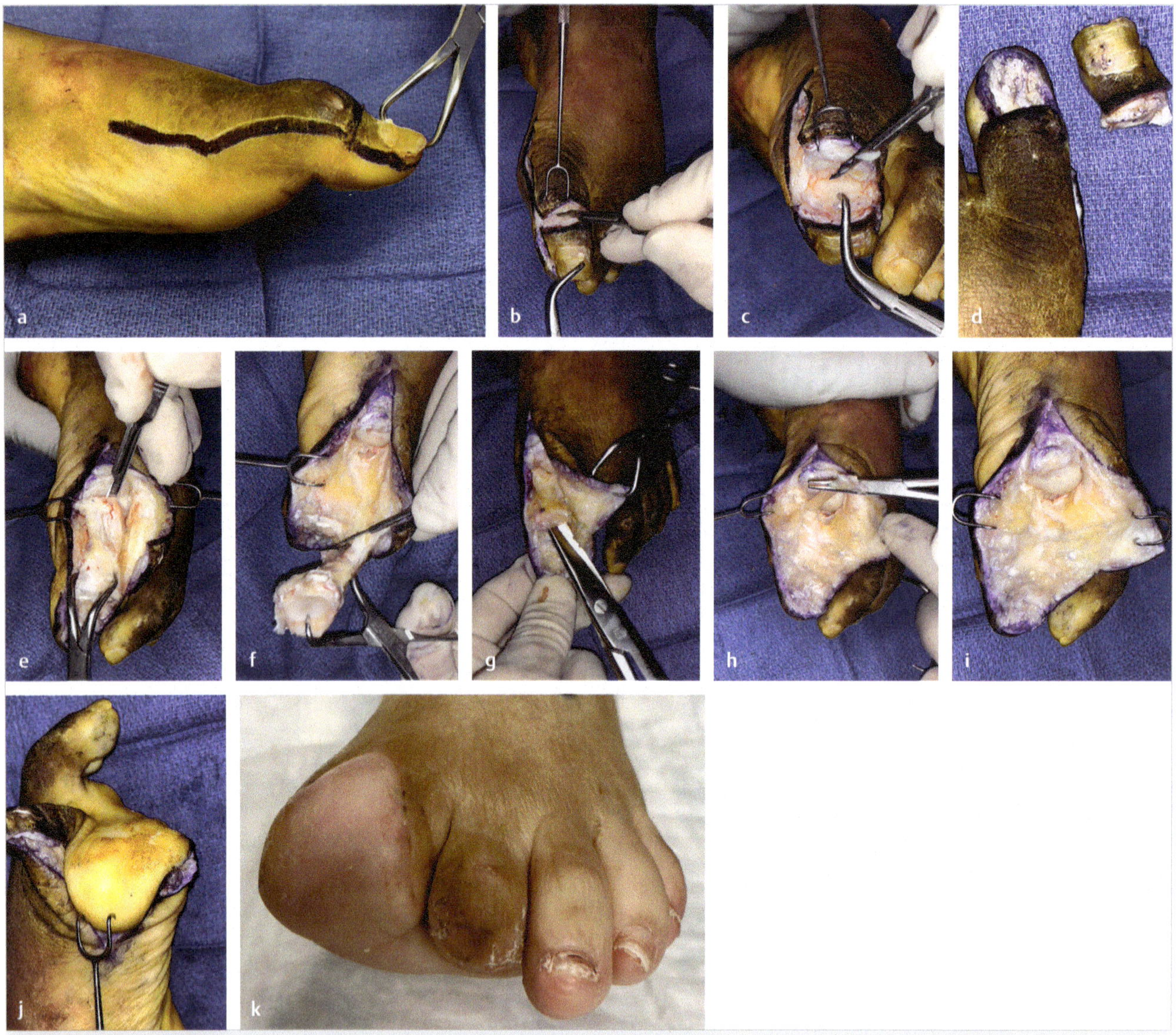

Fig. 7.1 Great toe fillet flap. **(a)** A line is drawn along the medial glabrous junction of the toe proceeding circumferentially to the lateral side, and then connecting the sides of this line dorsally just proximal to the germinal matrix of the nail bed. **(b)** The glabrous junction is incised, and then also the dorsal line proximal to the germinal matrix to expose the interphalangeal joint. **(c)** With the towel clamp grasping the distal phalanx, that can be flipped 180 degrees toward the surgeon while the bone is freed up from the underlying soft tissue from proximal to distal. **(d)** The distal phalanx has been removed from the hallux leaving the distal plantar tissue intact. **(e)** Similarly, the proximal phalanx has been freed from the overlying tissue and the metatarsophalangeal joint entered. **(f)** With the towel clamp now grasping the proximal phalanx, again it can be flipped 180 degrees toward the surgeon so that the bone can be freed from the underlying soft tissue with minimal damage. **(g)** Identify the volar plate with scissors by going into the flexor tendon sheath, cut it along its center, and remove both halves while carefully staying on the plantar volar plate surface to avoid damaging the proper digital arteries. **(h)** The flexor hallucis longus tendon is grasped and removed. **(i)** The now filleted great toe flap is stretched out and **(j)** rotated dorsally to cover the preserved hallux metatarsal head. **(k)** Clinical result of distal filleted hallux flap and concomitant second toe amputation that used a horizontal clamshell skin flap closure.

to cover the exposed bone to provide an adequate soft-tissue envelope (▶ Fig. 7.2g–j). This allows the foot to be longer so that the plantar surface area will endure a lower pressure in pounds per square inch through the gait cycle (▶ Fig. 7.2k, l).

At a secondary operation for a TMA, after the initial debridement, all exposed tissue is painted with blue dye and re-excised to clean healthy tissue (▶ Fig. 7.3a, b). The metatarsals are then cut in an arch with the second being the longest (as in ▶ Fig. 7.2e, f). The cuts are made generally in a direction perpendicular to the shaft, although some bias is preferable by beveling them so that the plantar side is slightly shorter. The first metatarsal and the fifth distal metatarsal are also cut with a slight proximal/distal bias so the distal end will be less prominent medially and laterally, respectively. The metatarsal heads are then removed by grasping the proximal cut metatarsal with a towel clip and flipping 180 degrees to free them up carefully from the underlying soft tissue that is separated without damaging the blood supply (▶ Fig. 7.3c). Generally, the volar plates are split in the middle and removed with care so as not to damage the underlying plantar metatarsal vessels (Fig. 7.3d). The sesamoids from the hallux are removed. Once the wound has been debrided thoroughly and is ready for closure, it is lavaged

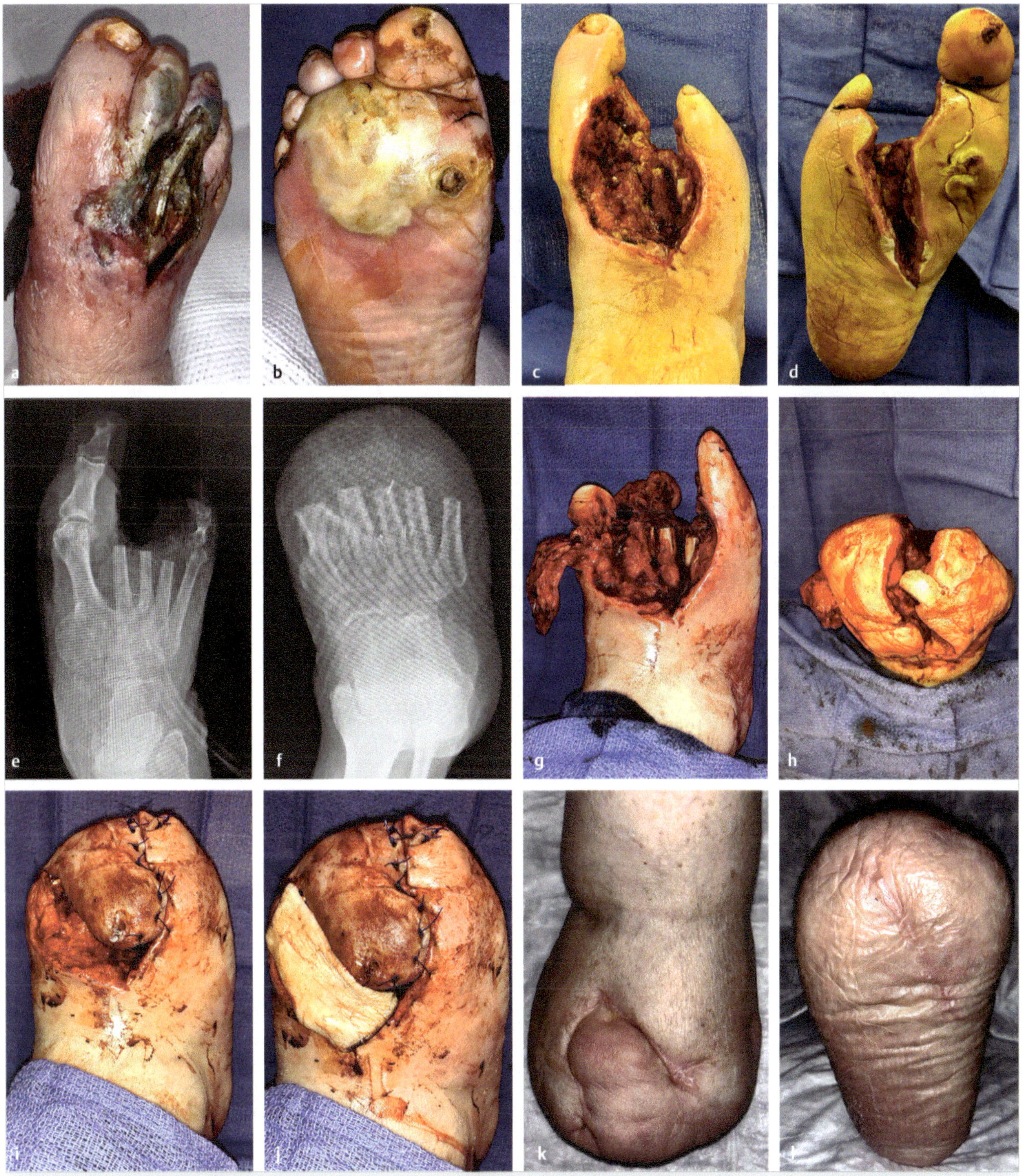

Fig. 7.2 Transmetatarsal amputation with toe fillet coverage. Necrotizing fasciitis involving both **(a)** the right dorsal and **(b)** the plantar mid forefoot. During the initial debridement of nonviable tissue, most of the hallux and fifth toe did not appear involved on the **(c)** dorsal and **(d)** plantar surfaces. They were preserved for the eventual reconstruction. **(e)** Radiograph of the right foot following soft-tissue and bony debridement. **(f)** A transmetatarsal amputation (TMA) was planned. The normal metatarsal head parabola was recreated by cutting across the proximal metatarsals with that of the second toe being the longest. Both the **(g)** first and **(h)** fifth toes were filleted so they could be used as soft-tissue flaps to help close the TMA while preserving length. **(i)** The toe fillet flaps were rotated dorsally to close the TMA defect. **(j)** A skin graft was placed on the remaining open medial dorsal aspect of the foot. **(k)** Dorsal and **(l)** plantar views of the healed TMA 3 months later.

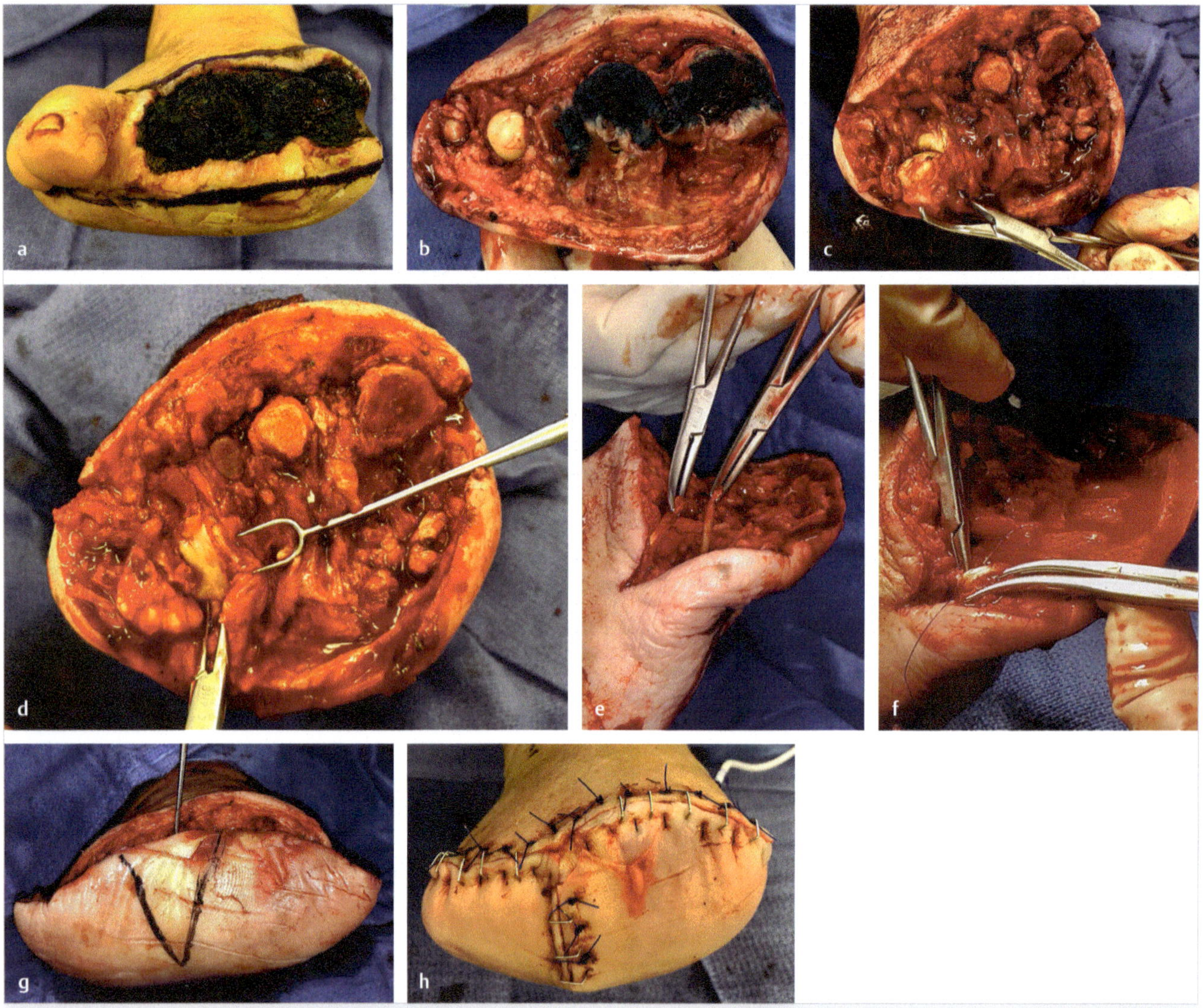

Fig. 7.3 Conventional transmetatarsal amputation (TMA). **(a)** Open area of debrided right foot has been painted with methylene blue to ensure that the secondary debridement is adequate prior to completion TMA, whose planned incision lines have also been marked. **(b)** The fourth and fifth toes have been disarticulated. **(c)** The cut fifth metatarsal head now grasped with a towel clip is freed up by vertically flipping 180 degrees toward the surgeon so that it can be dissected off the plantar soft tissue without destroying any underlying blood supply. Note that the rest of the foot has undergone excisional debridement. **(d)** The metatarsophalangeal joint volar plate is exposed by going into the flexor tendon sheath with a tonsil or scissor. It is then cut along its center and both halves are removed taking care to stay on the plantar side to avoid the digital arteries. Note that the metatarsals were recut to form a parabola with the second metatarsal being the longest. **(e)** To restore some dorsiflexion of the foot lost when the toe extensors were amputated, a tenodesis of the flexor and extensor tendon of the fifth toe was planned. Here they were located and placed on gentle traction, and **(f)** then sewn together to complete the tenodesis with the ankle maintained at 90 degrees or neutral position. **(g)** The plantar flap will usually have a longer arc than the dorsal flap. This inequality will lead to protruding dog ears on the medial and lateral sides of the stump. That can be circumvented by taking a large wedge from the center of the plantar flat to equalize the arcs. **(h)** A simple, smooth closure is then possible.

with the irrigation of choice, and new instruments are chosen to minimize contamination.

The foot will have lost a significant amount of its capability to dorsiflex because the deep and superficial extensors to the toes have been cut during the necessary debridement. The flexors of the foot, since overpowering, will cause the foot to slowly go into an equinovarus position with eventual breakdown of the lateral plantar foot under the fifth metatarsal. This can be prevented by a tenodesis of the flexor and extensor tendons of the fourth and fifth toes with the foot in neutral to restore some of that lost extension (▶ Fig. 7.3e, f). Alternatively, a percutaneous Achilles tendon lengthening will weaken the plantar flexion forces of the foot. Finally, the plantar flap will frequently have a larger diameter than the dorsal flap, so that when closed, dog-ears occur on either side. A wedge can be taken out of the center of the plantar flap so that the circumferences of both sides will be equal to avoid this (▶ Fig. 7.3g, h). Deep sutures are avoided if possible because they can potentiate infection.[7]

Postoperatively, the ankle is maintained in neutral with a well-padded posterior splint. Weight bearing is avoided until at least 3 weeks postsurgery. Staples remain for 1 week and sutures until 4 weeks. Only then will the patient be fitted for orthotics and accommodative shoe wear. However, the foot will remain in a cam walker when ambulatory for a total of 6 weeks

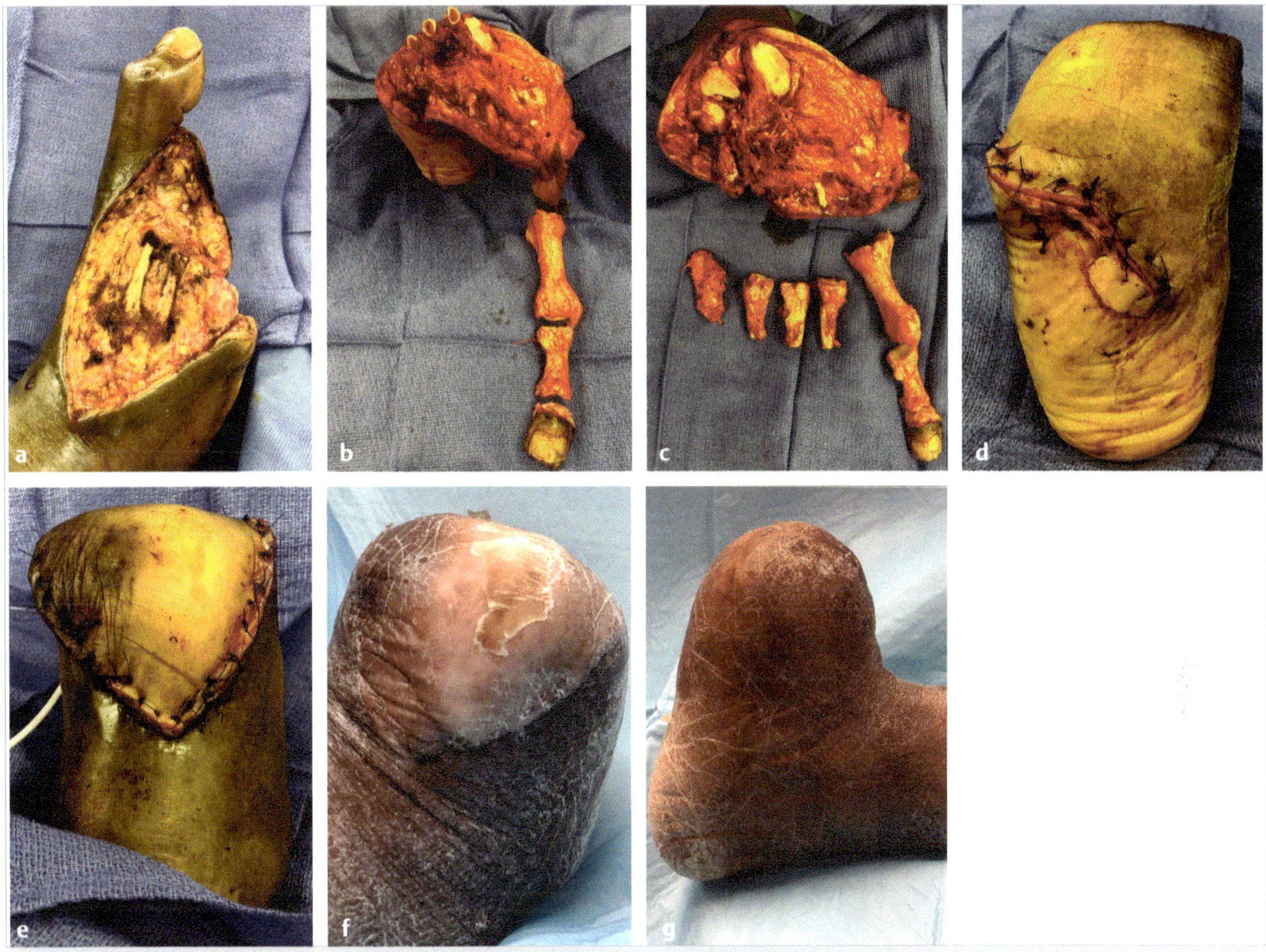

Fig. 7.4 Lisfranc amputation. **(a)** Necrotizing fasciitis of the lateral forefoot with uninvolved hallux. **(b)** The great toe was filleted. **(c)** All metatarsals were disarticulated at Lisfranc joint. **(d)** Plantar and **(e)** dorsal views of the great toe filleted flap rotated laterally to close the defect. **(f)** Three months postoperative, 2 cm of the distal Achilles tendon was also resected. **(g)** Medial view of the amputation stump shows prevention of equinovarus deformity.

from the date of surgery to protect the skin closure and the Achilles tendon (if it was percutaneously lengthened) from being overstressed and rupturing.

7.1.4 Lisfranc Amputation

If infection or tissue necrosis is proximal enough that a Lisfranc amputation will be necessary, again, the blood flow must be assessed to ensure that both the dorsal and plantar tissue have independent inflow. If that is not the case and either side depends on the arterial arch being open, then it is all the more important not to damage the arch during any dissection. To reiterate, that must be done by removing the first metatarsal medially without disturbing the arch, and then removing the second through fifth metatarsals laterally while also avoiding the arch soft tissues.

When determining which flap (dorsal or plantar) to trim to get an adequate closure, one should always preserve the tissue from the better vascularized side and trim the less well-vascularized side. The circumferences of the dorsal and plantar flaps may vary and create dog-ears at either side if closed directly. This can be circumvented either by removing the dog-ears in routine fashion or by taking a central wedge from the plantar flap wide enough so that the circumference of both sides is equal.

As should always be the case in the foot, all available viable tissue is preserved at the time of the initial debridement to provide the surgeon with the most possibly healthy soft tissue for later closure (▶ Fig. 7.4). The longest possible dorsal and plantar flaps are created, and the metatarsals are disarticulated at the Lisfranc joint. A proximal-to-distal approach is used to remove the metatarsal and thus minimize damage to the underlying tissue. The keystone proximal second metatarsal can be cut at the level of the cuneiforms for stability. Great care with that cut has to be taken if the vascular arch is to be preserved. When the flaps are brought together to close the amputation, always remove the less vascularized tissue in favor of the better vascularized tissue. Since obviously the glabrous plantar tissue is more resistant to repetitive trauma, that if at all feasible should be brought up to cover as much of the Lisfranc joint as possible.

The Achilles tendon with a Lisfranc amputation can be a real problem. Because it will be unopposed, it will cause an equinovarus deformity and lead to eventual skin breakdown over the distal cuboid. A frank tenectomy by removing 1 to 2 cm of the

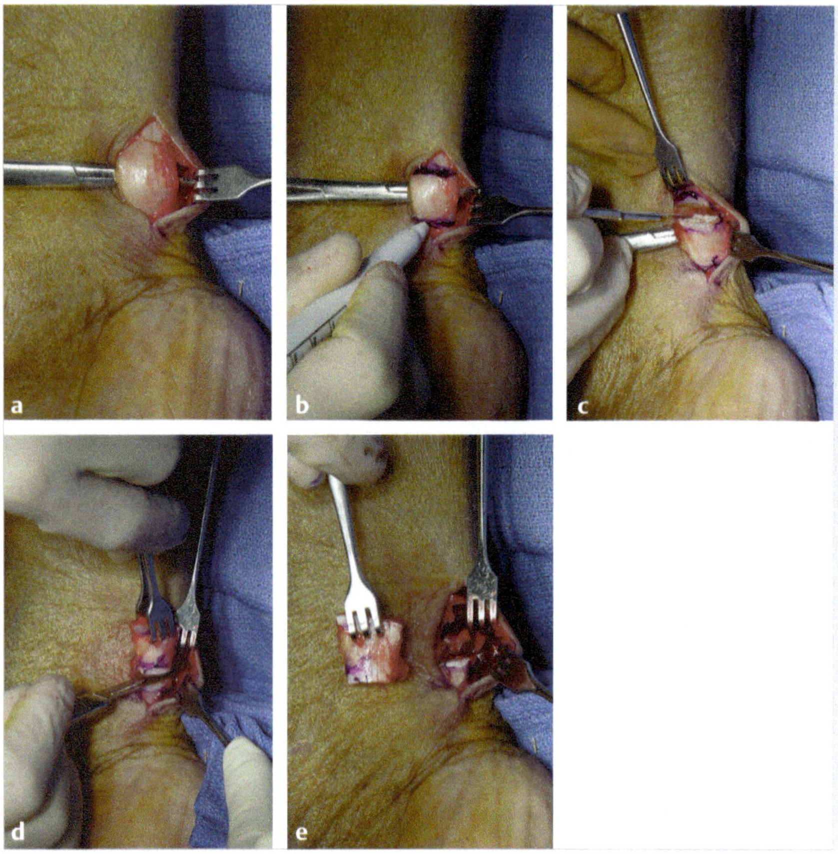

Fig. 7.5 Achilles tendon resection to prevent equinovarus deformity. **(a)** An incision is made just medial to the palpable Achilles tendon. The Achilles tendon is then isolated near its insertion using a clamp. **(b)** A 1.5-cm section of the Achilles tendon that will be resected is marked. **(c)** The superior mark is first incised, as the proximal tendon will then retract cephalad. **(d)** The distal Achilles tendon is then grasped with a clamp, and the distal mark is incised **(e)** to complete the segmental Achilles tendon resection.

distal Achilles tendon just above its insertion will be a solution for two reasons (▶ Fig. 7.5). The first is to prevent the equinovarus deformity from occurring at all. The second is to prevent the Achilles tendon from healing back together later and causing a delayed equinovarus deformity. In patients who are not infected, one can also consider reinserting the anterior tibial tendon by splitting it and attaching it to the lateral aspect to the cuboid using an anchor. This would strengthen dorsiflexion of the foot sufficiently to possibly help counterbalance the overwhelming plantar deflecting force from the Achilles tendon.

7.1.5 Chopart Amputation

A Chopart amputation is a very useful option in the patient who wants to be able to carry on with daily acts of living. It is not as functional for the athletic patient. It requires wearing an ankle foot orthosis (AFO). Given that there is such a small area left of the total plantar surface, it is easy to develop a pressure point. As a result, it has limited but useful functionality preferably in the less active patient.

As is always the situation with any planned foot amputation, blood flow must be reassessed to ensure both dorsal and plantar inflows. It may be harder to preserve an intact arch when such a proximal amputation is considered. The dorsal and plantar flaps are created by making an incision along their glabrous junction bilaterally. Both flaps are elevated by staying directly on bone. The dorsal dissection should be done first, as since thin it is easier; and then the bones are peeled off proceeding distally using towel clamps for retraction and flipping the bones 180 degrees so as to leave the plantar tissue as intact as possible. One then turns up as much of the plantar flap as possible, assuming it is well vascularized, to cover the anterior talus and calcaneus. The dorsal flap is cut where it meets with the plantar flap to create a well-tailored amputation stump. Again, preserve as much well-vascularized tissue (dorsal or plantar) as possible and sacrifice the less vascularized tissue when planning the closure. It is always preferable to preserve as much glabrous plantar tissue as possible, as it will better withstand repetitive trauma as in ambulation. Often the surgeon must be creative to use the best possible tissues to close the amputation (▶ Fig. 7.6). The Achilles tendon poses the same problems that it did in Lisfranc amputation in causing an equinovarus deformity. The best prevention would be to remove 1 to 2 cm of the Achilles tendon at its insertion to avoid a recurrence (▶ Fig. 7.5).

7.1.6 Syme Amputation

This is an excellent amputation[8] provided there is a prosthetist who is comfortable with this type of amputation. This amputation can be weight bearing without a prosthesis for short spurts and allows the patient to go to the bathroom without putting his or her prosthesis on. It does require stump maintenance, and will be difficult to create an articulating artificial ankle given the lack of room between the end of the stump and the floor. A Syme amputation usually requires patent calcaneal branches of the posterior tibial and peroneal arteries to ensure good inflow to the heel. The planned incision is made just anterior to the malleoli using the same pattern as that of a stirrup. The talus is removed by using a large bone clamp to twist it out

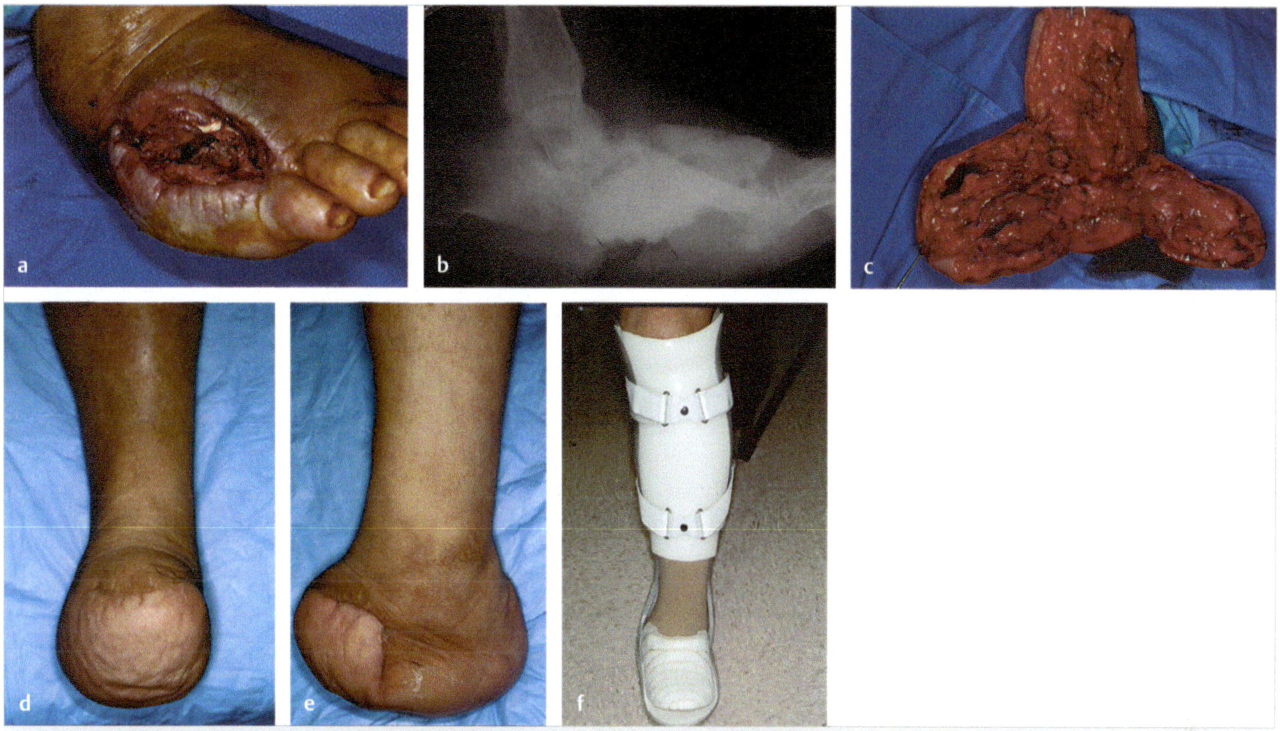

Fig. 7.6 Chopart amputation. **(a)** Extensive open wound extending into the right midfoot, **(b)** with chronic osteomyelitis and Charcot arthropathy as seen on X-ray. **(c)** The foot was filleted into three proximal-based flaps to simplify removal of all infected bone. Only an intact talus and calcaneus remained clean of infection. **(d)** The medial-based flap was used to close the anterior portion of the amputation, **(e)** lateral view. The other flaps were discarded. **(f)** An Achilles tenectomy was performed. At 6 months, walking was possible with an ankle foot orthosis.

of its position and cut the attachments without damaging the surrounding tissue. It may be hard to remove the calcaneus without damaging the surrounding soft tissue. This can be simplified by using a sagittal saw, and then in a crosshair pattern cutting it into four pieces. The pieces are twisted apart using a chisel, until each individually can be teased from the surrounding soft tissue without damaging the blood supply. The tibial plateau is removed 1 to 2.5 cm above the joint line, as well is the lateral malleolus to create a flat surface. Drills holes in the anterior portion of the tibia will be used to anchor the heel fat pad. The heel flap is rotated anteriorly and sewn to the anterior portion of the distal tibia so that it does not shift. Any dog-ears are trimmed of the cutaneous portion only while being very careful not to damage the calcaneal branches in the subcutaneous tissues (▶ Fig. 7.7).

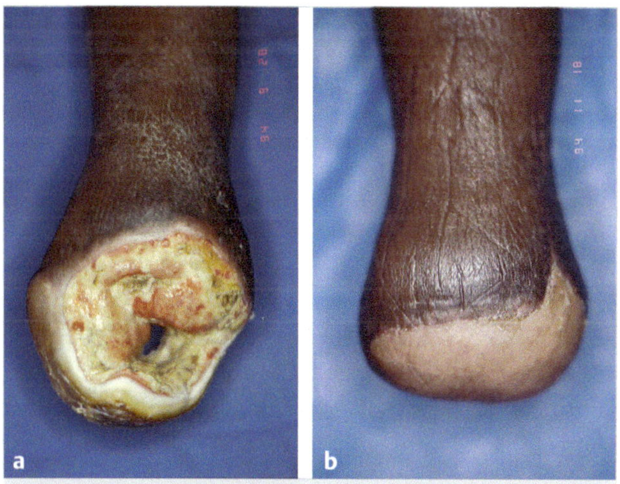

Fig. 7.7 Syme amputation. **(a)** This improperly performed Syme amputation remained open with residual talus. **(b)** The amputation stump was revised by removing the talus, the tibial plateau, and the lateral malleolus. The plantar tissue was redesigned so that it would cover the distal aspect of Syme amputation.

7.1.7 Below-Knee Amputation

The level of the BKA is dependent on the available viable soft tissue and bone after debridement or toileting amputation. If the leg is ischemic, review of the angiogram is helpful to better assess what angiosomes are well perfused. Even if the popliteal or superficial femoral artery is occluded, collateral flow can be adequate to heal a below-knee operation. The demarcation line of cold to warm tissue usually coincides with the level of ischemic pain. Choosing to perform the amputation above where the level of pain and temperature demarcate has proved to be remarkably accurate in determining amputation levels with only a 2% conversion rate of BKA to above-knee amputation (AKA).[9] It is also important that the patient meet with a prosthetist preoperatively so that the patient fully understands what is about to occur. The prosthetist can give invaluable feedback to the surgeon so that the ideal residual limb can be designed. If possible, it is also very helpful for the patient to meet with another amputee who has gone through what the patient is about to experience. This preamputation consultation is invaluable not only in allaying the fears of the patient but also in ensuring the most functional outcome.

Preoperative and perioperative medical management is as important as the surgical technique. Diabetes, end-stage renal disease (ESRD), coronary artery disease, any coagulopathy, and chronic anemia are associated with increased surgical complications and should be managed aggressively. Patients with ESRD should be dialyzed the day before the amputation. Betablockers should be taken the morning of surgery. Perioperative antibiotics should be current and redosed as needed. Glucose should be kept under 200 in the perioperative period.

The level of anesthesia may vary based on the planned procedure. Epidural anesthesia or regional blocks, with sedation, are preferred so that analgesia can be continued for 4 to 5 days postoperative. In our recent experience, regional nerve blocks, targeted motor nerve reinnervation (TMR; peroneal and posterior tibial nerves), and neurectomy (crushing the nerve 5 cm proximal to the nerve cut and burying the distal nerve stump deep along the original nerve path) have been very successful in controlling postoperative pain and minimizing phantom pain.

Amputations performed in the setting of infection should be done in two stages. Two-stage BKA for ischemic and infectious causes has been shown to significantly decrease reoperation rates.[10] This gives 24 to 48 hours for the lymphatic system to clear residual bacteria, and limits possible cross-contamination that can occur when done in a single stage. In addition, time for demarcation from suspected progression of soft-tissue ischemia or infection will be better evident. If only the foot is involved by the infection, the initial drainage amputation should be an ankle disarticulation. If the ankle is involved, a guillotine amputation is planned above the level of infection. When there is lymphedema in the leg, removing the infection will help decrease the swelling. In addition, a lymphedema wrap applied by physical therapy to the residual limb postdrainage amputation works remarkably well to get rid of the edema and make the tissue more pliable for the definitive amputation. The completion amputation is then performed at least 2 to 3 days after the drainage amputation and with a lymphedema wrap on the residual limb to decrease the swelling.

Bickel popularized the use of the posterior myocutaneous flap (PMF) in 1943. Burgess et al later modified it by recommending that the deep posterior compartment be removed to limit unnecessary bulk in the posterior flap and limit the amount of tissue dependent on presumably diseased posterior tibial and peroneal arteries.[11] Interestingly, in popliteal or trifurcation disease, the sural arteries that feed the gastrocnemius muscles are usually spared and provide the necessary blood flow to the superficial posterior flap. This is reflected in our series of 294 flaps where the ratio of BKA to AKA was 4:1 with a 2% eventual conversion rate from BKA to AKA. Our institution uses a PMF in which the superficial posterior compartment provides vascularized and durable coverage of the tibial/fibular osteotomy. Tenodesis and myodesis of the superficial posterior compartment serve several functions. The gastrocnemius muscle will continue to function as a knee flexor, and thus maintain soft-tissue bulk and prevent muscle atrophy. A second benefit of the PMF is preventing a suture line and future scar over the distal stump. A final benefit is that the retained musculature with insertion intact still functions as a venous pump to help prevent lower leg edema.

Technique

The componentry below the socket in the average below-knee prosthesis requires at least an 8-inch clearance from the ground. This leaves plenty of amputation length as it allows increased leverage of a longer moment arm, increased area of interaction of soft tissue with the socket, and provides additional tissue for an adequate revision BKA should it ever be required. After consulting with the prosthetist, each BKA is planned with a tibial osteotomy at 15 to 18 cm from the tibial tubercle if there is adequate distal soft tissue. Otherwise, the amputation is done at 12 cm (▶ Fig. 7.8a). The leg is elevated and a thigh tourniquet is inflated provided there is no counterindication (e.g., recent femoral–popliteal bypass). Coban is used to isolate the distal drainage wound or foot and prevent contamination of the field and proximal clean tissue.

An anterior line is drawn on the skin at the planned tibial osteotomy site encompassing approximately two-thirds the circumference of the leg (▶ Fig. 7.8b). The medial limit is just below the posterior tibia, and the lateral limit is at the fascia separating the lateral from the posterior compartment. This

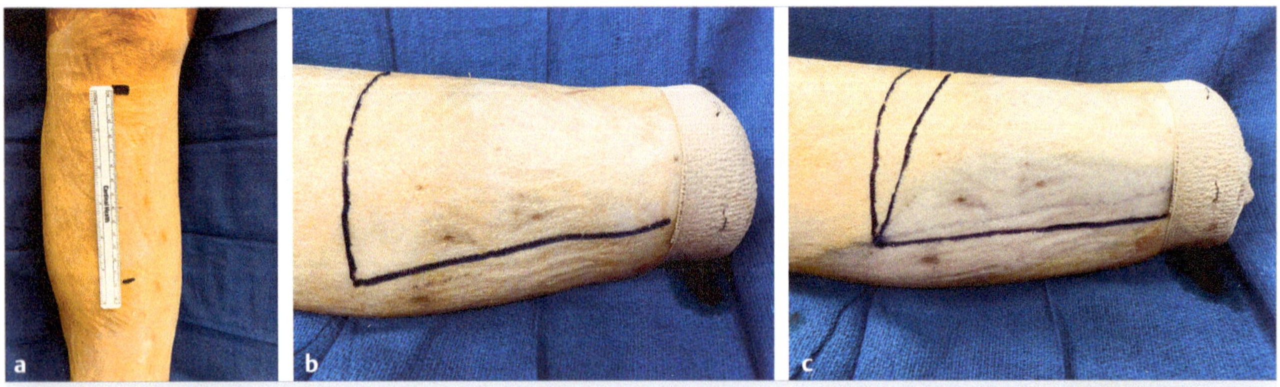

Fig. 7.8 Standard below-knee amputation design. **(a)** The length of the amputation is measured from the tibial tubercle. It should be anywhere between 12 and 15 cm in length. **(b)** A horizontal line marking the bone cut line is drawn. The medial margin of this line stops just below the posterior aspect of the tibia. The lateral margin will go all the way to the fascia separating the posterior from the lateral compartment. **(c)** The actual skin incision line is drawn 2 to 4 cm distal to the bone cut line so that the skin incision will not lie on the bone osteotomy.

gives a slightly skewed posterior flap with the medial side being more anterior than the lateral side. The actual skin incision line is then drawn so that it starts at the same point medially and laterally but extends 2 to 4 cm distal to the previously just drawn anterior skin line at the most anterior portion of the tibia (▶ Fig. 7.8c). This will ensure that the eventual skin suture line does not coincide with the level of the osteotomy site.

Medially and laterally, the skin incision will be carried distally with a slight anterior bevel toward the ankle. The skin cuts are through the deep fascia taking great care to ligate or clip the saphenous vein and small arteries and veins as encountered. The saphenous nerve is identified and preserved. The superficial peroneal nerve lies in the anterior intermuscular septum just lateral to the fascia separating the anterior from the lateral compartment and should be identified and preserved. Special attention is made to preserve the distal peroneus longus and brevis muscles in the lateral compartment that will be used for myodesis later. The anterior muscle compartment is then cut using electric cautery at the level of the planned bone cut. The anterior tibial artery and vein are identified and suture ligated. The deep peroneal nerve is isolated and cut as long as possible, then crushed 5 cm from its distal end and reburied in the anterior compartment as deeply as possible.

The tibia thereby becomes exposed and the planned osteotomy verified at the preplanned distance. An army-navy retractor is passed posterior to the tibia, and the osteotomy is made perpendicular to the longitudinal axis of the tibia (▶ Fig. 7.9). The fibular osteotomy next will be approximately 1.5 cm shorter with a bevel slightly oriented from lateral to medial (▶ Fig. 7.9).

After both osteotomies are completed, a bone hook into the open end of distal tibia provides anterior retraction to expose the deep posterior compartment. A no. 10 blade is used to sharply dissect the lateral and deep posterior compartment muscles off the distal tibia and fibula, respectively (▶ Fig. 7.10a, b). The distal leg is then amputated at a distance that guarantees sufficient posterior flap length when folded anteriorly to close the amputation (▶ Fig. 7.10c). After discarding the distal leg, the deep posterior compartment is dissected away along the transverse intermuscular septum from the superficial posterior compartment (▶ Fig. 7.10d, e) with careful ligation of the peroneal and posterior tibial branches to the latter. The posterior tibial and peroneal arteries are tied off distally and the posterior tibial nerve is preserved. The peroneal muscles are then freed from the superficial posterior compartment muscles all the way up to the cut fibula. Minor pedicles from the peroneal muscles must be tied off.

The anterior half of the tibial cortex is then beveled for about 1 cm using a sagittal saw (▶ Fig. 7.11a) taking great care to keep the remaining thickness of the cortex at least equal to that of the rest of the cut tibia. The bevel is then sanded down by brushing the sagittal saw over that area. Three holes are drilled into the anterior tibia extending from the anterior cortex into the medullary canal to be used later for the future tenodesis of the soleus and gastrocnemius muscles (▶ Fig. 7.11b). Two holes are drilled in the lateral tibial bone for tenodesis of the peroneal muscles.

The tourniquet is released and bleeding is controlled. Irrigation is then done to wash off bone dust. New gloves and sterile drapes are placed, while a clean table and set of instrumentation are used to avoid any possible contamination with the removed distal stump.

At this point, all nerve endings can be addressed. The saphenous nerve is crushed at 5 cm from the distal end and reburied in the anterior compartment as deeply as possible. A TMR of the superficial peroneal and tibial nerve to proximal motor branches can then be done. If a TMR is not performed, those nerves are also crushed 5 cm proximally and buried deep along the respective proximal nerve tract. Those areas are then also injected with Exparel (Pacira Pharmaceuticals, Parsippany, NJ) if the patient does not have a regional block for postoperative analgesia.

The peroneus muscles are next rotated medially and cut at the level of the lateral tibia, and then sewn onto the lateral tibial cortex using the predrilled holes and a running 2–0 monofilament (▶ Fig. 7.12). The most superior stitch is then run through the anterior tibial muscles with a running horizontal mattress suture so that the latter are myodesed to the freshly myodesed peroneal muscle(s). The inferior stitch is used to myodese the deep posterior compartment muscles in a similar fashion. This maneuver gives an insertion point to the anterior and deep posterior compartment muscles to minimize the loss of muscle

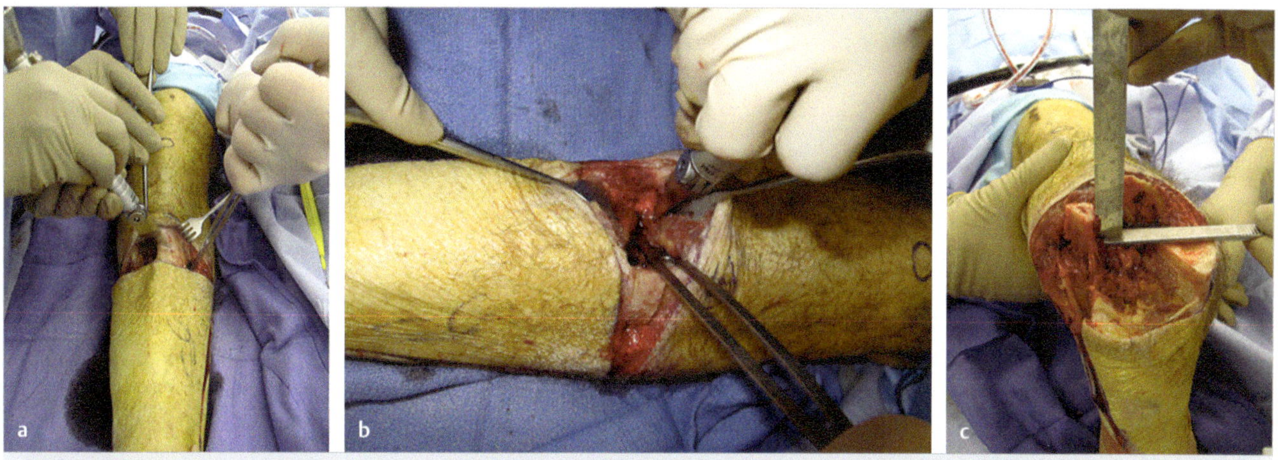

Fig. 7.9 Bone osteotomies. **(a)** With the anterior skin retracted, the tibia is cut **(b)** and next the fibula **(c)** with the latter approximately 1 to 2 cm shorter than the tibia.

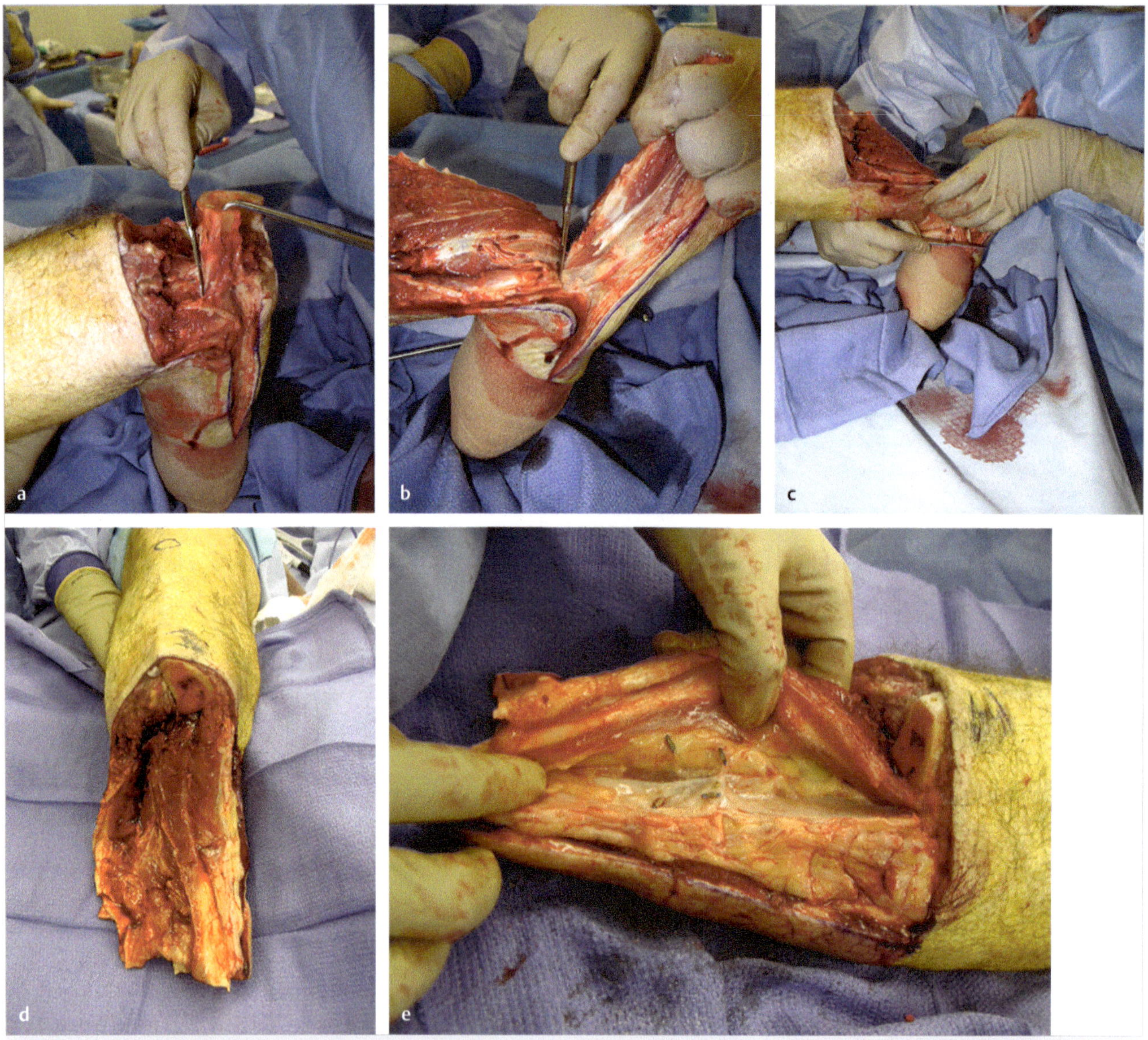

Fig. 7.10 Completion of leg amputation. **(a)** The posterior soft tissues are dissected off of the tibia and fibula **(b)** until reaching the designed length, taking great care to preserve the peroneal muscles. **(c)** The posterior flap is incised so that the distal leg can be cut off, done at a level where the posterior flap is long enough to easily reach the anterior soft tissues overlying the tibia for closure. **(d)** The deep posterior compartment is then separated along the transverse intermuscular septum from the superficial posterior compartment, **(e)** being careful to ligate all communicating branches.

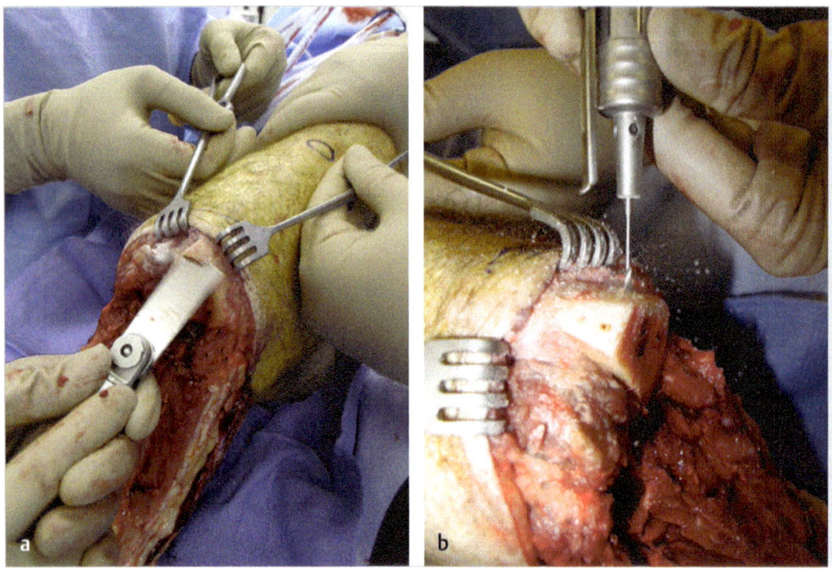

Fig. 7.11 Preparation of the distal tibia. **(a)** The anterior aspect of the distal tibia is beveled, and all sharp edges smoothed. Great care must be taken to ensure that the circumferential thickness of the tibial cortex is not compromised in any way. **(b)** Five holes are drilled through the cortex in the distal tibia: three on the medial and anterior surfaces, and two laterally.

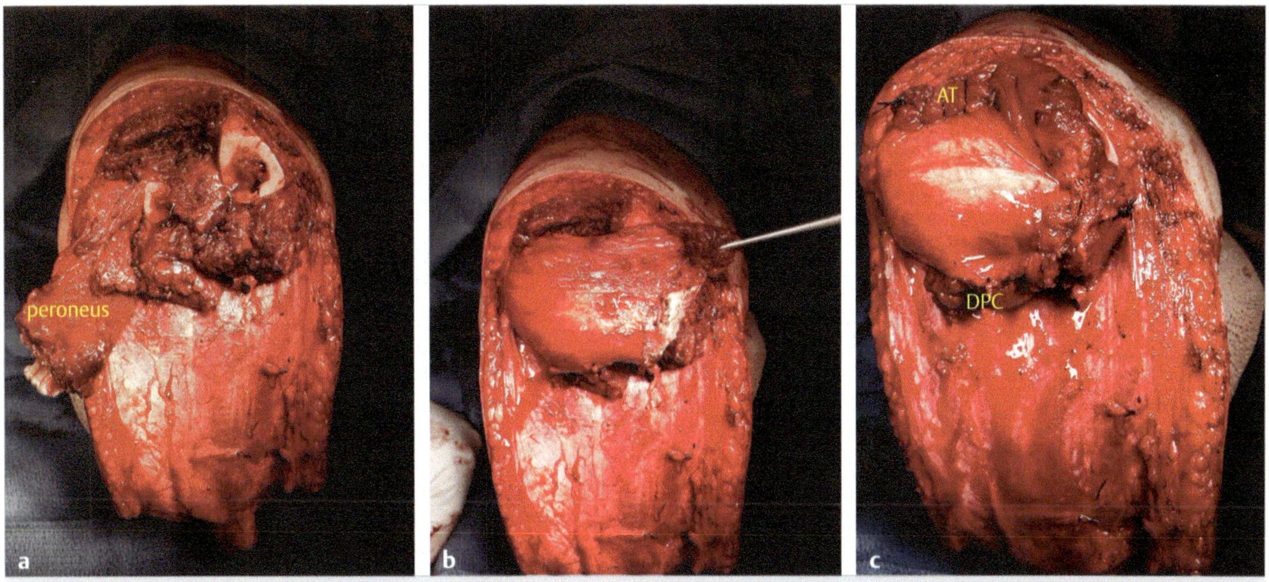

Fig. 7.12 Peroneal tenodesis and myodesis. **(a)** The peroneus longus and brevis muscles are cut at the length where they can reach **(b)** to be inserted into the lateral aspect of the tibia. **(c)** The peroneal muscles have been tenodesed to the lateral aspect of the tibia using the drill holes for fixation, and then the anterior tibial and muscles from the deep posterior compartment have been myodesed in turn to the peroneal muscles.

bulk over time. If the muscles are too bulky, the peroneus brevis is cut at the level to the fibula and only the longus is used for the myodesis. A tacking stitch would then be used to keep the residual peroneus brevis attached to the longus.

The remaining posterior flap is then swung up to the level of the anterior portion of the tibia, and a semilunar line is drawn on the soleus muscle to mark that junction (▸ Fig. 7.13a). One or two drains are placed along the base of the flap. The soleus muscle is then incised along the drawn line with cautery or no. 10 blade down to the Achilles tendon using a proximal to distal bevel (▸ Fig. 7.13b) so that when the posterior flap is rotated forward, the distal soleus muscle can be sewn to the anterior tibial cortex using the three predrilled holes with 0 monofilament suture (▸ Fig. 7.13c–e).

The skin and subcutaneous tissues are then dissected off the distal anterior stump fascia for a distance of about 2 ▸ Fig. 7.14a). The Achilles tendon and gastrocnemius tendon contribution and surrounding fascia are cut 1 to 2 cm distal to the distal end of the soleus tenodesis (▸ Fig. 7.14b) and then sewn to the anterior stump fascia with a running back and forth 0 monofilament (▸ Fig. 7.14c). The sural nerve and lesser saphenous vein will be located at the distal central end of the posterior flap. The nerve is crushed, buried deep, and injected with a long-term anesthetic. The lesser saphenous vein is clipped. The skin is closed with vertical mattress 2–0 monofilament, and skin staples are used between each stitch to ensure good skin edge eversion (▸ Fig. 7.14d). Dog-ears, if present at the medial and lateral edge of the closure, are removed and the suture line recontoured to create a smooth tapered end so that the leg is ready for a prosthesis as soon as the stitches are removed. The wound is then dressed and the leg is placed in a knee immobilizer to protect it from falls and prevent possible knee flexion that will result in a knee contracture. The skin staples are removed at 1 week, and the stitches after 4 weeks.

Evidence comparing PMF versus skew or sagittal flaps show no significant differences, although the level of evidence is poor.[12] In our hands, however, the PMF provides sufficient vascularized soft-tissue coverage over the tibial osteotomy to allow us to successfully perform BKAs in 80% of all patients who presented with an ischemic or a nonviable or nonfunctional foot. Eighty percent of those BKAs resulted in ambulatory patients. In addition, only 2% of the BKAs had to undergo a higher level amputation.[9] This is the highest rate of BKA success versus AKA conversion in the literature, suggesting that the vascular supply to the PMF may be superior to that of other flap designs.

Below-Knee Amputation Using the Ertl Technique

Alternatively, an Ertl modification to the standard BKA can be performed in patients who have the capacity of being very physically active. The Ertl modification for BKA involves placing a vascularized fibula bone graft between the distal tibia and fibula osteotomy sites to promote distal bony fusion between the two. The distal bone then forms a large "U," which allows better transfer of leg rotational torque to the artificial prosthetic ankle/foot.[13] It also allows the distal stump to be end bearing when not wearing a prosthesis.

The initial surgical technique and markings are identical as for a conventional BKA up to the planning of the fibular osteotomy. The distance between the tibia and fibula at the planned amputation point is measured (usually 1.5–2 cm). The first of two fibular osteotomies is marked distal to the tibial osteotomy so that the extra distance matches a little more than that of the width between the medial cortex of the fibula and the lateral cortex of the tibia (▸ Fig. 7.15a). The fibula is cut at that mark taking care to avoid traumatizing the peroneal artery and venae comitantes to maintain the vascularization of what will be a vascularized fibula bone graft. The peroneal vessels will be tied off at the level of that more distal fibular osteotomy, and then the distal leg is removed in the same fashion as described previously for the conventional BKA.

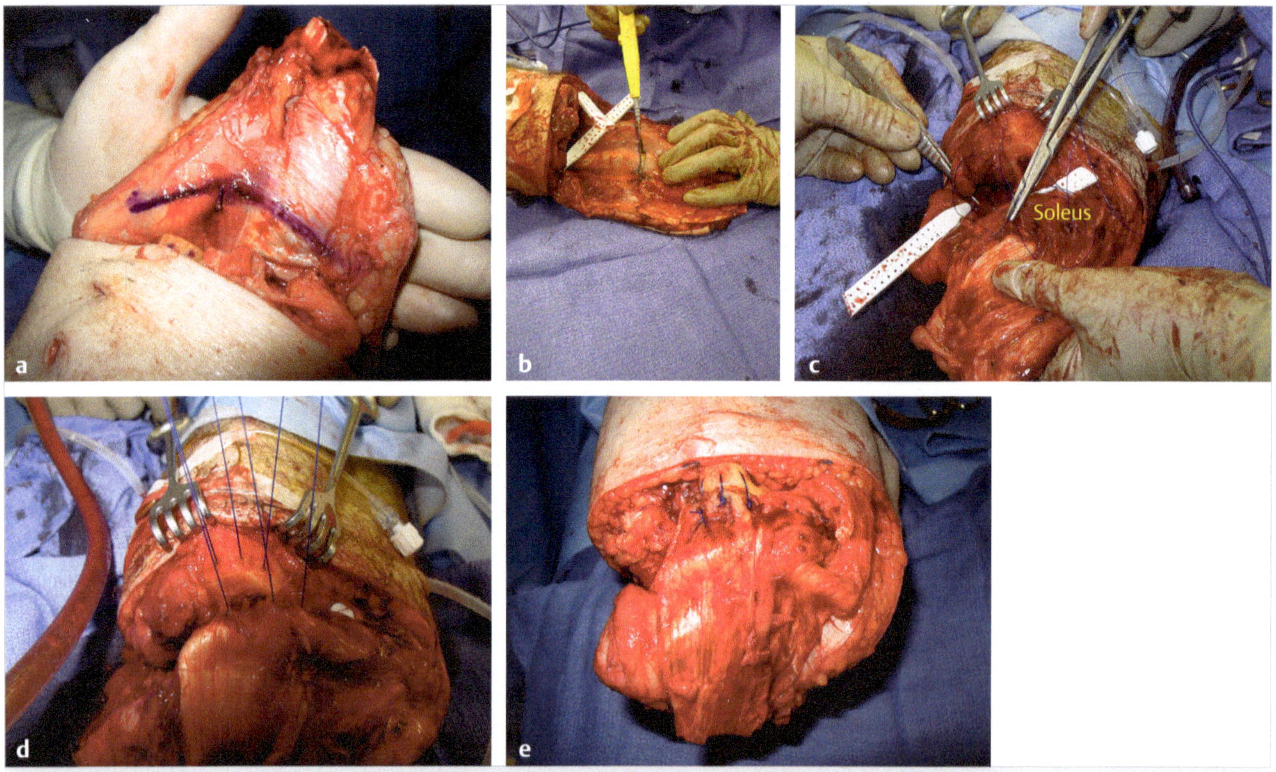

Fig. 7.13 Design of posterior flap and soleus tenodesis. **(a)** The remaining composite posterior flap is folded upward, and a line is drawn at the level where it will match the anterior fascia of the proximal leg without tension. **(b)** All soft tissue distal to the drawn posterior flap line is removed with either a bovie or a knife. Great care is taken to preserve the underlying Achilles tendon and fascia. **(c)** Three 0 monofilament dissolvable stitches are sutured into the soleus muscle and underlying fascia and **(d)** then passed through the predrilled anterior or medial tibial holes. **(e)** The soleus muscle and fascia are tenodesed to the anterior portion of the tibia.

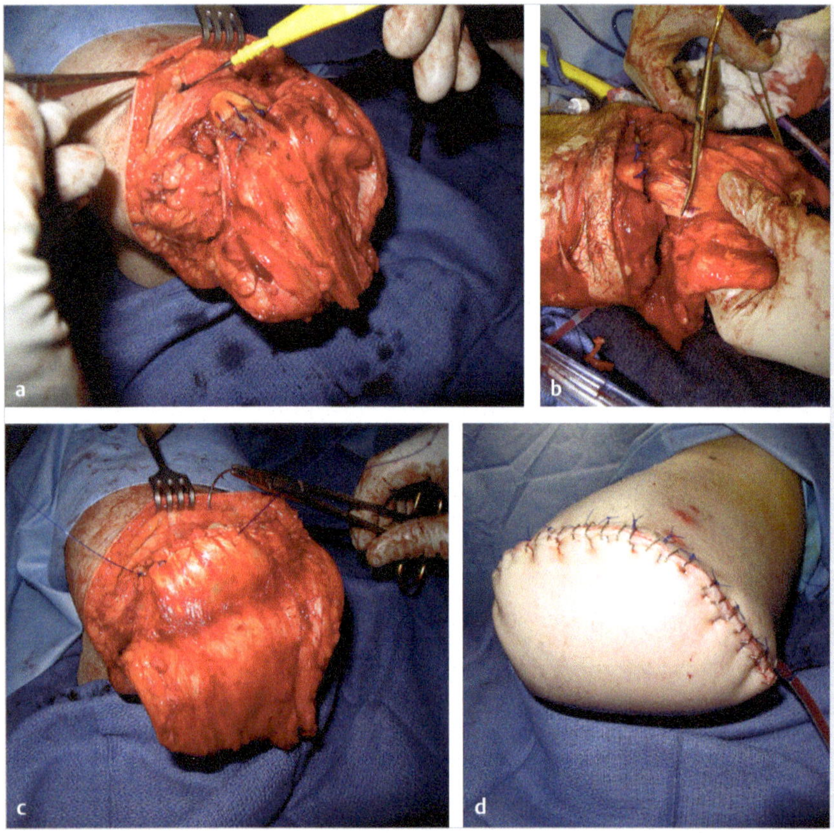

Fig. 7.14 Achilles anterior tenodesis. **(a)** The distal anterior skin and subcutaneous tissue are freed up from the underlying anterior fascia for a distance of about 2 cm. **(b)** The Achilles tendon and posterior fascia are cut 1 to 2 cm distal to where the soleus muscle has been tenodesed, so that they can be sewn into the anterior leg fascia without tension. **(c)** This final tenodesis is performed using a running 0 monofilament horizontal mattress suture. **(d)** The skin is closed in this case using vertical mattress sutures with intervening staples. Dog-ears are minimized so that the amputation stump is funneled to be more readily fitted for a prosthesis at the time of suture removal.

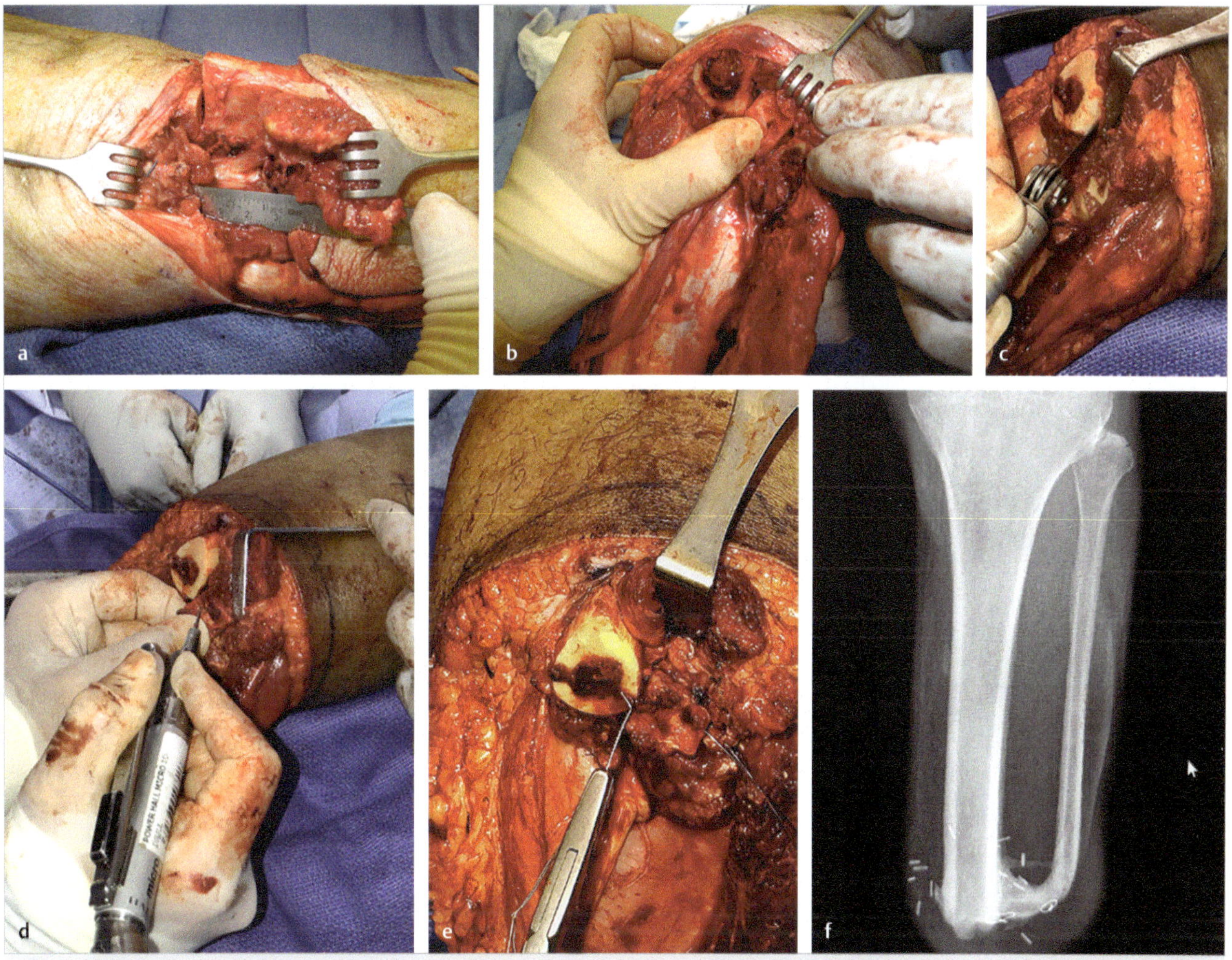

Fig. 7.15 Preparation and fixation of vascularized fibula strut. **(a)** The distance between the lateral surface of the tibia and medial fibula will determine the length of the initial distal cut of the fibula. **(b)** After the proximal cut of the fibula is done as in the standard below-knee amputation (BKA), the more distal segment, now a vascularized fibula bone graft, is checked for proper fit. **(c)** The lateral side of the tibia and the medial side of the fibula are smoothed down using a saw to ensure better contact and aid in fusion of the pedicled fibula bone graft. **(d)** Holes are drilled into the lateral tibia and medial fibula as well as the lateral and medial anterior aspect of the pedicled fibula bone graft. **(e)** The pedicled vascularized fibula bone graft is fixed to the medial fibula and lateral tibia using a no. 24 wire that must be twisted tightly into position, then cut and buried away from the end of the stump. **(f)** Fused fibula bone graft seen in this late X-ray of an Ertl BKA.

The proximal fibular osteotomy cut is performed after reconfirming the fibula bone graft length needed to equal the interosseous distance. We recommend a lateral approach to the fibular osteotomy with care when cutting the medial fibular cortex, such as by interposing a retractor, so as not to damage the peroneal vessels. The vascularized fibula bone graft is rotated into position between the tibia and fibula to make sure that it fits well (▶ Fig. 7.15b). The lateral cortex of the tibia (▶ Fig. 7.15c) and medial cortex of the distal fibula are then burred down so when juxtaposed to the fibula bone graft will provide a stable contact to aid in bony fusion. The vascularized fibula bone graft is finally interposed between the in situ distal fibula and tibia. Corresponding holes are drilled into both sides of the fibular strut graft, the medial distal fibula, and lateral distal tibia (▶ Fig. 7.15d). Twenty-four-gauge wires via these drill holes are used to fixate the vascularized fibula graft to the lateral tibia and the medial fibula (▶ Fig. 7.15e). Note that a cannulated screw used to be used, but it had to be later removed in over 50% of our patients. This had not been a problem using the suggested fine-wire fixation. Excellent fusion typically occurs between the fibula bone graft and distal fibula and tibia by 2 to 3 months (▶ Fig. 7.15f). Completion of the myodesis and skin closure is then the same as for the normal BKA.

7.1.8 Postoperative Care

Proper postoperative care is an essential component for all major lower extremity amputations. Pain control immediately following surgery typically involves intravenous narcotics via patient-controlled analgesia versus 5 days of epidural or regional blocks, if utilized. While a regional block is the best option, it is often not used if the patient is on any form of anticoagulation. Alternatively, the intraoperative use of long-lasting local anesthesia (Exparel) is strongly recommended, which should be infiltrated along the five nerves identified when performing the BKA.

After any lower extremity amputation, there is a significant disturbance in the patient's sense of balance as their center of gravity has been altered significantly. Nursing care and physical therapy play an important role in protecting the patient as they learn to transfer. Falls after amputation can be devastating and frequently lead to reoperation. Nearly one in five amputees will require amputation revisions due to postoperative falls. Thus, it is important to protect the residual limb. A knee immobilizer is placed immediately after each BKA to both protect the distal stump and prevent knee contracture until the patient is ready for a prosthesis.

Gentle compression in the immediate postoperative period aids with swelling, but should be balanced when there is a question of possible ischemia. Compression should be avoided in patients with severe ischemic disease. One can apply an incisional negative pressure device to the incision to protect it for 5 to 7 days postoperatively. Alternatively, the dressing is removed on day 2 to evaluate for signs of hematoma and ischemia. Drains should be observed and output recorded. Once the amount is less than 30 mL daily, the drain may safely be removed. Surgical staples are removed the day of discharge (5 days) and the sutures are typically removed at 4 weeks in clinic (6 weeks with renal failure patients).

7.1.9 Rehabilitation

Rehabilitation begins immediately after surgery in the hospital. Typically, each patient must be hospitalized 4 to 5 days for inpatient pain control and concomitant evaluation by physical therapy to assess each patient's strength and ability to transfer safely. Their evaluation will determine the amount of assistance needed and on this basis recommend acute, subacute, or home-based rehabilitation. Our strong preference is an acute rehabilitation facility that has a center that is familiar with and trained in caring for amputees. The medical complexity and need for frequent follow-up underscore the importance of open communication with the rehabilitation center, and use of a multidisciplinary approach to provide the best outcome.

Once the incision has healed, the prosthetist becomes the most important individual in the care of the amputee. Fitting of the prosthesis may commence once the sutures have been removed. Patients should also then be educated on care of the residual limb, compression devices, and the progression from initial prosthetic fitting to final prosthesis. We advocate for this fitting and ambulation as soon as it is safe for the patient. This prevents further deconditioning, minimizes the risk of injuries from falls, and promotes their return to a normal functional status.

7.1.10 Follow-up

Reoperation following an amputation is unfortunate, but it is relatively common as found to occur in up to 30% of amputations. Trauma, dehiscences, infection, wound-healing issues, and ischemia all contribute to these high reoperation rates. Follow-up is recommended at 2- and 4-week intervals. At 2 weeks, the residual limb can be examined for signs of infection, dehiscence, or progressive ischemia. At the 4-week visit, typically removal of sutures and arrangement for prosthetic fitting can be done. If the postoperative course is uneventful, our aim is to have each patient ambulating by 6 to 12 weeks.

7.2 Conclusion

The important lesson to learn when confronted with an impaired lower extremity is to always keep in mind what will be the function goal when making the decision to salvage or amputate a limb. Assuming biomechanical principles are followed, forefoot amputations will yield good function. To keep a foot that is as long as possible is the goal. The use of angiosome principles and flap techniques to ensure adequate soft-tissue perfusion is why plastic surgeons are uniquely positioned to excel in achieving this outcome in cooperation with our equally skilled orthopaedic and podiatry colleagues. With TMAs, one should not overlook the risk of equinovarus deformities. Shorter foot amputations (Lisfranc, Chopart, and Syme amputations) all require significant AFO devices in order to ambulate. For the less active patient, these foot amputations provide an excellent solution to allow them to perform daily activities of living and stay independent. For active patients, reliance on AFO devices may be too restrictive to allow them everything that they may want to do.

If the resulting function of the salvaged foot does not meet the patient's physical needs, then a major amputation should be performed. It has to be done with the same amount of care and attention to detail and function that would have been done for limb salvage, because the surgeon is actually creating a new, albeit shorter, limb. Focusing on myodesis and tenodesis techniques ensures that the residual muscles remain functional and that the residual limb does not loose mobility and strength. Attention spent in relocating the distal nerves is critical to minimize postoperative pain and phantom pain. The closure should have a smooth tapered design so that the patient can start wearing a prosthesis as soon as the stitches are removed, and the prosthesis is ready. Remember that it is our duty as reconstructive surgeons to give the patient the best possible leg (reconstructed or amputated) to return to as active a lifestyle as he or she may desire.

References

[1] Attinger C, Cooper P, Blume P, Bulan E. The safest surgical incisions and amputations applying the angiosome principles and using the Doppler to assess the arterial-arterial connections of the foot and ankle. Foot Ankle Clin. 2001; 6(4):745–799

[2] Janhofer, DE, Lakhiani, C, Kim, PJ, Naz, I, Black, CK, Tefera, EA, Akbari, C, Hashmi, A, Attinger, CE, Evans, KK, The Utility of Preoperative Venous Testing for Lower Extremity Flap Planning in Patients with Lower Extremity Wounds, Plast Reconstr Surg, 2020;145(1):164e–171e

[3] Endara M, Attinger C. Using color to guide debridement. Adv Skin Wound Care. 2012; 25(12):549–555

[4] Lipsky BA, Berendt AR, Cornia PB, et al. Infectious Diseases Society of America. 2012 Infectious Diseases Society of America clinical practice guideline for the diagnosis and treatment of diabetic foot infections. Clin Infect Dis. 2012; 54(12):e132–e173

[5] Mueller MJ, Sinacore DR, Hastings MK, Strube MJ, Johnson JE. Effect of Achilles tendon lengthening on neuropathic plantar ulcers. A randomized clinical trial. J Bone Joint Surg Am. 2003; 85(8):1436–1445

[6] Oliver NG, Attinger CE, Steinberg JS, Evans KK, Vieweger D, Kim PJ. Influence of hallux rigidus on re-amputation in patients with diabetes mellitus after partial hallux amputation. J Foot Ankle Surg. 2015; 54(6):1076–1080

[7] Edlich RF, Rodeheaver GT, Thacker JG, Edgerton MT. Technical factors in wound management. In: Hunt TK, Dunphy JE, eds. Fundamentals of Wound Management in the Surgery. South Plainfield, NJ: Chirugecom Inc.; 1977

[8] Pinzur MS, Morrison C, Sage R, Stuck R, Osterman H, Vrbos L. Syme's two-stage amputation in insulin-requiring diabetics with gangrene of the forefoot. Foot Ankle. 1991; 11(6):394–396

[9] Brown BJ, Iorio ML, Klement M, et al. Outcomes after 294 transtibial amputations with the posterior myocutaneous flap. Int J Low Extrem Wounds. 2014; 13(1):33–40

[10] Fisher DF, Jr, Clagett GP, Fry RE, Humble TH, Fry WJ. One-stage versus two-stage amputation for wet gangrene of the lower extremity: a randomized study. J Vasc Surg. 1988; 8(4):428–433

[11] Burgess EM, Romano RL, Zettl JH, Schrock RD, Jr. Amputations of the leg for peripheral vascular insufficiency. J Bone Joint Surg Am. 1971; 53(5):874–890

[12] Tisi PV, Than MM. Type of incision for below knee amputation. Cochrane Database Syst Rev. 2014(4):CD003749

[13] Brown BJ, Iorio ML, Hill L, Carlisle B, Attinger CE. Below-knee amputation with a vascularized fibular graft and headless compression screw. Plast Reconstr Surg. 2013; 131(2):323–327

8 Vascular Anatomy of the Lower Extremity: A Practical Guide to Vascular Territories, Perforators, and Selection of Recipient Vessels

Alison Wong and Steven F. Morris

Summary

In order to choose the appropriate flap donor site or recipient vessels in lower extremity reconstruction, it is important to have an understanding of vascular architecture and anatomy of individual perforators in the region. The lower extremity has 21 vascular territories or angiosomes, and can be divided into four anatomic subregions: (1) gluteal, (2) hip and thigh, (3) knee and leg, and (4) ankle and foot. Within these regions, there are about 180 perforators to the integument, which are highly variable in caliber or location, although they tend to cluster about the main source arteries. Each perforator angiosome is linked to those adjacent by choke anastomotic or true anastomotic vessels, with a longitudinal or proximal-to-distal orientation. The dimensions of the available vascular territory supplied by an individual perforator depend on the size of that perforator, subregion, and unpredictable intrinsic patient factors. Since venous congestion is a well-known phenomenon occurring with perforator flaps, variations in venous anatomy should also be appreciated. Note that the lower limb is drained by both a superficial and a deep venous network, the latter usually the mirror image of the arteries that they accompany, which are interdependent and interconnected. Each source artery as well as its perforators can potentially serve as the recipient site for any microvascular tissue transfer.

Keywords: vascular anatomy, angiosome, perforator angiosome, choke vessel, microvascular recipient site

8.1 Introduction

This review of the vascular anatomy of the lower extremity is intended to emphasize the details of the anatomy of greatest interest to the reconstructive surgeon. Since the lower extremity is a common site for trauma and for reconstruction, knowledge of the vascular architecture of the lower limb is critical before deciding on an appropriate flap donor site or the planning of recipient vessels. The status of the main arterial supply to the lower extremity as well as the general pattern of individual perforators will be helpful in this regard.

8.2 Vascular Territories and the Angiosome Concept

Taylor and Palmer introduced the angiosome concept, which has been a guide to our understanding of the vascular territories of the human body.[1] The word angiosome is derived from the Greek word *angeion*, which means vessel, and somite, which means segment of the body. The body can be divided into a series of angiosomes (vascular territories) based on the anatomy of the individual source artery to that angiosome. Each angiosome is a composite block of tissue all supplied by one main named source artery, and may consist of bone, muscle, fascia, and skin as well as other tissues. The main source vessel within the given angiosome gives off multiple branches or perforators, which in turn will be the vascular supply to each of its tissues. Individual angiosomes are linked to adjacent angiosomes via reduced caliber choke anastomotic vessels or true anastomotic vessels, which are subject to numerous physiologic influences (e.g., a delay procedure). The specific anatomy of a given angiosome and presence (or absence) of individual perforators or branches will then affect the survival of tissues harvested. A larger source artery with a larger angiosome and larger perforators may supply larger flaps and vice versa. The smallest division of the angiosome is that of an individual perforator that supplies a discrete region of tissue or perforator angiosome. The size of the vascular territory supplied by an individual perforator is dependent on a variety of factors including the size of the perforator, region of the body, and intrinsic patient factors, which may influence blood flow.

8.3 Arterial Territories

The integument of the human body can be divided into about 60 vascular territories that are supplied by about 400 perforators. However, the arterial framework of the body is actually a huge continuous interlocking arcade of vessels through all layers of all tissues. Arteries tend to give a branch to each structure they pass through, which has led to a myriad of terms such as fasciocutaneous, septocutaneous, and musculocutaneous perforators. The vessels that pierce the deep fascia and supply the skin may be *direct*, such as would be axial or septocutaneous perforators, or *indirect*, as those perforators which pass through other structures first en route to the skin such as would be musculocutaneous perforators. Note that there is roughly a 2/3:1/3 ratio of musculocutaneous to septocutaneous perforators throughout the body. The important point is to be able to identify the pattern of distribution of individual perforators in order to capture a suitable skin vascular territory in a flap.

The lower extremity has 21 vascular territories with a mean of about 180 perforators (▶ Table 8.1).[2,3] The location of these vascular territories in the lower extremity was summarized in a series of cadaver studies (▶ Fig. 8.1). As a rule, the named source vessels to these vascular territories are large consistent arteries with associated venae comitantes. These provide the vascular supply to numerous flaps in the body and also are available as recipient vessels for free microvascular tissue transfers. The individual cutaneous perforators to skin in the lower extremity are highly variable in terms of size and exact position, but tend to cluster around the main source vessels often with a longitudinal orientation, which allows some anticipation of their location.

Table 8.1 Vascular territories of the lower extremity[3]

Vascular territory		Source vessel	Perforator diameter (mm)	Superficial length (mm)	Total area (cm²)	No. of perforators ≥0.5 mm	Area/ perforator (cm²)	Ratio: MC/SC
SGA	Superior gluteal artery	Internal iliac artery, posterior	0.7 (±0.2)	23 (±8)	198 (±77)	9 (±4)	19 (±5)	1:0
IGA	Inferior gluteal artery	Internal iliac artery, anterior	0.6 (±0.1)	24 (±11)	221 (±54)	12 (±3)	18 (±3)	1:0
SFA	Superficial femoral artery	Common femoral artery	0.8 (±0.2)	38 (±24)	**427 (±70)**	11 (±3)	39 (±12)	2:3
SCIA	Superficial circumflex iliac artery	Femoral artery	1.0 (±0.1)	81 (±26)	66 (±20)	1 (±0.5)	52 (±25)	1:0
LCFA	Lateral circumflex femoral artery	Profunda femoris artery	0.7 (±0.3)	33 (±15)	362 (±121)	10 (±5)	38 (±22)	3:1
MCFA	Medial circumflex femoral artery	Profunda femoris artery	0.7 (±0.2)	34 (±25)	191 (±52)	4 (±2)	43 (±18)	1:0
PFA	Profunda femoris artery	Common femoral artery	0.8 (±0.3)	34 (±15)	296 (±118)	8 (±7)	38 (±18)	3:2
DGA	Descending genicular artery	Femoral artery	0.8 (±0.3)	46 (±23)	133 (±39)	3 (±1)	42 (±22)	1:1
PA	Popliteal artery	Femoral artery	0.9 (±0.2)	72 (±43)	160 (±30)	3 (±1)	55 (±30)	1:1
MSGA	Medial superior genicular artery	Popliteal artery	0.6 (±0.2)	27 (±14)	79 (±21)	2 (±1)	44 (±19)	0:1
LSGA	Lateral superior genicular artery	Popliteal artery	0.8 (±0.2)	39 (±22)	100 (±24)	2 (±1)	55 (±38)	0:1
MIGA	Medial inferior genicular artery	Popliteal artery	0.6 (±0.1)	33 (±22)	59 (±26)	1 (±1)	45 (±19)	0:1
LIGA	Lateral inferior genicular artery	Popliteal artery	0.6 (±0.2)	34 (±16)	57 (±27)	1 (±1)	48 (±17)	0:1
ATA	Anterior tibial artery	Popliteal artery	0.6 (0.2)	29 (±13)	187 (±66)	6 (±3)	33 (±8)	1:1
PNA	Peroneal artery	Posterior tibial artery	0.8 (±0.3)	35 (±19)	170 (±39)	5 (±2)	32 (10)	1:1
PTA	Posterior tibial artery	Popliteal artery	0.7 (±0.2)	32 (±17)	337 (±111)	10 (±4)	34 (±12)	2:1
MCA	Medial calcaneal artery	Posterior tibial artery	0.8 (± 0.2)	27 (±6)	54 (±15)	1 (±1)	42 (±16)	0:1
LCA	Lateral calcaneal artery	Peroneal artery	0.6 (±0.1)	21 (±9)	48 (±14)	1 (±1)	38 (±8)	1:4
MPA	Medial plantar artery	Posterior tibial artery	0.7 (±0.2)	42 (±10)	80 (±24)	1 (±1)	62 (±24)	1:2
LPA	Lateral plantar artery	Posterior tibial artery	1.1 (±0.5)	38 (±19)	83 (±11)	1 (±1)	83 (±11)	1:2
DPA	Dorsalis pedis artery	Anterior tibial artery	0.6 (±0.1)	22 (±15)	134 (±42)	1 (±1)	134 (±42)	1:1

Abbreviation: MC/SC, musculocutaneous/septocutaneous perforators.

8.4 Venous Drainage

The venous anatomy of the body has received relatively less attention, but is certainly equally important for successful reconstructive surgery. It is well known that perforator flap failure is often caused by venous insufficiency. The integument of the body is drained by a superficial and a deep venous network, which are interdependent and interconnected. The deep venous architecture generally mirrors that of the arterial tree and in most regions is duplicated. The superficial venous network is quite different and consists of long named venous channels that connect to the deep system via venae communicantes. Adjacent venous territories of the skin are interconnected via veins without valves, which are called oscillating or bidirectional veins (▶ Fig. 8.2).

8.5 Neurovascular Territories

The cutaneous nerves of the lower extremity are longitudinally arranged. Each cutaneous nerve is associated with an arterial

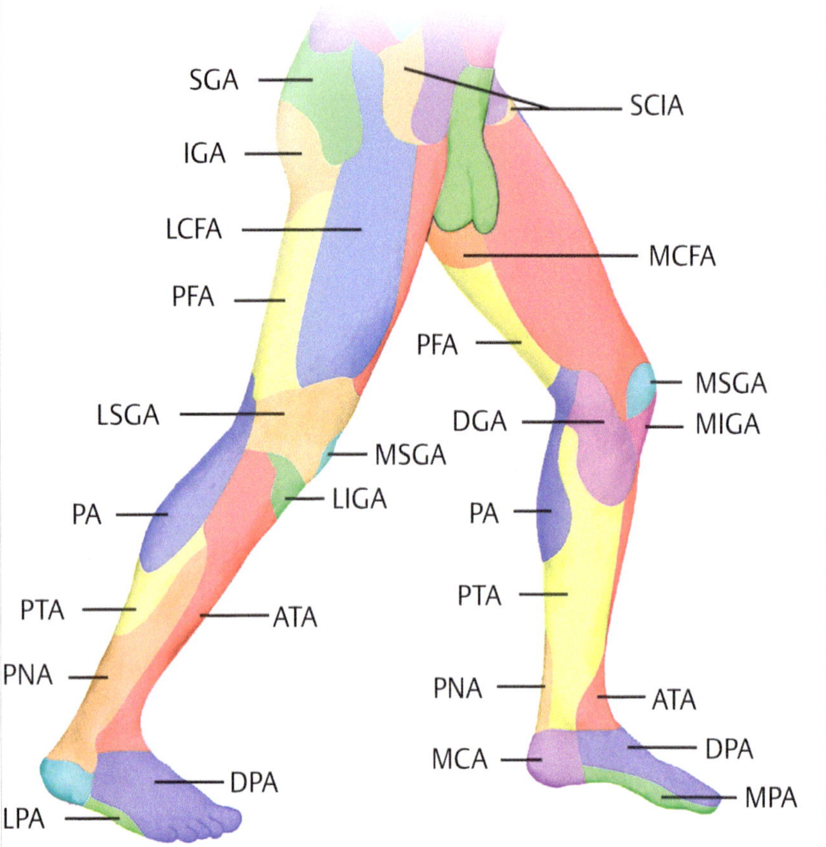

Fig. 8.1 Lower limb angiosomes derived from a series of angiograms in human cadavers. The vascular territories of the integument are shown in different colors according to the specific source artery. Abbreviations: ATA, anterior tibial artery; DGA, descending genicular [saphenous] artery; DPA, dorsalis pedis artery; FA, femoral artery; GT, greater trochanter; IGA, inferior gluteal artery; L, lateral epicondyle; LCA, lateral calcaneal artery; LCFA, lateral circumflex femoral artery; LIGA, lateral inferior genicular artery; LPA, lateral plantar artery; LSGA, lateral superior genicular artery; M, medial epicondyle; MCA, medial calcaneal artery; MCFA, medial circumflex femoral artery; MIGA, medial inferior genicular artery; MM, medial malleolus; MPA, medial plantar artery; MSGA, medial superior genicular artery; P, patella; PA, popliteal artery; PFA, profunda femoris artery; PNA, peroneal artery; PTA, posterior tibial artery; SCIA, superficial circumflex iliac artery; SGA, superior gluteal artery. (Adapted from Geddes CR, Tang M, Yang D, Morris SF. Anatomy of the lower extremity. In: Blondeel PN, Morris SF, Hallock GG, Neligan PC, eds. Perforator Flaps: Anatomy, Technique & Clinical Applications. St Louis, MO: Quality Medical Publishing; 2013:667–703.

supply that has a variety of orientations. For example, a series of small arterial branches can join the course of the nerve in a chain-linked pattern, or a single artery could run the full length of the nerve. In general, the cutaneous nerves have a well-vascularized longitudinal axis with indirect branches to the integument, which provides an opportunity to harvest local or regional neurocutaneous flaps (▶ Fig. 8.3).[4]

8.6 Vascular Anatomical Principles Applied to Flap Design

For decades, surgeons relied on dogma such as the length-to-width ratio and trial and error to try to predict flap survival. The so-called random flaps were commonly utilized to reconstruct defects with unpredictable results. Fasciocutaneous and musculocutaneous flaps gradually replaced random flaps, as these had a more specific source of circulation that allowed more consistent and reliable results. The more recent enthusiasm for perforator flaps has focused the spotlight on detailed descriptions of the anatomy of individual cutaneous perforators throughout the body, and particularly the lower extremity so that flap survival has been improved.

In addition to knowing the anatomy of cutaneous perforators, an awareness of the physiologic effects on the vascular supply of tissues is important. Cormack and Lamberty described this as the anatomic, dynamic, and potential flap anatomy (▶ Fig. 8.4). A flap based on a single perforator will completely survive if designed to include only its perforator angiosome, or anatomic territory. A flap that includes that same perforator and an adjacent perforator should also completely survive via flow-through choke or true anastomoses, except when a compromising physiologic condition exists, which is the dynamic territory. Capture of a potential territory by inclusion of a second adjacent perforator territory is possible with a delay procedure or equivalent maneuver (▶ Fig. 8.5).

The variable nature of perforator distribution, size, and behavior throughout the body is particularly evident in the lower limb. In many regions of the lower extremity, perforator territories are small, and consequently, reliable flaps are smaller. In addition, physiologic challenges to the dynamic or potential surviving territory of a flap are commonplace, including vascular compromise due to diabetes or peripheral vascular disease, dependent edema, and trauma. Thus, it is not surprising that historically a 1:1 length-to-width ratio for a cutaneous flap in the lower extremity was the rule.

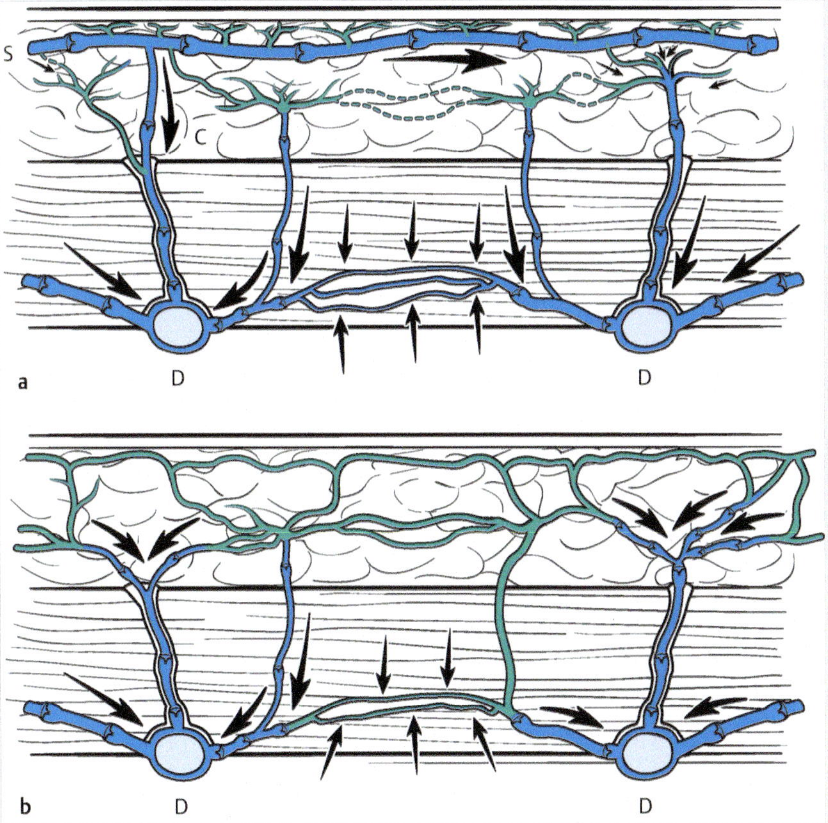

Fig. 8.2 Venous anatomy of the skin. **(a)** In the lower extremity, there are distinct superficial (S) and deep (D) venous networks that drain the skin and muscle. These are connected by valved venae communicantes (C), while venae comitantes provide secondary drainage. **(b)** Elsewhere in the body, there is only a deep system and venous drainage is predominantly from venae comitantes. In all areas of the body, oscillating veins (*small arrows*) link adjacent venous territories. (From Morris, SF, Davidson PG. Vascular basis of flaps and flap classification. In: Zenn MR, Jones G, eds. Reconstructive Surgery. Anatomy, Technique, and Clinical Applications. New York, NY: Thieme; 2012:35–80.)

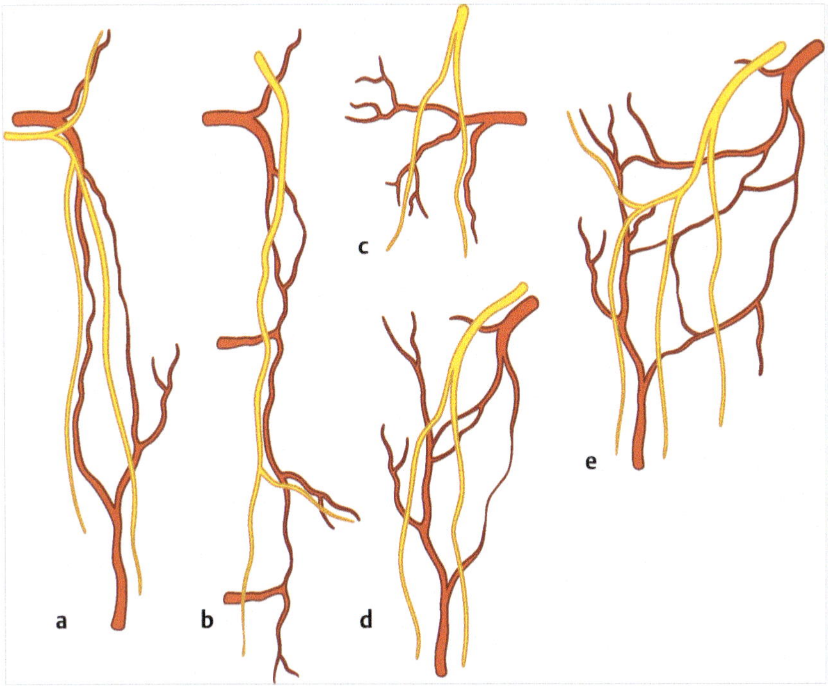

Fig. 8.3 The neurovascular patterns of the integument. **(a)** A long artery courses with the nerve, and here in addition there is a true anastomosis between perforator angiosomes. **(b)** A system of multiple arteries "hitchhike" with the nerve. **(c)** A nerve and artery pierce the fascia at separate sites, but unite distally. **(d)** A nerve diverges from its accompany artery and then descends toward the main trunk of another artery. **(e)** A nerve crosses the primary and secondary vascular arcades to then travel parallel to another artery. (From Morris, SF, Davidson PG. Vascular basis of flaps and flap classification. In: Zenn MR, Jones G, eds. Reconstructive Surgery. Anatomy, Technique, and Clinical Applications. New York, NY: Thieme; 2012:35–80.)

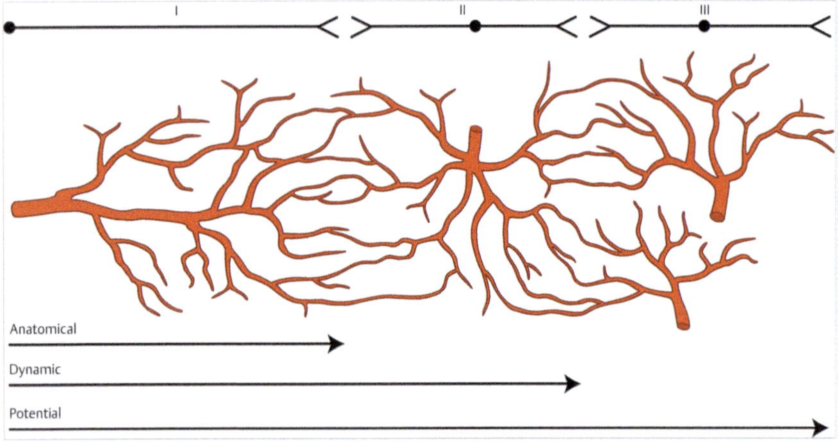

Fig. 8.4 Cormack and Lamberty's concept of the anatomic, dynamic and potential territories of flap design. (From Morris, SF, Davidson PG. Vascular basis of flaps and flap classification. In: Zenn MR, Jones G, eds. Reconstructive Surgery. Anatomy, Technique, and Clinical Applications. New York, NY: Thieme; 2012:35–80.)

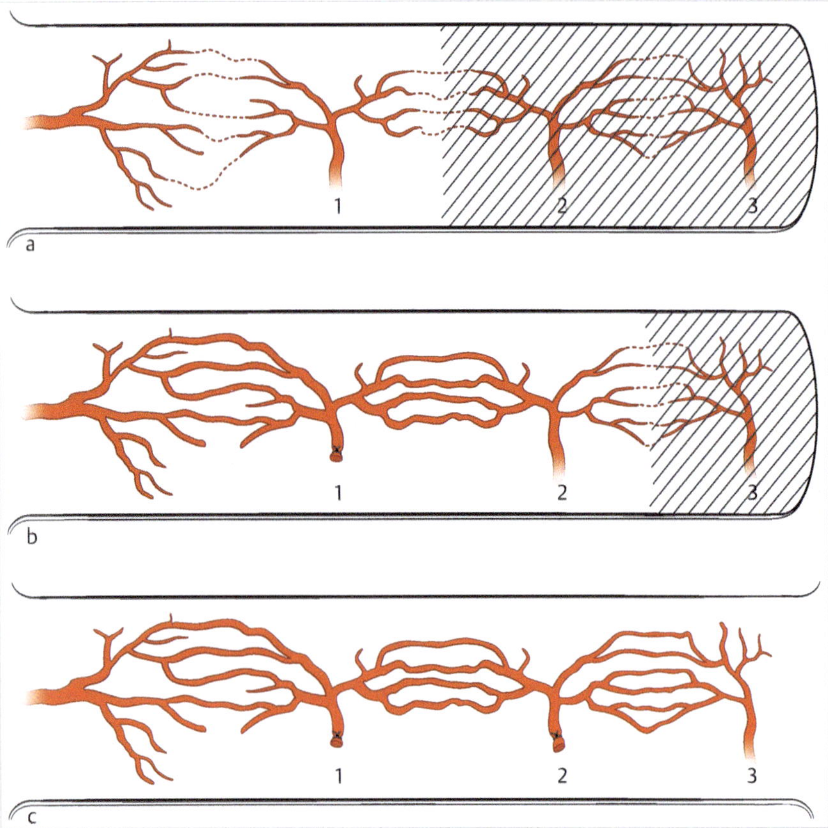

Fig. 8.5 **(a)** Flap elevated on a single perforator and including only the next perforator territory will completely survive consistently. **(b)** After delay of the next adjacent perforator angiosome, a flap will reliably and consistently survive including two territories. **(c)** A delay of perforators 1 and 2 will result in a large three-territory flap completely surviving. The shaded area represents flap necrosis. (From Morris, SF, Davidson PG. Vascular basis of flaps and flap classification. In: Zenn MR, Jones G, eds. Reconstructive Surgery. Anatomy, Technique, and Clinical Applications. New York, NY: Thieme; 2012:35–80.)

8.7 Main Source Vessels of the Lower Extremity

8.7.1 Arterial System

The blood supply to the lower extremity is predominantly a continuation of the external iliac, which proceeds all the way to the foot with name changes as it passes defined landmarks. After the external iliac enters the thigh deep to the inguinal ligament, it is referred to as the common femoral artery (FA). This continues as the superficial FA, popliteal artery (PA), tibioperoneal trunk, posterior tibial artery (PTA), and, ultimately, terminates as the medial and lateral plantar arteries (▶ Table 8.2). The other well-known arteries of the lower limb are branches arising from this main trunk (▶ Fig. 8.6).

The internal iliac artery also has a small contribution to the lower extremity via the gluteal vessels (superior and inferior), which are its terminal branches. The gluteal arteries supply the buttocks and form an anastomoses in the posterior thigh with the medial and lateral circumflex femoral vessels.

8.7.2 Venous System

The lower extremity circulation is drained by two venous systems: the superficial and the deep veins. The **deep venous system** travels with and is named after the arteries that it

Table 8.2 Arteries of the lower extremity and their anatomic location

	Main vessel (boundaries)	Primary branches (boundaries)	Secondary branches (boundaries)
Distal–Proximal	**Common iliac**	**>Internal iliac**	**>Superior gluteal** Exits pelvis through greater sciatic foramen, superior to the piriformis **Superficial branch** between gluteus maximus and medius, **deep branch** between gluteus medius and minimus **>Inferior gluteal** Exits pelvis through greater sciatic foramen inferior to piriformis Deep to gluteus maximus
	Sacroiliac joint		
	External iliac Medial border of the psoas major		
	Inguinal ligament		
	Femoral artery Within femoral sheath in femoral triangle bordered by sartorius, adductor longus and inguinal ligament	**>Profunda femoris** Proximal: adductor longus and brevis Distal: adductor longus and magnus	
	Sartorius		
	Superficial femoral artery Hunter's (adductor) canal: vastus medialis, sartorius, adductor longus, and magnus	**>Descending genicular** Adductor canal **Saphenous branch** between the sartorius and gracilis, accompanied by saphenous nerve	
	Adductor hiatus		
	Popliteal artery In popliteal fossa, midline, deep to all muscles	**>Anterior tibial artery** Between two heads of tibialis posterior, then lies on anterior surface of the interosseous membrane, deep to tibialis anterior **>Sural arteries** Deep to heads of the gastrocnemius at the level of the femoral condyles	**>Dorsalis pedis** Anterior to medial malleolus, lateral to the tendon of extensor hallucis longus tendon, overlying medial cuneiform
	Distal edge of popliteus		
	Tibial peroneal trunk Midline, deep to soleus	**>Peroneal** Lies of the posterior surface of the interosseous membrane between FHL and tibialis posterior	
	Posterior tibial Proximal: in interval between Achilles and flexor digitorum longus Distal: in tarsal tunnel posterior to medial malleolus		
	Medial malleolus		
	Medial plantar Proximal: deep to abductor hallucis Distal: lateral to abductor hallucis	**>Lateral plantar** Between superficial and middle layers of muscle; deep to abductor hallucis, flexor digitorum brevis, and abductor digiti minimi; superficial to quadratus plantae	

Abbreviation: FHL, flexor hallucis longus.

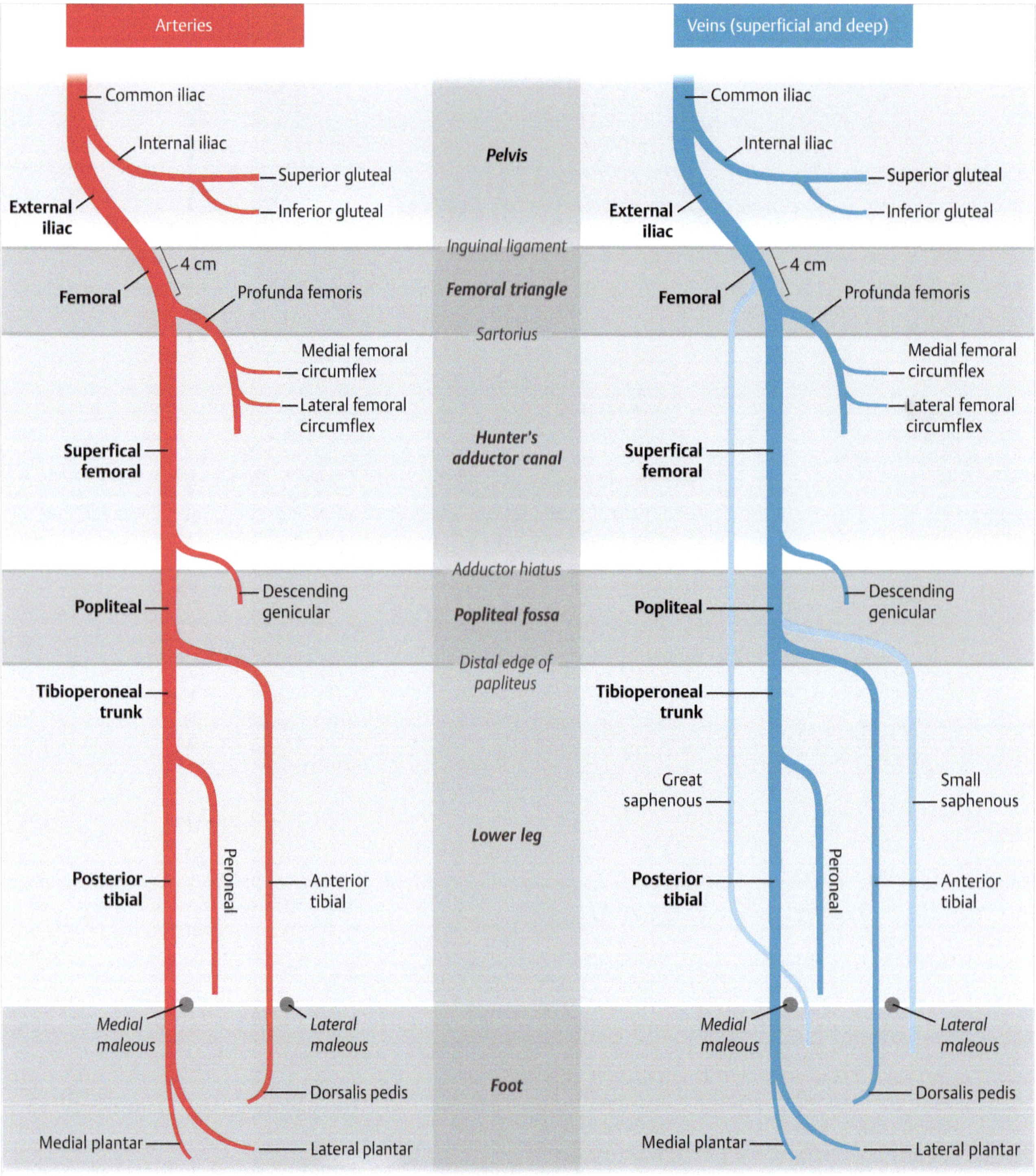

Fig. 8.6 Schematic diagram of the arterial and venous anatomy of the lower extremity showing important related anatomic landmarks.

accompanies, as described previously. The superficial venous system has two dominant veins: the great saphenous vein and the small saphenous veins, both of which run in the subcutaneous tissue (▶ Fig. 8.6). The **greater saphenous vein** is found medially, arising from the foot, passing anterior to the medial malleolus, and then traveling superiorly, to eventually enter the femoral triangle through the fossa ovalis to join the femoral vein. Through most of its course distal to the adductor canal of the thigh, it is accompanied by the *saphenous nerve*. The lateral portion of the foot and leg is supplied by the **small saphenous vein**, which exits the foot posterior to the lateral malleolus and then travels superiorly to pierce the crural fascia at a variable location to follow between the two heads of the gastrocnemius muscle until usually emptying into the popliteal vein. The *sural nerve* usually becomes superficial at the mid-calf level to join the small saphenous vein.

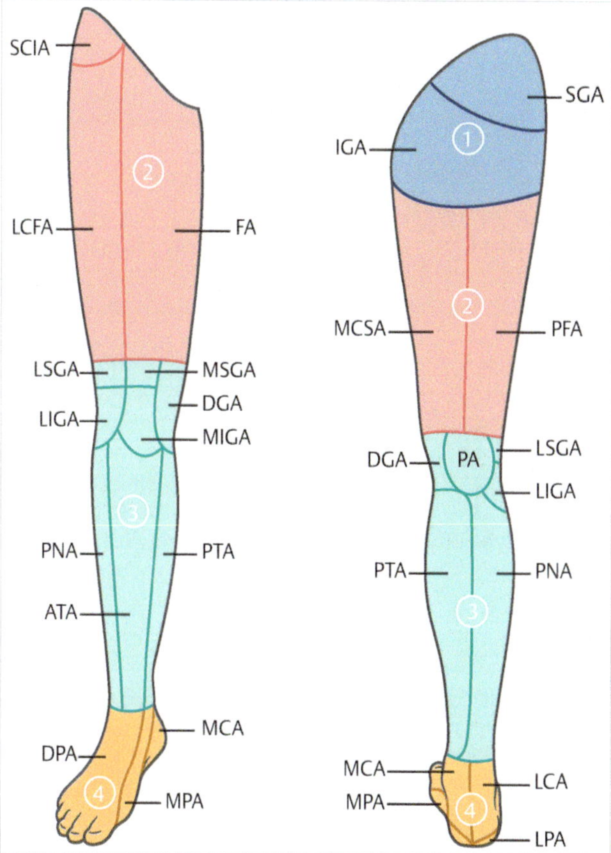

Fig. 8.7 The lower extremity can be divided into four anatomic subregions: (1) gluteal, (2) hip and thigh, (3) knee and leg, and (4) ankle and foot. Within these regions, there are 21 cutaneous vascular territories. See ▶ Table 8.1 to explain acronyms.

8.8 Regional Anatomy of Perforators of the Lower Extremity

Topographically, the lower extremity can be divided into four anatomic subregions: (1) gluteal, (2) hip and thigh, (3) knee and leg, and (4) ankle and foot (▶ Fig. 8.7). Within these subregions, there are 21 cutaneous vascular territories (▶ Fig. 8.1). The main source vessels are listed, and perforators in each major vascular territory can be described in terms of the area, size, location, and perforator course from the skin to the source vessel (▶ Table 8.1). Each source artery or its perforators could be potentially used to supply or serve as recipient vessels in microsurgical reconstruction of the lower extremity. In the following sections, perforators are described from their cutaneous location back to their source vessel.

8.9 Anatomical Regions

8.9.1 Gluteal Region

Introduction

The gluteal region extends from the iliac crest to the gluteal fold, posterior midline, and a line intersecting the anterior superior iliac spine and the greater trochanter. In total, the gluteal region constitutes 12% of the surface area of the lower extremity. The two main source arteries are the **superior** and **inferior gluteal arteries** (▶ Fig. 8.8). There are minor contributions from the fourth lumbar artery, lateral sacral artery, the internal pudendal artery, and the ascending branch of the lateral femoral circumflex artery (LCFA).

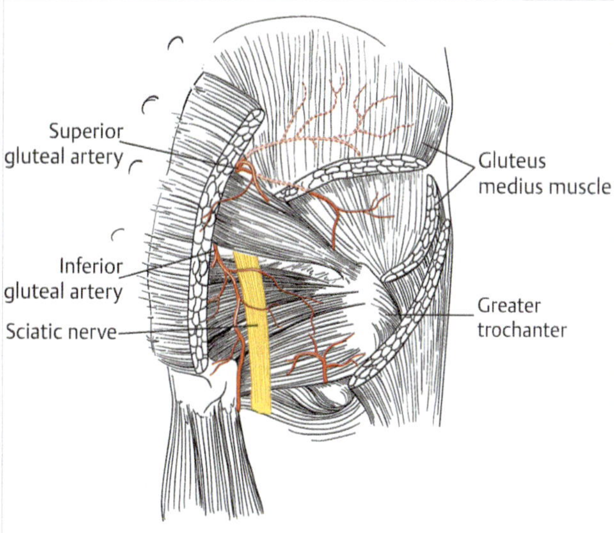

Fig. 8.8 The vascular supply of the gluteal region. (Adapted from Geddes CR, Tang M, Yang D, Morris SF. Anatomy of the lower extremity. In: Blondeel PN, Morris SF, Hallock GG, Neligan PC, eds. Perforator Flaps: Anatomy, Technique & Clinical Applications. St Louis, MO: Quality Medical Publishing; 2013:667–703.)

Superior Gluteal Region: Superior Gluteal Artery

The **superior gluteal artery** (SGA) supplies an area of about 200 cm^2 in size overlying the superior skin of the buttock. There are 8 to 10 perforators, which are all musculocutaneous passing through the gluteus maximus muscle, although some paramuscular perforators have been described. Perforators arise from the posterior or intermediate branches of the superficial branch of the SGA. The pedicle emerges from the greater sciatic foramen superior to the piriformis. The SGA also has a superficial anterior branch and a deep branch that only supply muscle.

Inferior and Lateral Gluteal Region: Inferior Gluteal Artery

The **inferior gluteal artery** (IGA) is the primary supply of skin in the gluteal region (60%), with a total area of skin about 220 cm^2 in size with 10 to 15 perforators. It supplies the **medial and inferolateral portions of the skin** overlying the **gluteus maximus** as well as a small region of skin on the posterior thigh. Like the SGA, all perforators pass through the gluteus maximus muscle. The medial skin is supplied by perforators from the medial branch of the IGA and the inferolateral skin is supplied by the lateral branch. There is a third branch that accompanies the posterior cutaneous nerve of the thigh and then anastomoses with perforators from the profunda femoris system. The perforators follow an intramuscular course through the gluteus maximus to join the IGA pedicle, which emerges from the inferior margin of the greater sciatic foramen, adjacent to the lower border of the piriformis and medial to the sciatic nerve.

8.9.2 Hip and Thigh Region

Introduction

The hip and thigh region extends from the inguinal ligament and gluteal fold proximally to a horizontal line along the superior pole of the patella. It is subdivided into four regions: (1) anteromedial thigh, (2) the anterolateral thigh and trochanteric region, (3) the posteromedial thigh, and (4) the posterolateral thigh (▸ Fig. 8.9). These regions are supplied by six principal source arteries, all branches of the superficial and profunda femoral arteries. The hip and thigh have a large number of perforators (about 50), some of which have large cutaneous territories and have become a preferred location for perforator flap donor sites due to both the number of large diameter perforators and relative ease of donor site closure.[2]

Anteromedial Thigh: Femoral Artery

The skin of the anteromedial thigh is supplied by the **FA**. There are 8 to 15 FA perforators, most of which are found in two rows of septocutaneous perforators, which emerge from the medial and lateral borders of the sartorius. The skin over the quadriceps tendon is supplied by distal musculocutaneous perforators that emerge from the vastus medialis muscle. The septocutaneous perforators have a long superficial pedicle after arising from the FA. The FA runs in the adductor (Hunter's) canal along with the saphenous nerve and nerve to the vastus medialis in the middle third of the thigh. In the proximal third, the FA is found within the femoral (Scarpa's) triangle, while the most proximal 4 cm of the FA are enclosed within the femoral sheath. Along with some direct perforators, proximally the FA also gives rise to the superficial inferior epigastric artery and the superficial external pudendal artery.

Anterolateral Thigh: Superficial Circumflex Iliac Artery

The **superficial circumflex iliac artery (SCIA)** supplies the skin of the proximal part of the anterolateral thigh, with one to two musculocutaneous perforators and usually a dominant superficial direct perforator. The deep perforator is usually found 3 cm medial to the anterior superior iliac spine and 1 cm inferior to the inguinal ligament. The vessel then runs medially, parallel to the inguinal ligament to then pierce the deep fascia of the sartorius and run deep to this muscle until it joins the superficial perforator and then ultimately the FA near the origin of the

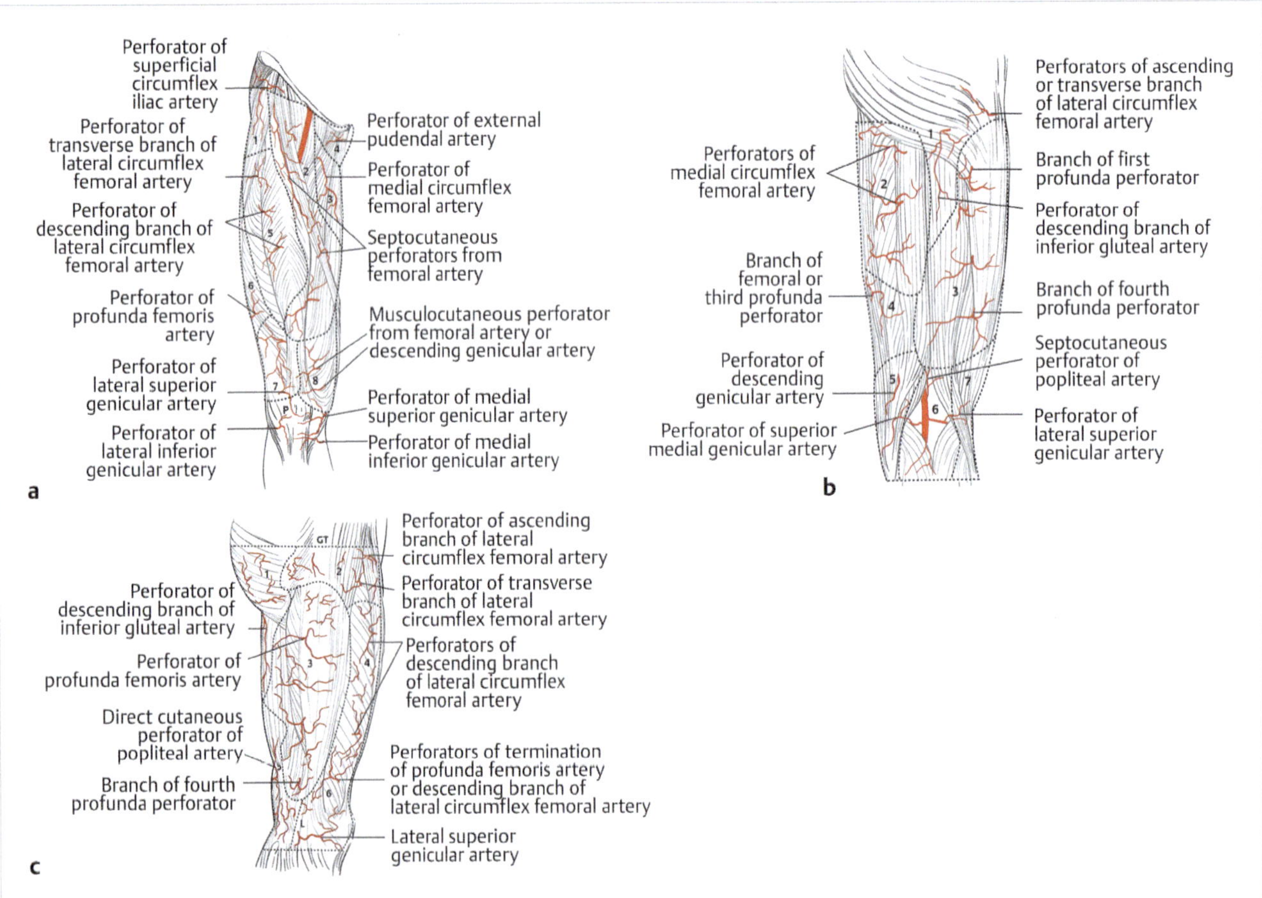

Fig. 8.9 The vascular supply of the hip and thigh regions. **(a)** Anterolateral and anteromedial thigh. **(b)** Posterior thigh. **(c)** Lateral thigh. (Adapted from Geddes CR, Tang M, Yang D, Morris SF. Anatomy of the lower extremity. In: Blondeel PN, Morris SF, Hallock GG, Neligan PC, eds. Perforator Flaps: Anatomy, Technique & Clinical Applications. St Louis, MO: Quality Medical Publishing; 2013:667–703.)

superficial inferior epigastric artery, although this may be in common with the latter.

Anterolateral Thigh: Lateral Femoral Circumflex Artery

The **LFCA** supplies the majority of skin of the anterolateral thigh. Proximally, the lateral aspect of the hip is supplied by three to five musculocutaneous perforators. These arise from the ascending branch of the LFCA and pierce the tensor fascia lata muscle. More distally, the lateral aspect of the thigh has both musculocutaneous and septocutaneous perforators that originate predominantly from the descending branch of the LFCA, with a small number of them sometimes from the transverse branch. Perforators may emerge along the anterior border of the vastus lateralis muscle as septocutaneous branches, arising from the intermuscular septum between the rectus femoris and vastus lateralis muscles. The transverse branch then courses laterally over the vastus intermedius, while the descending branch runs deep to the rectus femoris muscle, accompanied by the branch of the femoral nerve to the vastus lateralis. The LCFA finally passes horizontally between the divisions of the femoral nerve to usually join the **profunda femoris artery** (PFA) as its second branch after the medial circumflex femoral.

Posteromedial Thigh: Medial Circumflex Femoral Artery

The skin of the posteromedial thigh is supplied predominantly by the **medial circumflex femoral artery (MCFA)**. Musculocutaneous perforators from both its transverse and descending branches pierce the adductor magnus. These branches can be traced back to the MCFA, which is the first branch off the PFA, near its origin from the FA. The perforators have a superficial pedicle length of 2 to 5 cm and a deep pedicle length of almost 10 cm.

Posteromedial Thigh: Minor Vascular Contributions

Superiorly, the skin of the posteromedial thigh also receives a small contribution from the obturator artery. Distally the posteromedial thigh is supplied by perforators from the PFA and the PA.

Posterolateral Thigh: Profunda Femoris Artery

The **PFA** supplies the skin overlying the posterior compartment from the inferolateral margin of the gluteus maximus to the superior border of the popliteal fossa and the lateral intermuscular septum to a point slightly medial to the posterior midline. It is supplied by 5 to 10 perforators, which are a mixture of septocutaneous and musculocutaneous perforators. Septocutaneous perforators emerge predominantly from the posterolateral intermuscular septum between the vastus lateralis and the biceps femoris. There are also some septocutaneous perforators that emerge from between the biceps femoris and the semitendinosus and semimembranosus muscles at intervals of 5 to 8 cm to form a long perforator chain (with true anastomosis between adjacent perforator angiosomes) comprising two to three perforators from the PFA, accompanying the posterior femoral cutaneous nerve. Musculocutaneous perforators emerge from the short head of the biceps femoris muscle. Perforators can be traced back to one of the four deep branches of the PFA, traditionally called the first through fourth perforators. These then join the PFA, which lies on the medial side of the femur, lateral to the FA.

8.9.3 Knee and Leg Region

Introduction

The knee and leg region extends from a horizontal line around the superior pole of the patella to a circumferential line through the medial and lateral malleoli. The skin is supplied by approximately 30 perforators, with an equal ratio of musculocutaneous and septocutaneous perforators (▶ Fig. 8.10).

The knee joint and overlying skin has a rich vascular supply from musculocutaneous perforators from the FA and septocutaneous perforators from seven main arteries: (1) descending genicular, (2) medial superior genicular, (3) lateral superior genicular, (4) medial inferior genicular, (5) lateral inferior genicular, (6) anterior tibial recurrent, and (7) direct cutaneous branches of the popliteal. The arterial circle around the patella, known as the *patellar rete*, has contributions from the seven arteries listed and these all give off cutaneous branches.

Inferior to the knee, the leg is divided into five vascular territories: (1) descending genicular (saphenous), (2) popliteal (sural), (3) anterior tibial, (4) posterior tibial, and (5) peroneal.

Anteromedial Knee: Descending Genicular Artery, Saphenous Artery Branch

Though it branches from the FA in the thigh at the level of the adductor hiatus, the **descending genicular artery (DGA)** supplies a cutaneous territory about the knee through its superficial branch, known as the *saphenous artery*. This is an area of skin extending from the medial knee to the pes anserinus to the inferomedial border of the medial gastrocnemius muscle. Septocutaneous perforators emerge from between the vastus medialis and adductor magnus muscles with the saphenous nerve and vein. The perforators follow a direct course to join the DGA, which branches from the FA just before it passes through the opening of the adductor hiatus.

The DGA also has an articular branch that is part of the rich anastomotic network around the knee. As it descends anterior to the adductor magnus, it anastomoses with the medial superior genicular artery (MSGA) and the recurrent tibial artery. It then crosses the patella and anastomoses with the lateral superior genicular artery (LSGA). The saphenous artery is also part of the anastomotic network, anastomosing posteriorly with the sural artery, anteriorly with the anterior tibial artery (ATA), and inferiorly with the PTA.

Posterior Knee: Popliteal Artery and its Sural Branches

The **PA** supplies a large cutaneous area posteriorly in the midline of the knee and leg. Though there is a small contribution from direct PA perforators in the popliteal fossa, this area is largely supplied by the *superficial sural branches* of the PA with two to four perforators. One *lateral sural artery* musculocutaneous

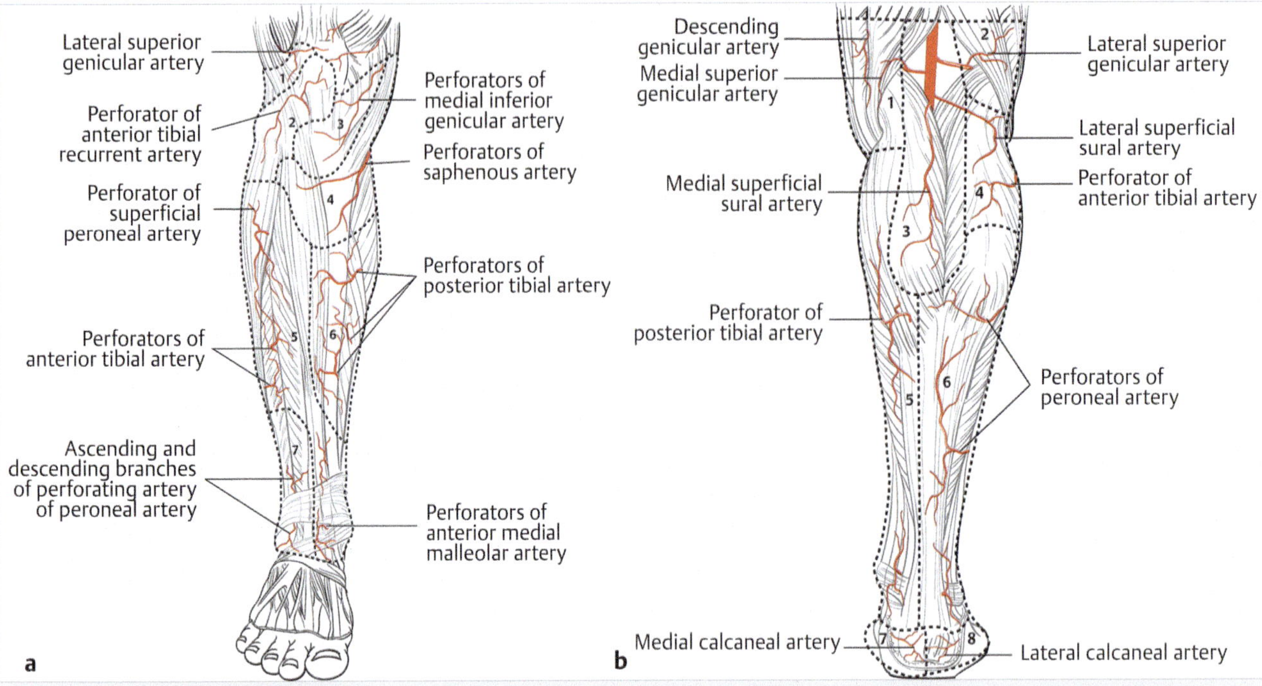

Fig. 8.10 The vascular supply of the knee and leg regions. **(a)** Anterior. **(b)** Posterior. (Adapted from Geddes CR, Tang M, Yang D, Morris SF. Anatomy of the lower extremity. In: Blondeel PN, Morris SF, Hallock GG, Neligan PC, eds. Perforator Flaps: Anatomy, Technique & Clinical Applications. St Louis, MO: Quality Medical Publishing; 2013:667–703.)

perforator is generally found over the lateral head of the gastrocnemius, while two to three *medial sural artery* perforators are found over the inferomedial part of the medial head. The medial superficial sural artery is usually accompanied by the small saphenous vein, medial sural cutaneous nerve, and sural nerve. It may have a large diameter (> 1.0 mm) and anastomoses medially with the lateral superficial sural artery. The lateral superficial sural artery accompanies the lateral cutaneous sural nerve. The medial and lateral deep sural arteries only supply muscles without a significant cutaneous contribution.

Medial Knee: Medial Superior Genicular Artery

The **MSGA** supplies the superomedial aspect of the suprapatellar area of skin with 2±1 septocutaneous perforators. The septocutaneous perforators emerge from the medial aspect of the popliteal fossa. The MSGA has two branches, the superior one supplies the distal vastus medialis and anastomoses with the descending genicular artery. The other branch travels anteriorly and laterally, anastomosing with the LSGA. The MSGA curves around the femur just superior to the medial femoral condyle until its branch point from the PA.

Lateral Knee: Lateral Superior Genicular Artery

The **LSGA** supplies the superolateral area of skin overlying the patella with one to three perforators. Septocutaneous perforators emerge from between the vastus lateralis and biceps femoris tendon. These perforators arise from the superficial branch of the LSGA, which also anastomoses with the descending branch of the LCFA, lateral inferior genicular artery (LIGA), perforators from the PFA, and musculocutaneous perforators from the vastus medialis muscle. The deep branch supplies the lower part of the femur and knee joint and forms an arch with the descending genicular and medial inferior genicular arteries. The common trunk of the LSGA lies just superior to the lateral femoral condyle, beneath the tendon of the biceps femoris. It joins the PA at the same level as the MSGA.

Medial Knee: Medial Inferior Genicular Artery

The **medial inferior genicular artery** (**MIGA**) supplies the inferomedial patella and the patellar tendon area of skin with one perforator. This septocutaneous perforator pierces the deep fascia near the pes anserinus, then runs deep to the medial head of the gastrocnemius muscle and the medial collateral ligament. The MIGA meets the PA at the level of the knee joint line.

Lateral Knee: Lateral Inferior Genicular Artery

The **LIGA** supplies the skin over the lateral inferior aspect of the knee with one perforator. This septocutaneous perforator is found inferolateral to the patella after travelling deep to the tendon of the biceps, fibular collateral ligament, and the lateral head of the gastrocnemius muscle. It then passes anterior to the knee joint, runs laterally above the head of the fibula, and joins the popliteal artery deep to the gastrocnemius at the same level as the MIGA. Distally, the LIGA terminates in branches that anastomose with the medial inferior and lateral superior genicular arteries and with the anterior recurrent tibial artery.

Anterior Leg: Anterior Tibial Artery

The **ATA** supplies the skin over the anterior compartment of the leg with four to eight perforators. There are two rows of perforators: the medial row is a combination of musculocutaneous from the tibialis anterior muscle or septocutaneous from between the tibialis anterior and extensor hallucis longus. The second row is more lateral, emerging from the anteromedial septum between the peroneus tertius and peroneus brevis muscles or from either of the two muscles. The musculocutaneous perforators have a very short course in the muscle. There is an especially large cutaneous perforator called the **superolateral peroneal branch** that accompanies the superficial peroneal nerve into the skin.

In the lower part of the leg, the perforators can be traced back to the ATA, where it lies on the tibia, deep to the tibialis anterior and extensor hallucis longus muscles. Proximally, the ATA lies on the anterior surface of the interosseous membrane, where it sends an **anterior recurrent branch** to pierce the deep fascia near the inferolateral border of the tibial tuberosity. Continuing proximally, the artery lies close to the medial side of the neck of the fibula. It then passes through the aperture at the border of the interosseous membrane, between the two heads of the tibialis posterior muscle; at the lower border of the popliteus muscle, the ATA arises from the bifurcation of the PA. At its distal end, the ATA courses anterior to the ankle, where it becomes the **dorsalis pedis artery** (**DPA**).

Lateral Leg: Peroneal Artery

The **peroneal artery** (**PNA**) supplies the fibula and muscles of the lateral compartment, along with the overlying skin including that overlying the Achilles tendon, with three to seven perforators. Perforators pierce the origin of the flexor hallucis longus muscle and emerge through the posterolateral septum between the peroneus longus and soleus muscles. A large, consistent branch pierces the interosseous membrane 5 cm above the lateral malleolus to reach the anterior leg, where it divides into ascending and descending branches. The ascending branch anastomoses with the superficial PNA to form the anterolateral arterial chain of the leg. Perforators can be traced back to the PNA where it is contained within a fibrous canal between the tibialis posterior and the flexor hallucis longus muscle on the posteromedial surface of the fibula. The PNA proximally arises from the tibioperoneal trunk, 3 cm below the inferior border of the popliteus. Distally, the PNA runs behind the tibiofibular syndesmosis and divides into lateral calcaneal branches.

Medial Leg: Posterior Tibial Artery

The **PTA** supplies the skin of the medial leg, with 6 to 12 perforators. Four to five septocutaneous perforators emerge from the intermuscular septum between the soleus and flexor digitorum longus muscles. These perforators anastomose superiorly with the *descending genicular artery* to form a long vascular chain that accompanies the *greater saphenous vein*. Three to four musculocutaneous perforators arise from the medial aspect of the soleus muscle. Other musculocutaneous perforators emerge from the posterior and lateral aspects of the soleus muscles and supply the skin around the region of the Achilles tendon.

The PTA begins at the lower border of the popliteus as the continuation of the tibioperoneal trunk, and extends obliquely down the medial aspect of the leg. In the lower part of the leg, the PTA is situated midway between the medial malleolus and the medial process of the calcaneal tuberosity. More distally, the PTA divides beneath the origin of the abductor hallucis muscle into the medial and lateral plantar arteries.

8.9.4 Foot and Ankle Region

Introduction

The foot and ankle region extends from circumferential line about the medial and lateral malleoli. This region has multiple anastomoses and arches that make it difficult to define discrete vascular territories. The PTA, ATA, and PNA all contribute to the foot; and at the ankle, the ATA becomes the dorsalis pedis (▶ Fig. 8.11). The PTA gives off the medial and lateral calcaneal arteries, then terminates as the medial and lateral plantar arteries. The PNA joins the lateral and medial calcaneal arteries through the calcaneal plexus. The dorsum of the foot is supplied by multiple small perforators from the DPA. The plantar surface of the foot is supplied by the medial and lateral plantar arteries.

Medial Ankle: Medial Calcaneal Artery

The **medial calcaneal artery** (**MCA**) supplies an area of skin posterior to the Achilles tendon, medial ankle, sole, and heel with one to two perforators. The MCA is not one, but multiple large arteries that arise from the PTA just before its final

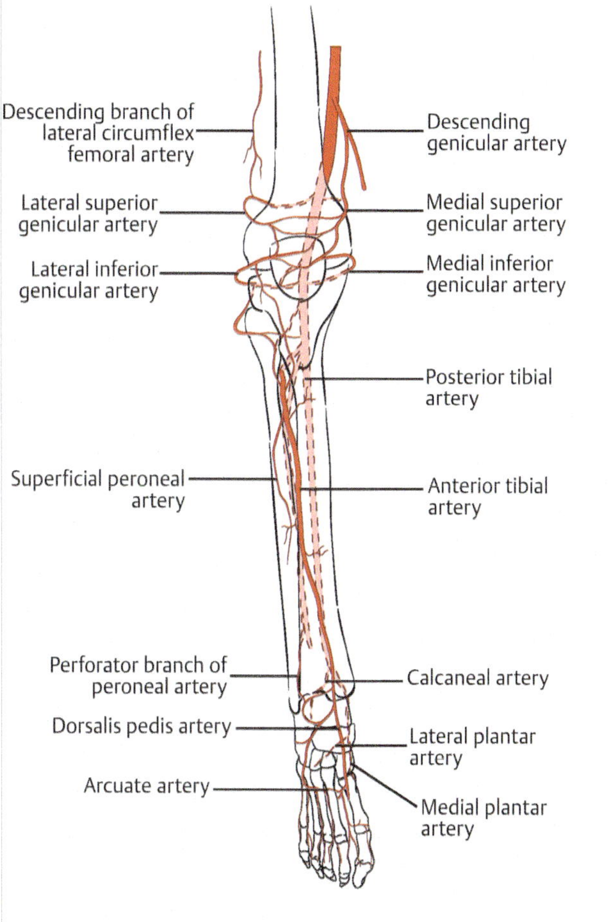

Fig. 8.11 Arteries of the leg and foot. (Adapted from Geddes CR, Tang M, Yang D, Morris SF. Anatomy of the lower extremity. In: Blondeel PN, Morris SF, Hallock GG, Neligan PC, eds. Perforator Flaps: Anatomy, Technique & Clinical Applications. St Louis, MO: Quality Medical Publishing; 2013:667–703.)

division. The perforators pierce the laciniate ligament and create multiple true anastomoses with the peroneal, medial malleolar, and lateral calcaneal arteries.

Lateral Ankle: Lateral Calcaneal Artery

The **lateral calcaneal artery** (**LCA**) supplies a small area of skin on the lateral ankle and heel with one to two perforators. The perforators can be found on the lateral side of the heel where the LCA arborizes into a plexus that anastomoses with the lateral calcaneal branches of the PTA. The LCA also gives rise to the anterior lateral malleolar artery that arises anteriorly and anastomoses with the DPA below the extensor retinaculum.

Medial Ankle: Medial Plantar Artery

The **medial plantar artery** (**MPA**) supplies skin along the medial aspect of the foot and plantar surface with one to two perforators. Perforators arise directly through the abductor hallucis muscle. The MPA courses between the abductor hallucis and the flexor digitorum brevis distally and is superficial to the abductor hallucis muscle more proximally. At the base of the first metatarsal, the MPA passes along the medial border of the first toe, anastomosing via an arch with the first dorsal metatarsal artery.

Lateral Foot: Lateral Plantar Artery

The **lateral plantar artery** (**LPA**) supplies the skin of the lateral sole with one to two perforators, which are a mix of septocutaneous and musculocutaneous perforators. These perforators run forward between the metatarsal bones, in contact with the interossei and divide into a pair of plantar digital arteries. At the point of division, each perforator sends a dorsal branch of plantar digital arteries upward to join the corresponding dorsal metatarsal artery. The LPA in the distal midfoot lies superficially between the flexor digitorum brevis and abductor digiti quinti muscles, covered by the plantar aponeurosis and skin. From the base of the fifth metatarsal moving proximally, it runs obliquely from lateral to medial, lying between the flexor digitorum brevis and quadratus plantae. At its origin from the PTA, on the medial ankle, the LPA is situated between the calcaneus and abductor hallucis. At the interval between the bases of the first and second metatarsals, the LPA unites with the deep plantar branch of the dorsalis pedis to complete the plantar arch.

Dorsum of Foot: Dorsalis Pedis Artery

The **DPA** supplies an area of skin on the dorsum of the foot with one to two perforators. The DPA is part of an extensive network anastomosing with perforators from the PNA and PTA. The DPA is a continuation of the ATA with three main branches. At the navicular bone, the first branch is the **lateral tarsal artery** that supplies the extensor digitorum brevis. A musculocutaneous perforator from this branch anastomoses with the anterior lateral malleolar artery and perforators of the PNA. Before reaching the metatarsals, the DPA gives rise to the **arcuate artery**, which arches laterally across the base of the metatarsals to anastomose with the lateral tarsal and lateral plantar arteries and gives rise to the metatarsal arteries. The DPA then continues to the proximal part of the first intermetatarsal space where it divides into two branches: the **first dorsal metatarsal artery** and the **deep plantar artery**. The deep plantar artery then completes the plantar arch by anastomosing with the LPA.

8.10 Selection of Recipient Vessels

8.10.1 General Principles

Preoperative planning is critically important in regional or free microsurgical reconstruction of the lower extremity. The selection of suitable recipient vessels for microsurgical reconstruction largely depends on the location of the defect and what vessel is in proximity to the wound. Arterial supply is generally the limiting factor, but venous drainage can sometimes be challenging as well. Ideally, the optimal recipient artery has robust flow, a good caliber (> 1 mm), and is out of the zone of injury.[5,6] If there are more than one vessel available in that location, it is important to consider the difficulty of dissection, including how the patient will be positioned for harvest of the donor flap. Usually, the closest source vessel will be the target recipient vessel so that the microsurgical reconstruction of the defect can be accomplished without the need for vein grafts.

Unless capable of supermicrosurgery, usually vascular anastomoses for a free tissue transfer should be outside of the **zone of injury**. Since so many lower extremity wounds are traumatic in nature, the appropriately named *zone of injury* is the injured, thrombogenic zone that extends beyond what macroscopically appears to be normal.[6] In this area, there is increased friability of vessels and an increased risk of thrombosis. Similarly, a previously radiated area carries many of the same risks.[7] It is important that the pedicle of the flap and the recipient vessel are beyond this zone of injury to improve flap survival.[7,8]

8.10.2 Preoperative Evaluation

Clinical Examination

First determine the extent of the defect and what needs to be covered. Manually check peripheral pulses. The absence of one or both of the dorsalis pedis or posterior tibial pulses warrants further investigation.[5,9]

Handheld Audible Doppler

A handheld Doppler can be used to further assess distal pulses in the lower extremity, but cannot differentiate between normal flow and nonocclusive atherosclerosis, proximal occlusion, and reconstitution, or anatomic variability.[10]

Computed Tomography Angiography

Computed tomography angiography (CTA) is a valuable tool to assess the vascular status of the lower limb. It is not only useful but also wise to order a CTA if there is a reason to suspect any vascular issues or if there is an inconclusive vascular status on clinical grounds. Appropriate indications include loss of one or more pedal pulses, neurologic deficit, compound fracture, or presence of peripheral vascular disease. A high-quality CTA is very useful for planning the reconstruction as it will show patency of the main arteries and veins, partial occlusions, reconstitution, and any anatomic variation. An added benefit is that a CTA will also demonstrate soft-tissue and bony defects and can even be used to generate a three-dimensional image.[10] It is important to communicate what information is needed to your radiologist to ensure a high-resolution CTA that can show these vessels in appropriate detail and to reduce radiation exposure to the patient.[11] Unlike conventional angiography, the contrast agent for a CTA is given as a venous, rather than, arterial bolus, reducing the risks of pseudoaneurysms, and thrombosis.[11] CTAs are not completely benign as they do carry a risk of radiation exposure, though the dosage is much lower with modern CT scanners. Some individuals can have allergies to the contrast dye, or not be candidates due to poor renal function.[10,12]

Magnetic Resonance Angiography

Magnetic resonance angiography (MRA) is another noninvasive imaging modality that can be used for better characterizing the lower extremity vasculature. It has the benefit of no radiation exposure and does not necessarily need a contrast agent. Early MRAs did not have as high a resolution as did the CTA, but this has improved.[11] The drawbacks to an MRA are the high costs and the long time needed to adequately perform a scan, which could be intolerable especially if the patient is claustrophobic. In addition, not all hardware or implanted devices are compatible with the magnet, so those patients may not be acceptable candidates.[12]

Conventional Angiography

Conventional angiography is not routinely used for characterization of recipient vessels or perforators as it is an invasive procedure requiring an arterial puncture and carries with it the risk of bleeding, thrombosis, pseudoaneurysm, a higher radiation dose, and the quality of images are not significantly better than those with newer CTA techniques.[10,11]

8.10.3 Recipient Vessels

Any of the main source vessels or perforators as already described (▶ Table 8.1) could potentially be used as recipient vessels depending on the extent of the defect and the vascular status of the extremity and those vessels. Historically, particularly to preserve distal flow to the foot, end-to-side anastomoses have been advocated for arterial anastomoses and end-to-end venous anastomoses. More recent literature has suggested that if the vascular configuration is intact in the lower extremity, or a vessel occluded distally, then an end-to-end arterial anastomosis can be performed without increased risk of thrombosis, flap failure, or limb ischemia.[13,14,15] The most important factor to consider is to have a complete map of the vascularity of the leg preoperatively to avoid iatrogenic limb ischemia, now or in the future.[14,16]

In addition to using the source vessels to specific angiosomes themselves as the recipient site,[17,18,19] which would also usually allow end-to-end anastomoses, increasingly, perforator vessels are being used as the recipient vessel with perforator-to-perforator anastomoses. The benefits of perforator-to-perforator reconstruction are the following: (1) less time is needed to elevate a flap as only a short pedicle is needed; (2) there is no need to sacrifice a main source vessel; and (3) risk for major vessel injury and disruption of circulation is minimized although perhaps a source of collateral circulation may be sacrifice. The details of this technique requiring supermicrosurgery skills are discussed in greater detail in Chapter 17.

References

[1] Taylor GI, Palmer JH. The vascular territories (angiosomes) of the body: experimental study and clinical applications. Br J Plast Surg. 1987; 40(2): 113–141

[2] Blondeel PN, Morris SF, Hallock GG, Neligan PC, eds. Perforator Flaps: Anatomy, Technique & Clinical Applications. Boca Raton, FL: CRC Press; 2013

[3] Geddes CR, Morris SF, Neligan PC. Perforator flaps: evolution, classification, and applications. Ann Plast Surg. 2003; 50(1):90–99

[4] Cormack GC, , Lamberty BG. A classification of fascio-cutaneous flaps according to their patterns of vascularisation. Br J Plast Surg. 1984; 37(1):80–7

[5] Wei F-C, Mardini S. Flaps and Reconstructive Surgery. New York, NY: Elsevier Health Sciences; 2009

[6] Dancey A, Blondeel PN. Technical tips for safe perforator vessel dissection applicable to all perforator flaps. Clin Plast Surg. 2010; 37(4):593–606, xi–vi

[7] Suh HS, Lee JS, Hong JP. Consideration in lower extremity reconstruction following oncologic surgery: patient selection, surgical techniques, and outcomes. J Surg Oncol. 2016; 113(8):955–961

[8] Hallock GG. Lower extremity muscle perforator flaps for lower extremity reconstruction. Plast Reconstr Surg. 2004; 114(5):1123–1130

[9] Neligan PC. Plastic Surgery. London: Elsevier Health Sciences; 2012

[10] Duymaz A, Karabekmez FE, Vrtiska TJ, Mardini S, Moran SL. Free tissue transfer for lower extremity reconstruction: a study of the role of computed angiography in the planning of free tissue transfer in the posttraumatic setting. Plast Reconstr Surg. 2009; 124(2):523–529

[11] Pratt GF, Rozen WM, Chubb D, Ashton MW, Alonso-Burgos A, Whitaker IS. Preoperative imaging for perforator flaps in reconstructive surgery: a systematic review of the evidence for current techniques. Ann Plast Surg. 2012; 69(1): 3–9

[12] Smit JM, Klein S, Werker PMN. An overview of methods for vascular mapping in the planning of free flaps. J Plast Reconstr Aesthet Surg. 2010; 63(9):e674–e682

[13] Cho EH, Garcia RM, Blau J, et al. Microvascular anastomoses using end-to-end versus end-to-side technique in lower extremity free tissue transfer. J Reconstr Microsurg. 2016; 32(2):114–120

[14] Cho EH, Garcia RM, Pien I, et al. Vascular considerations in foot and ankle free tissue transfer: analysis of 231 free flaps. Microsurgery. 2016; 36(4):276–283

[15] Tsai Y-T, Lin T-S. The suitability of end-to-side microvascular anastomosis in free flap transfer for limb reconstruction. Ann Plast Surg. 2012; 68(2):171–174

[16] Hong JP, Oh TS. An algorithm for limb salvage for diabetic foot ulcers. Clin Plast Surg. 2012; 39(3):341–352

[17] Hallock GG. The medial approach to the sural vessels to facilitate microanastomosis about the knee. Ann Plast Surg. 1994; 32(4):388–393

[18] Smith ML, Molina BJ, Dayan E, Kim JN, Kagen A, Dayan JH. Use of distal medial sural vessels as recipient vessels in free tissue transfer. J Reconstr Microsurg. 2017; 33(1):59–62

[19] Hallock GG. The vascular pedicle of the anterolateral thigh flap as an alternative recipient site for thigh free flaps. J Reconstr Microsurg. 2008; 24(2):131–136

9 Importance of Vascularity and Selecting the Recipient Vessels in Lower Extremity Reconstruction

Joon Pio Hong, Changsik John Park, and Peter Suh

Summary
Successful lower extremity reconstruction using free flaps begins by identifying a good recipient vessel and understanding the surrounding environment of the defect. One should consider multiple factors when selecting the recipient vessel, such as the status of the axial arteries, trying to preserve flow as much as possible, extent and severity of the defect, and ultimately choosing the ideal type of anastomosis. However, the ultimate decision should be made on the operating table during surgery when the actual artery or vein is exposed and it shows signs of good pulsation and flow.

Keywords: Microsurgery, selecting recipient vessels, vascular status of extremity

9.1 Introduction

Reconstructive microsurgery has played a pivotal role in achieving results where limb salvage reconstruction outcomes are similar to primary amputations.[1,2] Nevertheless, lower extremity reconstruction remains difficult due to multiple factors involved during reconstruction such as timing, wide zone of injury, infection, status of vascularity, and the long and complex process of healing till complete weight bearing. Now with the concept of reconstructive elevator to reach the ideal rung of reconstruction providing the best possible timely option to achieve aesthetic as well as functional outcome, it often requires the thinking and use of complex microsurgical procedures.[3] Despite the fact that normal function and appearance can be difficult to achieve, it may be warranted to support successful reconstruction leading to successful salvage of the extremity. Furthermore, microsurgical reconstruction of the lower extremity is now accepted as a safe process with acceptable rate of flap failures according to a meta-analysis by Xiong et al.[4]

The classical approach for lower extremity reconstruction using free flaps dictates the following: anastomose the vessel outside the zone of injury, make end-to-side arterial anastomosis and end-to-side or end-to-end venous anastomosis, and reconstruct the soft tissues first and then restore the skeletal support.[5] Although these teachings are still very valuable, they may not always be applicable to complex situations where vascular structures are poor and the zone of injury is complex and wide, making selection of recipient vessels complicated and confusing.

Once the decision is made for reconstructive microsurgery, complex or simple, selection of recipient vessels is one of the key factors in achieving successful outcomes. Once the recipient site is secured, one can choose the type of flap based on the pedicle length.[6] Inversely, one should consider where to select the recipient in regard to the flap that is chosen. In this chapter, we will review how to evaluate the lower extremity in regard to major vessels, select the recipient site, and the method of anastomosis.

9.2 Factors to Consider

9.2.1 Evaluating the Lower Extremity Vascular Status

After the decision is made to reconstruct the lower extremity, the first preoperative evaluation should start with vascular status. Without adequate vascular supply, microsurgical reconstruction will not be possible. This is especially true for ischemic conditions after trauma and ischemic chronic wounds. Most often, physical examination of palpable pulse, color, capillary refill, and turgor of the extremity allows us to assess the initial status. With the handheld Doppler examination, further information can be obtained.[7] The use of preoperative arteriography for lower extremity reconstruction is considered when physical/ Doppler examination reveals inconclusive vascular status or chronic vascular disease is suspected. It is usually performed for patients who have loss of one or more peripheral pulses, a neurologic deficit secondary to the injury, or a compound fracture of the extremity that has undergone reduction and either external or internal fixation.[8] In association with prior injuries to the lower extremity, the routine preoperative use of angiogram is controversial.[7,8,9,10,11,12,13] However, in our experience, 75 to 80% of lower extremity reconstruction that involves trauma, chronic wounds, and oncologic reconstruction may be indicated for detailed vascular evaluation. If angiogram is required, the simpler way is to obtain the vascular status by computed tomography (CT) angiography of the recipient region without the risk of complications from arterial puncture of the groin. In addition, it can provide vascular information of the donor flap when selected from the extremity, facilitating the planning and the surgical procedure.[11,14,15] ▶ Fig. 9.1 shows a patient with a diabetic foot having obstruction of both femoral artery and distal circulation being supplied by collateral vessels. This patient exhibited normal handheld Doppler findings and thus justifies the angiogram in patients with chronic conditions such as diabetes. It also shows the quality of the artery whether or not it is calcified proximal to the lesion, which may warrant angioplasty to improve distal flow. This can be frequently seen in patients with diabetes or other peripheral artery disease. Furthermore, it shows you whether or not calcification is present on the recipient artery, thus helping you to decide on selection of the artery near the defect. Finally, the CT angiogram when programed can see though the venous phase, detecting the superficial veins and the presence of deep vein thrombosis. However, in the cases where hardware is applied, it may distort the image. In these cases, although more invasive, classical angiogram will help the surgeon to determine the vascular status.

At this phase of evaluation, one should consider which major vessels are available to anastomose the flap: the anterior, posterior, or peroneal artery. One should remember that multiple variations of major vessels may be present. Some frequent variations are peroneus magna and distally intact (proximal

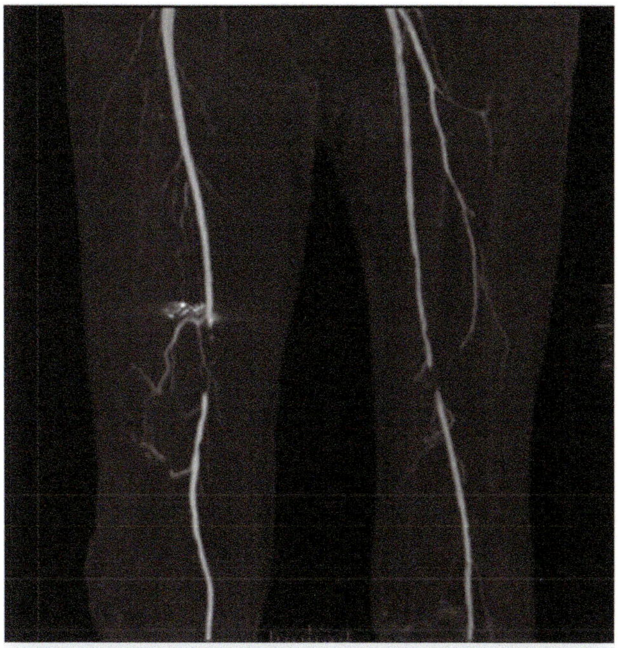

Fig. 9.1 A patient with a diabetic foot having obstruction of both femoral artery and distal circulation being supplied by collateral vessels. This patient exhibited normal hand-held Doppler findings and thus justifies the angiogram in patients with chronic condition such as diabetes. If one would harvest the anterolateral thigh flap without this knowledge, it would be catastrophic for the limb circulation as the major collateral vessel is the descending branch of the lateral circumflex femoral artery.

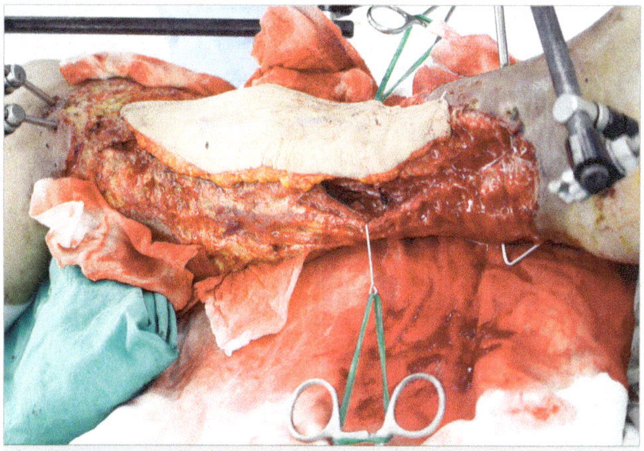

Fig. 9.2 One of the most important factors in selecting the recipient vessel may be the vascular quality itself and as long as the recipient vessels are healthy with pulsation and adequate outflow after opening the vessel, it can be presumed to be usable as seen in this figure where circumflex iliac artery perforator flap was used to anastomose end-to-side on the anterior tibial artery within the zone of injury.

injured) posterior or anterior artery by connecting the collaterals.[16] Taking all this into account, preoperative radiological evaluation of the major vessels will allow you to obtain good information and thus will allow you to facilitate the reconstruction process.

9.2.2 Zone of Injury

While burn and radiation injury may have a more definable zone of injury, many lower extremity wounds resulting from high-energy trauma have obscured zones of injury. The exact definition of the zone of injury still remains unclear and unreproducible.[17] However, this concept is clinically important as the thrombogenic zone is known to extend beyond what is macroscopically evident and failure to recognize the true extent of this zone is cited as a leading cause of microsurgical anastomotic failure.[9] This is more evident in the subacute period when usually the reconstructive consultation/transfer is made. Within this zone, perivascular changes such as increased friability of vessels and increased perivascular scar tissue may lead to difficult dissection of recipient vessels and higher incidence of thrombosis after anastomosis.[18] There have been many reports on how to avoid the zone of injury by going proximal to the zone of injury. Searching for the recipient vessel proximal to the zone makes a lot of sense as the vascular injury is usually within the zone and proximal vessels can be assumed to be normal.[19,20,21] Some studies even advocate using bypass grafts or arteriovenous (AV) loops linked to the proximal vessels to supply the vascularity to the flap to cover the defect.[22,23,24] If there are injured major vessel stumps close to the injury, one can explore the stump and often can see that it is quite usable. Using this stump will allow you to preserve maximal flow to the foot by avoiding sacrifice to the other major vessels, thus reducing the risk of developing ischemia in later life.[24,25,26] However, multiple studies show that anastomosing the flap distal to the zone of injury really makes no difference in outcome.[26,27,28,29] Thus, one must ask if one can make anastomosis in the zone of injury. Again, it is clinically very difficult to realize how extensive and what the zone of injury is. The zone of injury is not a two-dimensional concept but rather a three-dimensional concept and frequently deeper structures may be spared from injury with minimal or no injury to the vascular structures. The study by Isenberg and Sherman demonstrated that clinical presentation of the recipient vessel such as vessel wall pliability and the quality of blood from the transected end of the vessel was more important than the distance from the wound.[30] Park et al also concluded that the site of injury and vascular status of the lower extremity were the most important factors in choosing a recipient vessel.[28] This idea was further supported by successful anastomosis of the perforator adjacent to or within the zone of injury.[31] With advances in microscopes, microsurgery instruments, and techniques, one can dissect the scarred vessels within the zone of injury and utilize them. Based on these findings, one of the most important factors in selecting the recipient vessel may be the vascular quality itself and as long as the recipient vessels are healthy with pulsation and adequate outflow after opening the vessel, it can be presumed to be usable (▶ Fig. 9.2).

9.2.3 Type of Anastomosis

The classical debate on end-to-end versus end-to-side anastomosis has been shown to have no difference in achieving flap success and has been found to be equally effective.[25,32,33] If there is no difference in outcome, one should ask which one has more benefits for lower extremity reconstruction. Godina has advocated end-to-side anastomosis on extremity reconstruction

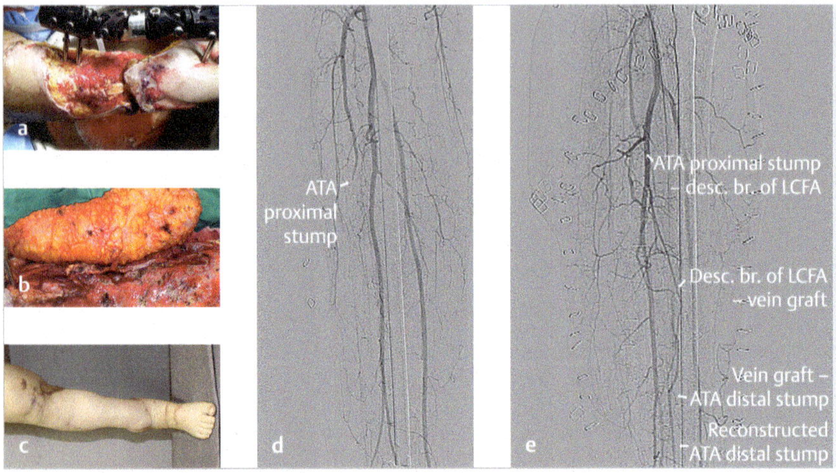

Fig. 9.3 **(a)** A patient with defect of the lower leg is shown with soft tissue defect, bone fracture, and a gap of missing anterior tibial artery. **(b)** An anterolateral thigh flap with a long descending branch with a vein graft was used to reconstruct the arterial defect achieving a flow-through reconstruction. **(c)** The patient at 3 years shows good results without any occurrence of bone infection. **(d)** Note the preoperative angiogram with a clear stump of anterior tibial artery (ATA). **(e)** Postoperative angiogram shows the reconstructed anterior tibial artery with good distal flow. Abbreviations: Desc. Br., descending branch; LCFA, lateral femoral circumflex artery.

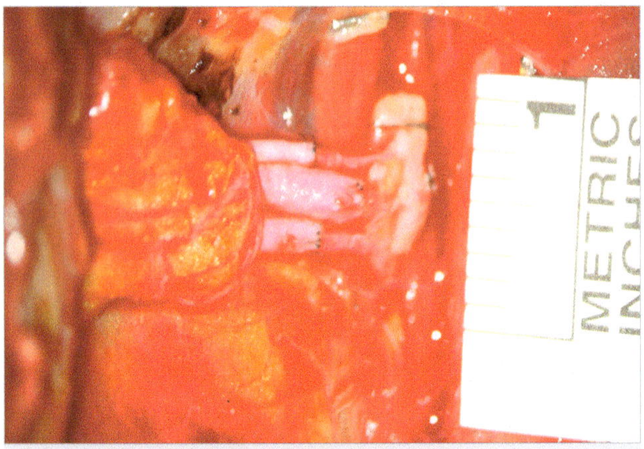

Fig. 9.4 The most important step is to identify a pulsating perforator under the microscope. An end-to-end anastomosis between the perforators of the recipient and the flap is shown.

based on advantages such as preservation of distal vasculature, avoidance of retraction and spasm of the recipient artery, and avoidance of flow disturbances from vessel mismatch.[17,34] Our practice has found this to be true and that it allows a better solution when there is anastomotic problem and increases the revision options by preserving the axial artery. Furthermore, the flap's vascular resistance plays a role in flap success. Reports have shown that muscle has less vascular resistance, while skin flaps have higher resistance, which implies when end-to-end anastomosis is performed one should use flaps with less resistance allowing the absorption of a high amount of flow into the flap.[35,36,37] In the days of perforator flaps and skin flaps, one should take this fact into consideration and perform end-to-side anastomosis to allow the best possible physiologic flow. Other than these two major types of anastomosis, T-shaped or flow-through anastomosis also plays an important role to preserve or to reconstruct distal flow.[38,39] In our experience, an extreme flow-through to reconstruct the injured major artery has shown to have a positive effect to combat infected wounds such as chronic osteomyelitis.[40] Thus, if a gap is noted in the axial artery, flow-through anastomosis or bypass for the artery defect should be considered for the best possible reconstruction[41,42] (▶ Fig. 9.3).

9.2.4 Perforators as Recipients

In lower extremity reconstruction, problems with axial arteries frequently arise; trauma may end up with single artery, elderly population and diabetics have poor perfusion from atherosclerosis, and steal phenomenon can lead to devastating outcome. Thus, the availability and reliability of the recipient artery are crucial in lower extremity reconstruction. Using the perforator vessel as the recipient can be an alternative to using major deep vessels that are difficult to reach and can avoid problems mentioned earlier.[31] Since a single perforator can provide adequate perfusion to a large territory of the skin, using the perforator as the recipient may be feasible to provide perfusion to a perforator flap while precluding the need for radical dissection to obtain recipient vessels as well as require long pedicles for a flap.[43] The key is to identify a good pulsating perforator. After locating the perforator under a loupe dissection, one can use the microscope to dissect further and confirm the pulse and flow of the perforator artery and vein (▶ Fig. 9.4). This minimal invasive approach to anastomose vessels can be especially useful when external fixators are in place, limiting the workspace.[31,44,45] With the perforator-to-perforator supermicrosurgery, the number of potential recipient vessels increases and is not limited to a few major vessels. The perforator artery is an end vessel with supply from multiple sources not only from the main artery but also from multiple branches. Even in the ischemic limb of the diabetic foot, the collateral forms the main artery, slowly undergoes arthrosclerosis, and is able to supply adequate perfusion to the perforator despite flow obstruction in major arteries.[46,47,48] Furthermore, the recipient pedicle may no longer require any predictable vessels other than a Doppler traceable perforator with an adequate caliber. Of course, there are limits to this approach such as using it as a recipient vessel for a reasonable perforator flap and not for a large flap or a chimeric flap that requires abundance of inflow.

9.3 Algorithm for Selecting Recipient Vessel

A successful lower extremity reconstruction using free flaps begins by identifying a good recipient vessel. In this chapter, we discussed various issues in regard to injured vessels, zone of injury, and the type of anastomosis. ▶ Fig. 9.5 shows an

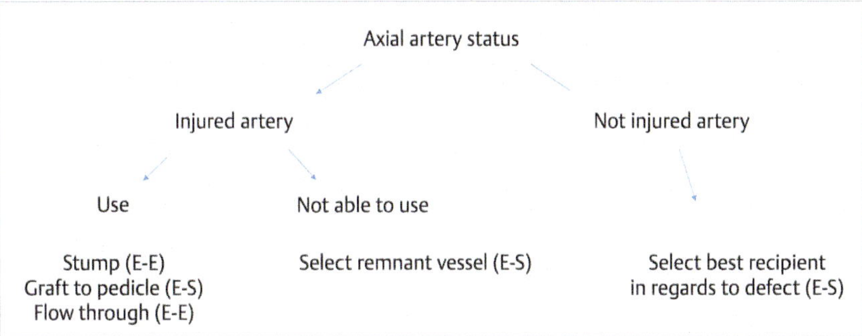

Fig. 9.5 An algorithm for selecting the axial artery as recipient is shown.

algorithm of approach. Note that all efforts are made to reconstitute the axial artery supply in case of artery defect and also to preserve the distal flow. Despite the concept of the zone of injury, wherever the recipient vessel is, the success of reconstruction after anastomosis depends on the quality of the recipient vascular status rather than the location. If angiogram is obtainable, one can better design the surgery by predicting the possible recipient candidates prior to surgery. One should also consider the composition of the flaps as the vascular resistance can be different and thus should avoid too much inflow to the flap. Using perforators allows us to avoid variables and may deliver an ideal flow to moderate-sized skin flaps while making the reconstruction minimally invasive. Since we started using this selection process, we were able to avoid using the cross-leg approach in the last 18 years of our practice. Nevertheless, the cross-leg approach, using the contralateral leg as the recipient, still remains the ultimate plan B.[49,50]

9.4 Conclusion

As mentioned, one should consider multiple factors when selecting the recipient vessel: status of the axial arteries, trying to preserve flow as much as possible, and extent and severity of the defect. However, the ultimate decision should be made on the table during surgery when the actual artery or vein is exposed and it shows signs of good pulsation and flow.

References

[1] Bosse MJ, MacKenzie EJ, Kellam JF, et al. An analysis of outcomes of reconstruction or amputation after leg-threatening injuries. N Engl J Med. 2002; 347(24):1924–1931

[2] Chung KC, Saddawi-Konefka D, Haase SC, Kaul G. A cost-utility analysis of amputation versus salvage for Gustilo type IIIB and IIIC open tibial fractures. Plast Reconstr Surg. 2009; 124(6):1965–1973

[3] Gottlieb LJ, Krieger LM. From the reconstructive ladder to the reconstructive elevator. Plast Reconstr Surg. 1994; 93(7):1503–1504

[4] Xiong L, Gazyakan E, Kremer T, et al. Free flaps for reconstruction of soft tissue defects in lower extremity: a meta-analysis on microsurgical outcome and safety. Microsurgery. 2016; 36(6):511–524

[5] Serafin D, Voci VE. Reconstruction of the lower extremity. Microsurgical composite tissue transplantation. Clin Plast Surg. 1983; 10(1):55–72

[6] Abdelfattah U, Power HA, Song S, Min K, Suh HP, Hong JP. Algorithm for free perforator flap selection in lower extremity reconstruction based on 563 cases. Plast Reconstr Surg. 2019; 144(5):1202–1213

[7] Lutz BS, Ng SH, Cabailo R, Lin CH, Wei FC. Value of routine angiography before traumatic lower-limb reconstruction with microvascular free tissue transplantation. J Trauma. 1998; 44(4):682–686

[8] Reddy V, Stevenson TR. MOC-PS(SM) CME article: lower extremity reconstruction. Plast Reconstr Surg. 2008; 121(4) Suppl:1–7

[9] Heller L, Levin LS. Lower extremity microsurgical reconstruction. Plast Reconstr Surg. 2001; 108(4):1029–1041, quiz 1042

[10] Dublin BA, Karp NS, Kasabian AK, Kolker AR, Shah MH. Selective use of preoperative lower extremity arteriography in free flap reconstruction. Ann Plast Surg. 1997; 38(4):404–407

[11] Duymaz A, Karabekmez FE, Vrtiska TJ, Mardini S, Moran SL. Free tissue transfer for lower extremity reconstruction: a study of the role of computed angiography in the planning of free tissue transfer in the posttraumatic setting. Plast Reconstr Surg. 2009; 124(2):523–529

[12] Haddock NT, Weichman KE, Reformat DD, Kligman BE, Levine JP, Saadeh PB. Lower extremity arterial injury patterns and reconstructive outcomes in patients with severe lower extremity trauma: a 26-year review. J Am Coll Surg. 2010; 210(1):66–72

[13] Wang Z, Yi X, He J, et al. Catheter-based computed tomography angiography in anterolateral thigh perforator mapping of Chinese patients. J Reconstr Microsurg. 2019; 35(3):221–228

[14] Mun GH, Lee SJ, Jeon BJ. Perforator topography of the thoracodorsal artery perforator flap. Plast Reconstr Surg. 2008; 121(2):497–504

[15] Masia J, Clavero JA, LarraC1aga J, Vives L, Pons G. Preoperative planning of the abdominal perforator flap with multidetector row computed tomography: 3 years of experience. Plast Reconstr Surg. 2008; 122(2):80e–81e

[16] Gaillard J, Bourcheix LM, Masquelet AC. Perforators of the fibular artery and suprafascial network. Surg Radiol Anat. 2018; 40(8):927–933

[17] Loos MS, Freeman BG, Lorenzetti A. Zone of injury: a critical review of the literature. Ann Plast Surg. 2010; 65(6):573–577

[18] Arnez ZM. Immediate reconstruction of the lower extremity: an update. Clin Plast Surg. 1991; 18(3):449–457

[19] CelikC6z B, Sengezer M, Isik S, et al. Subacute reconstruction of lower leg and foot defects due to high velocity-high energy injuries caused by gunshots, missiles, and land mines. Microsurgery. 2005; 25(1):3–14, discussion 15

[20] Godina M. Early microsurgical reconstruction of complex trauma of the extremities. Plast Reconstr Surg. 1986; 78(3):285–292

[21] Hallock GG. Liability of recipient vessels distal to the zone of injury when used for extremity free flaps. J Reconstr Microsurg. 1996; 12(2):89–92

[22] Freedman AM, Meland NB. Arteriovenous shunts in free vascularized tissue transfer for extremity reconstruction. Ann Plast Surg. 1989; 23(2):123–128

[23] Lin CH, Mardini S, Lin YT, Yeh JT, Wei FC, Chen HC. Sixty-five clinical cases of free tissue transfer using long arteriovenous fistulas or vein grafts. J Trauma. 2004; 56(5):1107–1117

[24] Yazar S, Lin CH. Selection of recipient vessel in traumatic lower extremity. J Reconstr Microsurg. 2012; 28(3):199–204

[25] Samaha FJ, Oliva A, Buncke GM, Buncke HJ, Siko PP. A clinical study of end-to-end versus end-to-side techniques for microvascular anastomosis. Plast Reconstr Surg. 1997; 99(4):1109–1111

[26] Stompro BE, Stcvcnson TR. Rcconstruction of thc traumatizcd lcg: usc of distally based free flaps. Plast Reconstr Surg. 1994; 93(5):1021–1025, discussion 1026-1027

[27] Kolker AR, Kasabian AK, Karp NS, Gottlieb JJ. Fate of free flap microanastomosis distal to the zone of injury in lower extremity trauma. Plast Reconstr Surg. 1997; 99(4):1068–1073

[28] Park S, Han SH, Lee TJ. Algorithm for recipient vessel selection in free tissue transfer to the lower extremity. Plast Reconstr Surg. 1999; 103(7):1937–1948

[29] Stranix JT, Borab ZM, Rifkin WJ, et al. Proximal versus distal recipient vessels in lower extremity reconstruction: a retrospective series and systematic review. J Reconstr Microsurg. 2018; 34(5):334–340

[30] Isenberg JS, Sherman R. Zone of injury: a valid concept in microvascular reconstruction of the traumatized lower limb? Ann Plast Surg. 1996; 36(3):270–272

[31] Hong JP. The use of supermicrosurgery in lower extremity reconstruction: the next step in evolution. Plast Reconstr Surg. 2009; 123(1):230–235
[32] Albertengo JB, Rodriguez A, Buncke HJ, Hall EJ. A comparative study of flap survival rates in end-to-end and end-to-side microvascular anastomosis. Plast Reconstr Surg. 1981; 67(2):194–199
[33] Cho EH, Garcia RM, Blau J, et al. Microvascular anastomoses using end-to-end versus end-to-side technique in lower extremity free tissue transfer. J Reconstr Microsurg. 2016; 32(2):114–120
[34] Godina M. Preferential use of end-to-side arterial anastomoses in free flap transfers. Plast Reconstr Surg. 1979; 64(5):673–682
[35] Takanari K, Kamei Y, Toriyama K, Yagi S, Torii S. Differences in blood flow volume and vascular resistance between free flaps: assessment in 58 cases. J Reconstr Microsurg. 2009; 25(1):39–45
[36] Sasmor MT, Reus WF, Straker DJ, Colen LB. Vascular resistance considerations in free-tissue transfer. J Reconstr Microsurg. 1992; 8(3):195–200
[37] Ono M, Takanari K, Toriyama K, et al. Effects of tissue component volumes on vascular resistance in free flaps. J Reconstr Microsurg. 2017; 33(1):32–39
[38] Kim JT, Kim CY, Kim YH. T-anastomosis in microsurgical free flap reconstruction: an overview of clinical applications. J Plast Reconstr Aesthet Surg. 2008; 61(10):1157–1163
[39] Verhelle NA, Heymans O. How to deal with difficult microsurgical end-to-side anastomoses. Microsurgery. 2005; 25(3):203–208
[40] Hong JPJ, Goh TLH, Choi DH, Kim JJ, Suh HS. The efficacy of perforator flaps in the treatment of chronic osteomyelitis. Plast Reconstr Surg. 2017; 140 (1):179–188
[41] Fernandez-Garrido M, Lopez Penha TR, Qiu SS. Flow-through flaps in the absence of an arterial gap for extremity defect reconstruction: minimizing the donor-site morbidity. J Reconstr Microsurg. 2019; 35(5):329–334
[42] Toia F, Zabbia G, Roggio T, Pirrello R, D'Arpa S, Cordova A. Vascular grafts and flow-through flaps for microsurgical lower extremity reconstruction. J Reconstr Microsurg. 2017; 33 S 01:S14–S19
[43] Saint-Cyr M, Wong C, Schaverien M, Mojallal A, Rohrich RJ. The perforasome theory: vascular anatomy and clinical implications. Plast Reconstr Surg. 2009; 124(5):1529–1544
[44] Kim KN, Hong JP, Park SW, Kim SW, Yoon CS. Overcoming the obstacles of the ilizarov device in extremity reconstruction: usefulness of the perforator as the recipient vessel. J Reconstr Microsurg. 2015; 31(6):420–425
[45] Hong JP, Koshima I. Using perforators as recipient vessels (supermicrosurgery) for free flap reconstruction of the knee region. Ann Plast Surg. 2010; 64 (3):291–293
[46] Suh HS, Oh TS, Lee HS, et al. A new approach for reconstruction of diabetic foot wounds using the angiosome and supermicrosurgery concept. Plast Reconstr Surg. 2016; 138(4):702e–709e
[47] Suh HP, Kim Y, Suh Y, Hong J. Multidetector computed tomography (CT) analysis of 168 cases in diabetic patients with total superficial femoral artery occlusion: is it safe to use an anterolateral thigh flap without CT angiography in diabetic patients? J Reconstr Microsurg. 2018; 34(1):65–70
[48] Suh HS, Oh TS, Hong JP. Innovations in diabetic foot reconstruction using supermicrosurgery. Diabetes Metab Res Rev. 2016; 32 Suppl 1:275–280
[49] Van Boerum MS, Wright T, McFarland M, Fiander M, Pannucci CJ. Cross-leg flaps for lower extremity salvage: a scoping review. J Reconstr Microsurg. 2019; 35(7):505–515
[50] Manrique OJ, Bishop SN, Ciudad P, et al. Lower extremity limb salvage with cross leg pedicle flap, cross leg free flap, and cross leg vascular cable bridge flap. J Reconstr Microsurg. 2018; 34(7):522–529

10 General Wound Preparation and Timing

Casey T. Kraft, Ibrahim Khansa, and Jeffrey E. Janis

Summary

With few exceptions, the lower extremity defect is rarely suitable for reconstruction at the time of initial presentation. Preoperative patient optimization such as by smoking cessation, assurance of adequate nutrition, diabetes management with glucose control, and correction of any vascular insufficiencies will allow superior wound healing and lessen the risk of complications. The timing of wound closure is then controversial, but preferably before the onset of the subacute phase and definitely not until initial irrigation to remove contaminants and lessen any risk of infection, followed by serial debridement that removes all nonviable elements and residual biofilm, has been completed.

Keywords: nutrition, debridement, biofilm, timing of wound closure

10.1 Introduction

Lower extremity reconstruction can be necessary for multiple reasons, ranging from traumatic injury to oncologic extirpation to infection and osteomyelitis. Except for immediate reconstruction after tumor resection, the wound is rarely ready for the final repair at the index presentation. Preparation of the wound and timing of the reconstruction are two variables of paramount importance to consider for optimizing outcomes.

10.2 Patient Optimization

Whenever possible, proper patient optimization can have a substantial positive impact on the outcome in the elective setting. For example, smoking is well known to be detrimental to wound healing and tissue vascularity.[1,2] Preoperative and postoperative smoking cessation has been shown to reduce surgical complication rates.[3] Patients should abstain from nicotine use for at least 4 weeks before and 4 weeks after any elective surgery in order to reduce complication rates to the lowest possible level, although it is never superior to that of the nonsmoker.[2]

Nutrition is also a critical consideration, as protein deficiency, particularly deficiencies of arginine and methionine, is known to have a substantial deleterious impact on wound healing. Preoperative nutritional support has been shown to reduce the rates of infectious and noninfectious surgical complications.[4,5] Therefore, serum nutritional markers should be checked and optimized preoperatively, with a goal for a serum albumin greater than 3.25 g/dL, and serum prealbumin greater than 15 mg/dL.[2]

In diabetic patients with lower extremity ulcers, perioperative glucose control is of paramount importance. The risk of surgical-site infections increases proportionately to serum glucose above 110 mg/dL,[6] and even a single perioperative instance of serum glucose greater than 200 mg/dL has been found to significantly increase the risk of wound dehiscence.[7] Hemoglobin A1c should be ≤ 7.5% before any elective surgery is undertaken to optimize outcomes.[2]

Patients with compromised vascular inflow into the lower extremity, whether due to medical comorbidities or trauma, must have a vascular profile of that limb meticulously evaluated and optimized before reconstruction is attempted. The potential for healing is enhanced when the periwound transcutaneous partial pressure of oxygen is 40 mm Hg or greater.[8]

Prior to any reconstruction in the trauma patient, stability of homeostatic mechanisms always takes precedence. A full standard trauma survey of all systems must be completed, and then repeated routinely. If lower limb vascular injuries are identified, a preoperative angiogram can provide invaluable diagnostic data, and ascertain the need for vascular surgery intervention. Depending on the circumstances and risk of a compartment syndrome, fasciotomies may be required. Fractures must next be reduced and stabilized. Finally, thorough irrigation and debridement of the wound bed is a fundamental and critical cornerstone for success. The ultimate choice of reconstructive modality must take into account the exposure of vital structures, such as tendon, bone, nerve, and blood vessel.

10.3 Timing of Lower Extremity Coverage after Trauma

Timing of posttraumatic lower extremity reconstruction has been debated in the literature for decades. A landmark study by Godina in 1986 dramatically influenced the timing of posttraumatic lower extremity reconstruction in open tibia–fibula fractures.[9] In this study, 532 patients were categorized into three groups based on timing of free flap reconstruction after trauma: less than 72 hours (acute), 72 hours to 3 months (subacute), and greater than 3 months (chronic). Godina found that coverage in the acute phase resulted in the lowest rates of postoperative infection, flap failure, bone healing time, and hospital length of stay. Coverage in the subacute period resulted in the worst outcomes. As a result, early flap coverage of open tibia–fibula fractures within 72 hours of injury has generally been proposed as the ideal time for reconstruction.

Similarly, Byrd et al emphasized the importance of thorough debridement and acute (defined as within 5 days) microsurgical coverage of open tibia–fibula fractures.[10] They classified open tibial fractures based on the amount of energy involved in the trauma, the degree of bone comminution, and the extent of soft-tissue injury. Higher-grade injuries were characterized by greater bone fragmentation and bacterial colonization, and thus had worse outcomes.

Other studies have sought to challenge the acute coverage paradigm. Francel et al argued that good surgical and functional outcomes are achievable when reconstruction is performed up to 15 days after Gustilo grade IIIB tibia–fibula fractures.[11] However, these good outcomes are predicated on meticulous wound debridement with excision of any necrotic tissue or debris, and serial washouts. Emphasis was placed on debridement of devitalized bone, which may otherwise form a sequestrum and subsequent nidus for infection. Recent military experience has also demonstrated that delaying reconstruction to the subacute time period, with intervening serial debridements, has an acceptable complication rate for reconstruction.[12,13,14]

Negative-pressure wound therapy (NPWT) is one of the advancements that have facilitated delayed lower extremity reconstruction. NPWT has been shown to promote granulation tissue formation, enhance wound contraction,[15,16,17] remove inflammatory cytokines and metalloproteinases,[18] and decrease bacterial burden.[19] By delaying reconstruction with the use of NPWT, tissue edema can decrease, and areas of necrosis are allowed to demarcate.[13,20] NPWT therefore serves as a valuable dressing between serial debridements, but always in the preparation for definitive reconstruction. A novel advance in NPWT is the addition of instillation therapy, whereby the negative suction is intermittently interrupted for a few minutes, and saline or a topical antiseptic is instilled into the wound, allowed to dwell, and then suctioned out. NPWT with instillation significantly reduces wound bacterial contamination.[21,22]

At the time of serial debridement, the surgeon should obtain quantitative bacterial tissue culture. A positive quantitative culture may warrant further debridement before reconstruction, as reconstruction in the setting of a positive culture has been shown to portend significantly higher complication rates.[23]

10.4 Wound Bed Preparation

Wound bed preparation is the most critical step to ensure successful lower extremity reconstruction. Multiple methods of cleansing wounds exist, but the fundamental principles of removing foreign bodies and debriding devitalized tissue are the ultimate focus of all methods of wound bed preparation.

Irrigation is the initial step in cleansing a contaminated or infected wound. It allows for the simple removal of foreign bodies and contaminated tissue. Normal saline is the most common solution used, and there is little evidence to suggest any sustained benefit to additives such as antibiotics or detergents.[24] The irrigation may be delivered to the wound under low pressure (1–15 psi), such as cystoscopy tubing, or under high pressure, such as pulsed lavage (35–70 psi).[25] Some literature has suggested that high-pressure irrigation may be more effective at reducing bacterial counts and wound infection rates.[26,27] However, there is also concern that high-pressure irrigation causes soft-tissue damage[28] and bacterial propagation into deeper tissues, such as bone.[29]

The second step in wound preparation is complete debridement of any necrotic tissue. The goal of debridement is to achieve residual tissues that are clean, viable, and free from contamination (▶ Fig. 10.1). A goal of debridement is also to address and remove bacterial biofilm. Bacteria encased in biofilm are especially resilient even in the face of antibiotic therapy.[30] Surgical debridement temporarily converts bacteria in the biofilm to a planktonic state, rendering them more susceptible to antimicrobial treatment.

Surgeons who are comfortable with reconstruction may be more aggressive at making a wound larger through debridement, knowing that they will be able to cover the resulting defect. In the traumatic wound, sharp excisional debridement is the most commonly used modality. This can be performed with conventional surgical instruments, such as scalpels, scissors,

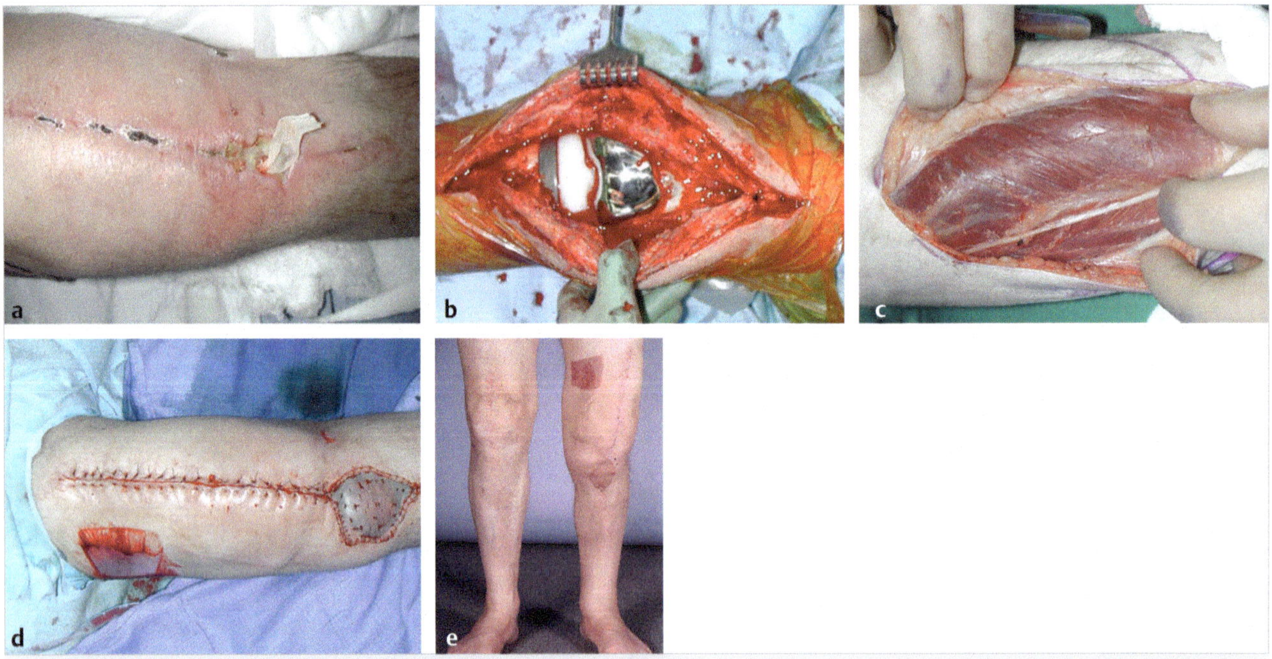

Fig. 10.1 Coverage of total knee arthroplasty wound compromise. **(a)** Following left total knee arthroplasty, the surgical incision became a nonhealing, draining wound. **(b)** The wound was excised sharply in its entirety. All necrotic tissue was radically excised. The original wound did track down to the implant, but the implant did not appear to be infected. The wound was then irrigated copiously with normal saline at low pressure. **(c)** A medial gastrocnemius muscle flap was chosen as the reconstructive modality. **(d)** The medial gastrocnemius flap after transposition provided healthy, well-vascularized tissue to cover the implant, and fill all dead space. A split-thickness skin graft was applied onto the muscle. **(e)** The patient healed uneventfully and was able to progress to normal ambulation.

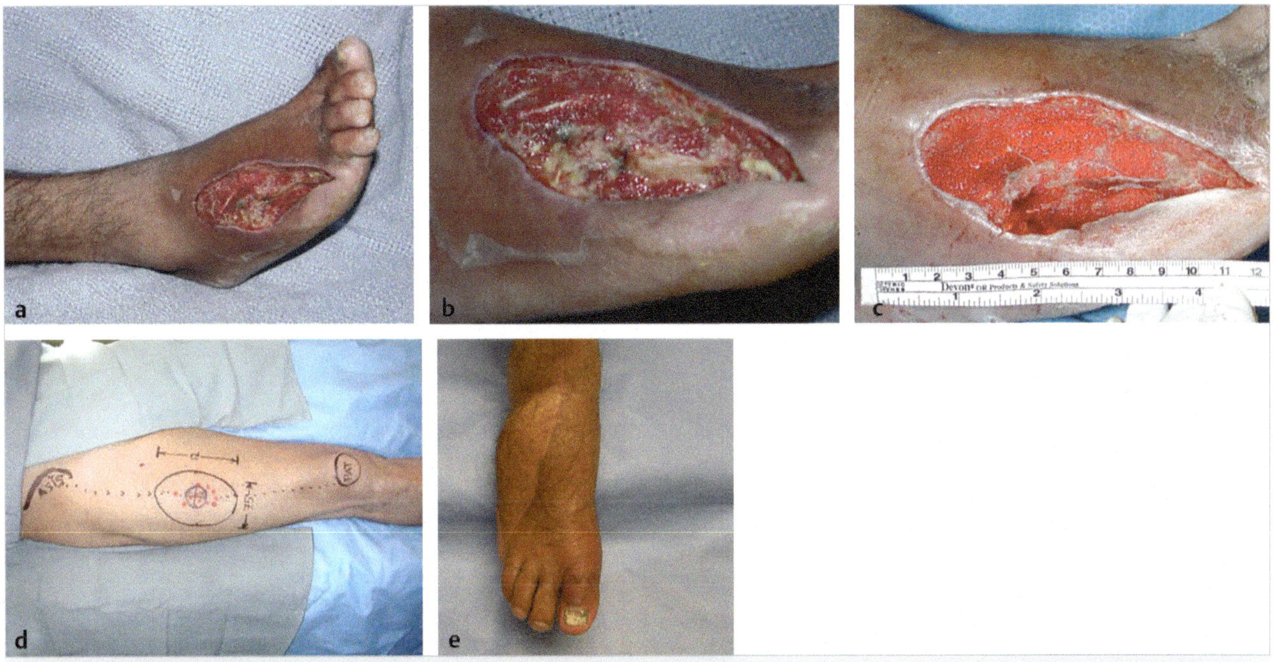

Fig. 10.2 Preparation and coverage of a diabetic foot ulcer. **(a)** This poorly controlled diabetic had had a previous small toe amputation. He then developed a nonhealing ulcer over the lateral aspect of his dorsal foot, with exposed metatarsal bone. **(b)** Closer evaluation of the wound revealed not only the exposed metatarsal bone, but also a moderate amount of necrotic tissue and fibrinous exudate. **(c)** After optimization of glucose control, all fibrinous and necrotic material in the wound was debrided with the use of a hydrosurgical debrider. The remaining wound bed was then cleaned, with healthy bleeding tissue at its base. **(d)** To cover the exposed bone, an anterolateral thigh free flap was chosen. **(e)** Healing was then uneventful, allowing ambulation with full weight bearing.

and curettes. Debridement can also be achieved with hydrosurgery (Versajet, Smith & Nephew, Cambridge, UK), which uses a high-speed stream of water to generate a localized vacuum via the Venturi effect (▶ Fig. 10.2), with the subsequent removal of nonadherent tissue.[31,32] Hydrosurgery has been found to be more efficient and result in less blood loss than conventional sharp debridement.[33] It also has been shown to more effectively address biofilm than mechanical debridement alone[34] or high-pressure pulsed lavage.[35]

In nontraumatic wounds, such as pressure ulcers, diabetic ulcers, and venous ulcers, sharp surgical debridement is also the mainstay of treatment. However, other nonsurgical options for debridement, such as enzymatic debridement using collagenase or papain urea, are available when surgery is not an option.[36,37]

10.5 Conclusion

Lower extremity reconstruction can be a challenge for even the most experienced reconstructive surgeon. Preparation and proper timing can have a significant impact on the overall success of the reconstruction. Fundamental principles of patient optimization, adequate debridement and clearance of infection, and expeditious reconstruction onto a healthy wound bed can lay the foundation for ultimate success.

References

[1] Krueger JK, Rohrich RJ. Clearing the smoke: the scientific rationale for tobacco abstention with plastic surgery. Plast Reconstr Surg. 2001; 108(4):1063–1073, discussion 1074–1077

[2] Harrison B, Khansa I, Janis JE. Evidence-based strategies to reduce postoperative complications in plastic surgery. Plast Reconstr Surg. 2016; 137(1):351–360

[3] Møller AM, Villebro N, Pedersen T, Tønnesen H. Effect of preoperative smoking intervention on postoperative complications: a randomised clinical trial. Lancet. 2002; 359(9301):114–117

[4] Veterans Affairs Total Parenteral Nutrition Cooperative Study Group. Perioperative total parenteral nutrition in surgical patients. N Engl J Med. 1991; 325(8):525–532

[5] Jie B, Jiang ZM, Nolan MT, et al. Impact of nutritional support on clinical outcome in patients at nutritional risk: a multicenter, prospective cohort study in Baltimore and Beijing teaching hospitals. Nutrition. 2010; 26(11–12):1088–1093

[6] Ramos M, Khalpey Z, Lipsitz S, et al. Relationship of perioperative hyperglycemia and postoperative infections in patients who undergo general and vascular surgery. Ann Surg. 2008; 248(4):585–591

[7] Endara M, Masden D, Goldstein J, Gondek S, Steinberg J, Attinger C. The role of chronic and perioperative glucose management in high-risk surgical closures: a case for tighter glycemic control. Plast Reconstr Surg. 2013; 132(4):996–1004

[8] Arsenault KA, McDonald J, Devereaux PJ, Thorlund K, Tittley JG, Whitlock RP. The use of transcutaneous oximetry to predict complications of chronic wound healing: a systematic review and meta-analysis. Wound Repair Regen. 2011; 19(6):657–663

[9] Godina M. Early microsurgical reconstruction of complex trauma of the extremities. Plast Reconstr Surg. 1986; 78(3):285–292

[10] Byrd HS, Spicer TE, Cierney G, III. Management of open tibial fractures. Plast Reconstr Surg. 1985; 76(5):719–730

[11] Francel TJ, Vander Kolk CA, Hoopes JE, Manson PN, Yaremchuk MJ. Microvascular soft-tissue transplantation for reconstruction of acute open tibial fractures: timing of coverage and long-term functional results. Plast Reconstr Surg. 1992; 89(3):478–487, discussion 488–489

[12] Pollak AN, Ficke JR, Extremity War Injuries III Session Moderators. Extremity war injuries: challenges in definitive reconstruction. J Am Acad Orthop Surg. 2008; 16(11):628–634

[13] Baechler MF, Groth AT, Nesti LJ, Martin BD. Soft tissue management of war wounds to the foot and ankle. Foot Ankle Clin. 2010; 15(1):113–138

[14] Kumar AR, Grewal NS, Chung TL, Bradley JP. Lessons from operation Iraqi freedom: successful subacute reconstruction of complex lower extremity battle injuries. Plast Reconstr Surg. 2009; 123(1):218–229

[15] Parrett BM, Matros E, Pribaz JJ, Orgill DP. Lower extremity trauma: trends in the management of soft-tissue reconstruction of open tibia-fibula fractures. Plast Reconstr Surg. 2006; 117(4):1315–1322, discussion 1323–1324

[16] DeFranzo AJ, Argenta LC, Marks MW, et al. The use of vacuum-assisted closure therapy for the treatment of lower-extremity wounds with exposed bone. Plast Reconstr Surg. 2001; 108(5):1184–1191

[17] Argenta LC, Morykwas MJ. Vacuum-assisted closure: a new method for wound control and treatment: clinical experience. Ann Plast Surg. 1997; 38(6): 563–576, discussion 577

[18] Mouës CM, van Toorenenbergen AW, Heule F, Hop WC, Hovius SER. The role of topical negative pressure in wound repair: expression of biochemical markers in wound fluid during wound healing. Wound Repair Regen. 2008; 16(4):488–494

[19] Morykwas MJ, Argenta LC, Shelton-Brown EI, McGuirt W. Vacuum-assisted closure: a new method for wound control and treatment: animal studies and basic foundation. Ann Plast Surg. 1997; 38(6):553–562

[20] Hou Z, Irgit K, Strohecker KA, et al. Delayed flap reconstruction with vacuum-assisted closure management of the open IIIB tibial fracture. J Trauma. 2011; 71(6):1705–1708

[21] Davis K, Bills J, Barker J, Kim P, Lavery L. Simultaneous irrigation and negative pressure wound therapy enhances wound healing and reduces wound bioburden in a porcine model. Wound Repair Regen. 2013; 21(6):869–875

[22] Phillips PL, Yang Q, Schultz GS. The effect of negative pressure wound therapy with periodic instillation using antimicrobial solutions on Pseudomonas aeruginosa biofilm on porcine skin explants. Int Wound J. 2013; 10 Suppl 1: 48–55

[23] Shuck J, Nolan J, Kanuri A, et al. The effect of positive post-debridement cultures on local muscle flap reconstruction of the lower extremity. Plast Reconstr Surg. 2015; 136 Suppl 4S:9–10

[24] Petrisor B, Sun X, Bhandari M, et al. FLOW Investigators. Fluid lavage of open wounds (FLOW): a multicenter, blinded, factorial pilot trial comparing alternative irrigating solutions and pressures in patients with open fractures. J Trauma. 2011; 71(3):596–606

[25] Sullivan SR, Engrav LH, Klein MB. Basic surgical and perioperative considerations: acute wound care. ACS Surgery: Principles and Practice. Philadelphia, PA: ACS; 2007

[26] Brown LL, Shelton HT, Bornside GH, Cohn I, Jr. Evaluation of wound irrigation by pulsatile jet and conventional methods. Ann Surg. 1978; 187(2):170–173

[27] Stevenson TR, Thacker JG, Rodeheaver GT, Bacchetta C, Edgerton MT, Edlich RF. Cleansing the traumatic wound by high pressure syringe irrigation. JACEP. 1976; 5(1):17–21

[28] Boyd JI, III, Wongworawat MD. High-pressure pulsatile lavage causes soft tissue damage. Clin Orthop Relat Res. 2004(427):13–17

[29] Hassinger SM, Harding G, Wongworawat MD. High-pressure pulsatile lavage propagates bacteria into soft tissue. Clin Orthop Relat Res. 2005; 439(439): 27–31

[30] Anghel EL, DeFazio MV, Barker JC, Janis JE, Attinger CE. Current concepts in debridement: science and strategies. Plast Reconstr Surg. 2016; 138(3) Suppl:82S–93S

[31] Janis J, Harrison B. Wound healing: Part II. Clinical applications. Plast Reconstr Surg. 2014; 133(3):383e–392e

[32] Klein MB, Hunter S, Heimbach DM, et al. The Versajet water dissector: a new tool for tangential excision. J Burn Care Rehabil. 2005; 26(6):483–487

[33] Liu J, Galiano JH, Chukwu CS, Krol J. Comparing the Versajet hydrosurgery system to conventional debridement techniques for the treatment of delayed healing wounds: a prospective, randomized clinical trial to investigate clinical efficacy and cost-effectiveness. Plast Reconstr Surg. 2012; 130:41

[34] Davis SC, Martinez L, Kirsner R. The diabetic foot: the importance of biofilms and wound bed preparation. Curr Diab Rep. 2006; 6(6):439–445

[35] Granick MS, Posnett J, Jacoby M, Noruthun S, Ganchi PA, Datiashvili RO. Efficacy and cost-effectiveness of a high-powered parallel waterjet for wound debridement. Wound Repair Regen. 2006; 14(4):394–397

[36] Lee LK, Ambrus JL. Collagenase therapy for decubitus ulcers. Geriatrics. 1975; 30(5):91–93, 97–98

[37] Alvarez OM, Fernandez-Obregon A, Rogers RS, Bergamo L, Masso J, Black M. A prospective, randomized, comparative study of collagenase and papain-urea for pressure ulcer debridement. Wounds. 2002; 14:293–301

11 The Pertinence of the Reconstructive Ladder and the Reconstructive Elevator

Patrick L. Reavey and Lawrence J. Gottlieb

Summary
If the goal in salvaging a lower limb were to just close the wound, then the stepwise approach beginning at the bottom rung of the reconstructive ladder that first chooses the simplest and least surgically morbid option would be considered, moving upward toward more complex alternatives only if unavoidable. Yet the reconstructive ladder is a flawed concept in that the goal initially should be instead the best *long-term* solution, and not just a solution. This can be best obtained by taking the reconstructive elevator to reach that floor where all the available choices can be scrutinized to allow an optimum selection process that will then obtain the desired durable, functional, as well as aesthetic outcome.

Keywords: reconstructive ladder, reconstructive elevator, long-term solution

11.1 Introduction

Descriptions and definitions of the *reconstructive ladder* permeate the literature and every discussion of reconstructive surgery. Medical students, surgical residents, and fellows are often still taught to approach wounds, traumatic injuries, and even congenital deformities within the framework of the reconstructive ladder (▶ Fig. 11.1). However, the reconstructive ladder is a flawed concept in that it implies that our reconstructive thought process should sequentially "go up" a ladder rather than directly to the best reconstructive option. The phrase *reconstructive elevator* was originally introduced to better describe the contemplative principles and practice of plastic surgery.[1] There are few, if any, areas of plastic surgery where the power and implications of the reconstructive elevator are as pertinent as in lower extremity reconstruction.

The difference between a *reconstructive ladder* and a *reconstructive elevator* may seem to be a mere nuance of semantics. However, semantics are important. They shape our perceptions and frame our discussions. When used appropriately, they expand our horizons. When used inappropriately, they limit them. Remember that the best *long-term* solution, not just a solution, should then be that chosen initially. And that requires consideration of ALL options, any of which can be reached best by using the *reconstructive elevator.*

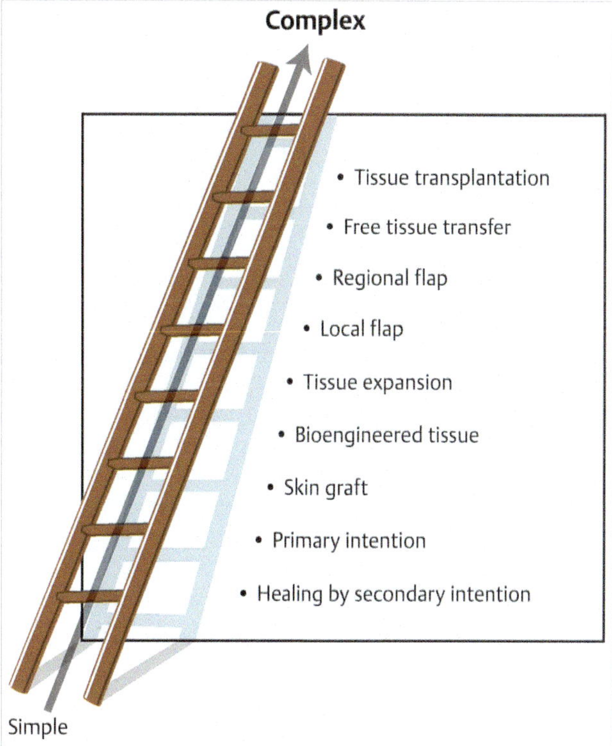

Fig. 11.1 The *reconstructive ladder* has a sequential approach to wound closure beginning with the simplest option adequate to close the wound starting at the bottom rung, then proceeding upward to more complex alternatives if indicated.

11.2 From Wound Closure to Reconstruction

To understand the flaws of the reconstructive ladder and the strengths of the reconstructive elevator, we must look at the origins of the terms. The reconstructive ladder is an improper extension of the well-known and appropriate concept of a *wound-closure* ladder. The wound-closure ladder signifies the stepwise algorithm used to decide on a wound-closure technique. It mandates starting with the simplest, least complex closure possibility, and then progress up the ladder only when required. For example, a clean, open wound that cannot be closed edge to edge would next be closed with a skin graft. If the wound bed would not support a skin graft, as if because of exposed bone without periosteum, then one would typically go up to the next rung of the wound-closure ladder and use a flap to close the wound.

This concept of wound-closure ladder has its roots with the ancient Egyptians. The Smith Papyrus, written sometime between 2,600 and 200 BC, taught methods to treat different types of wounds. The papyrus advised that simple wounds should be "drawn together with ydr [suture]." Other wounds should be closed with "awy" strips with gum adhesive, while the infected wound cannot be closed immediately and should be treated with topical dressings including honey and sycamore leaves.[2]

The move from just wound closure to true reconstruction began in India around 600 BC when Sushruta described the reconstruction of noses with skin pedicled from the forehead—the first description of a technique that has evolved into the modern forehead flap. Their concern for preserving both form and function is linked to these principles of the ancient Indians, and marked the beginning of the modern era of plastic surgery. Where the concept of a wound-closure ladder is as accurate today as it was for the ancient Egyptians, the notion of a reconstructive ladder became obsolete with the ancient Indians and remains so.

The evolution of true lower extremity reconstruction then followed advances in the understanding of wound healing and the development of advanced surgical techniques. Due to its complex anatomy and wide spectrum of injuries, lower extremity reconstruction has lagged behind other areas of the body. Lower extremity amputation was the rule for most significant lower extremity wounds from the time of Hippocrates (460–370 BC) to that of Ambroise Pare (1509–1590). Ollier (1825–1900) developed the "occlusive technique" utilizing plaster of Paris for rest of the injured extremity. During the first World War, Winnett Orr combined the "closed plaster treatment" with incisional drainage of wounds. Joseph Trueta, in the Spanish Civil War (1935–1938), expanded on the closed treatment by performing surgical debridement of the wound prior to the placement of a plaster splint. Change was slow. Wounds were left to granulate and heal by secondary intention. Amputation rates may have decreased significantly, but postfracture osteomyelitis occurred in nearly 80% of patients. During World War II, the availability of antibiotics when added to Trueta technique decreased the rate of osteomyelitis to 25%.[3]

These historically poor results demonstrate the inadequacy of the *reconstructive ladder* in the lower extremity. Wounds of the lower extremity often involved and still do underlying fractures, or the exposure of vital structures in an area with a paucity of redundant vascular soft tissue. While the wounds may have been "closed" with the Trueta approach, the final result was often less than satisfactory. Early methods to compensate for inadequate soft tissues included the cross-leg flap described by Hamilton and tubed pedicle flaps by Gilles. Yet these techniques were time-consuming, required multiple operations, and often resulted in joint contractures and inhibited ambulatory function that as an option may have been no better.

11.3 The Modern Era of Lower Extremity Reconstruction

It was not until the discovery of regional lower extremity flaps in the 1960s that true reconstruction of the lower extremity became practical. The development of microsurgery in the 1970s, reintroduction of lower extremity fasciocutaneous flaps in the 1980s,[4] and expansion of the angiosome concept[5,6] that led to perforator free flaps and local free-style perforator flaps[7,8,9,10,11] increased the options for flaps while decreasing donor site morbidity. Suprafascial thin adipocutaneous flaps and perforator-to-perforator free tissue transfer utilizing supermicrosurgical techniques are the ultimate extension of this experience.[12,13] In many cases, these now established techniques allow for the closure of lower extremity wounds that may otherwise have required amputation.

With the advent of local perforator flaps, and perforator-to-perforator free flaps, one could say that more rungs have been added to the reconstructive ladder. However, this advancement is more appropriately viewed as an adoption of parallel thinking required within the reconstructive elevator (▶ Fig. 11.2). When the goal is not to just close a wound but also to maximize form and function and minimize donor-site morbidity, pick the best floor possible by taking the reconstructive elevator to choose which of the similar yet different options would be the more suitable.

11.4 The Reconstructive Elevator and the Lower Extremity

To reiterate in this era when form *and* function must be the goal, the concept of the reconstructive elevator implies that simplest is not necessarily the best. To think sequentially about what is the next better reconstruction option no longer suffices. Modern technology and advanced techniques have made such thinking obsolete. Reconstructive surgery as we now know it requires parallel, creative thought processes rather than simple sequential thinking. The reconstructive surgeon must be capable of skipping a rung of the ladder and take the elevator up to the next floor or two when necessary.

When approaching a challenging lower extremity defect using the concept of the reconstructive elevator, the most important step for the surgeon is to consider the outcome possible due to surgical intervention for that specific patient. Is the goal of the surgery to get the wound closed with minimal additional morbidity or anesthetic time for the patient? Is the goal of the surgery to close the wound maximizing the aesthetic and functional result for the patient? Is the goal of the surgery to close the wound and reconstruct other vital structures such as tendon, bone, or nerve? The answers to these questions often depend not only on the characteristics of the wound, but also on factors specific to the patient such as their anesthetic risk, potential functional status, and need for future procedures or postoperative adjunctive therapy such as radiation.

Sometimes clinical examples will better clarify these points. Consider the case of a patient with a soft-tissue defect after tumor extirpation (▶ Fig. 11.3). If the only goal were to close the wound, the Trueta technique of letting it heal by secondary intention may be adequate. Alternatively, a skin graft could be used to shorten the healing time with less risk of scar contracture. However, if the goal is to not only close the wound but also to provide long-term stable coverage that best tolerates the shear forces that constantly impinge on the lower limb, restore an optimal soft-tissue contour, and minimize any potential of joint contracture, then it would be appropriate to skip the lower rungs of the ladder and jump on the elevator to proceed with the best flap coverage.

Consider also a patient who had an injury resulting in both a segmental loss of the distal Achilles tendon and the overlying soft tissue. A sequential plan using the reconstructive ladder might indicate a reverse sural flap to close the wound, but without tendon reconstruction, to be the most appropriate next step. This, however, could result in life-long use of an ankle foot orthotic or multiple secondary operations to reconstruct the Achilles tendon. Alternatively, one could jump on the elevator and both close the wound and reconstruct the Achilles tendon in a single stage using a conjoined anterolateral thigh free flap

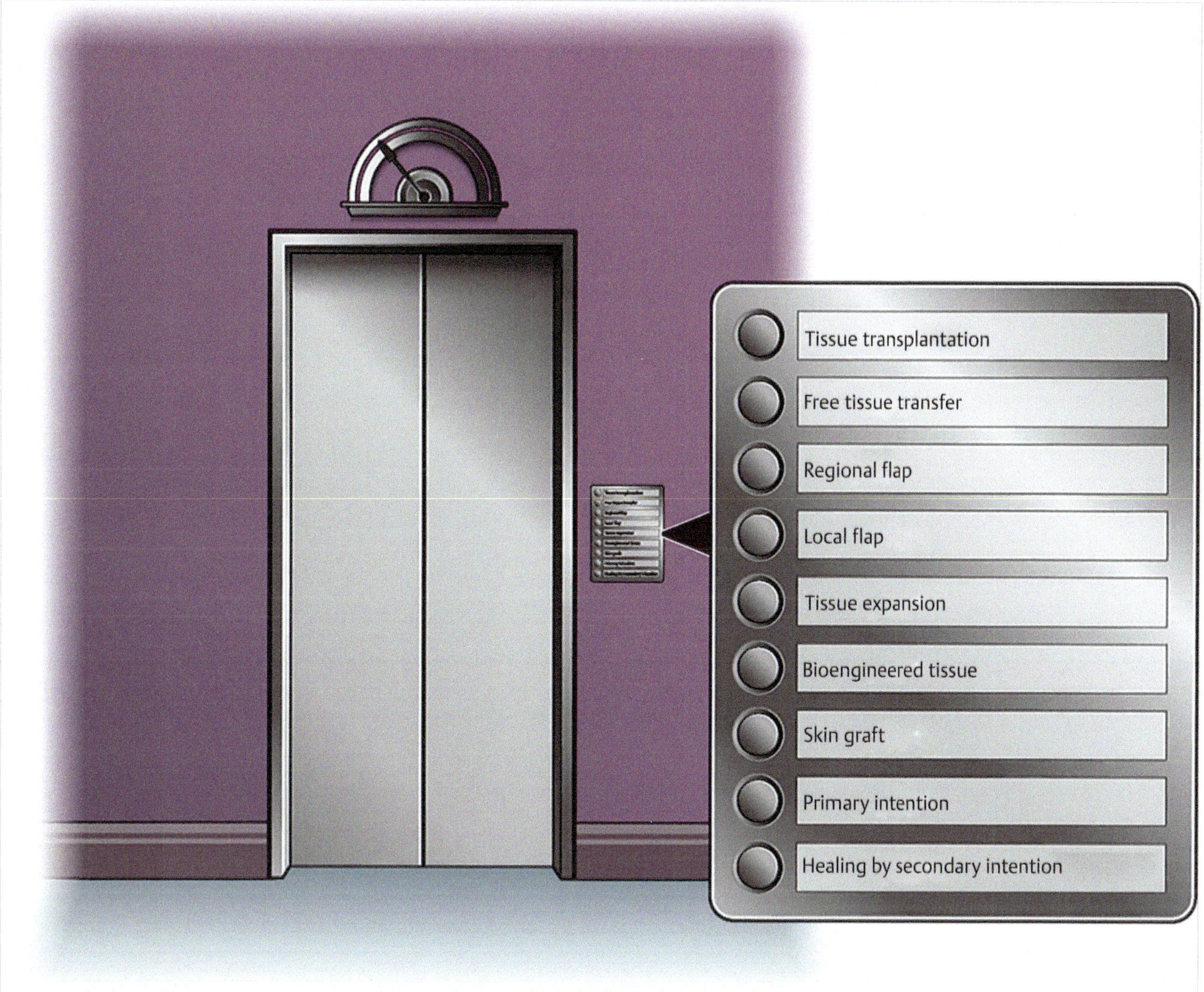

Fig. 11.2 Although options for reconstruction are arranged from simple to complex from the ground floor to the penthouse, multiple alternatives of similar complexity can be found on each "floor." One "takes the elevator up" to that floor where the surgical approach will best match the reconstructive goals.

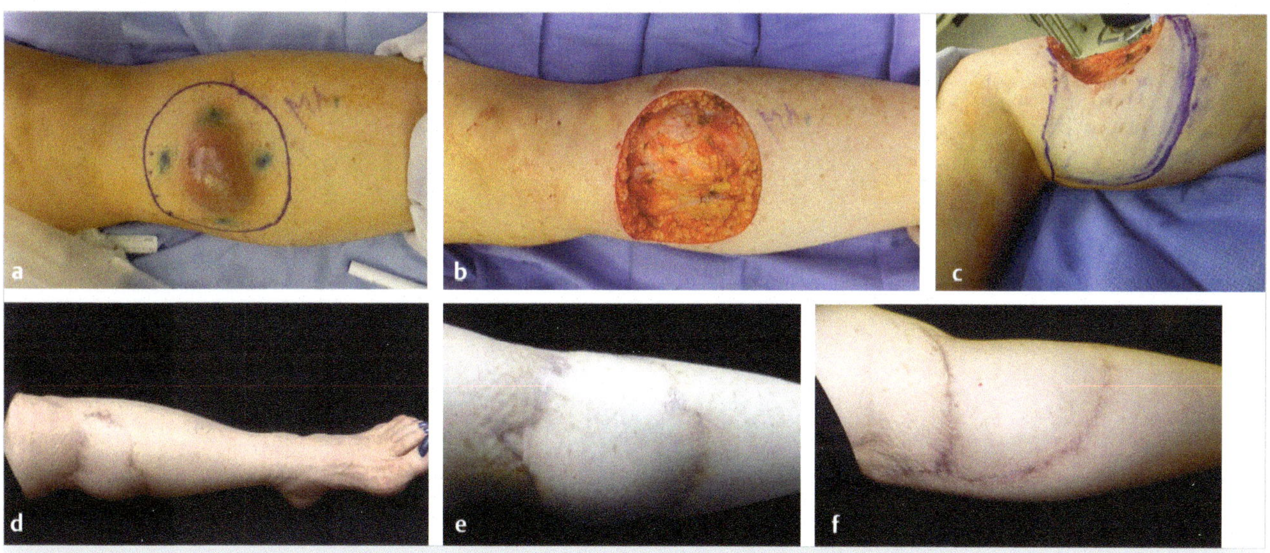

Fig. 11.3 An elderly woman with a melanoma of her left proximal pretibial area. **(a)** Planned resection. **(b)** resulting 10 × 12 cm defect overlying the tibia. **(c)** contour deformity seen on lateral view, with medial sural-based advancement flap designed to close the wound and restore the contour discrepancy. **(d–f)** Multiple views of stable result at 6 months. Using the *reconstructive ladder*, a skin graft would have provided adequate wound closure, but that would have provided inferior durability over the tibia as well as creating a nonaesthetic result.

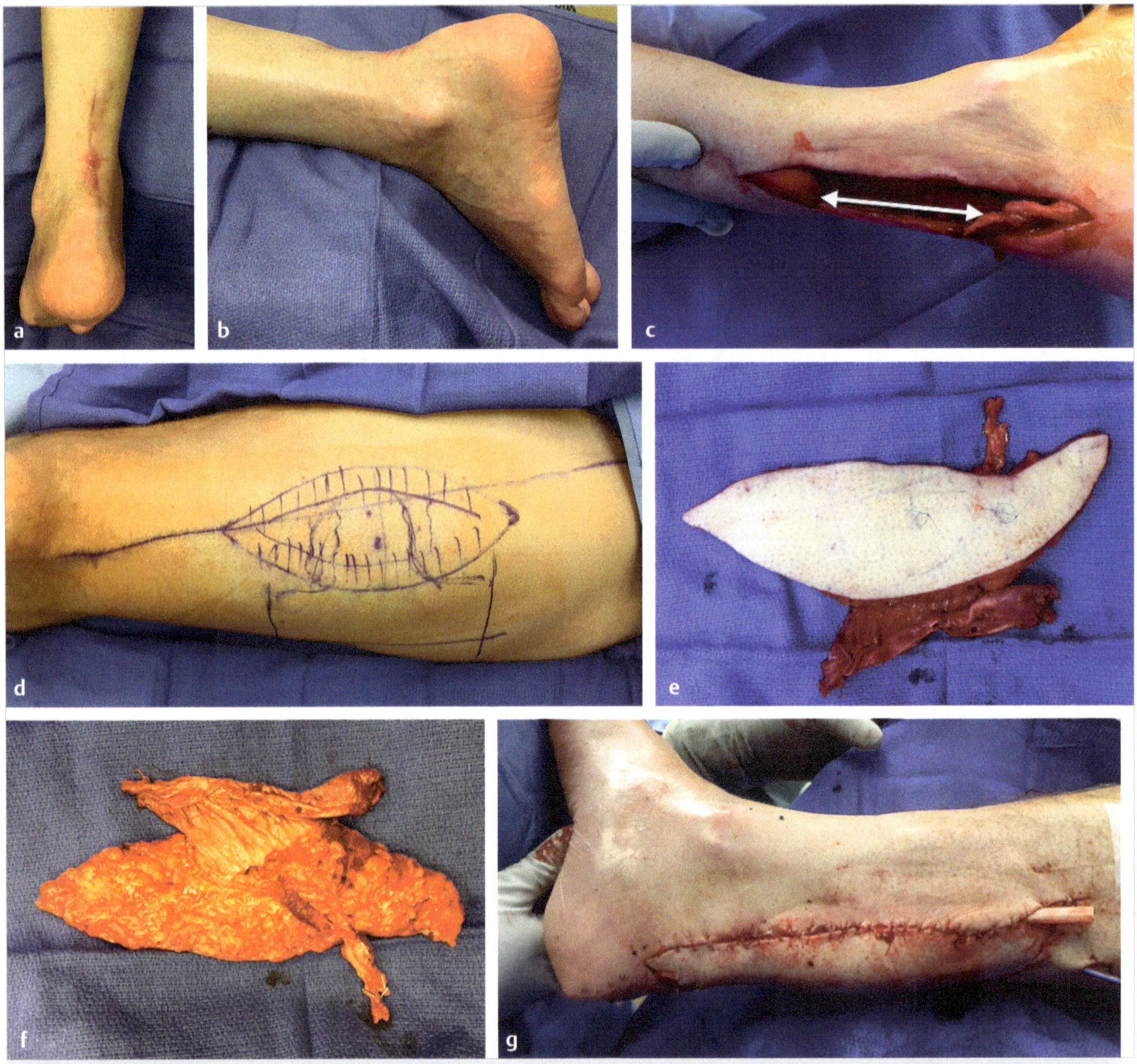

Fig. 11.4 (a, b) A middle-aged man who had primary Achilles tendon repair that got infected, requiring wide debridement and secondary wound closure that left a contour deformity. **(c)** After recreation of the defect. The *arrow* demonstrates an 8-cm Achilles tendon gap. **(d)** Design of conjoined anterolateral thigh (ALT) flap with attached rectangle of vascularized tensor fascia lata (TFL) inferiorly, intended to be then tubed to reconstruct the Achilles tendon. **(e, f)** Anterior and undersurface of thinned ALT free flap with attached TFL tube. **(g)** Flap inset.
If using the *reconstructive ladder* approach, the preoperative result **(a, b)** would be considered adequate, although the patient might later require an ankle orthotic for stability and to reasonably ambulate.

along with vascularized fascia lata (▶ Fig. 11.4, ▶ Fig. 11.5). In these examples, prioritizing both form and function necessitated choosing the better option, even if a simpler yet less ideal option was feasible.

11.5 Conclusion

When faced with a lower extremity defect or deformity of whatever etiology, priorities and goals for any planned reconstruction must be carefully scrutinized. Is the goal to close the wound or reconstruct the part? If the goal is simply to close the wound, then use the sequential thought process of the wound-closure ladder to choose the simplest and least morbid possible method. However, if the goal is to reconstruct a missing part, then the "best" method reached by using the elevator should be taken to obtain the desired aesthetic, functional, and mechanical outcome.

The intent of this textbook is to include a multitude of practical options for reconstructing defects of the lower extremity, and admittedly is organized in a sequential fashion from the simple to the complex. However, this arrangement is for the sake of simplicity, so do not be fooled in thinking that this implies one should always use a sequential or reconstructive ladder approach to lower extremity reconstruction. Strict adherence to the reconstructive ladder concept leaves the plastic surgeon handcuffed. The reconstructive elevator, in contrast,

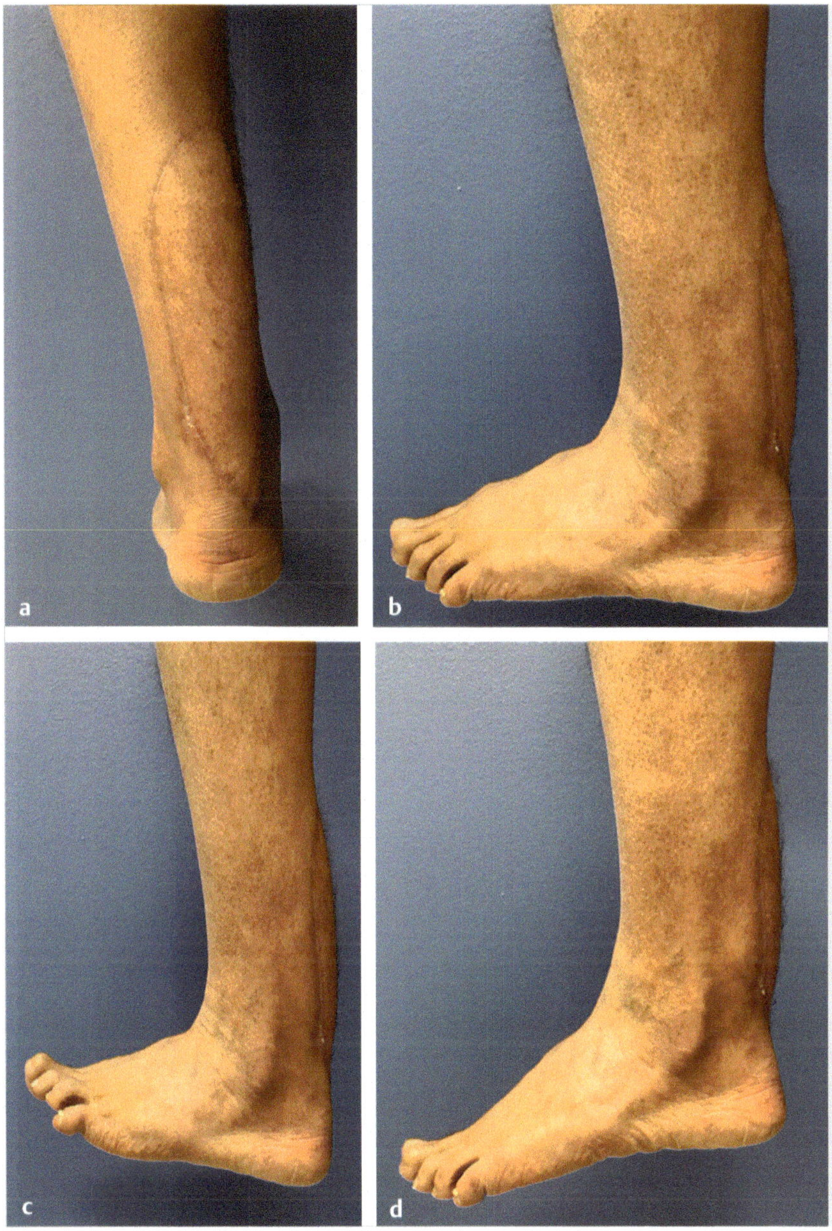

Fig. 11.5 At 1-year follow-up, the patient ambulated well and returned to his normal physical activity. **(a, b)** views of the healed flap with minimal bulk. **(c, d)** On ankle dorsiflexion and plantar flexion, range of motion demonstrates adequacy of Achilles function.
By instead using the *reconstructive elevator*, a secondary reconstruction with a conjoined free anterolateral thigh (ALT) and tensor fascia lata (TFL) flap restored not just Achilles function, but also lower leg contour and an improved quality of life for the patient.

accommodates a wider spectrum of options that often will give a superior outcome. This parallel thinking process is more complex and intense, as it requires a careful assessment of attributes and detriments of all options and encourages greater problem-solving skills. But only this way will optimal form and function be possible.

The reconstructive elevator is an especially important concept for students, residents, and fellows to absorb and understand. To train good thinkers, innovative problems solvers, and thus good reconstructive surgeons, teachers must make students aware of all the options open to them. Creativity and excellence must be stressed. Admittedly, it is difficult to train someone to be creative, but it is very easy to stifle the creativity of someone who has it. In today's era of exploding technology and rapidly advancing operative techniques, it would be a disservice to imprison the minds of the young reconstructive surgeons with the rigid and bounded dogma symbolized by the rungs of a ladder.

References

[1] Gottlieb LJ, Krieger LM. From the reconstructive ladder to the reconstructive elevator. Plast Reconstr Surg. 1994; 93(7):1503–1504

[2] Majno G. The Swnw (Egypt). In: The Healing Hand: Man and Wound in the Ancient World. Cambridge, MA: Harvard University Press; 1975

[3] Brown RF. The management of traumatic tissue loss in the lower limb, especially when complicated by skeletal injury. Br J Plast Surg. 1965; 18:26–50

[4] Pontén B. The fasciocutaneous flap: its use in soft tissue defects of the lower leg. Br J Plast Surg. 1981; 34(2):215–220

[5] Pan W-R, Taylor GI. The angiosomes of the thigh and buttock. Plast Reconstr Surg. 2009; 123(1):236–249

[6] Taylor GI, Pan W-R. Angiosomes of the leg: anatomic study and clinical implications. Plast Reconstr Surg. 1998; 102(3):599–616, discussion 617–618

[7] Hallock GG. Direct and indirect perforator flaps: the history and the controversy. Plast Reconstr Surg. 2003; 111(2):855–865, quiz 866

[8] Hallock GG. A paradigm shift in flap selection protocols for zones of the lower extremity using perforator flaps. J Reconstr Microsurg. 2013; 29(4):233–240

[9] Koshima I, Urushibara K, Inagawa K, Hamasaki T, Moriguchi T. Free medial plantar perforator flaps for the resurfacing of finger and foot defects. Plast Reconstr Surg. 2001; 107(7):1753–1758

[10] Koshima I, Nanba Y, Tsutsui T, et al. Superficial circumflex iliac artery perforator flap for reconstruction of limb defects. Plast Reconstr Surg. 2004; 113(1): 233–240

[11] Wei F-C, Jain V, Suominen S, Chen H-C. Confusion among perforator flaps: what is a true perforator flap? Plast Reconstr Surg. 2001; 107(3):874–876

[12] Hong JP. The use of supermicrosurgery in lower extremity reconstruction: the next step in evolution. Plast Reconstr Surg. 2009; 123(1):230–235

[13] Hong JP, Choi DH, Suh H, et al. A new plane of elevation: the superficial fascial plane for perforator flap elevation. J Reconstr Microsurg. 2014; 30(7):491–496

12 Nonflap Wound Closure Alternatives: Skin Graft, Skin Substitute, Skin Stretch, and Negative-Pressure Wound Therapy

Hyunsuk Peter Suh

Summary

The evolution of wound closure techniques has introduced different alternative methods of closing the wound. Nonflap-wound-closure methods can be applied to cover many types of the wound. Negative-pressure wound therapy has changed the way we approach reconstruction in terms of preparation and closure for some defects. Skin substitutes allow faster granulation and skin stretch devices allow us to close small wounds that are ambiguous for reconstruction. This chapter covers these alternative methods of healing wound. This chapter covers these alternative supporting approaches.

Keywords: negative-pressure wound therapy, skin stretching device, skin substitutes

12.1 Introduction

The skin is the largest organ of the human body with a surface area of 1.2 to 2.0 m^2 and 8% of total body weight.[1] The skin protects the body from pathogens and excessive water loss. It also controls body temperature, senses external stimuli, blocks ultraviolet rays, and serves an aesthetic function. It is a complex organ consisting of epidermis and dermis including hair follicle, sensory nerve, and sweat gland. When injury to the skin is deep to the dermis and the apocrine glands and the pilosebaceous unit is destroyed, the skin loses its generative capacity.[2]

The use of modalities of secondary healing with negative-pressure wound therapy (NPWT), primary closure, and skin graft is located at the lower part of the traditional reconstructive ladder.[3] Although it is at the lower step of the ladder, it can cause more complications than the modalities that is at the upper rungs of the ladder when the method is applied to the improper condition of the wound.

A small wound can be healed by secondary intention by wound contraction and epithelization from the wound margin. However, if the defect is full thickness and wide, it takes a long time to heal and eventually makes a wide scar with deformity and sometimes it becomes a nonhealing wound. Even when we close the wound with a primary suture, it does not heal well due to its tension and also produces unsightly scars. Therefore, if the wound is wide, skin graft or flap must be used to cover the wound.

Skin graft is the most common and simplest way to cover a superficial defect. The origin of the skin graft is an ancient technique. It was performed as early as 2500 BC to cover nasal skin defect.[4] Then, over the next few thousand years, only a few anecdotal descriptions report the use of grafts to cover the traumatic defects. In Bologna, in his famous treatise on medicine of 1597, Gaspare Tagliacozzi (1545–1599) mentions a cutaneous transplantation.[5] Although skin grafting has been known for centuries, it was not until the 19th century that grafting was rediscovered, improved, and then generalized.[6,7,8]

Skin grafts are indicated for covering of skin defect caused by trauma, burn, after excision of tumor, in case the primary closure of the defect is not possible, and wound bed is well granulated and vascularized.

12.2 Negative-Pressure Wound Therapy

NPWT is used for almost all wounds including pressure sores, soft-tissue injuries caused by trauma, burns, diabetic foot, and postoperative wounds. Despite its universal use of NPWT, there are still no randomized clinical trials (RCT) with high-certainty evidence that demonstrates its superior efficacy over conventional dressing,[9,10,11,12,13] but only few people suspect its efficacy. NPWT is being used for an increasingly wide range of applications with the primary purpose of promoting granulation tissue formation.

12.2.1 Indications of NPWT in Open Wounds

NPWT can be used for the following indications:

- Deep open wound.
- Wound bed preparation (▸ Fig. 12.1, ▸ Fig. 12.2):
  - Before split-thickness skin graft (STSG) or flap surgery.
- During the infected wound management:
  - Instillation system can be used.
  - Surgical wound dehiscence.
- If neither primary closure nor flap surgery is possible.

12.2.2 Protocols of NPWT for the Infected Wound with Necrotic Tissue

NPWT is a very effective method to remove a large amount of discharge and minimize the bacterial burden of the wound. During the early period of wound management for the infected wound with massive necrotic tissue, serial surgical debridement is needed along with proper antibiotics use and dressing. In between the serial debridement, NPWT can be applied as a wound dressing method. For infected wound, NPWT with instillation is better than standard NPWT,[14,15] and as an instillation solution, normal saline solution is as effective as other antiseptics.[16,17]

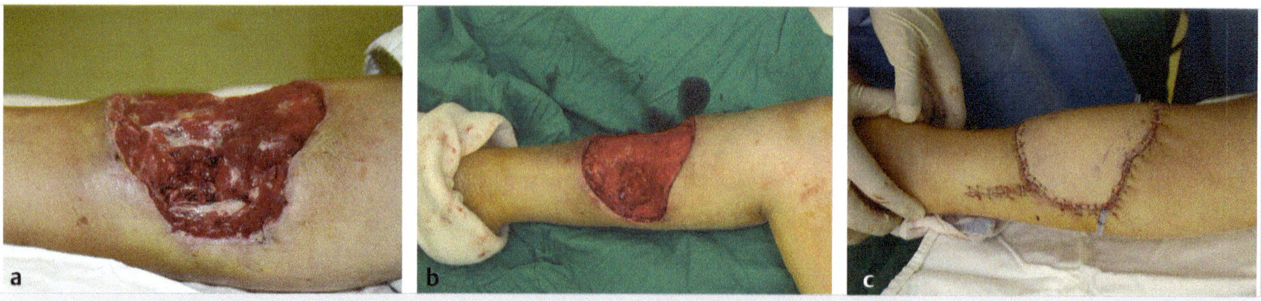

Fig. 12.1 (a) Necrotic tissue and biofilm remaining after first debridement of dog bite wound. (b) After applying negative-pressure wound therapy for the wound for a week, and (c) wound coverage with free perforator flap.

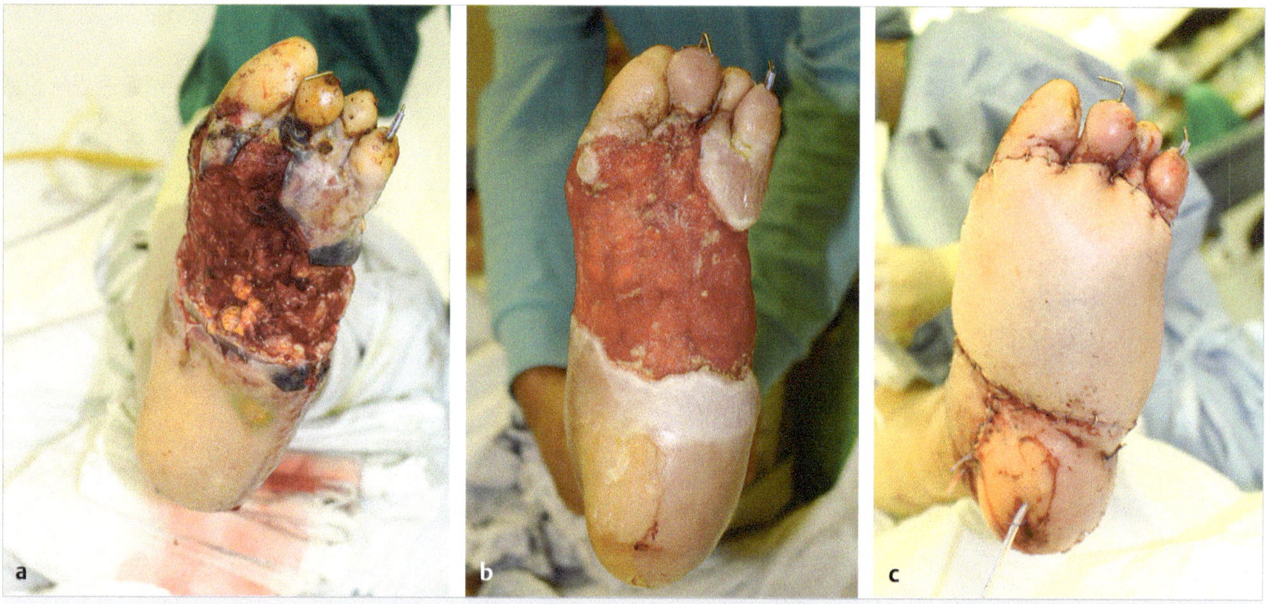

Fig. 12.2 (a) Necrotic tissue was seen on the surface after initial debridement. (b) Healthy granulation tissue was covering the surface following serial debridement and negative-pressure wound therapy after 11 days after initial debridement. (c) The wound was covered with free perforator flap.

12.2.3 Limitations

NPWT is only a dressing method bridging in between the surgical debridement. NPWT cannot replace scheduled wound evaluation or any surgical procedure including necrotic tissue removal and pus drainage. For example, in the early phase of infected diabetic wound care, daily surgical debridement is needed in the severely infected limb. The duration in between the debridement can be modified based on the condition of the wound.

12.2.4 Pitfalls of Negative-Pressure Wound Therapy

NPWT undoubtedly has the advantage of growing granulation tissue. Sometimes wounds that previously only could be covered with flaps can also be covered with secondary healing or skin grafts after using NPWT. As some of the reports could be easily found,[18,19,20,21,22] more and more people are using NPWT for deeper wounds. In some wounds with exposed bone or ligament, NPWT may make it covered by the granulation tissue and, finally, STSG could be applied with cosmetically or functionally undesirable result. If there was no sufficient granulation even after weeks of NPWT, eventually flap coverage is needed, which is already delayed and the cost of the wound care is inevitably increasing.

12.3 Split-Thickness Skin Graft

The recipient bed should have good vascular supply, with no devitalized tissue. Skin graft take is possible over the healthy granulation tissue, fat, muscle, and fascia, but skin graft will be necrotized over the cartilage or bone without periosteum or perichondrium and tendon without paratenon due to lack of nutrition. However, even if there is no vascular distribution, skin grafts can survive if the defective skin area is narrow. Up to a distance of 0.5 cm from the edge of the skin defect, the skin graft can be nourished by the bridge.[23] In practice, 0.5-cm-width cartilage or tendon without paratenon and perichondrium can be covered by skin graft alone. If there is a necrotic tissue in the recipient site, surgical debridement is needed. After the removal of the necrotic tissue, thorough hemostasis is essential. After debridement, a skin graft can be delayed until the granulation covers the defect.

12.3.1 Flap versus Skin Graft

The choice between skin graft and flap depends mainly on recipient status, defect size, location, and postsurgery aesthetics. The success of skin graft depends on the vascular status of the recipient site. A well-vascularized bed is the best indication for skin graft. In the cases where the bone or the implants are exposed or dead space in the defect is large, free tissue transfer or local flap, including propeller flap, is essential to fill and cover the defect (▶ Fig. 12.3).

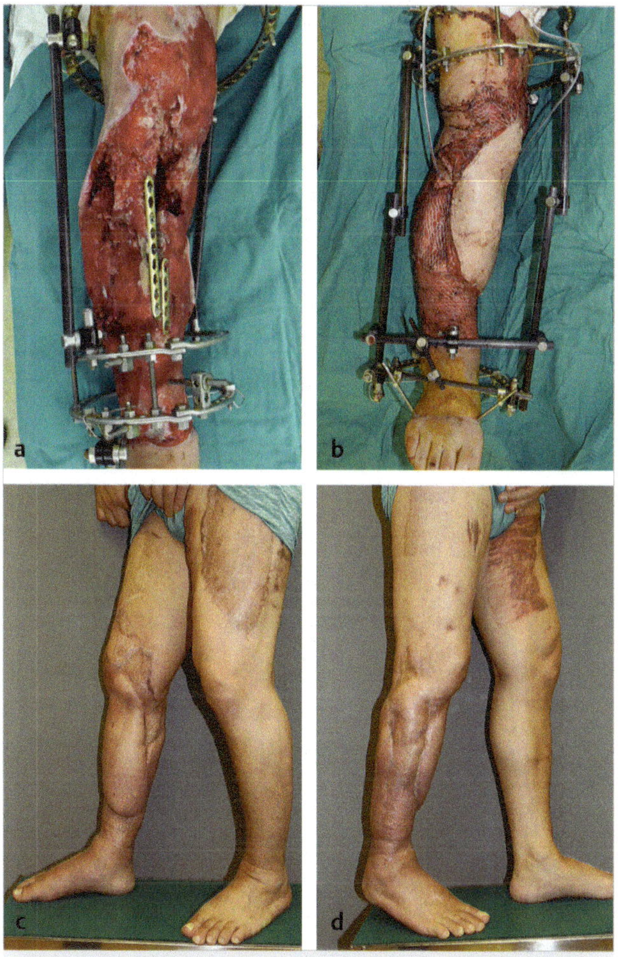

Fig. 12.3 Large wound with bone defect and muscle necrosis. **(a)** A free flap was used to cover the exposed bone and fill the dead space. **(b)** Split-thickness skin graft was used to cover the exposed muscle and granulation tissue. **(c, d)** Eighteen months after coverage, grafted skin and flap are stable, and hypertrophic scar on the skin graft donor site is observed.

Color and texture match of the skin graft and flap is also essential when we are considering wound coverage on the exposed body surface.

12.3.2 Advantages of Split-Thickness Skin Graft

The advantages of STSG are as follows (▶ Table 12.1):

- Possible to cover a large surface.
- Reharvest is possible on the same donor site after healing.
- The meshing of skin is possible to enlarge the graft and cover the larger defect.
- Short operation time.
- No microanastomosis or microdissection is needed.

12.3.3 Detriments of Split-Thickness Skin Graft

The detriments of STSG are as follows (▶ Table 12.1):

- Irregular texture.
- Lack of hair.
- Lack of dermal element.
- Less pliability and elasticity.
- More contracture.
- Wide donor site scar.
- The technical difficulty of harvesting skin in old patients and long-term steroid use.

12.3.4 Recipient Bed Preparation

One of the most important aspects of skin graft success is wound bed preparation. The wound must be free of devitalized tissue and inflammation or biofilm. Wound surface should be debrided if the wound was kept open for dressing especially in the case of a chronic wound. Pin-point bleeding from the entire bed is the most essential factor to ensure the well-vascularized bed and sufficient debridement. At the same time, meticulous hemostasis is essential to prevent hematoma under the graft (▶ Fig. 12.4).

12.3.5 Split-Thickness Skin Harvest

The most import thing in skin harvest is to get even thickness skin as we planned to harvest. The use of hand-held dermatome operated by air pressure with depth gauge is recommended. Choose the area that is easy to harvest. To minimize the visible scar, the buttock or the posterior thigh can be selected. The width of the harvested skin can be selected by changing the width plate. As the width plate has a few

Table 12.1 Characteristics of split-thickness skin graft (STSG) and full-thickness skin graft (FTSG)

		Thickness	Recipient site	Contracture	Donor site	Revascularization	Take
STSG	Thin STSG	8–12/1,000 inch	thigh, buttock, scalp, back, chest wall	More	Fast epithelialization	Fast	Easy
	Intermediate STSG	12–18/1,000 inch					
	Thick STSG	18–25/1,000 inch			Slow epithelialization		
FTSG		Different based on the donor site	Postauricular, groin, wrist, elbow	Less	Primary closure recommended	Slow	Difficult

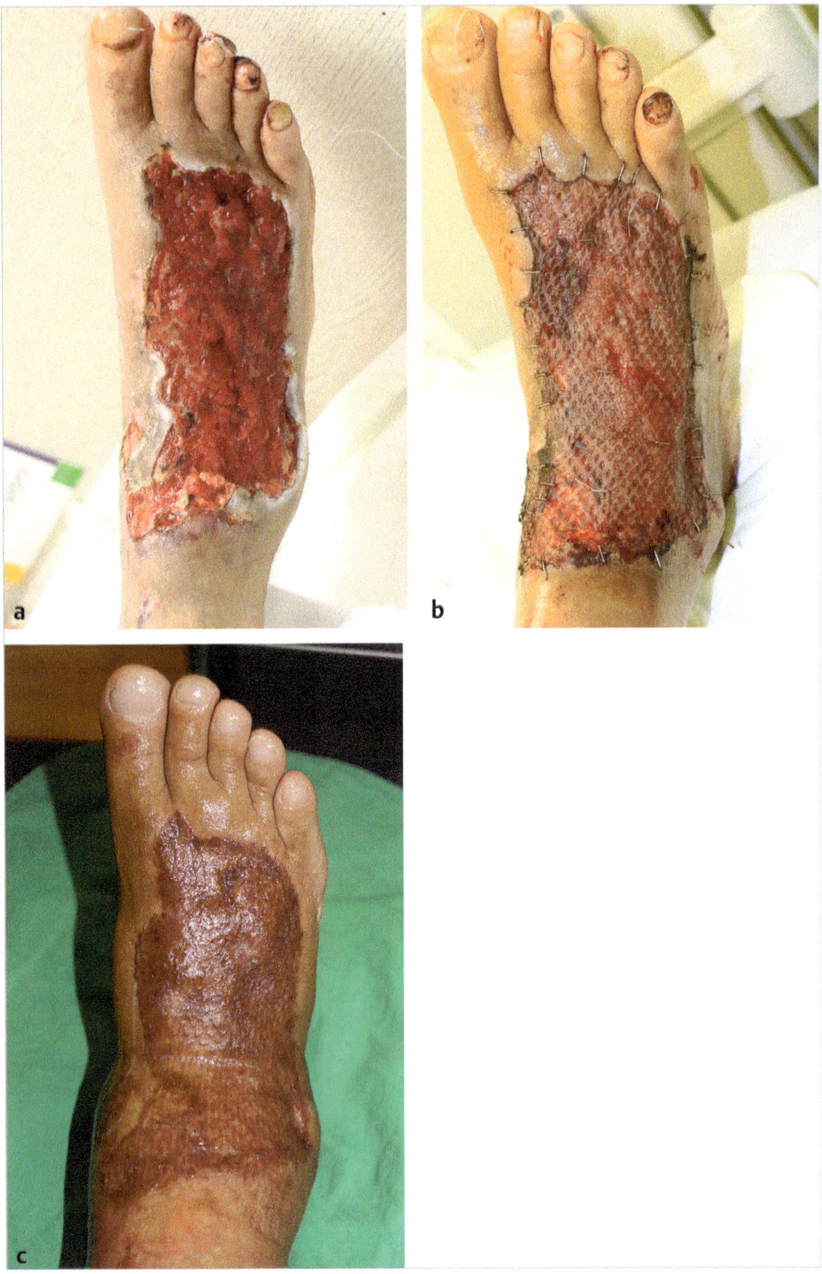

Fig. 12.4 The wound bed was covered with biofilm and nonviable tissue. **(a)** It was debrided before the coverage. **(b)** Two weeks after skin graft. **(c)** 4 months later coverage.

millimeters of thickness, the width of the harvested skin is narrower than the actual width marked on the width plate. The harvesting area is prepared with lubricating oil or jelly. The entire surface of the donor site should be on tension to make an even friction during the harvest. It is useful if the assistant can pull the lateral margin with gauze and use the nondominant hand of the operator to pull the skin to make a countertraction. After starting the dermatome, it is engaged to the donor site at a 45-degree angle and a firm and gentle amount of pressure is applied during the movement. The harvested skin can be seen over the blade during the harvest. If the donor skin is thin in an old patient or in patients with long-term steroid use, thickness gauge should be adjusted and extra caution should be made not to apply an excessive pressure during the harvest. At the completion, the dermatome is lifted while it is on, to detach graft from the donor site. If you are planning to mesh the skin, it is easier to stop the machine while it is kept attached to the donor site and locate the plastic skin graft carriers under the machine before spreading the skin over the carrier.

12.3.6 Meshing Split-Thickness Graft

By meshing the graft, you can enlarge the graft, minimize hematoma under the graft, and promote easier graft take. On the contrary, mesh graft heals with more scarring because of the secondary healing by epithelialization of the openings on the graft. Mesh graft is usually applied to large defect or defect of the unexposed body surface (▶ Fig. 12.5).

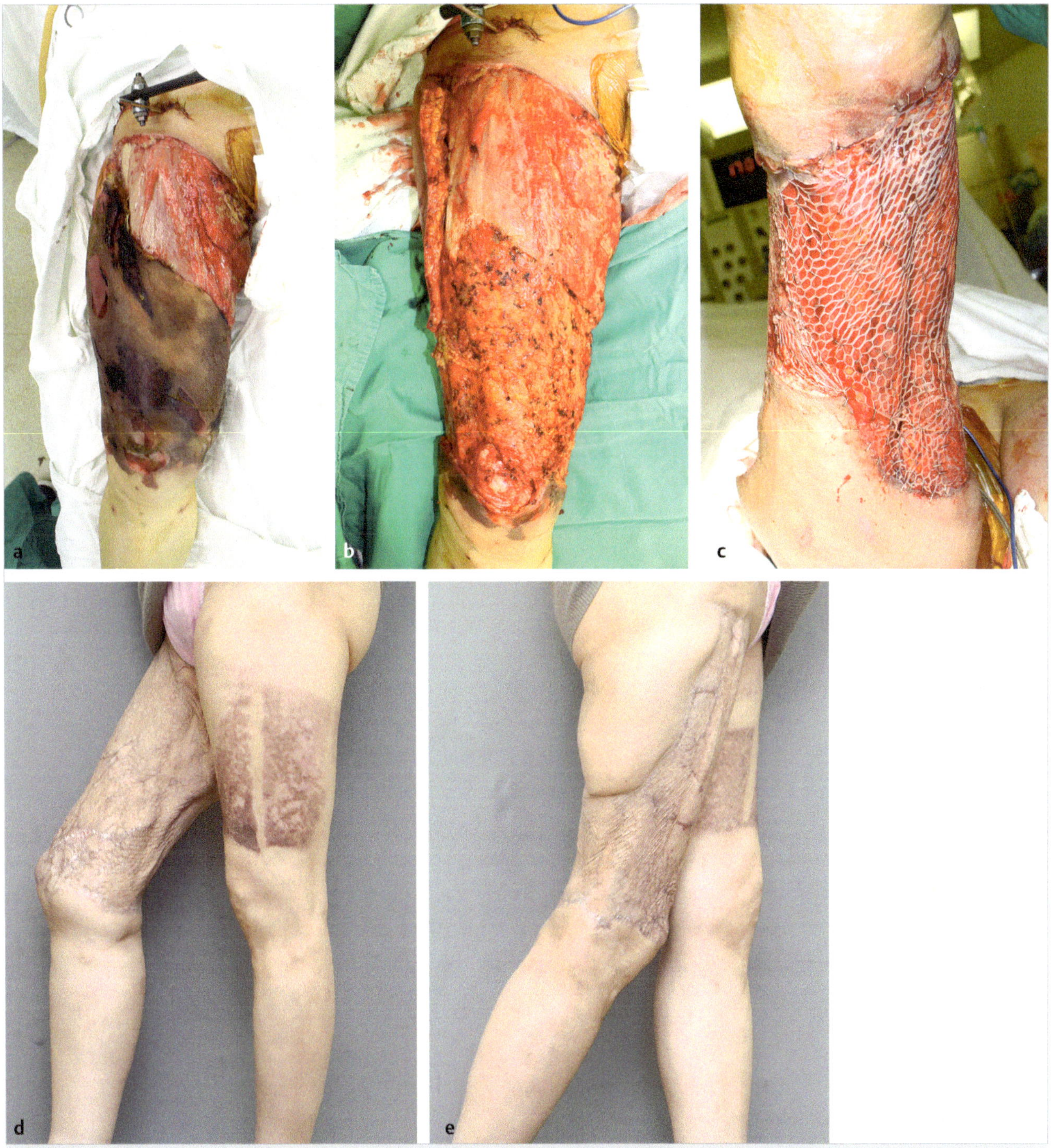

Fig. 12.5 Mesh graft can be effective in large wounds. **(a)** A 67-year-old patient had a degloving injury on her right thigh. **(b)** After the debridement, **(c)** 1:3 mesh graft was done over the wound mostly. **(d, e)** As most of the meshed graft was transferred over the fat tissue, there were minimal hypertrophy and tethering.

12.3.7 Graft Fixation and Immobilization

Harvested skin is transferred to the defect. The dermal side should face the defect. There should be no raw surface at the margin of the defect to minimize the hypertrophic scar. The graft can overlap on the skin margin. The graft can be fixed with suture or staples.

NPWT is an effective method to immobilize the graft.[24,25,26] Continuous mode with −125 mm Hg pressure is suitable for most of the wound. NPWT can be applied for 5 to 10 days after the graft. It is crucial to seal correctly. Leakage of air makes the graft wet or dry and makes it difficult to get the proper graft take. If it is not possible to use NPWT, especially wound is near the external fixator, tie-over dressing or bolster dressing with stapler and gauze is also possible and effective. The dressing should be maintained until the graft is revascularized and has a robust fixation on the wound bed. Usually, the first dressing change is done on day 5 and excessive care and sufficient time should be assigned not to detach the skin from the bed. If there is hematoma under the skin, compression and irrigation should be done to remove all the hematoma.

12.4 Skin Substitute for Additional Thickness

When the full-thickness wound is healed by secondary intention or covered by STSG, dermal regeneration is inevitably absent. To add the thickness and viscoelasticity of the grafted skin, a dermal substitute can be used. It can be used as an implant to work as a template and allow the ingrowth of the host fibroblast and gradually replaced by the host extracellular matrix. Allogenic dermal substitutes, including AlloDerm, Graftjacket, and Synthetic material including Integra and Matriderm, can be used to help dermal regeneration.[27,28,29,30] Some of the Xenograft and allogenic epidermis products are used as a biological dressing to protect the wound from fluid loss and infection (▶ Table 12.2).

The use of dermal substitutes with thin STSG has become common. Collagen is often used as the main component. To control interconnectivity and antigenic potential, the freeze-drying method can be used. The properties are determined by adjusting the substitutes with glycosaminoglycans and cross-linking.[28,29] Allogenic and animal-derived dermal substitutes are commercially available.[31] One-stage graft is also possible for most of the dermal substitutes and it is also possible to use NPWT for immobilization (▶ Fig. 12.6, ▶ Video 12.1).[24]

12.5 Serial Closure of the Wound

When skin graft or flap surgery is not available or possible, the wound can be closed serially by staged closure. By mechanical creep (skin stretch under continuous stretching force) and stress relaxation, the skin will stretch and enable tension-free closure after days or weeks.[32,33] There are commercially available products in Europe and show good result of closing large soft-tissue defect without graft or flap surgery.[34] Simple rubber traction or serial tightening of wire suture can also be used.[35] As the wound remains open for days to weeks, there is a higher chance that wound infections will need a more frequent outpatient visit and there are chances of device failure or skin ulceration during the stretching.

12.6 Skin Graft for a Chronic Ulcer

In venous ulceration, additional compression is essential besides the skin graft before and after the procedure. Compression is also essential even when the defect is covered with the flap in the venous ulcer. In diabetic ulcer, ischemia and osteomyelitis are factors that make the skin graft success difficult.

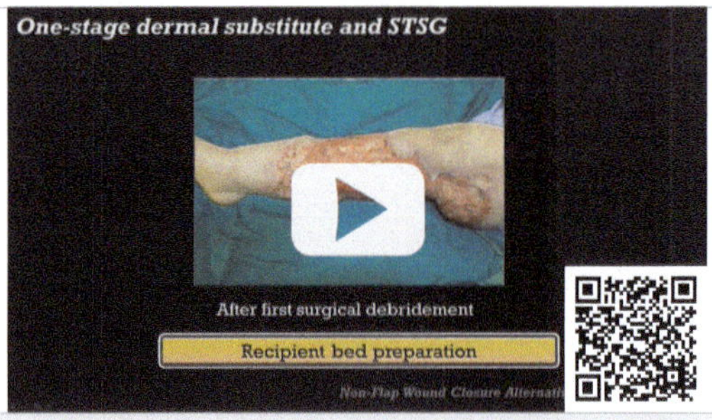

Video 12.1 Application of One Stage Dermal Substitutive with Skin Graft. https://www.thieme.de/de/q.htm?p=opn/cs/20/7/12265262-1f735bbd

Table 12.2 Definition based on the origin of the donor

Tissue origin	Graft donor	Type	Products	Function/mechanism	Risk
Autograft	Same subject			Graft take	
		Epidermis	Epicel, Laserskin, Cell Spray	Graft take or replaced by host epithelium	Graft loss
Isograft	Same gene (twin)			Graft take	
Allograft	Same species	Acellular	AlloDerm, Graftjacket, GammaGraft, DermaMatrix, Neoform	Template for tissue ingrowth	Disease transmission
		Epidermis	StrataGraft	Biologic dressing	
		Fibroblast	Dermagraft		
Xenograft	Different species		Biobrane, EZ-derm, Permacol, Oasis Matrix	Biologic dressing	Disease transmission
		Acellular collagen	Matrierm, Integra	Template for tissue ingrowth	
Xenograft + allograft		Allogenic epidermis with acellular bovine collagen	Apligraf	Acellular bovine works as a template	Disease transmission

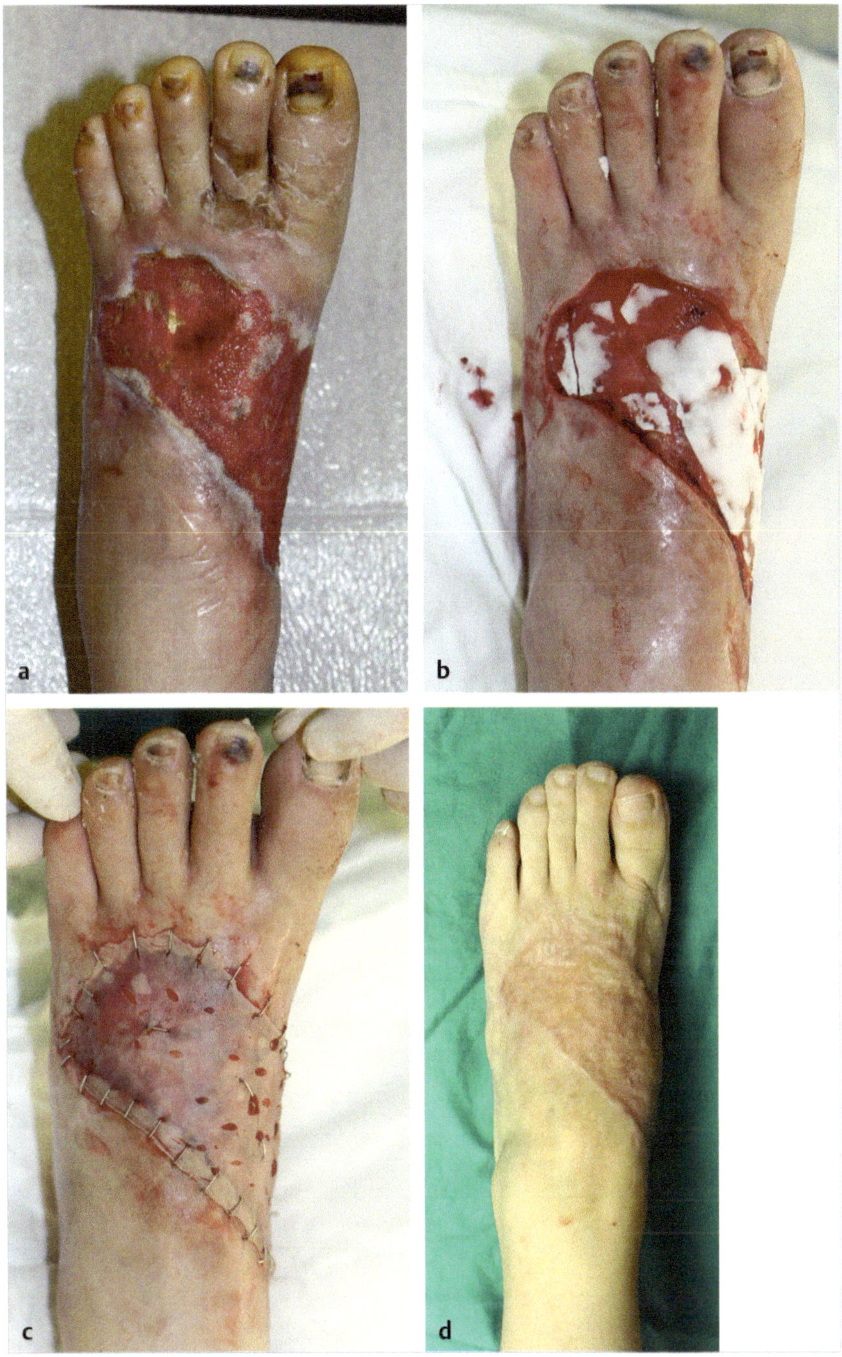

Fig. 12.6 **(a)** Wound on the dorsum of foot has exposed tendons. **(b)** After debridement of wound bed and margin, synthetic xenograft was used as a one-stage graft **(b)** Split-thickness skin graft was applied over the dermal substitute. **(c)** Graft was carefully located to cover the entire defect and margin to minimize the hypertrophic scar from the raw surface and secondary healing of it. **(d)** Six months after graft, it shows no hypertrophy on the margin.

12.7 Conclusion

Skin graft and NPWT is a simple method but may cause more complications, delay wound healing, and increase cost of treatment if it is applied to the deep wound without proper wound preparation. Reconstruction methods, including skin graft or NPWT, should be selected base on the defect size location/ depth and chose the right approach for each wound.

References

[1] Millington P, Wilkinson R. Skin (Biological Structure and Function Books). Cambridge: Cambridge University Press; 2009

[2] Gantwerker EA, Hom DB. Skin: histology and physiology of wound healing. Clin Plast Surg. 2012; 39(1):85–97

[3] Gottlieb LJ, Krieger LM. From the reconstructive ladder to the reconstructive elevator. Plast Reconstr Surg. 1994; 93(7):1503–1504

[4] Davis JS. Address of the president: the story of plastic surgery. Ann Surg. 1941; 113(5):641–656

[5] Tagliacozzi G. De curtorum chirurgia per insitionem. Venice: Gaspare Bindoni; 1597

[6] Hauben DJ, Baruchin A, Mahler A. On the history of the free skin graft. Ann Plast Surg. 1982; 9(3):242–245

[7] Boudana D, Wolber A, Coeugniet E, Martinot-Duquennoy V, Pellerin P. History of skin graft. Ann Chir Plast Esthet. 2010; 55(4):328–332

[8] Singh M, Nuutila K, Collins KC, Huang A. Evolution of skin grafting for treatment of burns: Reverdin pinch grafting to Tanner mesh grafting and beyond. Burns. 2017; 43(6):1149–1154

[9] Liu Z, Dumville JC, Hinchliffe RJ, et al. Negative pressure wound therapy for treating foot wounds in people with diabetes mellitus. Cochrane Database of Systematic Reviews. 2018; 10

[10] Dumville JC, Owens GL, Crosbie EJ, Peinemann F, Liu Z. Negative pressure wound therapy for treating surgical wounds healing by secondary intention. Cochrane Database Syst Rev. 2015; 6(6):CD011278

[11] Dumville JC, Land L, Evans D, Peinemann F. Negative pressure wound therapy for treating leg ulcers. Cochrane Database Syst Rev. 2015(7):CD011354

[12] DeFranzo AJ, Argenta LC, Marks MW, et al. The use of vacuum-assisted closure therapy for the treatment of lower-extremity wounds with exposed bone. Plast Reconstr Surg. 2001; 108(5):1184–1191

[13] Anghel EL, Kim PJ. Negative-pressure wound therapy: a comprehensive review of the evidence. Plast Reconstr Surg. 2016; 138(3) Suppl:129S–137S

[14] Kim PJ, Attinger CE, Steinberg JS, et al. The impact of negative-pressure wound therapy with instillation compared with standard negative-pressure wound therapy: a retrospective, historical, cohort, controlled study. Plast Reconstr Surg. 2014; 133(3):709–716

[15] Anghel EL, Kim PJ, Attinger CE. A solution for complex wounds: the evidence for negative pressure wound therapy with instillation. Int Wound J. 2016; 13 Suppl 3:19–24

[16] Kim PJ, Attinger CE, Oliver N, et al. Comparison of outcomes for normal saline and an antiseptic solution for negative-pressure wound therapy with instillation. Plast Reconstr Surg. 2015; 136(5):657e–664e

[17] Brinkert D, Ali M, Naud M, Maire N, Trial C, Téot L. Negative pressure wound therapy with saline instillation: 131 patient case series. Int Wound J. 2013; 10 Suppl 1:56–60

[18] Robert N. Negative pressure wound therapy in orthopaedic surgery. Orthop Traumatol Surg Res. 2017; 103 1S:S99–S103

[19] Shaheed N, Chowdhury AJ, Mondal AR, et al. Negative pressure wound therapy (NPWT) in open wound management: a study of 16 cases in Orthopaedic Department of Faridpur Medical College Hospital. Faridpur Med Col J. 2012; 7 (2):63–66

[20] Lahouel N, Mokwatlo P, Ndobe E. Coverage of extensive tibial bone exposure in burn patients with three local flaps. S Afr J Surg. 2016; 54(4):58–64

[21] González Alaña I, Torrero López JV, Martín Playá P, Gabilondo Zubizarreta FJ. Combined use of negative pressure wound therapy and Integra® to treat complex defects in lower extremities after burns. Ann Burns Fire Disasters. 2013; 26(2):90–93

[22] Verbelen J, Hoeksema H, Pirayesh A, Van Landuyt K, Monstrey S. Exposed tibial bone after burns: flap reconstruction versus dermal substitute. Burns. 2016; 42(2):e31–e37

[23] van Wingerden JJ, Lapid O, van der Horst CM. Bridging phenomenon: simplifying complex ear reconstructions. Head Neck. 2014; 36(5):735–738

[24] Kim EK, Hong JP. Efficacy of negative pressure therapy to enhance take of 1-stage allodermis and a split-thickness graft. Ann Plast Surg. 2007; 58(5):536–540

[25] Webster J, Scuffham P, Stankiewicz M, Chaboyer WP. Negative pressure wound therapy for skin grafts and surgical wounds healing by primary intention. Cochrane Database Syst Rev. 2014(10):CD009261

[26] Suh H, Hong JP. One Stage Allogenic Acellular Dermal Matrices (ADM) and Split-Thickness Skin Graft with Negative Pressure Wound Therapy. London: IntechOpen; 2013

[27] Harley BA, Leung JH, Silva EC, Gibson LJ. Mechanical characterization of collagen-glycosaminoglycan scaffolds. Acta Biomater. 2007; 3(4):463–474

[28] Widjaja W, Tan J, Maitz PKM. Efficacy of dermal substitute on deep dermal to full thickness burn injury: a systematic review. ANZ J Surg. 2017; 87(6):446–452

[29] van der Veen VC, Boekema BK, Ulrich MM, Middelkoop E. New dermal substitutes. Wound Repair Regen. 2011; 19 Suppl 1:s59–s65

[30] Schneider J, Biedermann T, Widmer D, et al. Matriderm versus Integra: a comparative experimental study. Burns. 2009; 35(1):51–57

[31] Sando IC, Chung KC. The use of dermal skin substitutes for the treatment of the burned hand. Hand Clin. 2017; 33(2):269–276

[32] Mustoe TA, Bartell TH, Garner WL. Physical, biomechanical, histologic, and biochemical effects of rapid versus conventional tissue expansion. Plast Reconstr Surg. 1989; 83(4):687–691

[33] Liu Z, Yeung K. The preconditioning and stress relaxation of skin tissue. J Biomed Pharmaceut Eng. 2008; 2(1):22–28

[34] Topaz M, Carmel NN, Topaz G, Li M, Li YZ. Stress-relaxation and tension relief system for immediate primary closure of large and huge soft tissue defects: an old-new concept: new concept for direct closure of large defects. Medicine (Baltimore). 2014; 93(28):e234

[35] Cheng LF, Lee JT, Hsu H, Wu MS. Simple skin-stretching device in assisted tension-free wound closure. Ann Plast Surg. 2017; 78(3) Suppl 2:S52–S57

13 The Process for Flap Selection by Region of the Lower Extremity

Geoffrey G. Hallock

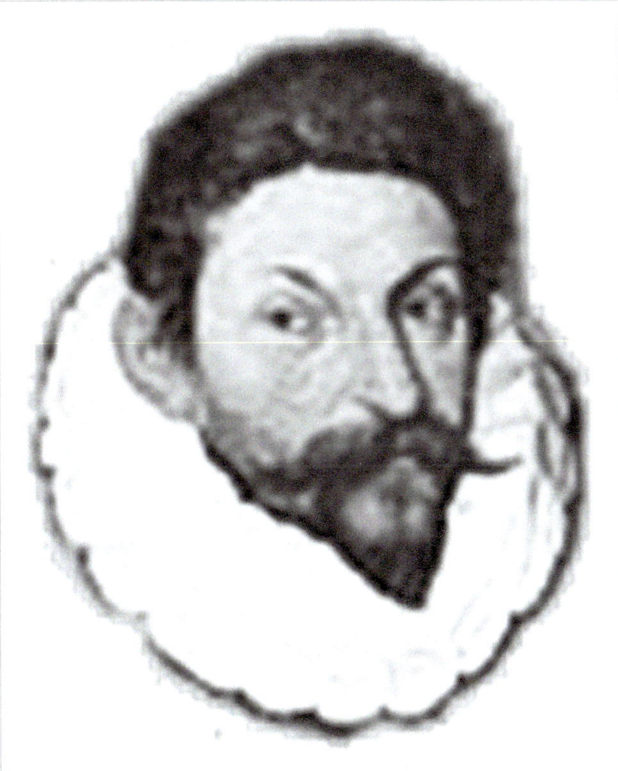

Fig. 13.1 Tagliocozzi: a pioneer in Reconstructive Surgery.

We restore, rebuild, and make whole those parts which nature hath given, but which fortune has taken away. Not so much that it may delight the eye, but that it might buoy up the spirit, and help the mind of the afflicted.

—Gaspare Tagliocozzi (▶ Fig. 13.1)[1]

Summary
A wound requiring repair, or a defect that must be restored, may often be solved even without the need for a vascularized flap. The exact solution indeed must be a process requiring first a careful preoperative analysis of the complexity of the patient's problem and any rate-limiting comorbidities, and by having an astute awareness of the given institution's technological capabilities and also that of the reconstructive surgeons themselves. The completion of every such assessment after scrutinizing all these parameters will thus always be unique for that individual patient. For the same reason, if the planned optimum strategy requires a flap, that too must be individualized. Whether muscle, integument, bone, or perhaps some other soft tissues are required as a flap, the exact choice must not only best fit the requirements of the recipient site but also simultaneously minimize donor site deformity. The expanded lower extremity zone concept, unlike traditional dogma, knows no arbitrary boundaries and tailors a flap selection process to be determined by specific factors such as recipient site size and complexity, whether function must be restored, what choices are available, and a realization that the final appearance may be just as important a factor for the patient who seeks as close as possible the restoration of normalcy.

Keywords: reconstructive ladder, reconstructive elevator, reconstructive matrix, expanded zone concept, chimeric flap

13.1 Introduction

The correction of any wound involving the lower extremity requires repair of disrupted parts, while a defect will always require the restoration of missing components.[2] Traditionally, the method to accomplish either of these objectives adhered to the reconstructive ladder, beginning in the basement with the simplicity of a secondary closure, then stepwise in a sequential fashion proceeding upward with increasing complexity through skin grafts and dermal matrices until reaching the available assortments of flaps.[2,3] Levin expanded his orthoplastic ladder to also include the appropriate steps for management of bone injury or gaps.[4] Gottlieb and Krieger[5] challenged this conventional approach with their reconstructive "elevator" that allowed them to jump at will to whatever level they considered the best solution not only for the immediate problem but also for the long term. The reconstructive matrix may be the best model of all as it emphasizes all aspects of the critical preoperative decision-making analysis necessary to provide the best overall result[6]; that will be unique in the lower limb, as this must assure not only bony stability and adequate soft-tissue coverage but also, most importantly, the maintenance of function and mobility.[7] Closer inspection of this matrix reveals a three-dimensional structure with its axes corresponding to the technological capabilities available at the given institution, which may somewhat correspond to the rungs of the reconstructive ladder, patient surgical risk factors such as comorbidities, and the complexity of the problem that needs to be solved (▶ Fig. 13.2).[6] A simultaneous assessment of how all of these parameters interconnect will be essential for each individual patient to permit formulation of their optimal reconstructive strategy.[8] Thus, if a vascularized flap is indicated, the exact choice will never be the same for every patient, as the product of all these parameters will have an infinite variability necessitating that the final selection always be individualized so that the best outcome can be anticipated.

Rausky et al[9] believed that the goals of lower limb reconstruction must include timely intervention to better ensure function preservation, creation of no impediment in the use of shoe wear, and the provision ultimately of a reasonable appearance, while causing minimal donor site morbidity. A properly selected flap may be the only alternative that is possible to fulfill all these prerequisites. The possible options for bone deficits

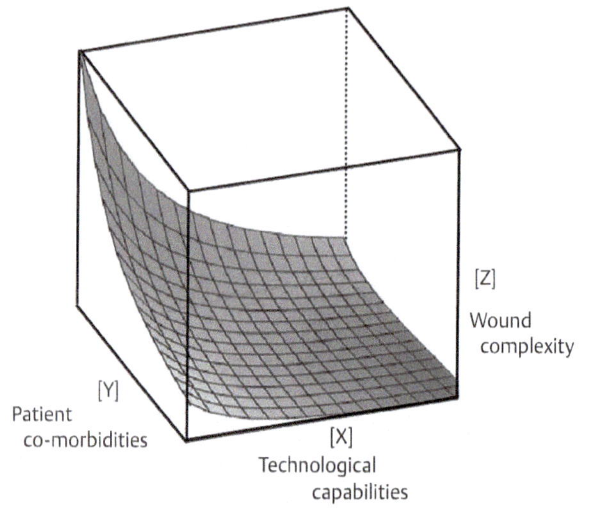

Fig. 13.2 The optimal reconstructive strategy must be individualized for each patient using the reconstructive matrix. This requires that the surgeon assess the complexity of the wound or defect, then consider all possible modalities including flaps needed for restoration, while also considering the limitations of the patient's inherent risk factors. The three-dimensional hyperbola within this matrix represents the optimal outcomes possible after consideration of the individual components of these three variable parameters. (Following the guidelines of Erba et al.[6])

will be better discussed in Chapter 23. Soft-tissue requirements are the more common need anyway in this region, and hereafter the most practical or workhorse flaps will be emphasized (▶ Fig. 13.3), recognizing that a "laundry list" of all available flaps would be an impossibility and that notable satisfactory exceptions exist that may rely instead on a surgeon's familiarity and particular preferences.[10]

Comparable rates of primary fracture and skin healing, time to ambulation, and thus limb salvage are similar regardless of whether a muscle or fasciocutaneous flap is used.[11,12] The latter includes the genre of perforator flaps, which many consider provide a superior aesthetic result, the potential for later elevation to allow secondary procedures as a better option than a muscle flap, and, since no muscle is included, minimize function loss at the donor site (▶ Table 13.1). The adoption of this concept of perforator flaps has rapidly seen an increase in the use of local or so-called freestyle[13,14] flaps throughout the lower extremity in lieu of free flaps, perhaps a consequence of the fact that the latter may be riskier, especially in patients with multiple comorbidities, and certainly require a greater allocation of resources and time as well as technical expertise that may not be universal. However, even a small defect may still be better resurfaced with a microsurgical tissue transfer if adjacent tissues have been damaged and perforators are unavailable or unreliable[15]; and it certainly will always be a solution for all zones of the lower extremity even if some might think that choice inappropriate (▶ Fig. 13.4).

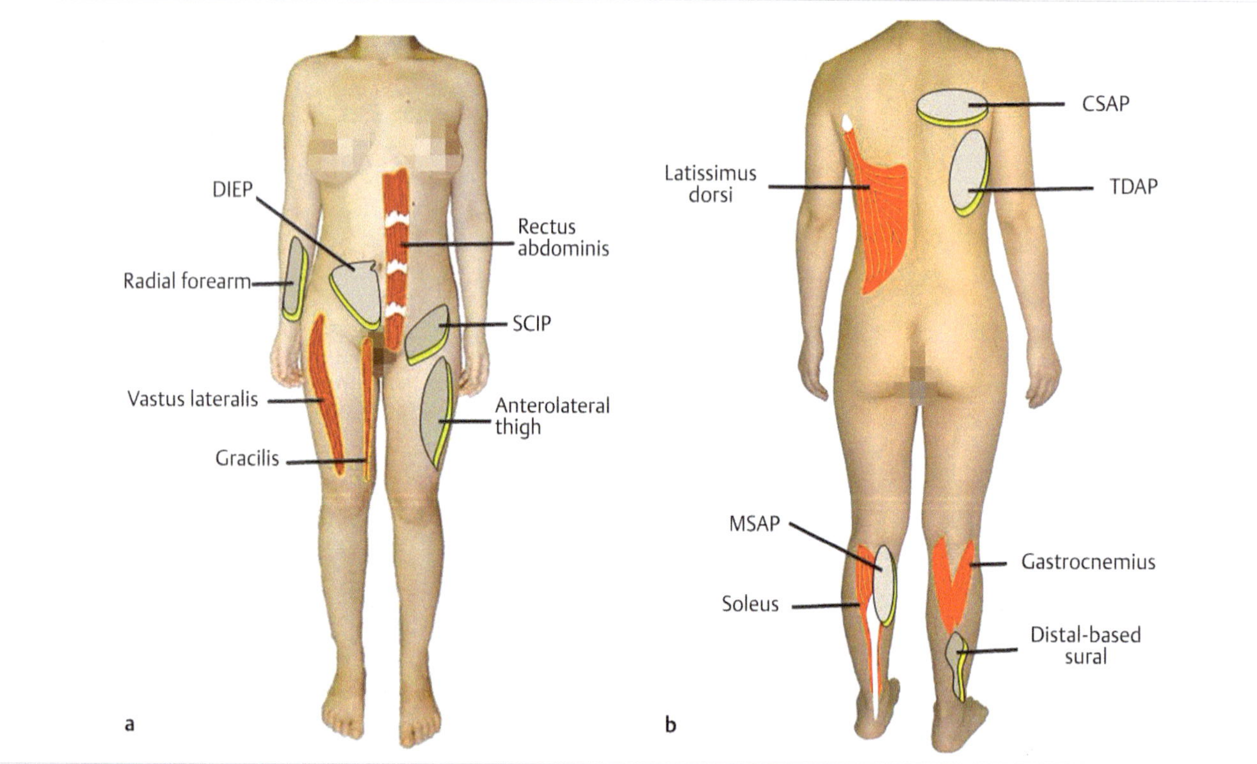

Fig. 13.3 The named pragmatic and workhorse flaps commonly used in the lower extremity. **(a)** Anterior donor sites. **(b)** Posterior donor sites (CSAP, circumflex scapular artery perforator; DIEP, deep inferior epigastric artery perforator; MSAP, medial sural artery perforator; SCIP, superficial circumflex iliac artery perforator; TDAP, thoracodorsal artery perforator).

Table 13.1 Attributes of commonly used perforator flaps

	ALT	CSAP	DIEP	Distal-based sural	Keystone	MSAP	Peninsular	Propeller	Radial forearm	SCIP	TDAP
Ease of harvest	Difficult	Moderate	Difficult	Moderate	Facile	Difficult	Facile	Moderate	Moderate	Difficult	Difficult
Anatomic anomalies	Yes	Minimal	Yes	Minimal	No	Yes	No	Yes	No	Yes	Yes
Surface area	Large	Large	Huge	Moderate	Variable	Small	Moderate	Small	Small	Moderate	Large
Pedicle length	Long	Medium	Long	Short	n/a	Long	n/a	Short	Long	Short	Long
Pedicle caliber	Large	Large	Large	n/a	n/a	Medium	n/a	Small	Medium	Small	Large
Lower limb local flap	Yes	No	No	Yes	Yes	Yes	Yes	Yes	No	Yes	No
Arc of rotation	Large	n/a	Large	Moderate	n/a	Large	Small	Large	n/a	Large	n/a
Lower limb free flap	Yes	Yes	Yes	No	No	Yes	No	No	Yes	Yes	yes
Combined flap	MSBFL	MSB	MS	MS	No	MS	No	No	No	MSFL	MSB
Best indication	All zones	Thigh/proximal leg	Thigh	Foot and ankle	Mobile skin regions	Knee, foot, and ankle	All zones	All zones	Foot and ankle	All zones	All zones
Workhorse	Yes	No	No	Maybe	Yes	Maybe	Yes	Maybe	No	Maybe	Yes
Donor site morbidity	Minimal	None	Maybe	Maybe	None	Moderate	Maybe	Maybe	May be significant	None	None

Abbreviations: ALT, anterolateral thigh; B, bone; CSAP, circumflex scapular artery perforator (scapular and parascapular flaps); DIEP, deep inferior epigastric artery perforator; FL, fascia lata; M, muscle; MSAP, medial sural artery perforator; n/a, not applicable; S, skin; SCIP, superficial circumflex iliac artery perforator; TDAP, thoracodorsal artery perforator.

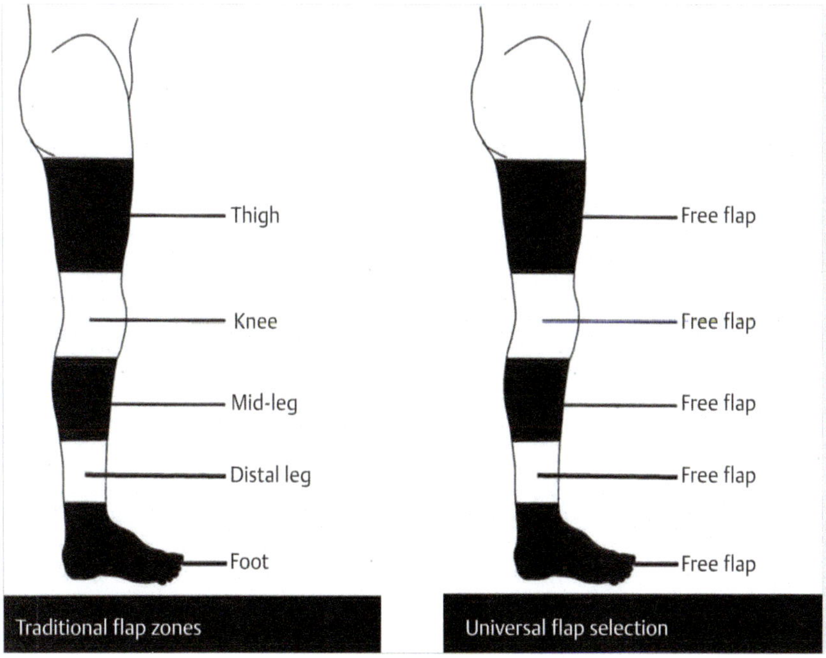

Fig. 13.4 With the lower extremity divided into the traditional zones, selection of a "free flap" can be a universal, if not unrealistic, solution for all regions if a flap is needed.

13.2 Selection According to the Recipient Site

Formerly, the lower extremity was divided into regional zones (▶ Fig. 13.4) where the flap choice would be either a pedicled flap available from that zone or a free flap.[16] Mathes and Nahai[17] in their original book on muscle flaps listed some 22 available muscles in the lower limb as possible local flaps, but most were too diminutive or had an unreliable pattern of circulation. Those still commonly in use include the vastus lateralis or tensor fascia lata[18] muscle for the trochanteric area; gracilis and rectus femoris[19] for the groin, or occasionally also the sartorius,[8] but its vascular supply may be unreliable; gastrocnemius for the knee and proximal third of the leg; and soleus for the middle third (see Chapter 14; ▶ Table 13.2). The rectus abdominis muscle, although a distant flap, can still reach the upper thigh and groin, but at the potential price of causing abdominal wall incompetence.[20] A paradigm shift has recently evolved for the utilization of local cutaneous flaps instead throughout the lower limb, whether based on perforators or not (▶ Fig. 13.5).[21] These have included propeller, peninsular, island, or advancement flaps including keystone flaps (see Chapter 15). Many would consider the distal-based sural flap, which many prefer for more acral defects as a substitute for a free flap, to be a peninsular flap or even a propeller flap, depending on the method of elevation.[22,23]

A better way to evaluate lower limb soft-tissue requirements has been proselytized by Lachica[24] who has introduced an "expanded zone concept" (▶ Fig. 13.6). Again, because of the advent of perforator flaps, the traditional zone idea has become too restrictive as it lacked specificity with regard to wound size and complexity as well as type of tissue loss.[24] The "expanded lower extremity zones" are not restricted by arbitrary boundaries, and are differentiated according to soft-tissue anatomical and functional requirements throughout this region, which in turn determines appropriate flap selection (▶ Table 13.3).[24] Areas densely surrounded by muscle such as the thigh and calf have no functional restrictions, and, although a skin graft or muscle flap would suffice, a thin perforator flap would give a superior aesthetic result,[20,24] replacing "like with like."[25] Most of the rest of the leg also requires soft-tissue replacement only, and that usually best as a perforator flap (▶ Table 13.3). Any flap in the knee area must allow unrestricted motion and the patella, since pressure bearing, must also have a more durable, resilient coverage.[24,26] Following the subunit principle for foot and ankle soft-tissue restoration,[27,28] all areas are similar in that a thin flap is mandatory to allow proper fit of shoes, while the plantar heel and forefoot differ in that any flap must be durable as these will be subjected constantly to weight bearing and the strains of ambulation.[24]

If for any reason a local flap is not available, a free flap may be the next option. Restricting the donor site to the same extremity if possible will minimize the overall scarring and burden on the rest of the body. The anterolateral thigh flap has become the "ideal" soft-tissue free flap to fulfill these requirements[29] (▶ Table 13.1), as this donor site can be prefabricated,[30] can undergo thinning to the proper contour,[31] can have gigantic dimensions or split into multiple smaller flaps,[32] has a long and reliable vascular pedicle, and can even be used in combination with other adjacent tissue components such as fascia lata or muscle if desired.[33] The medial sural artery perforator free flap

Table 13.2 Attributes of commonly used muscle flaps

	Gastrocnemius	Gracilis	LD	Rec abd	Rec fem	Sartorius	Soleus	TFL	Vas lat
Ease of harvest	Moderate	Moderate	Moderate	Difficult	Facile	Moderate	Moderate	Difficult	Moderate
Anatomic anomalies	No	No	No	No	No	Yes	Variable	No	Perhaps
Surface area	Small	Smaller	Large	Small	Small	Smaller	Small	Small	Moderate
Pedicle length	Short	Medium	Long	Long	Medium	Short	Short	Short	Long
Pedicle caliber	Medium	Medium	Large	Large	Large	Small	Small	Medium	Large
Lower limb local flap	Yes	Yes	No	Yes	Yes	Yes	Yes	Yes	Yes
Arc of rotation	Moderate	Wide	n/a	Wide	Moderate	Narrow	Moderate	Moderate	Wide
Lower limb free flap	No	Yes	Yes	Yes	No	No	No	Maybe	Yes
Combined flap	No	No	MSB	MS	No	No	No	FL	MSFL
Best indication	Proximal 1/3 leg	Groin, free flap	Large free flap	Groin, free flap	Groin	Groin	Middle 1/3 leg	Hip	Hip, groin, free flap
Workhorse	Yes	Yes	Yes	No	No	No	Yes	No	No
Donor site morbidity	Minimal	None	Minimal	Maybe	Maybe	None	Moderate	Maybe	Minimal

Abbreviations: B, bone; FL, fascia lata; LD, latissimus dorsi; M, muscle; n/a, not applicable; Rec abd, rectus abdominis; Rec fem, rectus femoris; S, skin; TFL, tensor fascia lata; Vas lat, vastus lateralis.

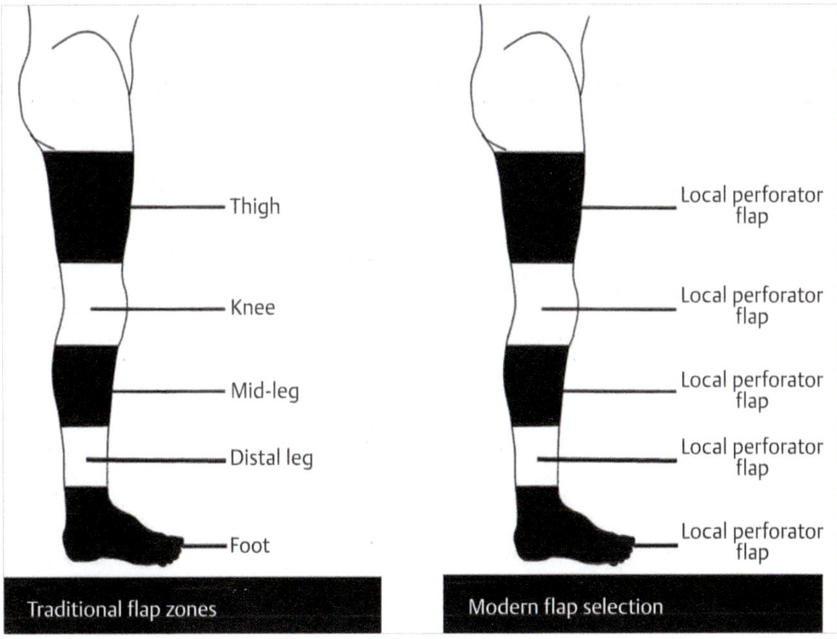

Fig. 13.5 With the advent of perforator flaps, a modern approach to flap selection in the lower extremity for all zones may possibly be by the choice of a local perforator flap.

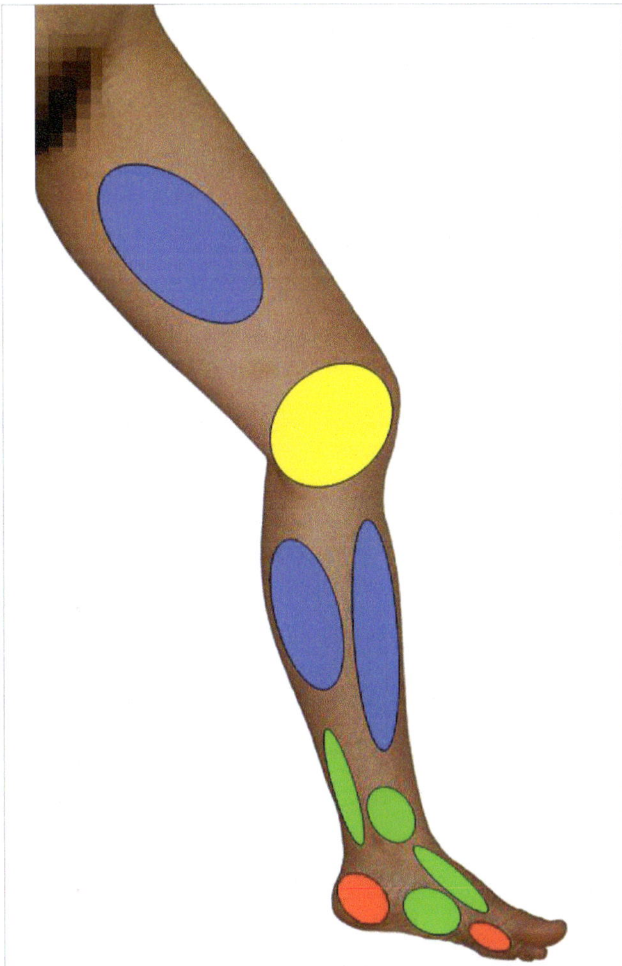

Fig. 13.6 The extended zone concept has no rigid anatomical boundaries, but the choice of flap is determined throughout the lower extremity by considering similarities in soft-tissue requirements for the given region as well as concomitant functional demand.

Table 13.3 Workhorse Soft Tissue Alternatives According to Defect Size for the Expanded Zones of the Lower Extremity

Thigh, Calf, Anterior tibial

SMALL—Keystone, peninsular, propeller, soleus [mid-pretibial], gracilis, vastus lateralis [thigh]
LARGE—ALT, TDAP, SCIP, LD

Knee

SMALL—peninsular, propeller, MSAP, gastrocnemius
LARGE—ALT, TDAP, SCIP, LD

Achilles, non-weight bearing foot & ankle

SMALL—Keystone, propeller, peninsular, gracilis, Distal-based sural
LARGE—ALT, TDAP, SCIP, LD

Weight bearing foot

SMALL—Keystone, peninsular, gracilis, radial forearm
LARGE—thinned ALT or TDAP

All flaps listed in descending order of preference.
ALT = anterolateral thigh; LD = latissimus dorsi muscle;
MSAP = medial sural artery perforator; SCIP = superficial circumflex iliac artery perforator; TDAP = thoracodorsal artery perforator.

is another option specifically for smaller defects, as it also has a potentially long pedicle to reach any available recipient vessels to thereby avoid use of vein grafts, with still moderately large caliber vessels.[34] The radial forearm flap similarly has a long pedicle, and may be the only thin cutaneous flap in the obese patient encountered most often in the western hemisphere, albeit sometimes this can create significant donor site compromise.[20,23,35] As an alternative for the morbidly obese, muscle flaps may still be preferable for proper contour and logistical reasons, with the "workhorse" flaps being the latissimus dorsi (LD) for large defects or the gracilis for smaller ones (▶ Table 13.2). Other cutaneous flaps from the dorsal thoracic fascia such as the circumflex scapular artery perforator flaps (also known as the scapular[36] or parascapular flaps[37]) or the thoracodorsal artery perforator (TDAP) flap may be just as versatile as the LD muscle, but the former offers function preservation if important. Note also that many prefer the TDAP flap over the scapular or parascapular flap, as the vascular pedicle is easier to dissect and can be longer (see Chapter 16).

If three-dimensional fill is required or more extensive soft-tissue coverage is necessary, multiple flap combinations incorporating diverse tissue types may instead be the proper choice.[38] The chimeric flap that has multiple adjoining flaps connected only by a common source vessel would be the best example, as each component can be independently inset wherever needed.[39] This option can also relieve the risk of tension on insetting of a solitary flap, or cover an exposed microanastomosis.[40] Another advantage of chimeric flaps is that only a single

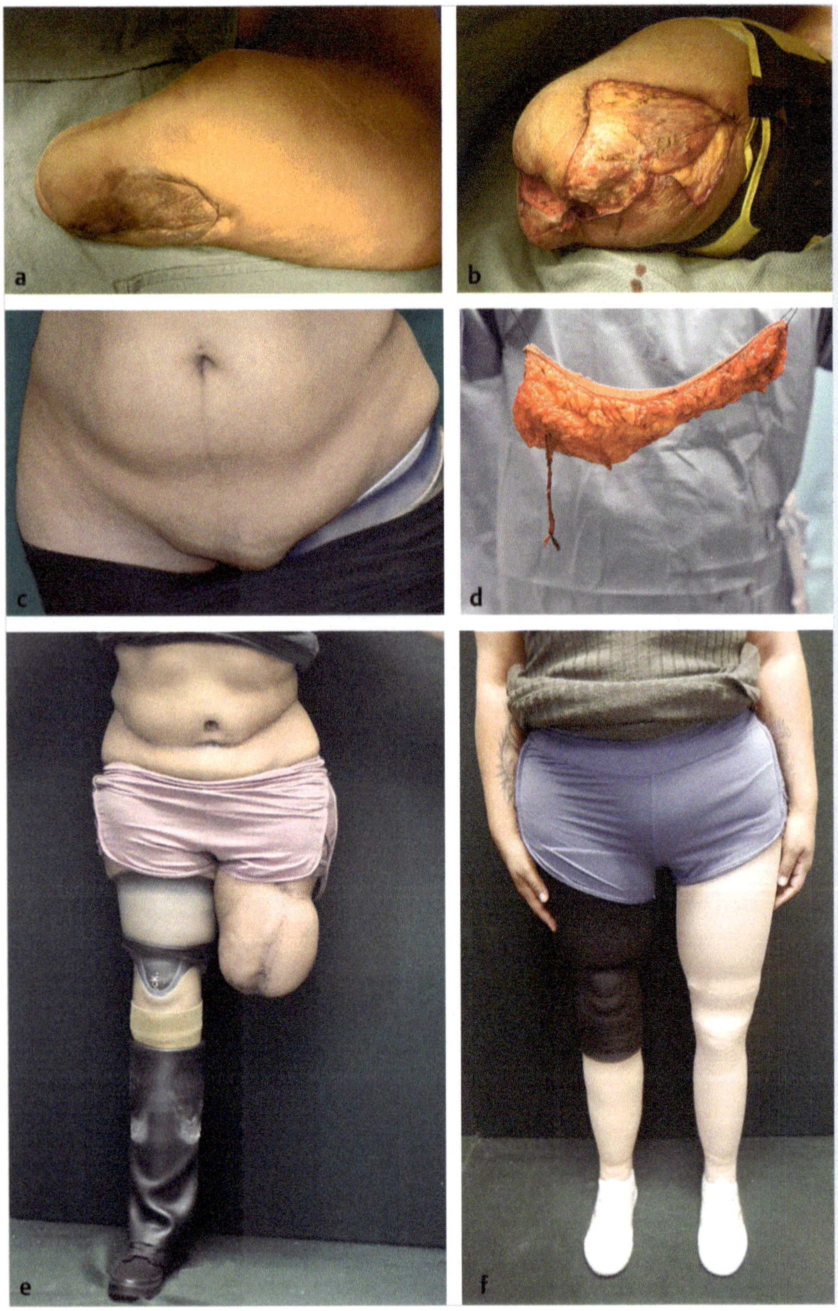

Fig. 13.7 Pragmatic or workhorse flaps may not always be the best choice in unusual circumstances, which require flexibility in flap selection. For example, this young woman had had a traumatic right below-knee as well as left above-knee amputation at age 8. **(a)** She now complained of pain in her left thigh where a skin graft used for initial coverage about the distal femur had become unstable due to rubbing by her prosthesis. **(b)** Radical removal of all attenuated tissues left a large defect. **(c)** Her lower abdominal pannus was selected as a unique donor site for obtaining a large flap that could provide sufficient soft-tissue padding. This donor site also had a long pedicle to allow reach to the descending branch of the lateral femoral circumflex vessels as the recipient site. **(d)** The left hemiabdomen was the source of a deep inferior epigastric artery perforator free flap, **(e)** with ultimate well-padded coverage of her left thigh stump, and actually improvement of the donor site after a "cosmetic" abdominoplasty, **(f)** allowing pain-free ambulation again with her left above-knee prosthesis.

recipient site is needed for microanastomoses to the combination's solitary source pedicle, often essential in the dysvascular or traumatized patient. Hong et al[41] have used a chimeric muscle and perforator flap for treating osteomyelitis, with the muscle filling the void after bony debridement, and the perforator flap then completing skin closure. The subscapular[40] and lateral circumflex femoral systems[42] are the most versatile donor sites for chimeric flaps. In addition, any perforator flap that is supplied by a musculocutaneous perforator, since that muscle after the latter's dissection remains relatively intact, could include both in a relatively straightforward way as a chimeric muscle–perforator flap!

13.3 Selection According to the Donor Site

Since there is such an abundance of flap choices in the lower extremity now, greater attention to minimize donor site morbidity has become fashionable. If the only sequela were a linear scar, then that would be the gold standard. That is usually obtainable with the harvest of every muscle flap, but the drawback is loss of function even with function preservation techniques.[43] The advantage of perforator flaps is that no muscle needs to be included, but if an intramuscular dissection of the perforator is required, there will still be some function loss, albeit minimal.[44] However, if the width of a perforator flap or the skin paddle of a musculocutaneous flap exceeds that allowing primary donor site closure, a skin graft will be necessary, resulting in a less than appealing appearance. This might even be considered, preoperatively, a contraindication for use of the medial sural artery perforator flap especially in women.[34] An acceptable alternative could be the deep inferior epigastric artery perforator (DIEAP) flap, not just because the potential flap surface area is the largest possible but also because the primary donor site closure via a cosmetic abdominoplasty actually improves the donor site appearance (▶ Fig. 13.7).[45] The superficial circumflex iliac artery perforator (SCIP) flap may even have a better donor site scar in the groin that is readily hidden by clothing (see Chapter 22).

The harvest of additional flaps to close the initial donor site just to avoid the appearance of a skin graft always results in more total scarring (see Chapter 16).[46] Conversely, the "kiss" principle using multiple narrow chain-linked chimeric perforator flaps may allow less of a donor site deformity by allowing a primary closure, but causes greater irregularities and scarring at the recipient site where the separate flaps are inset together.[47] Nevertheless, chimeric flaps in general may be the only way to obtain multiple flaps and yet create only a single donor site deformity, if that were to be an important consideration.

References

[1] Tagliacozzi G. De Curtorum Chirurgica per Insitionem. Venetiis: G Bindonus; 1597

[2] Lineaweaver WC. Problem analysis in reconstructive surgery: up and beyond the reconstructive ladders. In: Wei, FC, Mardini, S, eds. Flaps and Reconstructive Surgery. Philadelphia, PA: Saunders Elsevier; 2009:3–6

[3] Janis JE, Kwon RK, Attinger CE. The new reconstructive ladder: modifications to the traditional model. Plast Reconstr Surg. 2011; 127 Suppl 1:205S–212S

[4] Levin LS. The reconstructive ladder. An orthoplastic approach. Orthop Clin North Am. 1993; 24(3):393–409

[5] Gottlieb LJ, Krieger LM. From the reconstructive ladder to the reconstructive elevator. Plast Reconstr Surg. 1994; 93(7):1503–1504

[6] Erba P, Ogawa R, Vyas R, Orgill DP. The reconstructive matrix: a new paradigm in reconstructive plastic surgery. Plast Reconstr Surg. 2010; 126(2): 492–498

[7] Patel KM, Mantell M, Sosin M, Ramineni P. Chimeric functional latissimus flap transfer to restore ankle dorsiflexion following a traumatic defect of the lower leg: a case report. J Reconstr Microsurg. 2014; 30(4):279–282

[8] Töpel I, Betz T, Uhl C, Steinbauer MG. The impact of superficial femoral artery (SFA) occlusion on the outcome of proximal sartorius muscle transposition flaps in vascular surgery patients. J Vasc Surg. 2011; 53(4):1014–1019

[9] Rausky J, Binder JP, Mazouz-Dorval S, Hamou C, Revol M. Perforator-based chimaeric thoracodorsal flap for foot reconstruction. J Plast Reconstr Aesthet Surg. 2013; 66(12):1798–1800

[10] Hallock GG. Flap selection. In: Wei, FC, Mardini, S, eds. Flaps and Reconstructive Surgery. Philadelphia, PA: Saunders Elsevier; 2009:17–29

[11] Cho EH, Shammas RL, Carney MJ, et al. Muscle versus fasciocutaneous free flaps in lower extremity traumatic reconstruction: a multicenter outcomes analysis. Plast Reconstr Surg. 2018; 141(1):191–199

[12] Hallock GG. Utility of both muscle and fascia flaps in severe lower extremity trauma. J Trauma. 2000; 48(5):913–917

[13] Mardini S, Tsai FC, Wei FC. The thigh as a model for free style free flaps. Clin Plast Surg. 2003; 30(3):473–480

[14] D'Arpa S, Cordova A, Pignatti M, Moschella F. Freestyle pedicled perforator flaps: safety, prevention of complications, and management based on 85 consecutive cases. Plast Reconstr Surg. 2011; 128(4):892–906

[15] Hwang KT, Kim SW, Sung IH, Kim JT, Kim YH. Is delayed reconstruction using the latissimus dorsi free flap a worthy option in the management of open IIIB tibial fractures? Microsurgery. 2016; 36(6):453–459

[16] Mathes S, Nahai F. Clinical Applications for Muscle and Musculocutaneous Flaps. St. Louis, MO: Mosby; 1982:3

[17] Mathes SJ, Nahai F. Vastus Lateralis, Clinical Atlas of Muscle and Musculocutaneous Flaps. St. Louis, MO: C.V. Mosby; 1979:7–307

[18] Ishida LH, Munhoz AM, Montag E, et al. Tensor fasciae latae perforator flap: minimizing donor-site morbidity in the treatment of trochanteric pressure sores. Plast Reconstr Surg. 2005; 116(5):1346–1352

[19] Chatterjee A, Kosowski T, Pyfer B, Fisher CS, Tchou JC, Maddali S. A cost-utility analysis comparing the sartorius versus the rectus femoris flap in the treatment of the infected vascular groin graft wound. Plast Reconstr Surg. 2015; 135(6):1707–1714

[20] Soltanian H, Garcia RM, Hollenbeck ST. Current concepts in lower extremity reconstruction. Plast Reconstr Surg. 2015; 136:815e–829-e

[21] Hallock GG. A paradigm shift in flap selection protocols for zones of the lower extremity using perforator flaps. J Reconstr Microsurg. 2013; 29(4):233–240

[22] Parrett BM, Pribaz JJ, Matros E, Przylecki W, Sampson CE, Orgill DP. Risk analysis for the reverse sural fasciocutaneous flap in distal leg reconstruction. Plast Reconstr Surg. 2009; 123(5):1499–1504

[23] Hallock GG, Morris SF. Skin grafts and local flaps. Plast Reconstr Surg. 2011; 127(1):5e–22e

[24] Lachica RD. Evidence-based medicine: management of acute lower extremity trauma. Plast Reconstr Surg. 2017; 139(1):287e–301e

[25] Millard DR Jr. Tissue losses should be replaced in kind. In: Principalization of Plastic Surgery. Boston, MA: Little, Brown & Co; 1986:191–228

[26] Li Z, Li P, Tan Q. Reconstruction of soft tissue defects around the knee with pedicled perforator flaps. Ann Plast Surg. 2018; 81(4):462–467

[27] Hollenbeck ST, Woo S, Komatsu I, Erdmann D, Zenn MR, Levin LS. Longitudinal outcomes and application of the subunit principle to 165 foot and ankle free tissue transfers. Plast Reconstr Surg. 2010; 125(3):924 934

[28] Hallock GG. Evidence-based medicine: lower extremity acute trauma. Plast Reconstr Surg. 2013; 132(6):1733–1741

[29] Wei FC, Jain V, Celik N, Chen HC, Chuang DCC, Lin CH. Have we found an ideal soft-tissue flap? An experience with 672 anterolateral thigh flaps. Plast Reconstr Surg. 2002; 109(7):2219–2226, discussion 2227–2230

[30] Hallock GG. The preexpanded anterolateral thigh free flap. Ann Plast Surg. 2004; 53(2):170–173

[31] Kimura N, Satoh K, Hasumi T, Ostuka T. Clinical application of the free thin anterolateral thigh flap in 31 consecutive patients. Plast Reconstr Surg. 2001; 108(5):1197–1208, discussion 1209–1210

[32] Tsai FC, Yang JY, Mardini S, Chuang SS, Wei FC. Free split-cutaneous perforator flaps procured using a three-dimensional harvest technique for the

reconstruction of postburn contracture defects. Plast Reconstr Surg. 2004; 113(1):185–193, discussion 194–195
[33] Wei FC, Celik N, Jeng SF. Application of "simplified nomenclature for compound flaps" to the anterolateral thigh flap. Plast Reconstr Surg. 2005; 115(4): 1051–1055, discussion 1056–1057
[34] Hallock GG. Medial sural artery perforator free flap: legitimate use as a solution for the ipsilateral distal lower extremity defect. J Reconstr Microsurg. 2014; 30(3):187–192
[35] Weinzweig N, Davies BW. Foot and ankle reconstruction using the radial forearm flap: a review of 25 cases. Plast Reconstr Surg. 1998; 102(6):1999–2005
[36] Rautio J, Asko-Seljavaara S, Laasonen L, Härmä M. Suitability of the scapular flap for reconstructions of the foot. Plast Reconstr Surg. 1990; 85(6):922–928
[37] Nassif TM, Vidal L, Bovet JL, Baudet J. The parascapular flap: a new cutaneous microsurgical free flap. Plast Reconstr Surg. 1982; 69(4):591–600
[38] Kuo YR, Kuo MH, Chou WC, Liu YT, Lutz BS, Jeng SF. One-stage reconstruction of soft tissue and Achilles tendon defects using a composite free anterolateral thigh flap with vascularized fascia lata: clinical experience and functional assessment. Ann Plast Surg. 2003; 50(2):149–155
[39] Hallock GG. The chimera flap: a quarter century odyssey. Ann Plast Surg. 2017; 78(2):223–229
[40] Hallock GG. Permutations of combined free flaps using the subscapular system. J Reconstr Microsurg. 1997; 13(1):47–54
[41] Hong JPJ, Goh TLH, Choi DH, Kim JJ, Suh HS. the efficacy of perforator flaps in the treatment of chronic osteomyelitis. Plast Reconstr Surg. 2017; 140(1): 179–188
[42] Koshima I, Yamamoto H, Hosoda M, Moriguchi T, Orita Y, Nagayama H. Free combined composite flaps using the lateral circumflex femoral system for repair of massive defects of the head and neck regions: an introduction to the chimeric flap principle. Plast Reconstr Surg. 1993; 92(3):411–420
[43] Mathes SJ, Nahai F. Muscle flap transposition with function preservation: technical and clinical considerations. Plast Reconstr Surg. 1980; 66(2):242–249
[44] Kimata Y, Uchiyama K, Ebihara S, et al. Anterolateral thigh flap donor-site complications and morbidity. Plast Reconstr Surg. 2000; 106(3):584–589
[45] Hallock GG. Abdominoplasty as the patient impetus for selection of the deep inferior epigastric artery perforator free flap for knee coverage. Microsurgery. 2014; 34(2):102–105
[46] Marsh DJ, Chana JS. Reconstruction of very large defects: a novel application of the double skin paddle anterolateral thigh flap design provides for primary donor-site closure. J Plast Reconstr Aesthet Surg. 2010; 63(1):120–125
[47] Zhang YX, Hayakawa TJ, Levin LS, Hallock GG, Lazzeri D. The economy in autologous tissue transfer: part 1. The kiss flap technique. Plast Reconstr Surg. 2016; 137(3):1018–1030

14 The Basic Practical Lower Limb Muscle Local Flaps

Geoffrey G. Hallock

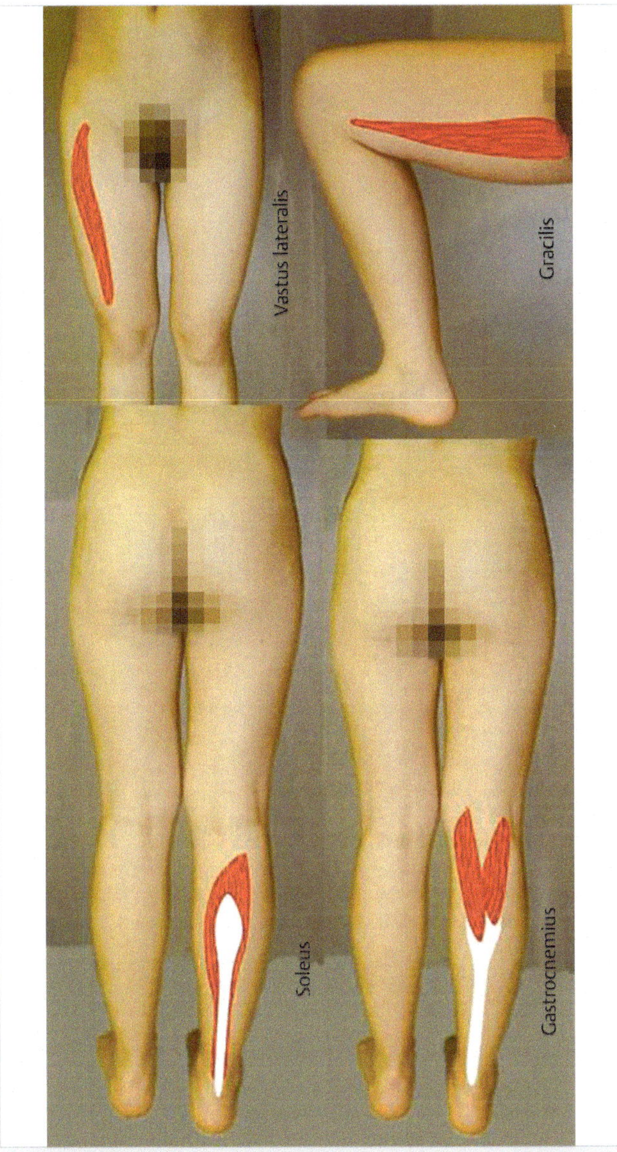

Fig. 14.1 The fundamental intrinsic lower limb muscles.

Summary

Outcome studies of functional lower limb salvage cite no difference if a muscle or cutaneous flap were used. Muscle flaps will never be obsolete, inarguably when, for example, a dynamic tissue transfer were indicated! Muscles are highly malleable, facilitating three-dimensional insetting. Since they are relatively nonbulky, the ultimate contour will not be obtrusive. Their vascular anatomy has few anomalies so that harvest of a muscle flap is a relatively simple process. Historically, the gracilis, gastrocnemius, and soleus muscles have been proven to be extraordinarily efficacious as local flaps in the lower extremity. The vastus lateralis muscle is invariably well known due to its intimate connection with the "workhorse" anterolateral thigh flap. Although many other lower limb muscle flap options exist, these four should necessarily be a part of the repertoire of every reconstructive surgeon.

Keywords: gracilis, medial and lateral gastrocnemius, soleus, vastus lateralis, muscle flaps

14.1 Introduction (▶ Fig. 14.1)

Many might say that muscle flaps have become obsolete[1] now that there has been a paradigm shift in the selection of perforator flaps instead for lower extremity soft-tissue reconstruction.[2] But the reconstructive matrix should remind us that the *optimal* reconstructive strategy must take into consideration more than just what will be the flap that will be chosen.[3] There should be a realization that multiple factors are intertwined including the surgeon's capabilities and preferences, the availability of technological resources, and proper evaluation of the patient's own comorbidities and specific tissue requirements that must be completely understood.[3,4]

If the ultimate goal is functional limb salvage, note that outcome studies have shown no difference whether muscle or skin flaps are used.[5,6] However, the number one absolute indication for selection of a muscle flap, that is inarguable, is if a dynamic transfer is indicated (see Chapter 20).[1,7] Muscle flaps are highly malleable and relatively nonbulky, allowing easier contouring for three-dimensional insetting.[1] The vascular pedicle for muscle flaps is more anatomically consistent, compared to perforator flaps where anomalies are always anticipated.[1] This fact alone allows a more expeditious harvest of a muscle flap, which may be most important in the critically ill patient.[1] In fact, in general the overall elevation of a muscle flap is comparatively simple. Usually, donor site morbidity is less, except for the loss of that muscle function; as always, a primary closure leaving a linear scar is possible.[8] Muscle flaps are also important in combination with their corresponding perforator flap to capture all the advantages of chimeric flaps.[9] Finally, if a perforator flap based on a musculocutaneous perforator is unsuccessful, the muscle that had the requisite intramuscular dissection by definition should have had enough function preservation that it could then be the back-up flap option.[10,11]

A step back in history to review the inaugural book on muscle flaps by Mathes and Nahai[12] reveals the anatomy and how to use 22 intrinsic muscles as flaps in the lower limb. Over time, the majority have been proven to be too small or have segmental or variable blood supplies, and so they are unreliable for most of the lower extremity problems.[13] For valid reasons, some flaps that many surgeons may prefer in their practices will not be discussed in this chapter. Is the distal-based peroneus brevis muscle flap always reliable?[14,15] Will not the segmentally supplied sartorius muscle be at risk in the patient with significant peripheral vascular disease?[16,17] Does not use of the rectus femoris muscle result in a loss of 15 degrees of knee extension, which would be problematic in the athlete?[16] Are there not better alternatives to the rectus abdominis flap,[18,19] such as the anterolateral thigh flap where the high risk of hernia or other abdominal wall morbidity can be altogether avoided?[4,20] Is not the tensor fascia lata perforator flap without muscle better for the ambulatory patient?[11] At least from a traditional standpoint, the gastrocnemius[21] and soleus[22] muscles as local flaps for the lower leg have long proven their value as basic flaps that must be part of the repertoire of every reconstructive surgeon. The gracilis muscle is a "workhorse" flap not just for the lower extremity,[23] but also throughout the body, with special emphasis deserved for its dynamic versatility.[24] The overwhelming adoption of the anterolateral thigh flap as the "ideal soft-tissue flap,"[25] requires an intimate knowledge of the vastus lateralis muscle through which its perforators are closely aligned. For these reasons, this chapter is intended to provide enough that is basic to allow a fundamental understanding of the role of lower limb muscles for lower limb reconstruction.

References

[1] Hallock GG. In an era of perforator flaps, are muscle flaps passé? Plast Reconstr Surg. 2009; 123(4):1357–1363

[2] Hallock GG. A paradigm shift in flap selection protocols for zones of the lower extremity using perforator flaps. J Reconstr Microsurg. 2013; 29(4):233–240

[3] Erba P, Ogawa R, Vyas R, Orgill DP. The reconstructive matrix: a new paradigm in reconstructive plastic surgery. Plast Reconstr Surg. 2010; 126(2): 492–498

[4] Soltanian H, Garcia RM, Hollenbeck ST. current concepts in lower extremity reconstruction. Plast Reconstr Surg. 2015; 136(6):815e–829e

[5] Cho EH, Shammas RL, Carney MJ, et al. Muscle versus fasciocutaneous free flaps in lower extremity traumatic reconstruction: a multicenter outcomes analysis. Plast Reconstr Surg. 2018; 141(1):191–199

[6] Hallock GG. Utility of both muscle and fascia flaps in severe lower extremity trauma. J Trauma. 2000; 48(5):913–917

[7] Hallock GG. Restoration of quadriceps femoris function with a dynamic microsurgical free latissimus dorsi muscle transfer. Ann Plast Surg. 2004; 52(1):89–92

[8] Hallock GG. Relative donor-site morbidity of muscle and fascial flaps. Plast Reconstr Surg. 1993; 92(1):70–76

[9] Hallock GG. Simultaneous transposition of anterior thigh muscle and fascia flaps: an introduction to the chimera flap principle. Ann Plast Surg. 1991; 27(2):126–131

[10] Hallock GG. Sequential use of a true perforator flap and its corresponding muscle flap. Ann Plast Surg. 2003; 51(6):617–620, discussion 621–622

[11] Ishida LH, Munhoz AM, Montag E, et al. Tensor fasciae latae perforator flap: minimizing donor-site morbidity in the treatment of trochanteric pressure sores. Plast Reconstr Surg. 2005; 116(5):1346–1352

[12] Mathes SJ, Nahai F. Vastus Lateralis, Clinical Atlas of Muscle and Musculocutaneous Flaps. St. Louis, MO: C.V. Mosby; 1979:7–307

[13] Hallock GG. Sagittal split tibialis anterior muscle flap. Ann Plast Surg. 2002; 49(1):39–43

[14] Eren S, Ghofrani A, Reifenrath M. The distally pedicled peroneus brevis muscle flap: a new flap for the lower leg. Plast Reconstr Surg. 2001; 107(6): 1443–1448

[15] Barr ST, Rowley JM, O'Neill PJ, Barillo DJ, Paulsen SM. How reliable is the distally based peroneus brevis muscle flap? Plast Reconstr Surg. 2002; 110(1): 360–362

[16] Chatterjee A, Kosowski T, Pyfer B, Fisher CS, Tchou JC, Maddali S. A cost-utility analysis comparing the sartorius versus the rectus femoris flap in the treatment of the infected vascular groin graft wound. Plast Reconstr Surg. 2015; 135(6):1707–1714

[17] Töpel I, Betz T, Uhl C, Steinbauer MG. The impact of superficial femoral artery (SFA) occlusion on the outcome of proximal sartorius muscle transposition flaps in vascular surgery patients. J Vasc Surg. 2011; 53(4):1014–1019

[18] Qi F, Gu J, Shi Y. Difficult groin reconstruction using contralateral rectus abdominis myocutaneous flap. Plast Reconstr Surg. 2008; 121(3):147e–148e

[19] Combs PD, Sousa JD, Louie O, Said HK, Neligan PC, Mathes DW. Comparison of vertical and oblique rectus abdominis myocutaneous flaps for pelvic, perineal, and groin reconstruction. Plast Reconstr Surg. 2014; 134(2):315–323

[20] LoGiudice JA, Haberman K, Sanger JR. The anterolateral thigh flap for groin and lower abdominal defects: a better alternative to the rectus abdominis flap. Plast Reconstr Surg. 2014; 133(1):162–168

[21] Arnold PG, Mixter RC. Making the most of the gastrocnemius muscles. Plast Reconstr Surg. 1983; 72(1):38–48

[22] Hallock GG. Getting the most from the soleus muscle. Ann Plast Surg. 1996; 36(2):139–146

[23] Hussey AJ, Laing AJ, Regan PJ. An anatomical study of the gracilis muscle and its application in groin wounds. Ann Plast Surg. 2007; 59(4):404–409

[24] Zuker RM, Bezuhly M, Manktelow RT. Selective fascicular coaptation of free functioning gracilis transfer for restoration of independent thumb and finger flexion following Volkmann ischemic contracture. J Reconstr Microsurg. 2011; 27(7):439–444

[25] Wei FC, Jain V, Celik N, Chen HC, Chuang DC, Lin CH. Have we found an ideal soft-tissue flap? An experience with 672 anterolateral thigh flaps. Plast Reconstr Surg. 2002; 109(7):2219–2226, discussion 2227–2230

14.2 Chapter 14A: The Medial and Lateral Gastrocnemius Muscle Flaps

Geoffrey G. Hallock

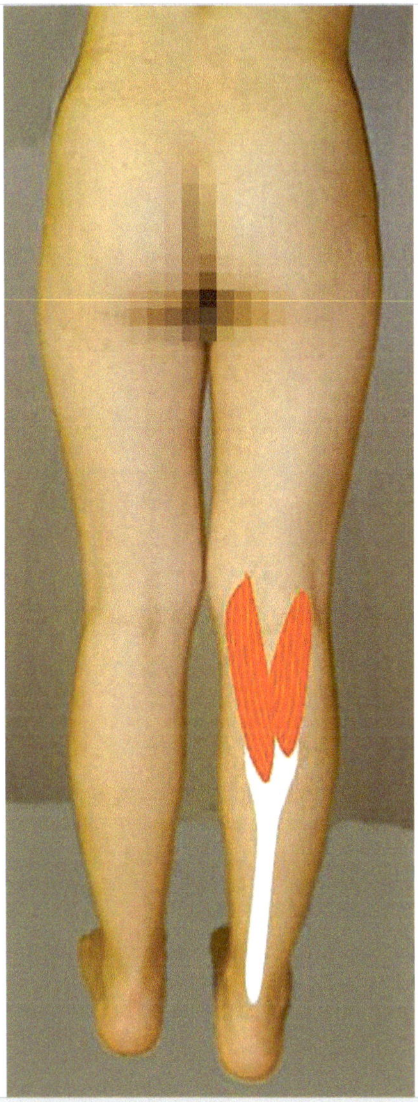

Fig. 14.2 The gastrocnemius muscle.

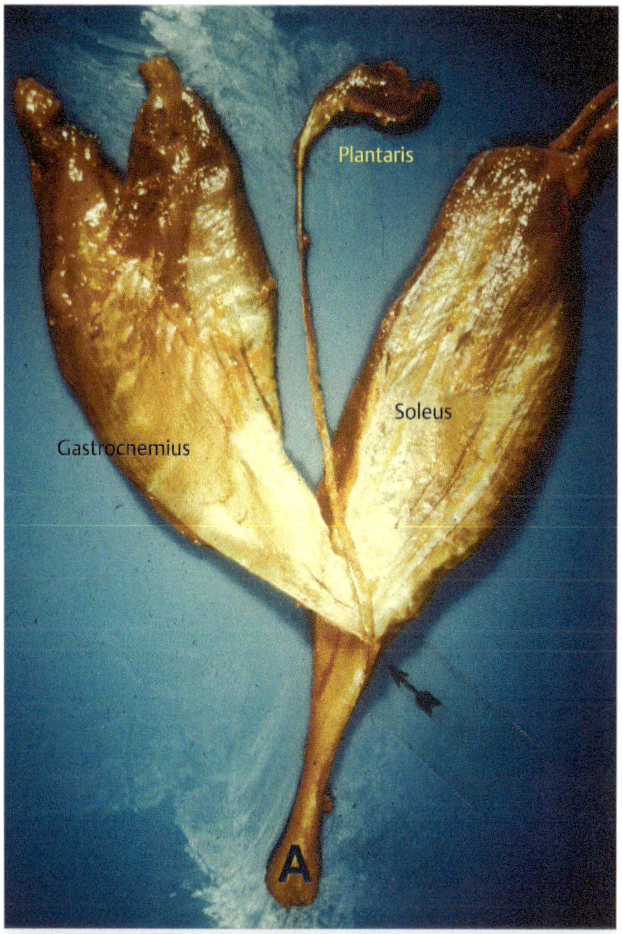

Fig. 14.3 The aponeuroses of the gastrocnemius and soleus muscles join to form the triceps surae (*arrow*), which continues as the Achilles (A) tendon. Note the plantaris tendon sandwiched between these two muscles.

14.2.1 Introduction to the Medial and Lateral Gastrocnemius Flap

Over the past half century, many would say that the gastrocnemius (▸ Fig. 14.2) and soleus muscles have been the "dynamic duo" (▸ Fig. 14.3) when considering coverage of the lower leg.[1] In actuality, the medial and lateral heads of the gastrocnemius muscle alone have been a "dynamic duo" and deserve their appellation as lower leg "workhorse" flaps.[2,3] Long before this achievement, Stark[4] had recognized the value of the pedicled gastrocnemius muscle for treatment of infected compound fractures, but only after similar repetitive reports by Barfod and Pers[5] as well as Ger and Efron[6] were surgeons convinced of their efficacy. McCraw et al[7] defined their reliable musculocutaneous territory, and believed as such were more versatile since reach was significantly extended. The gastrocnemius muscle has even been used in cross-leg fashion as a regional flap.[7,8] With the acquisition of microsurgical capabilities, this muscle soon proved useful under special circumstances as a free flap donor site for the more distal lower limb.[9,10] Neurovascular anastomoses have even permitted dynamic transfers for forearm function restoration.[9,11] Indeed, similarly an innervated pedicled gastrocnemius muscle flap has been attempted as an even simpler way to correct foot drop.[3]

The medial head of the gastrocnemius (MHG) muscle, since usually larger and longer (▸ Fig. 14.4),[1,12,13,14] has traditionally been selected to correct problems of the distal thigh, region of the patella and knee joint, and proximal third of the leg itself (▸ Fig. 14.5).[1,15] The less often used lateral head of the gastrocnemius (LHG) muscle still is important and a better choice for lateral knee or defects around the proximal fibula (▸ Fig. 14.6).[3,16] The gastrocnemius muscle as a whole not only assists plantar flexion of the foot but also is a knee flexor and stabilizer.[17,18] Yet the soleus muscle is a more powerful agonist with regard to

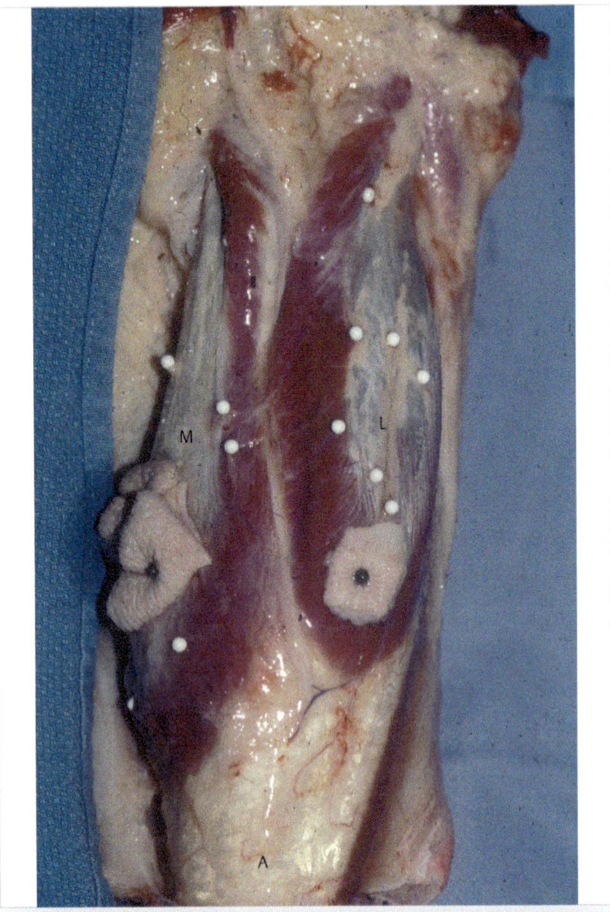

Fig. 14.4 In this posterior view of the gastrocnemius muscle in a fresh amputation specimen, as is not unusual, the muscle fibers of the medial head (M) have a more distal insertion than those of the lateral head (L) upon the aponeurosis that becomes the Achilles (A) tendon.

ankle movement; so, many patients even after transfer of both gastrocnemius heads can ambulate normally, suggesting that either or both heads are expendable.[2] However, Daigeler et al[7] in an extensive review of their experience found that patients had some restrictions in basic activities like walking upstairs, standing, or jumping on tiptoes, and especially running—even if only a single head had been used as a flap.

14.2.2 Attributes and Detriments

Attributes

- Local option for distal-third thigh, knee region, and proximal-third leg coverage.
- Expendable.
- Straightforward harvest.
- Possible Achilles tendon repair.
- Minimal donor site deformity.

Detriments

- Not suitable for athlete.
- Musculocutaneous versions leave nonaesthetic donor site residue.
- Lateral head risks peroneal nerve palsy.

14.2.3 Anatomical Considerations

Literally the "belly of the calf," the gastrocnemius muscle is the most superficial muscle of the posterior compartment of the leg.[13] There are two distinct heads, each with a discreet neurovascular supply. The medial head originates from the popliteal surface of the femur just superior to the medial condyle, whereas the lateral head arises from the lateral epicondyle of the femur.[3,18] The proximal portion of each head forms the

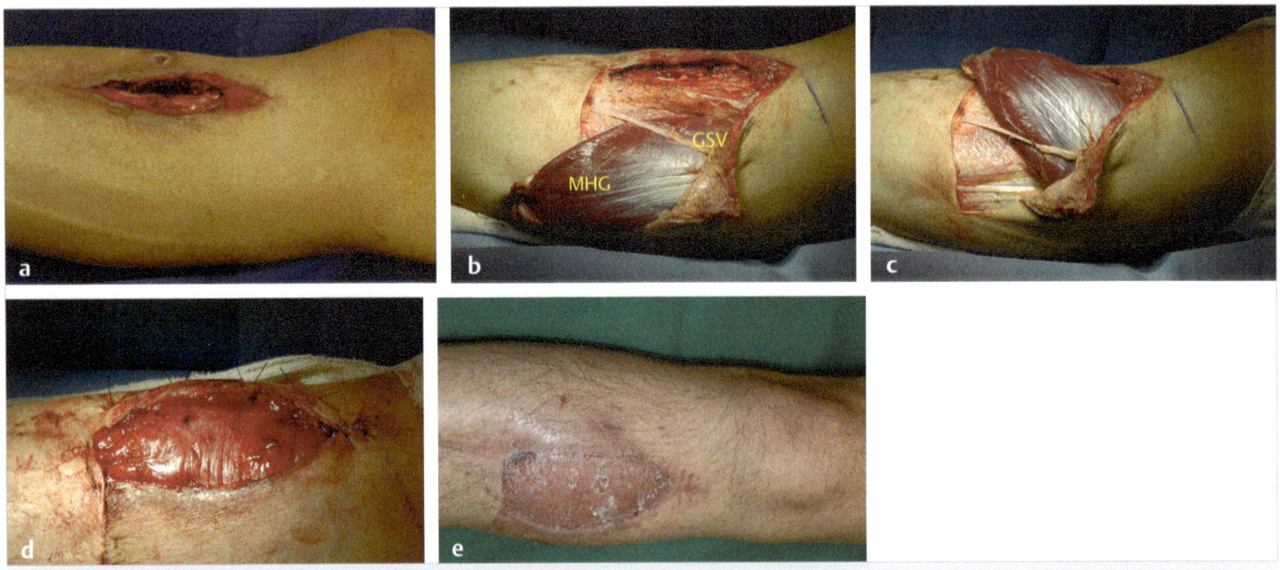

Fig. 14.5 **(a)** Chronic osteomyelitis of the right proximal tibia. **(b)** Transverse subfascial incision dropped from the distal margin of the open skin wound to the posterior midline (with preservation of the greater saphenous vein [GSV] and saphenous nerve) allowed access to the medial head of the gastrocnemius (MHG) muscle, taken with a short cuff of aponeurosis around the distal insertion of its muscle fibers. **(c)** MHG then rotated anteriorly under the GSV to fill the bony defect. **(d)** Perimeter of muscle inset as a safety factor underneath all the skin defect margins while covering the exposed bone in its entirety. **(e)** Healed skin grafted MHG flap.

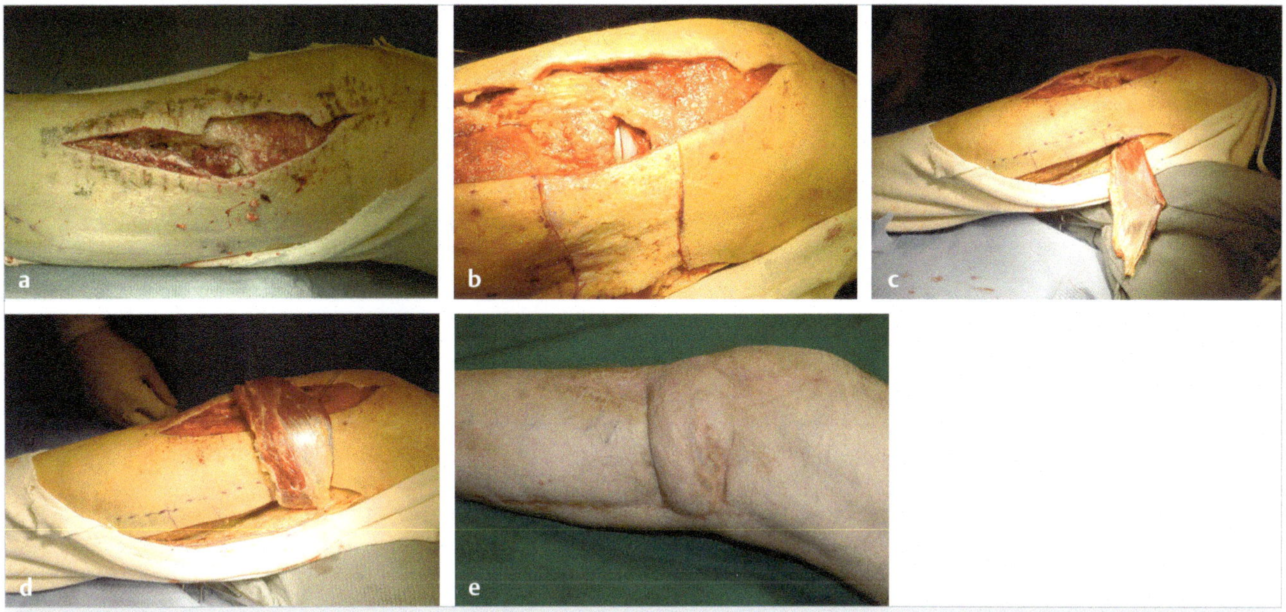

Fig. 14.6 **(a)** Debrided lateral parapatellar incision used for total knee replacement. **(b)** Implant exposed in lateral opening into joint capsule. Note area of skin de-epithelialization extending immediately inferiorly to the open joint to join the incision posteriorly used to harvest the lateral head of the gastrocnemius (LHG) muscle, which was selected since this head was the closest to the area needing coverage. **(c)** LHG withdrawn from incision that had proceeded longitudinally 2 to 3 cm below the fibula (marked by *dotted line*). **(d)** LHG transposed over the de-epithelialized skin to avoid the risk of compression in a subfascial tunnel in this thin individual, with tension-free coverage of the joint capsule. **(e)** Healed skin grafted LHG flap with prosthesis preservation. The donor site was closed primarily.

borders of the lower triangle of the popliteal fossa.[3] Distal to this, the two heads are fused together at a midline raphe that can be indistinguishable if not for the presence of the medial sural cutaneous nerve and accompanying branch of the lesser saphenous vein that traverse a groove between the two.[18] The muscle fibers of each head again become distinct when they insert on the posterior aspect of its aponeurosis (▶ Fig. 14.4) that joins its counterpart from the soleus muscle to form the triceps surae (▶ Fig. 14.3). This conjoined aponeurosis becomes the Achilles tendon that ultimately inserts on the calcaneus. Most consider the medial head to be the larger and longer of the two,[1,12,13,14] although Andejeklov et al[19] in a recent anatomical study of fresh cadavers suggest that there is really no significant difference between them.

The arterial supply to each head of the gastrocnemius muscle always arises from the posterior surface of the popliteal artery just above the knee joint, but may bifurcate from a single common vessel or have double pedicles.[9] Most often, however, there is a distinct solitary branch to each head, making each a type I muscle as defined by Mathes and Nahai.[20] The caliber of these arteries at their takeoff is about 2 to 3 mm, and potential pedicle length is 2 to 5 cm.[18,21] Soon after entering the hilum of each muscle, each source vessel bifurcates into two or more branches that run longitudinally throughout the length of the muscle,[18] and is the basis for safely splitting the muscle.[22] Communicating branches between the heads through the more distal fusion of the muscles will provide sufficient circulation such that one head can survive on that supplied by the other.[23,24] Major musculocutaneous perforators from the longitudinal branches typically are found in the more proximal half of the muscle.[25] Numerous venae comitantes accompany the arteries until eventually emptying into the popliteal vein.[18,21]

Motor innervation of the gastrocnemius muscle is by a distinct branch from the medial popliteal nerve that accompanies the dominant vascular pedicle into the hilum of each head.[18] According to Taylor et al,[26] this is a type III mode of innervation, since having multiple branches from the same nerve trunk to the gastrocnemius muscle as a whole, but an argument could be made that each head if considered individually would have a solitary unbranched nerve entering that muscle, and thus be a type I muscle. Especially when assessing the use of the LHG, it must be understood that the common peroneal nerve will be found near the head and neck of the fibula superficial to that muscle and deep to the biceps femoris.[12]

14.2.4 Anatomical Variants and Potential Pitfalls

Musculocutaneous Flaps

Perforasomes

The perforasome for each head of the gastrocnemius muscle approximately corresponds to the dimensions of that component. For the MHG muscle, this would stretch from the posterior midline to the medial tibial border, in contradistinction to the LHG muscle that would proceed from the posterior midline to the lateral border of the fibula.[7] Any distal extension beyond the point of insertion of the MHG or LHG muscle at the triceps surae will be safest if the Achilles tendon sheath or loose layer overlying that tendon and more proximally the involved muscle is kept attached to the subfascial layer under the cutaneous component of this composite flap,[27] as otherwise that portion would behave like a random flap where survival of a length-to-width ratio greater than 1:1 would be unlikely.[21] As a musculocutaneous flap, McCraw et al,[7] even without inclusion of the tendon sheath, found that the cutaneous portion of the MHG musculocutaneous flap could extend up to 5 cm above the medial malleolus, or the LHG up to 10 cm proximal to the lateral malleolus. This has provided enhanced reach of these flaps even to the mid-third of the tibia. Agarwal et al[28] after a series of delay tactics used an LHG musculocutaneous flap to even reach the midlateral femur.

Donor Site Morbidity

Although there may be some minor ways to improve the appearance of the usually bulky musculocutaneous flap,[29] the donor site for this variation is aesthetically unacceptable to most,[2,13,18,22] and rightfully so if the Achilles tendon itself would become exposed. Pico et al[30] also found that there was an increased risk of peripheral edema and cutaneous sensory loss compared to a muscle flap alone. Elghamry[27] avoided the latter concern by using a "myotendon sheath flap" that had no cutaneous component. This had a shorter reach than the musculocutaneous flap, but sufficed sometimes also for midleg coverage.

Split Flaps

Since the respective sural arteries at the least bifurcate soon after entering each head of the gastrocnemius muscle, segmental vertical splitting of either head about a longitudinal branch is possible.[22] This allows transfer of a smaller muscle portion if adequate, the creation of multiple flaps for multiple defects, or retention of a segment to allow some function preservation. The most proximal division of these segments requires an awareness of the branching pattern of each head's source artery, as that could be in the proximal third or not even until reaching the upper half of the muscle. Inadvertent division of a branch puts at risk devascularization of that segment.

Inferior-Based Flaps

Numerous vascular bundles or branches communicate as collaterals across the raphe between the two fused heads of the gastrocnemius muscle.[23,24] If only the most inferior branch or two were kept intact, one muscle head could be elevated independent of its dominant pedicle and turned over for more distal reach to the mid-tibia.[24,31] That head would then survive via perfusion through these branches originating from the contralateral head. Incorrect estimation of potential flow through these small connecting branches puts at risk ischemia of the transposed muscle head if inaccurate.

Chimeric Flaps

A cutaneous flap based on a musculocutaneous perforator of either head of the gastrocnemius muscle can be simultaneously elevated with the muscle flap.[3,32] Perforators of the LHG are often unreliable, so the medial head will more often be used with a medial sural artery perforator (MSAP) flap.[32] The separate pedicle to the MSAP flap can be lengthened as far as necessary as long as branches to the muscle component remain. The muscle, since more malleable, can then be used for fill or three-dimensional contouring, followed by independent insetting of the perforator flap to restore skin coverage.

Achilles Tendon Repair

Linton[33] has described using the combined attachment of the gastrocnemius muscle heads to the triceps surae with an extension of this aponeurosis for Achilles tendon reconstruction. This required a V-Y advancement of essentially a large island musculocutaneous flap, which might be limited in just how far advancement is possible. Another issue is how much donor Achilles tendon would be available, although the plantaris tendon under the gastrocnemius muscle, since now exposed, could be used as a reinforcing graft.

Extending Flap Reach

Even for the traditional role of providing coverage around the knee, reach of either gastrocnemius muscle head may be difficult. A simple way to extend the length and even width of the muscle flap would be to make incisions into or remove the investing fascia of the muscle.[2] Splitting the muscle into smaller segments may extend reach,[22] but would be limited by exactly where the circulation enters that segment, which is often uncertain. An inferior-based flap based on communicating branches from the contralateral head may also be precarious.[24] Division of the pes anserinus may allow some more minor proximal transposition of the MHG with limited function disturbance.[15] Rotating the LHG under the common peroneal nerve may similarly extend reach.[1] Probably the most reliable and best way to enhance reach is to take down the origin of each head, with subsequent dissection and release of the vascular pedicle, albeit with some risk of its injury.[1,15,34] Several analyses of the arc of rotation of the muscle heads have shown that a 30 to 50% increase in reach can be expected if this was done.[15,34]

Function Sequela

Sacrifice of either head of the gastrocnemius or even both as a muscle flap has traditionally been considered not to be an issue.[2] The muscle(s) is(are) therefore theoretically expendable. Yet Daigeler et al[17] in their review of several hundred cases showed some unexpected long-term findings, as confirmed by others.[30] Exercise-dependent activities like jumping, standing on tiptoes, and walking upstairs were restricted. Only 42% of their patients had no problems running.[17] Maximum plantar flexion force at the ankle joint was 25% weaker than that of the unoperated leg.[17] The take-home message is that every muscle has a function, and, therefore, there should always be a consideration to save the muscle if possible.

Peroneal Palsy

If the LHG muscle is the selected flap, an awareness of the location and proximity to the common peroneal nerve is essential during flap harvest. Even only raising the nerve to allow passage of the LHG underneath can result in a transient peroneal palsy. Daigeler et al[17] had a 4.5% incidence of peroneal palsy when the LHG was used as a muscle flap, which was sometimes permanent.

14.2.5 Flap Design

The defect requiring reconstruction will dictate the flap design, beginning with which head should be selected. Except in the obese individual, having the patient preoperatively stand on their tiptoes with the ankle joint maximally plantar flexed usually allows visualization of the outline of each head as they insert into the triceps surae. The muscle chosen will usually be the longer and that most likely to reach the defect.

Donor site morbidity is limited if only muscle is taken as the flap, but composite, chimeric, or other variations are possible; an overview on these anatomical variants has already been given in the preceding section. Both muscle heads and their vascular sources are readily approached using a stocking seam incision that is marked to crisscross the popliteal crease before continuing vertically distally along the midportion of the calf up to the triceps surae.[34] This is easiest with the patient in the prone position, but most parapatellar and proximal third leg defects are more amenable to having the patient in the supine position, which also simplifies the administration of anesthesia and nursing staff preparation. Depending on the margins of the defect (▶ Fig. 14.5), a curvilinear line starting at the knee joint and continued longitudinally to the level of the triceps surae about 2 cm posterior to the medial posterior border of the tibia will, in this position, most readily allow access to the medial head. The lateral head will require a similar line drawn (▶ Fig. 14.6), but instead 2 cm posterior to the lateral border of the fibula.

14.2.6 Flap Harvest

Proper markings for harvesting the gastrocnemius as a muscle flap will depend on the location of the defect, patient position on the operating table, and which head will be utilized, as described in the preceding section on flap design. In the majority of cases, the patient can be in the supine or lateral decubitus position to allow independent elevation of either head only, which will minimize donor site functional morbidity. Use of a mid-thigh tourniquet with the leg exsanguinated will provide the clearest assessment of anatomical details.

Medial Gastrocnemius

For proximal tibia and medial knee region defects, the medial head since usually longer will have the best reach (▶ Fig. 14.4). The patient, if supine on the table, should have the hip flexed 70 degrees, thigh abducted, and knee flexed where comfortable (▶ Video 14.1). A somewhat curved then longitudinal incision is made 2 to 3 cm below the posteromedial border of the tibia, extending from the medial knee joint to the calf where the muscle fibers inserting into the triceps surae often can be marked preoperatively with the patient standing on their tiptoes. The incision is immediately made through the deep fascia, which is kept with the overlying subcutaneous tissues. Usually, a rim of fat along the medial border of the MHG distinguishes it from the more anterior soleus muscle. A relatively bloodless subfascial dissection, except for a few musculocutaneous perforators that must be ligated or coagulated, extends superficial to the muscle to be ceased near the posterior midline when the paired medial sural cutaneous nerve and accessory branch of the lesser saphenous vein are found. The latter structures are important, as they will continue proximally superficial to the raphe where the medial and lateral heads have fused together.

The most distal extent of the medial head will be distinguished by the oval shape of its muscle fibers that have inserted onto the triceps surae (▶ Fig. 14.4). Preceding proximally along its anterior border, finger dissection in the loose areolar plane beneath it will separate it from the underlying soleus muscle as needed. More careful elevation begins distally by sharp incision of a few centimeters of the cuff of the triceps surae aponeurosis about its muscle fiber insertion (▶ Fig. 14.5), which facilitates traction during handling while being a tough material that will hold sutures during the eventual flap insetting.

With traction on this cuff, the only restraint for more proximal mobilization of the muscle is its decussation with the lateral head along the raphe. Muscle fibers must be sharply divided while being careful to protect the medial sural cutaneous nerve. Once the inferior triangle of the popliteal fossa is reached, this separation is easier as the two heads once again become distinct entities.

The amount of proximal dissection stops once the defect can be reached without tension. Although transverse incisions in the muscle fascia will provide some additional stretch,[2] this cannot be counted on. If the pes anserinus is obstructing flap rotation, it can be divided with marginal functional impairment.[15] Pulling it under or repairing the pes anserinus can be detrimental if it compresses the underlying muscle. A definite method to enhance reach is the division of the muscle origin from the popliteal surface of the femur.[15,34] The more anterior vascular pedicle may be nearby, so this can be a risky and not-so-easy a maneuver. Begin by severing the most aponeurotic appearing portion seen at the origin, and as proximal as possible, while always being wary of the vascular hilum on the muscle undersurface. Once the origin has been completely divided, this becomes an island flap allowing easier identification and freeing of the vascular pedicle. Pico et al[30] suggested dividing the medial sural nerve as well, as the denervated muscle is less likely to dehisce acutely from muscle spasms, atrophies eventually to minimize bulging and results in a better contour deformity, and eliminates pain that otherwise could occur during plantar flexion of the foot. The islanded muscle may reach up to 30 to 50% farther to allow the desired insetting,[15,34] best done with the knee joint extended to ensure a tensionless closure regardless of the patient position. Direct closure of the donor site incision should be possible.

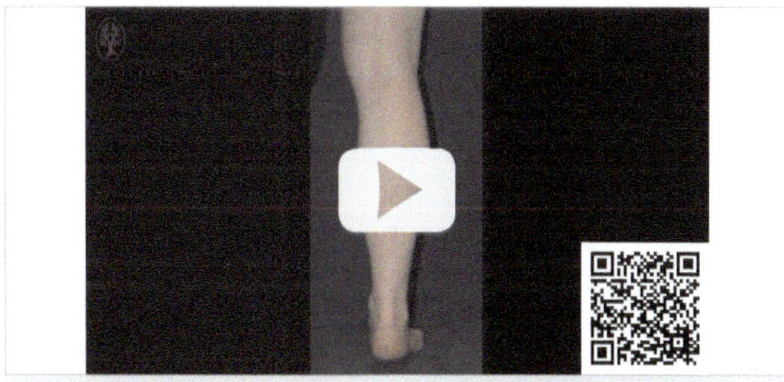

Video 14.1 Medial Head Gastrocnemius Muscle Flap. https://www.thieme.de/de/q.htm?p=opn/cs/20/7/12265265-ad3519f8

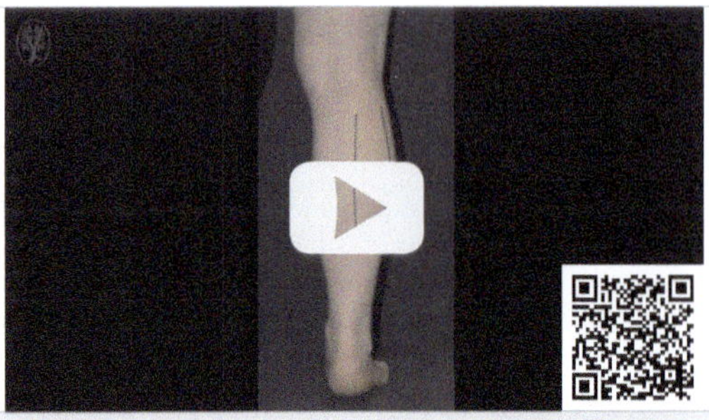

Video 14.2 Lateral Head Gastrocnemius Muscle Flap. https://www.thieme.de/de/q.htm?p=opn/cs/20/7/12265264-026e8167

Lateral Gastrocnemius

For lateral knee or proximal fibular region defects, the LHG will have better reach (▶ Video 14.2). With the patient in the supine position, or if better the lateral decubitus position with the contralateral side down, the LHG is approached by a longitudinal incision 2 to 3 cm posterior to the fibula, which should extend from the lateral knee joint to its point of insertion onto the triceps surae (▶ Fig. 14.6). Subsequent dissection is almost identical, albeit in mirror image fashion, to that as previously described for the MHG. A major difference that must be appreciated is that near the head and neck of the fibula the common peroneal nerve must always be identified and protected before proceeding with any more proximal LHG dissection. Additional reach may be sufficient by carefully pulling the muscle under the common peroneal nerve without excess traction on the latter before insetting. This approach will also prevent a compression neuropathy if it were to be left superficially. Of course, even more reach is possible if the LHG origin is released from the lateral epicondyle of the femur. If possible, division of the lateral sural nerve will result in a denervated muscle with the advantages as discussed already for the MHG.[30] Again, insetting with the knee extended will limit the risk of lower limb hyperextension causing flap dehiscence. Direct closure of the donor site incision should be possible.

14.2.7 Postoperative Care Protocols

Usually a suction drain left to collapse the void created by removal of either head of the gastrocnemius is a reasonable routine. Especially if the origins remain intact, or the muscle has been transposed across the knee joint, a posterior splint with the knee extended is essential until healing appears satisfactory, to prevent inadvertent knee joint flexion or hyperextension causing flap dehiscence. Care should be taken to also keep the ankle joint in a neutral position to prevent a subsequent equinus deformity of the foot.

14.2.8 Conclusion

The gastrocnemius muscle has two heads with distinct neurovascular pedicles that allow either or both to be used as a flap for reliable coverage of the distal thigh, knee, or proximal-third leg regions. Although considered expendable, there can sometimes be a considerable functional deficit left afterward, preventing common exercise activities. Design and harvest of either head as a flap is straightforward, as the muscle has a superficial location in the calf with a fairly reliable anatomy. Use as a musculocutaneous flap has virtually been abandoned primarily because of aesthetic concerns at the donor site and recipient site contour irregularities. Although possible to use as a regional or free flap donor site, the greatest efficacy in using the gastrocnemius muscle remains as a local pedicled flap.

References

[1] Hallock GG, Morris SF. Skin grafts and local flaps. Plast Reconstr Surg. 2011; 127(1):5e–22e

[2] Arnold PG, Mixter RC. Making the most of the gastrocnemius muscles. Plast Reconstr Surg. 1983; 72(1):38–48

[3] Masquelet AC, Sassu P, Innocenti M. Gastrocnemius flap. In: Wei FC, Mardini S, eds. Flaps and Reconstructive Surgery. Edinburgh: Elsevier; 2017:570–580

[4] Stark WJ. The use of pedicled muscle flaps in the surgical treatment of chronic osteomyelitis resulting from compound fractures. J Bone Joint Surg Am. 1946; 28:343–350

[5] Barfod B, Pers M. Gastrocnemius-plasty for primary closure of compound injuries of the knee. J Bone Joint Surg Br. 1970; 52(1):124–127

[6] Ger R, Efron G. New operative approach in the treatment of chronic osteomyelitis of the tibial diaphysis. A preliminary report. Clin Orthop Relat Res. 1970; 70(70):165–169

[7] McCraw JB, Fishman JH, Sharzer LA. The versatile gastrocnemius myocutaneous flap. Plast Reconstr Surg. 1978; 62(1):15–23

[8] de Roche R, Vögelin E, Regazzoni P, Lüscher NJ. How does a pure muscle cross-leg flap survive? An unusual salvage procedure reviewed. Plast Reconstr Surg. 1994; 94(3):540–543

[9] Potparić Z, Colen LB, Sućur D, Carwell GR, Carraway JH. The gastrocnemius muscle as a free-flap donor site. Plast Reconstr Surg. 1995; 95(7):1245–1252

[10] Keller A, Allen R, Shaw W. The medial gastrocnemius muscle flap: a local free flap. Plast Reconstr Surg. 1984; 73(6):974–976

[11] Liu XY, Ge BF, Win YM, Jing H. Free medial gastrocnemius myocutaneous flap transfer with neurovascular anastomosis to treat Volkmann's contracture of the forearm. Br J Plast Surg. 1992; 45(1):6–8

[12] Mathes SJ, Nahai F. Gastrocnemius, Clinical Atlas of Muscle and Musculocutaneous Flaps. St. Louis, MO: C.V. Mosby; 1979:141–155

[13] Cohen BE, Ciaravino ME. Gastrocnemius muscle and musculocutaneous flaps. In: Strauch B, Vasconez LO, Herman CK, Lee BT, eds. Grabb's Encyclopedia of Flaps. 4th ed. Philadelphia, PA: Wolters Kluwer; 2016:1358–1364

[14] Zenn MR, Jones G. Gastrocnemius Flap, Reconstructive Surgery: Anatomy, Technique, and Clinical Applications. St. Louis, MO: Quality Medical Publishing; 2012:1682–1705

[15] Veber M, Vaz G, Braye F, et al. Anatomical study of the medial gastrocnemius muscle flap: a quantitative assessment of the arc of rotation. Plast Reconstr Surg. 2011; 128(1):181–187

[16] Elsahy NI. Cover of the exposed knee joint by the lateral head of the gastrocnemius. Br J Plast Surg. 1978; 31(2):136–137

[17] Daigeler A, Drücke D, Tatar K, et al. The pedicled gastrocnemius muscle flap: a review of 218 cases. Plast Reconstr Surg. 2009; 123(1):250–257

[18] Serafin D. The gastrocnemius flap. In: Atlas of Microsurgical Composite Tissue Transplantation. Philadelphia, PA: W.B. Saunders; 1996:303–310

[19] Andjelkov K, Atanasijevic TC, Popovic VM, Sforza M, Atkinson CJ, Soldatovic I. Anatomical aspects of the gastrocnemius muscles: a study in 47 fresh cadavers. J Plast Reconstr Aesthet Surg. 2016; 69(8):1102–1108

[20] Mathes SJ, Nahai F. Classification of the vascular anatomy of muscles: experimental and clinical correlation. Plast Reconstr Surg. 1981; 67(2):177–187

[21] Feldman JJ, Cohen BE, May JW, Jr. The medial gastrocnemius myocutaneous flap. Plast Reconstr Surg. 1978; 61(4):531–539

[22] Moscona RA, Fodor L, Har-Shai Y. The segmental gastrocnemius muscle flap: anatomical study and clinical applications. Plast Reconstr Surg. 2006; 118(5): 1178–1182

[23] Tsetsonis CH, Kaxira OS, Laoulakos DH, Spiliopoulou CA, Koutselinis AS. The arterial communication between the gastrocnemius muscle heads: a fresh cadaveric study and clinical implications. Plast Reconstr Surg. 2000; 105(1): 94–98

[24] Tsetsonis CH, Kaxira OS, Laoulakos DH, Spiliopoulou CA, Koutselinis AS. The inferiorly based gastrocnemius muscle flap: anatomic aspects. Plast Reconstr Surg. 2000; 106(6):1312–1315

[25] Hallock GG. Anatomic basis of the gastrocnemius perforator-based flap. Ann Plast Surg. 2001; 47(5):517–522

[26] Taylor GI, Gianoutsos MP, Morris SF. The neurovascular territories of the skin and muscles: anatomic study and clinical implications. Plast Reconstr Surg. 1994; 94(1):1–36

[27] Elghamry AH. The medial gastrocnemius muscle with an Achilles tendon sheath extension flap as a versatile myo-tendon sheath flap for coverage of the upper two-thirds of the tibia and pre-tibial area: a preliminary report. J Plast Reconstr Aesthet Surg. 2014; 67(2):252–256

[28] Agarwal RR, Broder K, Kulidjian A, Bodor R. Lateral gastrocnemius myocutaneous flap transposition to the midlateral femur: extending the arc of rotation. Ann Plast Surg. 2014; 72 Suppl 1:S2–S5

[29] Kroll SS, Marcadis A. Aesthetic considerations of the medial gastrocnemius myocutaneous flap. Plast Reconstr Surg. 1987; 79(1):67–71

[30] Pico R, Lüscher NJ, Rometsch M, de Roche R. Why the denervated gastrocnemius muscle flap should be encouraged. Ann Plast Surg. 1991; 26(4):312–324

[31] Bashir AH. Inferiorly-based gastrocnemius muscle flap in the treatment of war wounds of the middle and lower third of the leg. Br J Plast Surg. 1983; 36 (3):307–309

[32] Hallock GG. Chimeric gastrocnemius muscle and sural artery perforator local flap. Ann Plast Surg. 2008; 61(3):306–309

[33] Linton PC. The combined medial and lateral gastrocnemius musculocutaneous V-Y island advancement flap. Plast Reconstr Surg. 1982; 70(4):490–493

[34] Lamaris GA, Carlisle MP, Durand P, Couto RA, Hendrickson MF. Maximizing the reach of the pedicled gastrocnemius muscle flap: a comparison of 2 surgical approaches. Ann Plast Surg. 2017; 78(3):342–346

14.3 Chapter 14B: The Gracilis Local Muscle Flap

Geoffrey G. Hallock

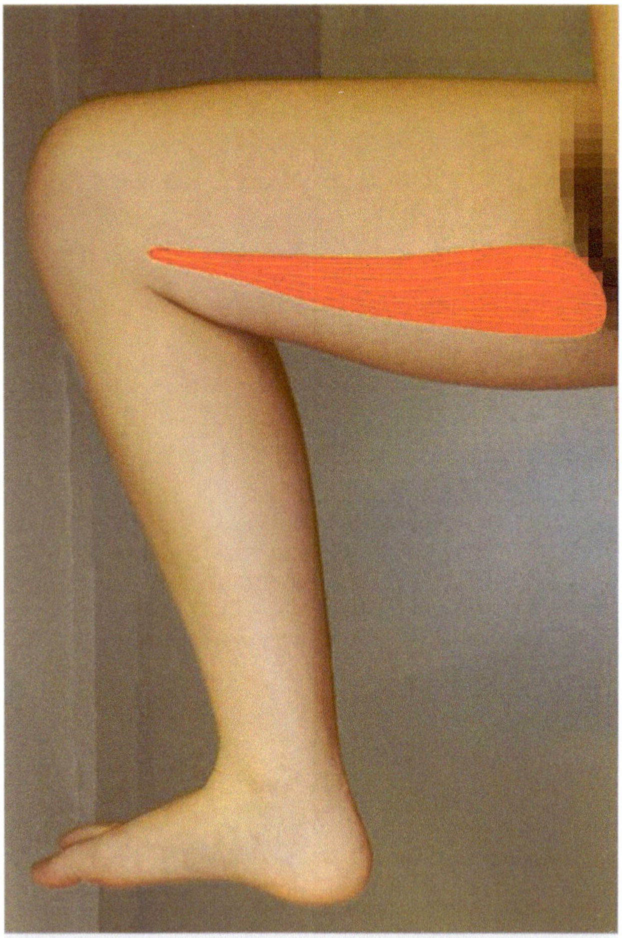

Fig. 14.7 The gracilis muscle.

14.3.1 Introduction to the Gracilis Local Muscle Flap

The history of muscle and musculocutaneous flaps has been marked by numerous yet sporadic precedents. The gracilis muscle as a flap has been no exception (▶ Fig. 14.7). Pickrell et al[1] used this as an option for recreating a rectal sphincter. Notably, the rebirth of the entire genre of muscle flaps in the 1970s and 1980s followed quickly after Orticochea[2] showed that large skin peninsular flaps could be safely raised without the need for any delay maneuvers. The trick was to include muscle underneath during the skin flap elevation, which he did by keeping the gracilis muscle attached to form a composite flap that then provided staged coverage of an ankle.[2] Orticochea claimed that perforators from the muscle allowed better perfusion to sustain a larger skin flap, although he used that word without a true understanding of their anatomical course.[2]

The gracilis muscle has truly become a "workhorse flap" found to solve all conceivable problems within the "skin and its contents," the realm of the true reconstructive surgeon. As a local flap, it can provide coverage for the genitalia,[3] perineum,[1,4] pubis,[5] groin,[6,7] ischium,[5] and sometimes if distal based even for the knee.[8] The muscle functions as a thigh adductor, knee and hip flexor, and medial hip rotator,[9] but only a minimal deficit is noted if absent, so it is considered expendable.[10] Potential donor site morbidity is minimal, and scarring on the medial thigh usually can be well hidden.[10,11,12] These characteristics demand that complete knowledge of this donor site be mastered by all who could potentially use it!

14.3.2 Attributes and Detriments

Attributes

- Versatile "workhorse flap."
- Expendable.
- Consistent anatomy.
- Expeditious harvest.
- Coverage of small and medium-sized defects about the upper thigh.
- Harvest possible in supine, lithotomy, or prone positions.
- Reliable to approach even in the morbidly obese.
- Virtually nonexistent donor site morbidity.
- Hidden donor site scar.

Detriments

- Often found far more posterior in the medial thigh than believed possible.
- Not suitable for large defects.
- Hyperesthesias of the medial distal thigh if the cutaneous branch of the obturator nerve is injured.
- Inconsistent reliability of vertical cutaneous paddle if musculocutaneous version is selected.

14.3.3 Anatomical Considerations

The gracilis muscle is found in the more posterior aspect of the medial thigh. It is the most superficial of the muscles of the adductor compartment, extending longitudinally for some 30 cm from its aponeurotic origin at the symphysis pubis and pubic arch to where its tendon inserts as part of the pes anserinus on the medial tibial condyle, found inferior to that of sartorius and above semitendinosus.[5,9] The width of the muscle may be up to about 7 cm at the level of the major vascular hilum,[6] then tapers distally toward its long tendon, forming overall a somewhat triangular shape (▶ Fig. 14.8).

The dominant vascular supply to the gracilis muscle is most commonly considered to be the medial circumflex femoral artery (MCFA),[5] although others state it may be the adductor branch or even the first profunda perforator,[6,8] but in essence always ultimately arising from the profunda femoris.[6,13] The MCFA then courses medially between the adductor longus and magnus muscles before entering the anterolateral undersurface of the gracilis at a point about 10 cm (range: 5–14 cm[6]) inferior to the pubic tubercle.[14] The artery caliber varies from 1.5 to 3 mm,[8] and venae comitantes that are larger are always present. The potential pedicle length is about 7 cm.[8] As with most muscles, minor pedicles may be found near the origin and insertion. For example, Tremp et al[15] describe a more proximal pedicle that was a

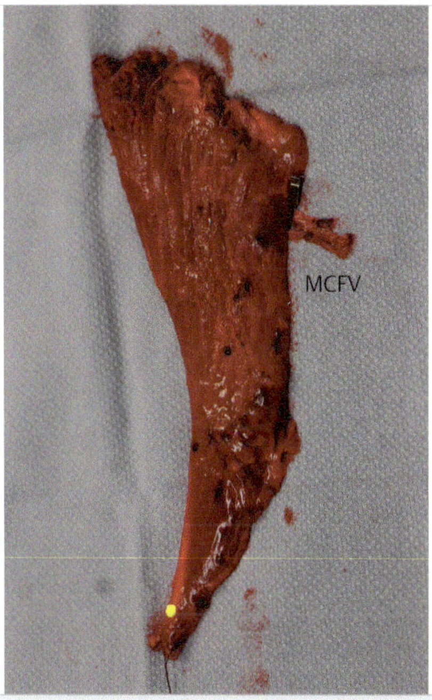

Fig. 14.8 The gracilis muscle has a triangular shape extending from a wide base at its origin until narrowing around its tendon distally (*yellow dot*). Here the medial circumflex femoral vessels (MCFV) were the dominant vascular pedicle.

deep branch of the MCFA. Cavadas et al[8] found a mean 2.2 distal secondary pedicles that arose from the superficial femoral or descending genicular arteries, with the most proximal of these commonly near the midportion of the muscle. Since circulation to the entire muscle is routinely satisfactory via just its dominant pedicle in spite of these minor pedicles, this would be considered a type II muscle using the classification of Mathes and Nahai.[16]

Motor innervation of the gracilis muscle is via the anterior branch of the obturator nerve.[9] That takes an oblique course between the adductor longus and magnus muscles before entering the gracilis muscle just superior to its dominant vascular hilum.

After entry into the muscle, the nerve splits into branches allowing segmental functional muscle transfers, making this a type I muscle according to the mode of innervation following the schema of Taylor et al.[17]

14.3.4 Anatomical Variations and Potential Pitfalls

Pedicle Lengthening

Many consider the vascular pedicle length of the gracilis muscle to be very short. However, a reasonable extension of perhaps a few centimeters is possible if the vascular origin at the profunda femoris vessels themselves can be reached. Exposure to allow this is best achieved following the advice of Hasen et al,[18] where after a subfascial dissection above the adductor longus muscle at the level of the observed gracilis pedicle, the sartorius and vastus medialis muscles are then retracted laterally to expose the source vessel origin from the profunda femoris vessels.

Skin Perforators and Gracilis Perforasome

Both septocutaneous and musculocutaneous perforators to the skin overlying the gracilis muscle exist, and are found predominantly about the vascular hilum.[19] A single and then usually large musculocutaneous perforator will often arise from the muscle over the entry point of the dominant pedicle,[5,14,20] and is a good clue as to its whereabouts. Unfortunately, in the more typical case, multiple perforators are present and of smaller caliber that are difficult to individually dissect.[19] It is far better to include all the fascia between the adductor longus and gracilis muscle to ensure inclusion of all perforators if a cutaneous flap is considered. Historically, long vertical skin paddles have been taken with the gracilis muscle with inevitable necrosis of their distal portion.[4,20] However, if the described fascial preservation is carefully observed, a vertically oriented flap at least to the mid-thigh level is usually reliable. Remember also that Yousif et al[14] showed in cadaver and then clinical studies that the true perforasome of the gracilis skin perforators had a transverse orientation extending anteriorly from the sartorius and adductor longus muscles to the posterior mid-thigh in its upper third. This more reliable skin orientation is the rationale for the transverse upper gracilis (TUG)[5] or anatomically identical transverse myocutaneous gracilis (TMG)[21] flap.

Secondary Pedicles and Segmental Muscle Flaps

The gracilis muscle can be split into multiple segmental muscle flaps, with at least one segment based on a secondary vascular pedicle. For example, Cavadas et al[8] have turned down the proximal half of the muscle that remained attached to the most proximal secondary pedicle to serve as a local flap for knee coverage.

14.3.5 Flap Design

If the patient is in a supine position, with the hip and knee flexed and thigh abducted, except in the most obese patient, the course of the adductor longus muscle can be palpated from the pubic tubercle to the medial condyle of the femur. The gracilis muscle itself will be found posterior to a vertical line drawn between these two points.[22] If a vertical-oriented musculocutaneous flap is required, the skin paddle should be planned below this line, centered over the gracilis muscle, and of a width that allows primary donor site closure. A transverse elliptical design should extend no more anteriorly than the hollow overlying the profunda femoris vessels, found just lateral to the anterior border of the adductor longus.[21] The upper border of the ellipse should be a few centimeters below the groin crease so as not to distort it, continuing posteriorly to the gluteal crease to almost the ischial tuberosity. The lower border of this flap will correspond to the amount of skin that can be pinched together to also permit direct donor site closure.[21]

14.3.6 Flap Harvest

While the lithotomy position would be preferable to reach perineal wounds, for problems confined to the lower extremity, the supine position with the hip and knee flexed and thigh abducted is adequate for harvest and use of the gracilis muscle as a local flap. Since the gracilis muscle lies almost immediately posterior to the adductor longus muscle, which corresponds to a line drawn from the pubic tubercle to the medial condyle of the femur, a lengthy longitudinal incision just inferior to this line along the medial thigh, or instead a transverse incision paralleling the groin crease as if performing an upper thigh lift, will allow adequate exposure of almost the entire muscle.[15] However, the scar length can be better minimized by first making a short vertical incision just proximal to the knee joint in the more posterior aspect of the medial thigh[23] (▶ Fig. 14.9; see ▶ Video 14.3). This approach is extended down through the deep fascia to usually expose the sartorius muscle fibers that can be seen to run parallel to the femur. If the greater saphenous vein is first seen in the subcutaneous tissues, the dissection should proceed even more inferiorly, remembering that the gracilis muscle will be more posterior just below the sartorius at this level. A circumferential finger dissection below the sartorius muscle permits retrieval of the gracilis tendon much like when grabbing the vas deferens during an inguinal herniorrhaphy.

A Penrose drain wrapped around the gracilis tendon, when distracted medially and distally, causes movement of the gracilis muscle that can be observed in the proximal thigh. This location is marked on the skin, as well as an arrow above it at about 10 cm distal to the pubic tubercle as a good estimate of where to anticipate the location of the requisite dominant pedicle. Only a short

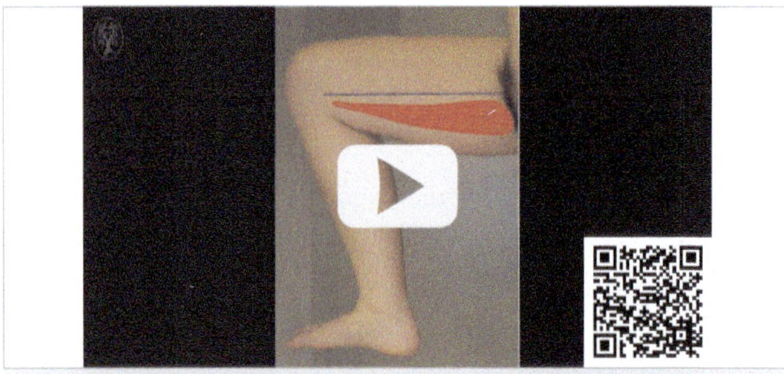

Video 14.3 The Gracilis Muscle Local Flap. https://www.thieme.de/de/q.htm?p=opn/cs/20/7/12265263-9c9a5e50

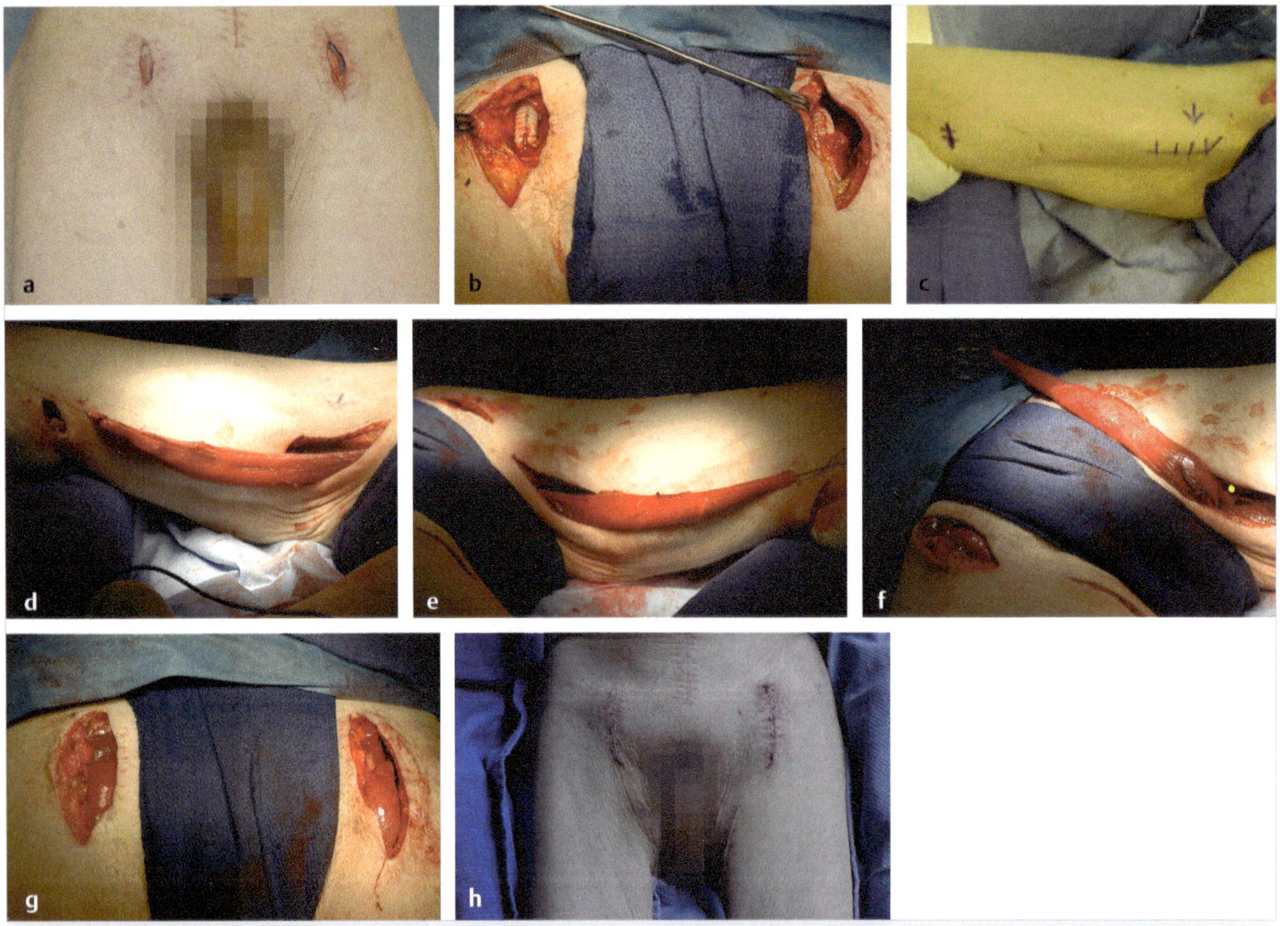

Fig. 14.9 **(a)** Status post aortobifemoral bypass for aortoiliac occlusive disease, with bilateral groin wound dehiscence. **(b)** Bilateral exposed femoral prosthetic limbs. **(c)** Plan to approach the gracilis muscle drawn on the posteromedial thigh—distal vertical incision will be to expose the gracilis tendon; *arrow* marks the expected region of the vascular hilum. **(d)** Available length of the right gracilis muscle after freed up only to the medial circumflex femoral vessels (MCFV) in proximal incision. **(e)** Similar dissection of the left gracilis muscle. **(f)** Ample reach of the left gracilis muscle that exceeds the superior aspect of the left groin wound, restrained only by its MCFV pedicle (*yellow dot*). **(g)** Bilateral femoral prosthetic limbs after they are wrapped around by the respective ipsilateral local gracilis muscles that were passed via a subcutaneous tunnel into the groin. **(h)** Early uninfected wound healing after bilateral local gracilis muscle flaps.

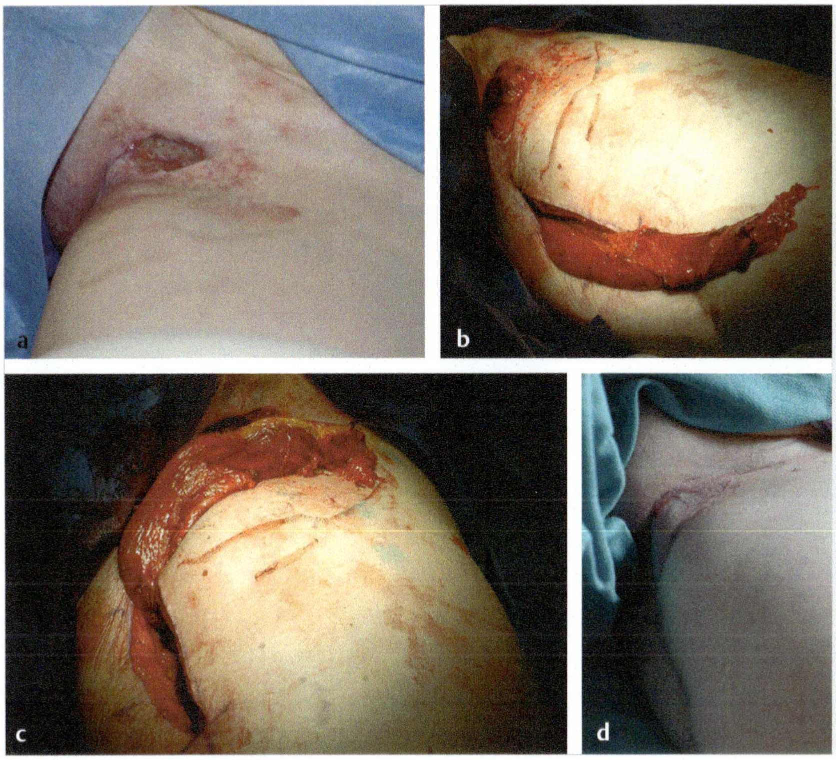

Fig. 14.10 **(a)** Left groin radiation ulcer. **(b)** Extent of harvested gracilis muscle, stopping proximally at the dominant vascular pedicle. **(c)** Since local tissues were indurated, the muscle had to be turned directly over the de-epithelized skin to reach the debrided ulcer. **(d)** Skin grafted local gracilis muscle flap permitted healing of the left groin.

longitudinal incision centered about this point once through the deep fascia allows access to confirm the anterior border of the muscle. With medial muscle retraction, by careful dissection the exact location of the vascular hilum is identified. The incision can then be extended as far proximally in a curvilinear fashion upward toward the groin crease to better expose the origin or the adductor longus muscle only if necessary.

For most local flaps, only the muscle distal to the vascular pedicle needs to be carefully freed circumferentially from any fascial connections. The incision needs to be extended distally until blunt finger dissection around the more distal unexposed muscle is completely possible via the two incisions that have been made. Often this will expose a prominent secondary pedicle that will have to be ligated. A long silk suture is sewn to the tendon with its free ends then brought with a long gooseneck clamp through the subfascial tunnel so created into the proximal incision. The tendon is divided distally, and traction on the suture will bring the distal muscle into the proximal wound.

The gracilis muscle often can then be placed directly where needed (▶ Fig. 14.10) or via a spacious subcutaneous tunnel that avoids compression (▶ Fig. 14.9), without having to lengthen the vascular pedicle or even performing any more proximal muscle dissection toward its origin. If additional reach is needed, release of the posterior border of the adductor longus muscle allows it to be retracted medially for exposure of the medial circumflex femoral vessels coursing under it and any anterior branches to the adductor longus that must be divided to gain length. If still unsatisfactory, as for a more lateral defect, the gracilis pedicle will have to be dissected back to its origin from the profunda femoris vessels.[7,18] This requires a subfascial dissection over the adductor longus muscle so that it can be retracted medially, while the sartorius and vastus medialis are drawn laterally to expose the profunda femoris. The gracilis muscle must next be divided proximal to its vascular hilum along with the obturator nerve. Now as an island flap, the muscle can be drawn under the adductor longus into the space so created over the profunda femoris to facilitate more tension-free insetting as desired.

14.3.7 Postoperative Care Protocols

Traction on the inset local gracilis muscle such as by hip movement must be avoided. If the muscle has been passed via a subcutaneous or subfascial tunnel, care must be observed to offload any external pressure that would compress the muscle or its vascular pedicle.

14.3.8 Conclusion

If a small to moderately sized local flap that needs to be extremely flexible for three-dimensional insetting is desired in the upper part of the lower extremity, the gracilis muscle has proven to be highly versatile. This may commonly resolve sequela of vascular dissections in the region of the femoral triangle or after inguinal lymph node surgical or radiation-induced residue. The vascular supply to this muscle is consistent, and usually outside the zone of injury of any proposed recipient site. Even in the presence of severe atherosclerotic peripheral vascular disease, circulation still remains sufficient to allow a reliable transfer as an island flap, often not true with alternatives like the type IV sartorius muscle or perhaps nearby perforator flap options.

References

[1] Pickrell K, Masters F, Georgiade N, Horton C. Rectal sphincter reconstruction using gracilis muscle transplant. Plast Reconstr Surg (1946). 1954; 13(1): 46–55

[2] Orticochea M. The musculo-cutaneous flap method: an immediate and heroic substitute for the method of delay. Br J Plast Surg. 1972; 25(2):106–110

[3] Ulrich D, Roos J, Jakse G, Pallua N. Gracilis muscle interposition for the treatment of recto-urethral and rectovaginal fistulas: a retrospective analysis of 35 cases. J Plast Reconstr Aesthet Surg. 2009; 62(3):352–356

[4] Persichetti P, Cogliandro A, Marangi GF, et al. Pelvic and perineal reconstruction following abdominoperineal resection: the role of gracilis flap. Ann Plast Surg. 2007; 59(2):168–172

[5] Zenn MR, Jones G. Gracilis and TUG/TMG flaps. In: Reconstructive Surgery: Anatomy, Technique, and Clinical Applications. St. Louis, MO: Quality Medical Publishing; 2012:1418–1465

[6] Hussey AJ, Laing AJ, Regan PJ. An anatomical study of the gracilis muscle and its application in groin wounds. Ann Plast Surg. 2007; 59(4):404–409

[7] Ducic I, Dayan JH, Attinger CE, Curry P. Complex perineal and groin wound reconstruction using the extended dissection technique of the gracilis flap. Plast Reconstr Surg. 2008; 122(2):472–478

[8] Cavadas PC, Sanz-Giménez-Rico JR, Landín L, Martínez-Soriano F. Segmental gracilis free flap based on secondary pedicles: anatomical study and clinical series. Plast Reconstr Surg. 2004; 114(3):684–691

[9] Zuker RM, Bains RD. Gracilis flap. In: Wei FC, Mardini S, eds. Flaps and Reconstructive Surgery. Edinburgh: Elsevier; 2017:559–569

[10] Huemer GM, Larcher L, Schoeller T, Bauer T. The free gracilis muscle flap in Achilles tendon coverage and reconstruction. Plast Reconstr Surg. 2012; 129(4):910–919

[11] Carr MM, Manktelow RT, Zuker RM. Gracilis donor site morbidity. Microsur. 1995; 16:598–600

[12] Deutinger M, Kuzbari R, Paternostro-Sluga T, et al. Donor-site morbidity of the gracilis flap. Plast Reconstr Surg. 1995; 95:1240–1244

[13] King IC, Obeid N, Woollard AC, Jones ME. Maximizing length and safety in gracilis free flap dissection. J Plast Reconstr Aesthet Surg. 2016; 69(10):1452–1453

[14] Yousif NJ, Matloub HS, Kolachalam R, Grunert BK, Sanger JR. The transverse gracilis musculocutaneous flap. Ann Plast Surg. 1992; 29(6):482–490

[15] Tremp M, Oranges CM, Wang WJ, et al. The "nugget design": a modified segmental gracilis free flap for small-sized defect reconstruction on the lower extremity. J Plast Reconstr Aesthet Surg. 2017; 70(9):1261–1266

[16] Mathes SJ, Nahai F. Classification of the vascular anatomy of muscles: experimental and clinical correlation. Plast Reconstr Surg. 1981; 67(2):177–187

[17] Taylor GI, Gianoutsos MP, Morris SF. The neurovascular territories of the skin and muscles: anatomic study and clinical implications. Plast Reconstr Surg. 1994; 94(1):1–36

[18] Hasen KV, Gallegos ML, Dumanian GA. Extended approach to the vascular pedicle of the gracilis muscle flap: anatomical and clinical study. Plast Reconstr Surg. 2003; 111(7):2203–2208

[19] Hallock GG. The medial circumflex femoral (gracilis) local perforator flap–a local medial groin perforator flap. Ann Plast Surg. 2003; 51(5):460–464

[20] Serafin D. The gracilis muscle—musculocutaneous flap. In: Atlas of Microsurgical Composite Tissue Transplantation. Philadelphia, PA: W.B. Saunders; 1996:293–299

[21] Fattah A, Figus A, Mathur B, Ramakrishnan VV. The transverse myocutaneous gracilis flap: technical refinements. J Plast Reconstr Aesthet Surg. 2010; 63(2): 305–313

[22] Hallock GG, Morris SF. Skin grafts and local flaps. [CME]. Plast Reconstr Surg. 2011; 127(1):5e–22e

[23] Hallock GG. Minimally invasive harvest of the gracilis muscle. Plast Reconstr Surg. 1999; 104(3):801–805

14.4 Chapter 14C: The Soleus Muscle Flap

Geoffrey G. Hallock

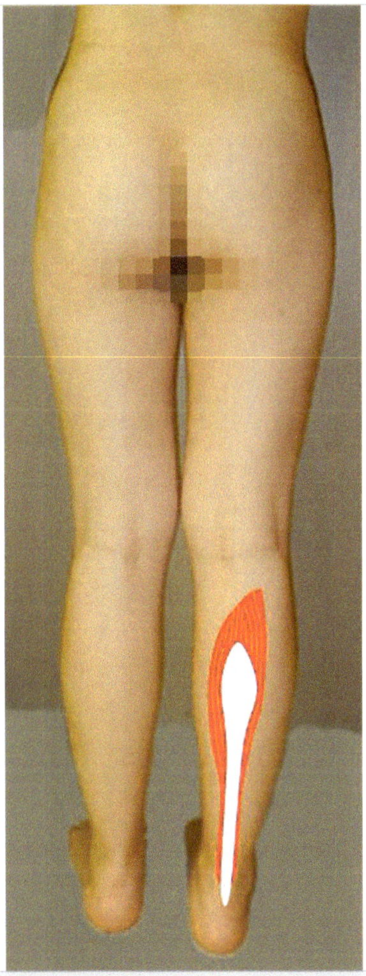

Fig. 14.11 The soleus muscle.

14.4.1 Introduction to the Soleus Muscle Flap

Indications for selection of the soleus muscle flap have declined significantly since perforator flaps have instead become a reasonable alternative that simultaneously maximizes function preservation. The primary function of the soleus muscle is plantar flexion of the foot while also providing ankle joint stabilization that prevents inadvertent dorsiflexion.[1] However, synergists that include the gastrocnemius, flexor hallucis longus, flexor digitorum longus, and tibialis posterior muscles are quite capable in maintaining that function, so it should be considered expendable (▶ Fig. 14.11).

Even though Stark[2] had earlier used the soleus muscle as a pedicled flap, many consider Ger[3,4] two decades later responsible for making this the traditional flap of choice for middle-third leg defects (▶ Fig. 14.12), including transposition to encompass the exposed Achilles tendon itself. In an acute wound, the pliable muscle can even be wrapped around the tendon without being disinserted (▶ Fig. 14.13), which better maintains the vascular integrity.[5] If distal minor pedicles exist, an inferior-based[6] or segmental island flap[7] can be designed to reach some portions of the distal third of the leg in lieu of a microsurgical tissue transfer. The soleus muscle has also been used as a regional cross-leg flap,[8] and as a composite fibular osteocutaneous–muscle flap for a large lower limb defect.[9] It can also be transferred as a dynamic free muscle flap, as shown to restore upper extremity function.[10] However, today its major role has become a secondary option if a cutaneous flap or free flap were not available to provide coverage of the middle third and perhaps sometimes upper distal third of the lower leg.[11,12]

14.4.2 Attributes and Detriments

Attributes

- Middle-third leg coverage.
- Occasionally proximal distal-third leg coverage.
- Expendable.
- Large potential surface area.
- Superficial location readily accessed.
- Reliable vascular anatomy.
- Proximal dominant pedicles maximize reach while maintaining circulation.
- Hemisoleus flap preserves some function.
- Minimal donor site morbidity.

Detriments

- Function loss may be a concern in an athlete.
- Reversed or distal-based flaps may be unreliable.
- Musculocutaneous flap may cause significant donor site deformity.
- Injury to superficial peroneal or sural nerve; lesser saphenous vein possible if using lateral hemisoleus flap.

14.4.3 Anatomical Considerations

The soleus muscle is the largest muscle of the lower leg, and is found in the superficial posterior compartment just anterior to the gastrocnemius muscles with the plantaris tendon running lateral to medial between them.[13,14] This is a bipenniform muscle whose lateral head originates from the posterior surface of the head and upper one-third of the shaft of the fibula, the tendinous arch coursing between the fibula and tibia to the soleal line of the tibia to join the medial head attached to the medial border of the middle third of the tibia.[15] While both subunits are fused proximally, after joining the aponeurosis of the gastrocnemius muscles at the triceps surae to form the tendo calcaneus, a vertical intramuscular raphe of variable distinction separates them more distally until the muscle fibers insert on the undersurface of the Achilles tendon (▶ Fig. 14.14, ▶ Fig. 14.15).[13] The location of this tendon insertion can be quite variable, ranging from 12 cm above the ankle joint to

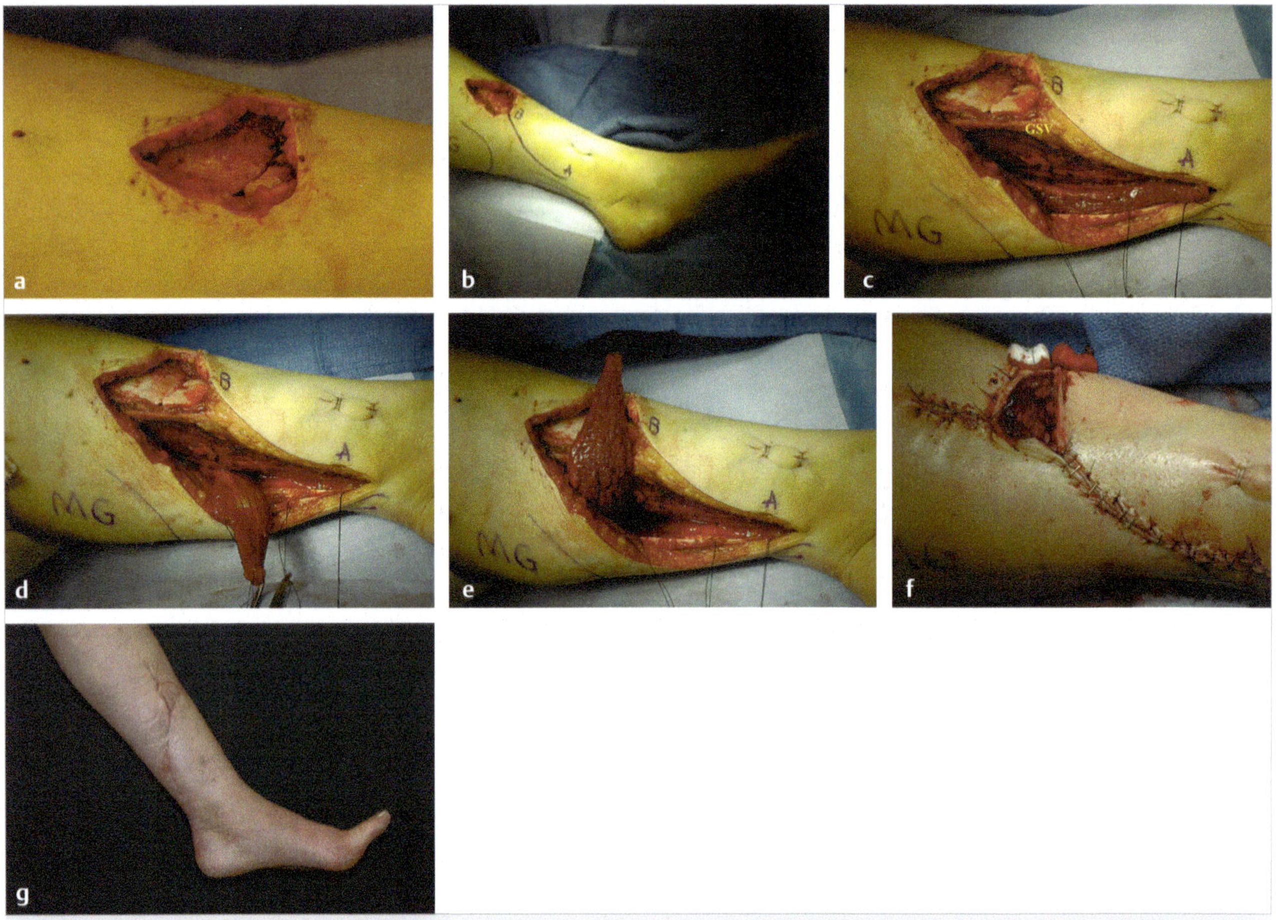

Fig. 14.12 **(a)** Left lower leg crush injury with open mid-tibia fracture and exposed intramedullary rod. **(b)** Incision marked on the medial lower leg curving from the distal posterior border of the defect (point B) to a horizontal line just anterior to the Achilles tendon (point A), terminating well proximal to the medial malleolus. **(c)** Medial hemisoleus subunit resting on the Achilles tendon (GSV = greater saphenous vein that was preserved). **(d)** Following disinsertion of fibers from Achilles tendon. **(e)** Adequate rotation over the tibial fracture. **(f)** Tension-free insetting of medial hemisoleus muscle over fracture site with primary donor site closure. **(g)** Healed skin grafted left leg showing plantar flexion ability of the foot.

almost the calcaneus below it, with usually the soleus muscle having a similar variability.[16]

The neurovascular supply to the paired soleus subunits is distinctly separate (▶ Fig. 14.14), which is the basis for reliability when used as hemisoleus flaps.[17] Baudet et al[14] describe three different levels to consider that can be quite tedious to understand in detail. Basically, the upper level of the lateral head has a dominant pedicle from the popliteal artery and innervation by the medial popliteal nerve.[14] The midportion has branches from the tibioperoneal trunk or peroneal artery that most often continue in an axial pattern distally to the inferior muscle, as minor segmental braches there are often absent.[14] The medial head in its midportion and distally is supplied by the posterior tibial artery and branches of the tibial nerve.[14] Minor branches to the inferior muscle territory are more common to the medial head than lateral,[7] but still frequently absent.[13,14] Numerous intramuscular connections allow cross-collateralization between the two heads. On the basis of this vascular supply, this would be a type II muscle pattern according to Mathes and Nahai.[18] Venae comitantes that follow the arterial pattern are adequate for venous outflow. Since the mode of innervation is via multiple branches of external nerve trunks, this would be a type III muscle using the schema of Taylor et al.[19]

14.4.4 Anatomical Variants and Potential Pitfalls

Insuring Adequacy of Circulation

A thorough assessment of the vascular status of the lower limb is essential to verify adequacy of circulation to the soleus muscle before it can be selected. Oftentimes just the gross appearance of the muscle, as in a traumatic wound, may justify its not being considered if there is any chance that its perfusion has been compromised. With the same fears, the relatively soft muscle once rotated into a defect through a subcutaneous tunnel could risk compression and necrosis. Connecting the defect in a curvilinear fashion to the distal horizontal incision routinely used for flap harvest avoids the creation of a bipedicled flap next to it as well as acute angles at skin margins that are both prone to vascular embarrassment, while simultaneously raising fasciocutaneous flaps that will lie without pressure on the inset muscle.

Extended Proximal Reach

If orthograde circulation via dominant branches has been selected, and the flap still cannot reach the defect, transverse

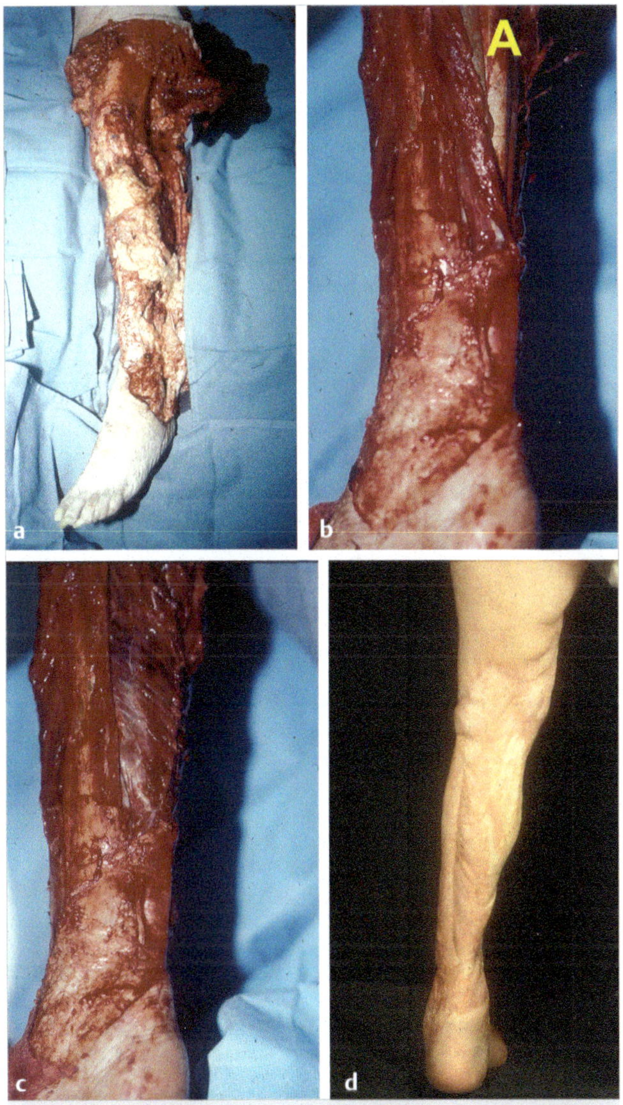

Fig. 14.13 **(a)** A female patient's horrific degloving injury of the left leg from the popliteal fossa to the ankle that occurred after being dragged when her walker got caught in the bumper of a bus. **(b)** No perforator flaps were available, and comorbidities precluded using a free flap to cover the exposed Achilles tendon (A). **(c)** Still malleable medial and lateral borders of the soleus muscle could be sewn together around the Achilles tendon for coverage, without the need to release any muscle fibers from their insertion. **(d)** Skin grafts were then enough to accomplish left leg healing and her return to using a walker.

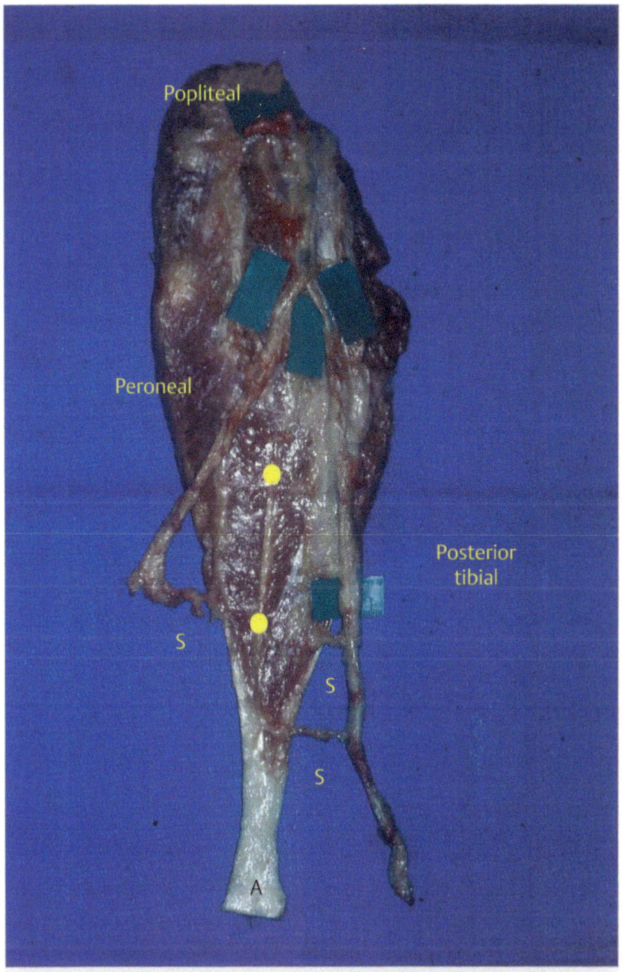

Fig. 14.14 Anterior (ventral) surface of the right soleus muscle, showing all dominant pedicles, including the popliteal to the upper level, peroneal to the middle level of the lateral subunit, and posterior tibial to the middle level of the medial subunit. Two minor segmental branches (s) from the posterior tibial artery were found to the lower level of the medial subunit. In this atypical example, a single branch to the lower level of the lateral subunit was also found, arising from the peroneal source vessel. Note the prominent vertical intramuscular raphe (between *yellow dots*) that distally separates the medial and lateral subunits, and that muscle fibers from the medial subunit insert more distally on the Achilles tendon (A) such that a medial hemisoleus flap would have greater reach than a lateral hemisoleus flap.

incisions in the epimysium will allow some stretch of the muscle.[20] This will also enhance skin graft take. A hemisoleus flap will have greater reach from the outset, as it will not be hampered by connections to origins or vascular branches remaining attached to its opposite subunit. Interosseous transfer of the flap between the tibia and fibula may increase reach, but this is not a simple maneuver and could result in compression similar to passage through subcutaneous tunnels.

Reversed Flap

Extended reach to a more distal defect has also been accomplished by transfer of the proximal muscle in a turnover or propeller fashion about a distal minor pedicle at the lower level of the muscle (▸ Fig. 14.14).[6,7,14,21] These are frequently absent from the peroneal artery, but quite often found arising from the posterior tibial artery as Yajima et al[7] reported to be a mean of 11.2 mm (range 6–14.5 mm) from the tip of the medial malleolus. The amount of muscle chosen to depend on that branch will determine if the vessel is adequate to provide the required circulation. As a general rule, if a reasonably simpler or safer option is available, the reversed flap should be the secondary option.

Composite Flap

Musculocutaneous

The soleus muscle usually is utilized purely as a muscle flap, but a musculocutaneous version is possible as musculocutaneous perforators of the soleus muscle do exist. Their perforasome

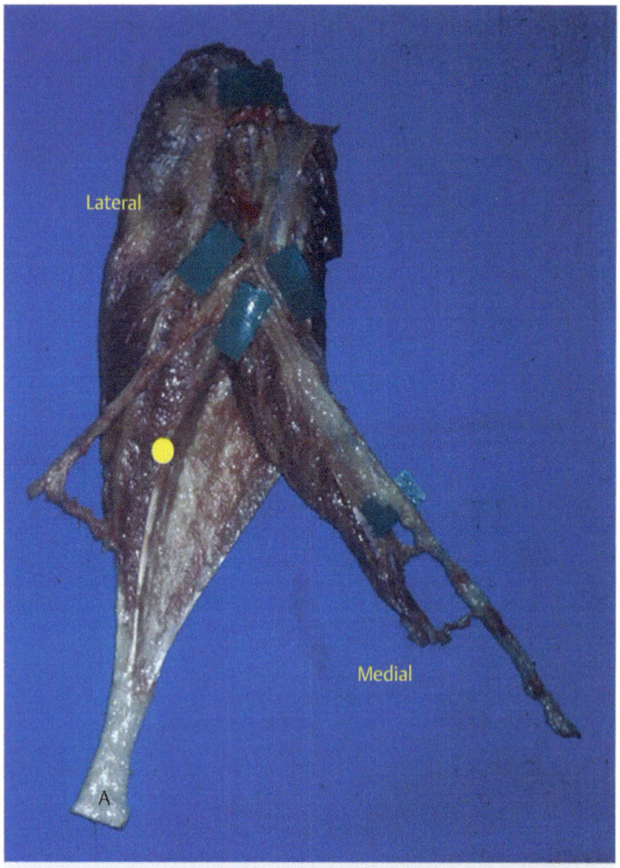

Fig. 14.15 Anterior (ventral) view of the right soleus muscle where a medial hemisoleus flap has been raised from the Achilles tendon (A) demonstrates the vertical intramuscular raphe (below *yellow dot*) that separates the medial from the lateral soleus subunit.

extends about each subunit from the posterior midline medially or laterally to near the respective septa separating the superficial and deep compartments.[22] However, primary donor site closure will be difficult, risking exposure of the tibia or fibular bone and Achilles tendon itself. This would be unwarranted.

Osteomuscular

A composite flap that also includes the fibula can provide vascularized bone as well as the soleus muscle adequate soft-tissue padding.[9,10,23] This will require sacrifice of the peroneal vessels as with any fibular free flap. That vessel would have adequate caliber, unlike the small branches to the soleus muscle that basically are relatively short and would make reach to a recipient site difficult as a free muscle flap alone.

14.4.5 Flap Design

The size of the defect and location will determine whether the soleus muscle is an appropriate choice. Although the mean width of the soleus muscle is variable (range 11–17 cm[14]), since during rotation the muscle always assumes an obtuse angle to the defect, greater coverage than expected is possible. A narrower defect may allow use of either hemisoleus subunit[17]; but if found not wide enough during that planned harvest, conversion to a total muscle flap would still be an option. Also variable is the distal site of insertion of muscle fibers on the ventral side

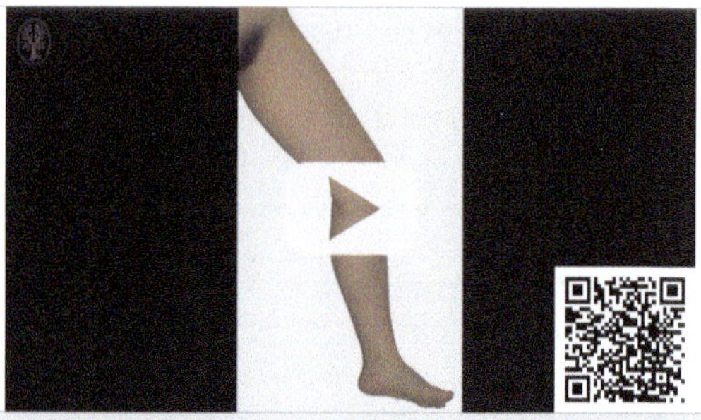

Video 14.4 Soleus Muscle Flap Harvest. https://www.thieme.de/de/q.htm?p=opn/cs/20/7/12265266-385a111f

of the Achilles tendon. Preoperative MRI can pinpoint this location.[16] The more distal this location, the more likely a more distal leg defect can be reached. If a reversed or island flap is desired based on distal minor branches,[7] they must first be explored for evaluation.[14] If unsatisfactory, at least this could serve as the recipient site for a free flap.

Most often, the medial approach to the flap is sufficient. A line from the posterior aspect of the distal border of the defect is drawn in a curvilinear fashion to ultimately join a horizontal line placed about 2 cm posterior to the palpable medial and posterior border of the tibia (▶ Fig. 14.12). This should stay anterior to the Achilles tendon so that donor site closure will not overlie it and result in tendon exposure if there would be a wound dehiscence. A lateral approach is also possible with the same horizontal line marked 2 cm posterior to the posterolateral border of the fibula, which more proximally will extend obliquely toward the popliteal fossa.[14]

14.4.6 Flap Harvest

Total Soleus Flap

As a local muscle flap for the lower leg, the patient will usually be in the supine position with the hip flexed slightly, thigh abducted, and knee flexed upon a pillow. A mid-thigh tourniquet is used to improve visibility during the dissection. The medial lower leg approach is the simplest and most commonly used. A curvilinear line is drawn from the posterior aspect of the distal border of the defect until it connects distally with a horizontal line about 2 cm posterior to the palpable posteromedial edge of the tibia, extending to just above the flare of the medial malleolus (▶ Fig. 14.12). Beginning posterior to the defect, a subcutaneous plane is followed until the greater saphenous vein and saphenous nerve can be isolated. Then the deep fascia is entered more posteriorly, and a relatively bloodless plane allows the skin to be swept away until the Achilles tendon is identified (▶ Video 14.4). The soleus muscle will be just anterior to this, and next the adjacent septum separating the superficial and deep posterior compartments of the lower leg easily found.

Staying posterior to the aforementioned septum, the soleus muscle can be bluntly pushed away as proximally as necessary except for minor branches encountered from the posterior tibial artery medially and peroneal artery laterally, if any are found. This then allows visualization of the medial and lateral subunit muscle fibers as they insert distally onto the undersurface of the Achilles tendon (▶ Fig. 14.14). Sharp dissection of these fibers releases them from the tendon, and this is continued in a cephalad direction until flap rotation is sufficient to cover the defect. If insufficient and even more proximal dissection is necessary, this may require separation of the soleus contribution to the triceps surae, which when released allows entry into a loose plane under the gastrocnemius muscle that can easily be separated even with a finger. However, the corresponding dissection on the anterior muscle surface will require a more difficult release of muscle fibers from their origin on the tibia and fibula. Once adequate, smooth, tension-free rotation is eventually possible without kinking, the muscle is inset. The donor site can always be closed primarily.

Medial Hemisoleus

The approach is identical to that for total soleus muscle harvest using the same medial lower leg incision format. Often, a vertically oriented intramuscular raphe can be seen on the posterior aspect invaginating upward from the Achilles tendon that separates the two soleus subunits (▶ Fig. 14.14, ▶ Fig. 14.15).[13] If not readily seen, the width of the flap needed will determine where the subunits are separated longitudinally as far as necessary, as intramuscular vascular connections are ubiquitous so total survival even if including some of the lateral subunit would be expected. The medial portion is then separated sharply from the Achilles tendon (▶ Fig. 14.15), and further dissection continues proximally just like for the total muscle harvest until reach is adequate for proper insetting, except no longer will there be attachments to the fibular origin.

Lateral Hemisoleus

The approach will follow that as per raising a medial hemisoleus flap except using a horizontal line 2 cm posterior to the fibula. Placing the patient in the supine position will be more difficult with the hip flexed and internally rotated, thigh adducted and elevated, and knee flexed as much as when harvesting a free fibula flap. Again, if the vertical intramuscular raphe is not obvious, as much muscle as needed to create a wide enough flap is taken proceeding medially as far as necessary. Proximal reach may require release from the fibular origins until adequate insetting can be achieved. Care during this dissection should be taken to avoid the lesser saphenous vein and sural nerve superficially, and the superficial sensory branch of the peroneal nerve near the fibula.[24]

14.4.7 Postoperative Care Protocols

If a local soleus muscle flap has not been totally released from the Achilles tendon, movement of the foot in either plantar or dorsiflexion will move the tendon and cause stretch on the inset muscle, potentially leading to disruption. A loose fitting, not compressive dressing, and posterior leg splint positioned to minimize an equinus deformity will in addition prevent ankle movement. Otherwise, no unusual postoperative precautions need to be made.

14.4.8 Conclusion

Although rarely considered today, the traditional role of the soleus muscle flap for coverage of the middle third of the lower leg stills remains a reliable secondary option as long as the muscle has not suffered itself as part of a traumatic injury, or its vascular supply interrupted by whatever cause. Either subunit as a hemisoleus flap may also be sufficient to allow some function preservation. In unusual circumstances, reach to traditional proximal and distal zones of the lower leg may be possible. Although descriptions for use as a dynamic muscle transfer or rudimentary free flap exist, the primary use of this muscle best serves for local wound coverage when other options do not exist or comorbidities preclude more complex alternatives.

References

[1] Magee WP, Jr, Gilbert DA, McInnis WD. Extended muscle and musculocutaneous flaps. Clin Plast Surg. 1980; 7(1):57–70

[2] Stark WJ. The use of pedicled muscle flaps in the surgical treatment of chronic osteomyelitis resulting from compound fractures. J Bone Joint Surg Am. 1946; 28:343–350

[3] Ger R. The operative treatment of the advanced stasis ulcer. A preliminary communication. Am J Surg. 1966; 111(5):659–663

[4] Ger R. The technique of muscle transposition in the operative treatment of traumatic and ulcerative lesions of the leg. J Trauma. 1971; 11(6):502–510

[5] Hallock GG. Multiple, synchronous ipsilateral soleus muscle flaps, including the Achilles' "wraparound" flap. Ann Plast Surg. 1998; 41(1):46–51

[6] Townsend PLG. An inferiorly based soleus muscle flap. Br J Plast Surg. 1978; 31(3):210–213

[7] Yajima H, Tamai S, Ishida H, Fukui A. Partial soleus muscle island flap transfer using minor pedicles from the posterior tibial vessels. Plast Reconstr Surg. 1995; 96(5):1162–1168

[8] Ladas C, Nicholson R, Ching V. The cross-leg soleus muscle flap. Ann Plast Surg. 2000; 45(6):612–615

[9] Baudet J, Panconi B, Caix P, Schoofs M, Amarante J, Kaddoura R. The composite fibula and soleus free transfer. Int J Microsurg. 1982; 4:10–26

[10] Chuang DCC, Chen HC, Wei FC, Noordhoff MS. Compound functioning free muscle flap transplantation (lateral half of soleus, fibula, and skin flap). Plast Reconstr Surg. 1992; 89(2):335–339

[11] Beck JB, Stile F, Lineaweaver W. Reconsidering the soleus muscle flap for coverage of wounds of the distal third of the leg. Ann Plast Surg. 2003; 50(6):631–635

[12] Hallock GG. A paradigm shift in flap selection protocols for zones of the lower extremity using perforator flaps. J Reconstr Microsurg. 2013; 29(4): 233–240

[13] Hallock GG. Getting the most from the soleus muscle. Ann Plast Surg. 1996; 36(2):139–146

[14] Baudet J, Pelissier P, Casoli V, Caix P, Farías FJ, Pawlikowski WD. Soleus flap. In: Wei FC, Mardini S, eds. Flaps and Reconstructive Surgery. 2nd ed. Edinburgh: Elsevier; 2017:581–595

[15] Serafin D, ed. The fibula flap. In: Atlas of Microsurgical Composite Tissue Transplantation. Philadelphia, PA: W.B. Saunders; 1996:552

[16] Hallock GG, Lutz DA, Osborne MA. Nonoperative estimation of the soleus musculotendinous junction using magnetic resonance imaging. Plast Reconstr Surg. 1997; 100(4):896–899

[17] Tobin GR. Hemisoleus and reversed hemisoleus flaps. Plast Reconstr Surg. 1985; 76(1):87–96

[18] Mathes SJ, Nahai F. Classification of the vascular anatomy of muscles: experimental and clinical correlation. Plast Reconstr Surg. 1981; 67(2):177–187

[19] Taylor GI, Gianoutsos MP, Morris SF. The neurovascular territories of the skin and muscles: anatomic study and clinical implications. Plast Reconstr Surg. 1994; 94(1):1–36

[20] Mathes SJ, Nahai F. Soleus. In: Clinical Atlas of Muscle and Musculocutaneous Flaps. St. Louis, MO: C.V. Mosby; 1979:157–177

[21] Unluer Z, Al-Ajam Y, Al-Benna S. Functional outcome after reconstruction of traumatic soft tissue defects in the lower half of the leg with distally based medial hemisoleus muscle flaps: a case series and literature review. Ann Plast Surg. 2018; 81(4):468–471

[22] Tobin GR. Soleus flaps. In: Strauch B, Vasconez LO, Herman CK, Lee BT, eds. Grabb's Encyclopedia of Flaps. 4th ed. Philadelphia, PA: Wolters Kluwer; 2016:1368–1373

[23] Kuo YR, Shih HS, Chen CC, et al. Free fibula osteocutaneous flap with soleus muscle as a chimeric flap for reconstructing mandibular segmental defect after oral cancer ablation. Ann Plast Surg. 2010; 64(6):738–742

[24] Zenn MR, Jones G. Soleus flap. Reconstructive Surgery: Anatomy, Technique, and Clinical Applications. St. Louis, MO: Quality Medical Publishing; 2012:1628–1653

14.5 Chapter 14D: The Vastus Lateralis Muscle Flap

Geoffrey G. Hallock

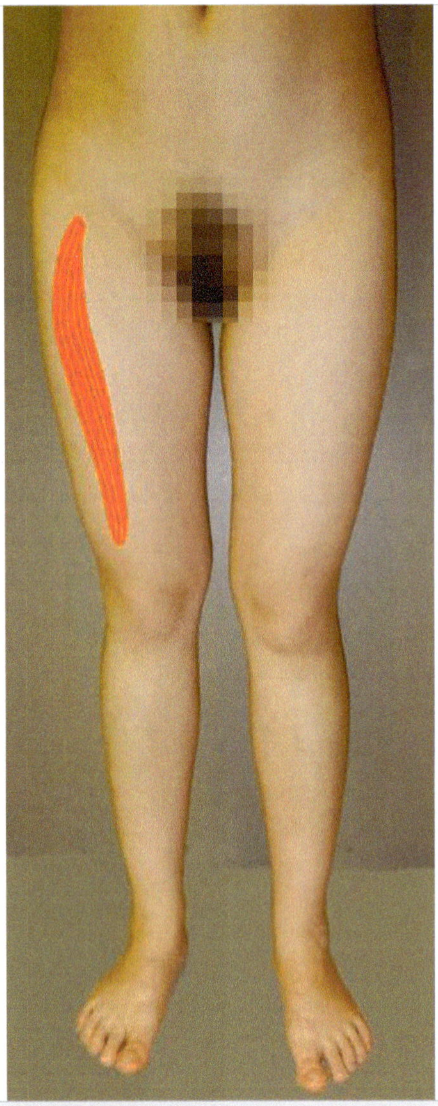

Fig. 14.16 The vastus lateralis muscle.

14.5.1 Introduction to the Vastus Lateralis Muscle Flap

Most of us are quite familiar with the location and quite ample dimensions of the vastus lateralis muscle (▸ Fig. 14.16), as that "ideal soft-tissue flap"[1] known as the anterolateral thigh flap overlies it. The latter often requires a tedious intramuscular dissection of the more commonly found musculocutaneous perforators through that very vastus lateralis muscle to ultimately reach its "mother" vessel. Yet the muscle itself is somewhat under-recognized for its ability to also be a useful flap. Actually, its recorded history predates that of the anterolateral thigh flap.[2] Ger and Levine[3], well known as one of the pioneers of muscle flaps, used the vastus lateralis muscle for coverage of trochanteric pressure ulcers. Mathes and Nahai's[4] classic book on muscle flaps supplied all the rudimentary and correct concepts for using the vastus lateralis muscle, with the exception of the statement that "This muscle may not be used as a musculocutaneous flap." Bovet et al[5] soon proved that was not a true statement using indeed a vastus lateralis musculocutaneous flap, also for trochanteric coverage.

The function of the vastus lateralis muscle, important as the largest of the quadriceps femoris,[6] is its major role in ambulation in being more than just a lower leg extensor or lateral knee stabilizer.[7] Some consider it expendable if the rectus femoris and tensor muscles remain intact.[7] If true, the possibility of creating a very long pedicle with large caliber vessels allows reach as a local flap to the groin,[7,8] acetabulum fossa,[9,10] ischium,[7,11] buttock,[4] and abdomen.[4] A distal-based flap can even reach the knee.[7,12] Its intimate connection with the anterolateral thigh flap allows formation of a chimeric perforator–muscle flap, where often the muscle independently can be used, to wrap around the exposed vessels in the groin while the perforator flap completes durable skin closure.[13] Sometimes either component of these chimeric flaps can be sensate, as the muscle alone has proven to be of value in unusual circumstances for paraplegic ischial pressure sores for restoration of protective sensibility.[14] Huge pelvic wounds can be filled with chimeric flaps consisting of muscle only, that is, the vastus lateralis combined with the vastus intermedius and rectus femoris, as they can all derive circulation from branches of the same source vessel.[15]

The large surface area dimensions, long pedicle, and large vessel caliber of the vastus lateralis muscle are also ideal qualities for a free flap donor site. Wolff and Grundmann[16] long ago reported this possibility. Yet Cavadas et al[17] later pointed out that there have been few reports using it specifically for the lower extremity, even though the aforementioned characteristics are similar to the more commonly used latissimus dorsi muscle; and yet the patient can be more conveniently kept in a supine position!! Today with muscle-sparing techniques, only a portion of the vastus lateralis needs to be transferred as a flap while still permitting preservation of function.[6]

14.5.2 Attributes and Detriments

Attributes

- Local flap that can reach from the lower pelvis to mid-thigh for coverage of groin, perineum, ischium, and trochanter.
- Expendable.
- Very large potential surface area.
- Very large three-dimensional fill capability.
- Large, easily dissected solitary source vessel.
- Supine position.
- Chimeric flap combinations, especially with anterolateral thigh perforator flap.
- Potential as reliable free muscle flap.

Detriments

- Function loss may not be suitable for an athlete.
- Variations in innervation pathways can make vascular pedicle dissection difficult.
- Both components of a musculocutaneous flap do not have guaranteed viability if oblique vascular branch exists.
- Distal-based flaps may be unreliable.

14.5.3 Anatomical Considerations

Classically, the vastus lateralis has been described as a single belly muscle supplied in toto by the descending branch of the lateral circumflex femoral vessels with minor pedicles at its origin and insertion, making this a type II muscle according to the schema of Mathes and Nahai.[18] The femoral nerve just before entering the muscle divides into multiple motor branches,[19] which would be a type II muscle according to its mode of innervation.[20] Recently, Toia et al[6] have better defined the segmental anatomy of this muscle in exquisite cadaver dissections, which has allowed clinical muscle-sparing flap harvest and some function preservation.

As Toia et al[6] have shown in perhaps overwhelmingly intricate detail, the vastus lateralis muscle has three clearly distinct muscle parts associated with two aponeuroses. The former for simplicity have been termed the superficial, intermediate, and deep partitions, corresponding to their position going from anterior to posterior in the lateral thigh.[6] The superficial aponeurosis originates from the greater trochanter and covers the proximal vastus lateralis muscle. The superficial partition is the largest, arising from the deep surface of the superficial aponeurosis, and laterally from the lateral intermuscular septum that separates the muscle from the bicep femoris. The intermediate partition is muscular proximally from its origin from the greater trochanter while then underlying the superficial aponeurosis until continuing in its middle third as the deep aponeurosis. It is the only partition that runs the entire muscle length, to insert on the patella. The superficial partition attaches distally on the deep aponeurosis and the rectus femoris tendon. The deep partition originates from the lateral lip of the linea aspera of the femur and the lateral intermuscular septum. It also inserts on the vastus lateralis tendon, as well as the lateral border of the patella and lateral retinaculum.[6] The deep aponeurosis separates it from the other partitions as does an adipose layer distally from the superficial partition. An adipose layer is also found between the superficial and intermediate partitions.

Each partition has a distinct vascular supply, although there are an abundance of interconnections throughout. The superficial partition is supplied by the descending branch of the lateral circumflex artery, which is found on its medial surface and runs into the adipose layer separating it from the intermediate partition.[6] The intermediate partition is supplied proximally by the transverse branch of the lateral circumflex femoral vessels, whereas the deep partition receives perforating branches from the profunda femoral artery and distally the deep branch of the superior lateral genicular artery, the basis for collateral supply to distal-based flaps.[6] Usually the descending branch is dominant, with the others only minor pedicles, which is why this has been classified as a type II muscle.[18]

Innervation usually is via a common branch of the femoral nerve that divides into multiple branches before entering the muscle, making this a type II muscle according to Taylor et al's classification schema.[20] The most lateral branch(es) proximally proceed to the intermediate partition and next in turn to the superficial partition, both following the vascular branches of the lateral circumflex femoral artery. The most medial branch(es) course to the deep partition. In 30% of cases, separate branches directly from the femoral nerve go to each partition, which would make that variation a type III muscle.[20]

14.5.4 Anatomical Variations and Potential Pitfalls

Oblique Branch Reach Limitations

There is one very important anomaly with regard to the vascular supply to the vastus lateralis muscle. The group from Chang Gung with its emphasis on the anterolateral thigh flap found that in 35% of their cases there was the so-called *oblique branch*, with the dominant perforator of that flap arising from it 14% of the time rather than from the descending branch.[21] The oblique branch was always found between the transverse branch and the descending branch,[21] but sometimes ran an intramuscular course through the entirety of what would be considered probably the intermediate partition by Toia et al.[6] In our unreported experience, sometimes this is the dominant pedicle to the vastus lateralis muscle, as the descending branch is diminutive or even absent. If either of the latter is true, the length of the vascular pedicle of a local vastus lateralis muscle flap may have insufficient reach compared to what would normally be anticipated.

Oblique Branch Chimeric and Musculocutaneous Flap Limitations

The oblique branch arises from the descending branch in 35% of cases and the transverse branch of the lateral circumflex femoral in 52% of cases.[21] Therefore, only in 87% of the time a chimeric flap consisting of an anterolateral thigh perforator flap and vastus lateralis muscle flap is conceivable without difficulty. Note also that if a musculocutaneous flap is planned, if the skin musculocutaneous perforators arise from the oblique branch, but only the descending branch to the muscle is kept, then the skin portion could necrose while the muscle remains viable.[21] Therefore, in this situation, it is always wisest to carefully ascertain the course and origin of the skin perforators without injuring the muscle vascular branches before completion of elevation of such a flap.

14.5.5 Flap Design

Although knowledge of the intricate segmental anatomy of the vastus lateralis muscle is important,[6] the actual planning for use as a local flap is far simpler. For all alternatives, the descending branch of the lateral circumflex femoral should serve as the vascular pedicle. If an extremely large flap is needed, the entire muscle including all three partitions can be detached from all origins and insertions, to form an island flap based on the descending branch leash. Reach will then be limited to how far proximally the latter can be dissected, which, even if including the lateral circumflex femoral vessel itself, will rarely be more than 10 cm.[7] More likely, the superficial partition, and that rarely in its entirety, will have ample muscle for most defects. Once the location where the descending branch enters the superficial partition is determined, the boundaries of the proposed flap of desired dimensions and bulk can be outlined about it. If the flap is designed eccentrically with the vessel entry point at its proximal border, and/or with even some dissection of the vascular pedicle into the muscle itself, this will allow a more extended reach.[17] Of course, what length is needed depends on the location of the defect, as if only mid-thigh, the superficial partition muscle can be raised en bloc without even dissection of the vascular pedicle itself (▶ Fig. 14.17). These same maneuvers can be followed to use this muscle as a free flap of required size, pedicle length, and vessel caliber.

If desired as a chimeric flap, most commonly as a combination with the anterolateral thigh perforator flap (▶ Fig. 14.18), the requisite musculocutaneous perforator to the skin component must first be isolated (see the discussion on anterolateral thigh flap for details in chapter 16A) to see if practical. If so, this perforator usually has its origin from the descending branch. The descending branch can be dissected further distal to the perforator takeoff point or other muscular side branch until long enough to capture the desired muscle component while still allowing independent insetting, with the muscle then raised as aforementioned.

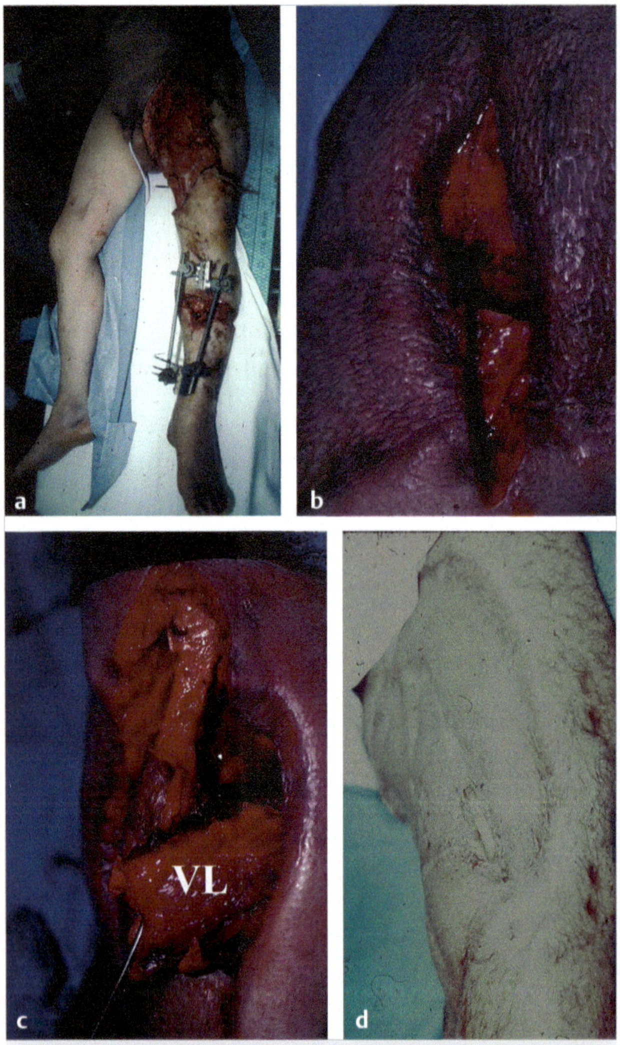

Fig. 14.17 **(a)** Traumatic left mid-tibia and femur fracture, with medial thigh skin avulsion that was initially skin grafted. **(b)** The femur fracture became exposed through the skin graft region. **(c)** A peninsular flap using the adjacent vastus lateralis (VL) muscle was raised, then rotated over the bone, **(d)** with the skin-grafted VL muscle flap allowing ultimate skin closure.

14.5.6 Flap Harvest

Probably the easiest approach to the vastus lateralis muscle is identical to that of the more familiar anterolateral thigh flap (▶ Video 14.5). A longitudinal line is drawn from the anterosuperior iliac spine to the superolateral margin of the patella. This line is incised in its midportion through the fascia lata. A ribbon of yellow adipose tissue usually demarks the intersection of the rectus femoris and vastus lateralis muscles. The rectus femoris muscle and the septum between these muscles are retracted medially to expose the descending branch of the lateral circumflex femoral vessels running along the medial side of the vastus lateralis. The descending branch is dissected proximally according to the operative plan. If possible, the branch to the rectus femoris muscle is spared. Care is taken to also preserve the motor nerve and its branches accompanying these vessels.

If the entire muscle must be used, it must be separated from its origins from the greater trochanter, lateral intermuscular septum, and femur, as well as its insertions on the quadriceps tendon, lateral patella, and lateral retinaculum. Usually, a much smaller muscle flap is indicated, and this need is served well by using the superficial partition into which the descending branch enters normally distal to the midpoint of the thigh, simplifying identification of its location. The descending branch can be dissected into the superficial partition muscle as far as necessary to extend the vascular pedicle, as long as large muscular branches are not violated. The flap borders now eccentric to this new entry point are incised beginning medially and distally even as deep as the deep aponeurosis, depending on the desired flap thickness. Muscular insertions into this aponeurosis will have to be divided sharply. The important point then during proximal dissection is to make sure the base of the flap as chosen is beneath the vascular pedicle, while the branches into the deep aponeurosis are appropriately ligated. Once this is ensured, the lateral border also can be elevated as dissection continues proximally until an island flap is formed. If it is to be used as a local flap, then the flap is passed through a subcutaneous tunnel to reach more lateral defects. For more medial defects, if passed under the rectus femoris and sartorius muscles, greater reach will be possible for insetting.

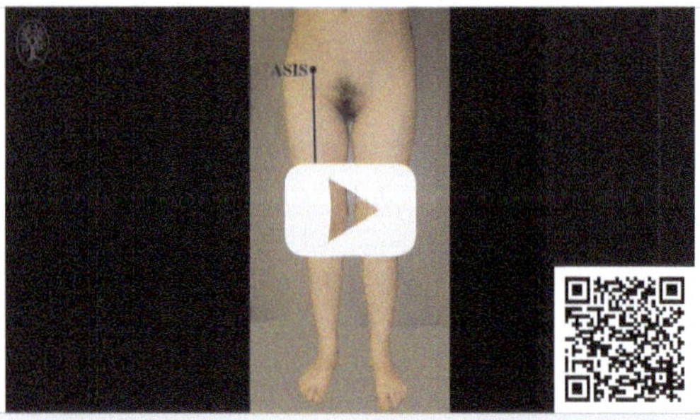

Video 14.5 Vastus Lateralis Muscle Flap Harvest. https://www.thieme.de/de/q.htm?p=opn/cs/20/7/12265267-5f81d6cf

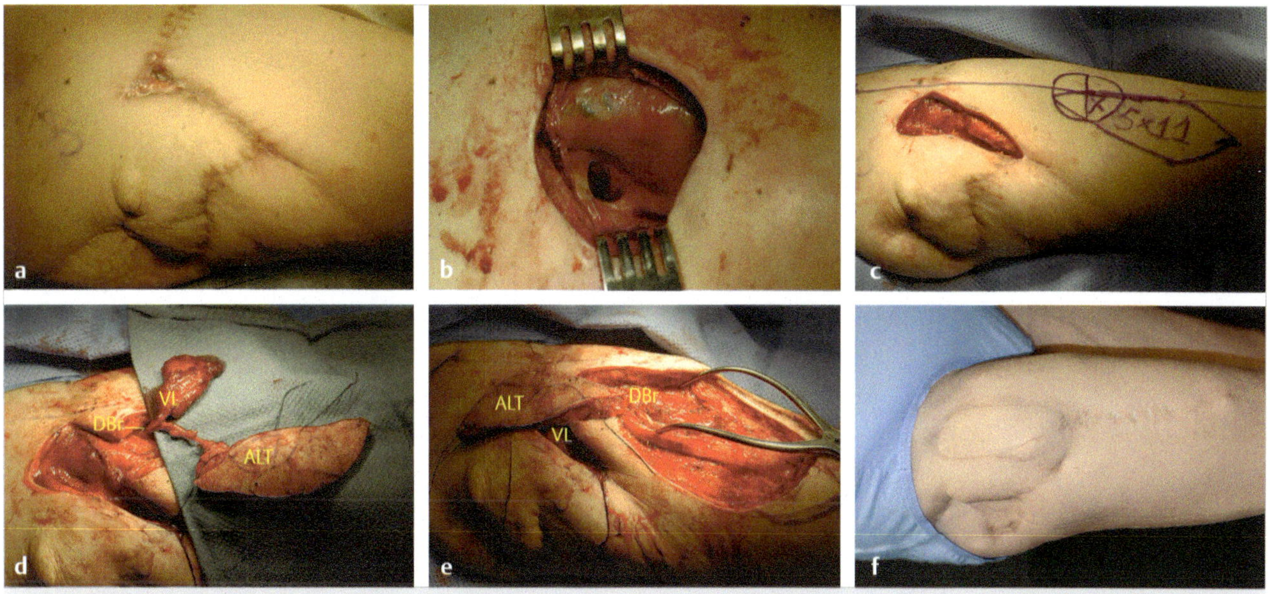

Fig. 14.18 **(a)** Purulent drainage over right total hip replacement after failed bilobed tensor fascia lata perforator flap. **(b)** Deep void existing around implant. **(c)** Skin deficit created over hip after completion of debridement, with anterolateral thigh flap (ALT) of identical size designed eccentric about perforator "x." **(d)** Chimeric ALT perforator flap and vastus lateralis (VL) muscle flap in situ with independent branches originating in common from the descending branch of the lateral circumflex femoral source vessel (DBr). **(e)** Combination transposed proximally on the DBr vascular leash, and inset with the more malleable VL muscle filling the deep cavity around the hip prosthesis, and the ALT flap independently transposed to complete the overlying skin closure. **(f)** Healed right hip a year later.

14.5.7 Postoperative Care Protocols

The patient must always be positioned to prevent pressure on a local flap as well as any tunnel through which its vascular pedicle passes, as otherwise that can be easily compressed. The mobility of the patient will determine how long this restriction is necessary, remembering that neovascularization to skin flaps is usually faster than for muscle flaps,[22] so that the time period before vastus lateralis flap circulation is pedicle independent will be longer.

With similar fears, tension on the vascular pedicle must also be avoided. Some redundancy in pedicle length prior to insetting is always advantageous. Excessive flexion, extension, or even rotation at the hip joint can hamper venous outflow of a pedicled flap, leading to its demise; this should be avoided.

14.5.8 Conclusion

The vastus lateralis muscle has the same vascular pedicle as the better known anterolateral thigh flap. Many consider its function to be expendable. If the advantages of a muscle flap are sought, this can be a bulky flap with a large surface area having a long vascular pedicle of large caliber. These intrinsic characteristics make it a suitable free flap donor site and can be used with the patient in the supine position. If it is used as a local flap, reach is sufficient to solve problems from the ischium laterally and the perineum medially. The vastus lateralis muscle can also be combined with the overlying anterolateral thigh flap or other quadriceps muscles as a chimeric flap that creates even more versatility.

References

[1] Wei FC, Jain V, Celik N, Chen HC, Chuang DC, Lin CH. Have we found an ideal soft-tissue flap? An experience with 672 anterolateral thigh flaps. Plast Reconstr Surg. 2002; 109(7):2219–2226, discussion 2227–2230

[2] Song YG, Chen GZ, Song YL. The free thigh flap: a new free flap concept based on the septocutaneous artery. Br J Plast Surg. 1984; 37(2):149–159

[3] Ger R, Levine SA. The management of decubitus ulcers by muscle transposition. An 8-year review. Plast Reconstr Surg. 1976; 58(4):419–428

[4] Mathes SJ, Nahai F. Vastus lateralis. In: Clinical Atlas of Muscle and Musculocutaneous Flaps. St. Louis, MO: C.V. Mosby; 1979:51–61

[5] Bovet JL, Nassif TM, Guimberteau JC, Baudet J. The vastus lateralis musculocutaneous flap in the repair of trochanteric pressure sores: technique and indications. Plast Reconstr Surg. 1982; 69(5):830–834

[6] Toia F, D'Arpa S, Brenner E, Melloni C, Moschella F, Cordova A. Segmental anatomy of the vastus lateralis: guidelines for muscle-sparing flap harvest. Plast Reconstr Surg. 2015; 135(1):185e–198e

[7] Zenn MR, Jones G. Vastus lateralis flap. In: Reconstructive Surgery: Anatomy, Technique, and Clinical Applications. St. Louis, MO: Quality Medical Publishing; 2012:1534–1551

[8] Ver Halen J, Yu P. Reconstruction of extensive groin defects with contralateral anterolateral thigh-vastus lateralis muscle flaps. Plast Reconstr Surg. 2010; 125(3):130e–132e

[9] Shieh SJ, Jou IM. Management of intractable hip infection after resectional arthroplasty using a vastus lateralis muscle flap and secondary total hip arthroplasty. Plast Reconstr Surg. 2007; 120(1):202–207

[10] Larson DL, Machol JA, IV, King DM. Vastus lateralis flap reconstruction after Girdlestone arthroplasty: thirteen consecutive cases and outcomes. Ann Plast Surg. 2013; 71(4):398–401

[11] Lee JT, Cheng LF, Lin CM, Wang CH, Huang CC, Chien SH. A new technique of transferring island pedicled anterolateral thigh and vastus lateralis myocutaneous flaps for reconstruction of recurrent ischial pressure sores. J Plast Reconstr Aesthet Surg. 2007; 60(9):1060–1066

[12] Sahasrabudhe P, Panse N, Baheti B, Jadhav A, Joshi N, Chandanwale A. Reconstruction of complex soft-tissue defects around the knee joint with distally based split vastus lateralis musculocutaneous flap: a new technique. J Plast Reconstr Aesthet Surg. 2015; 68(1):35–39

[13] Scaglioni MF, Franchi A, Giovanoli P. Pedicled chimeric sensitive fasciocutaneous anterolateral thigh (ALT) and vastus lateralis muscle (VLM) flap for groin defect reconstruction: a case report. Microsurg. 2018; 38(4):423–426

[14] Simón E, Pérez-García A, Lorca-García C, Safont J. Sensate vastus lateralis muscle flap for reconstruction of complex ischial sore. Microsurgery. 2013; 33(2):164–165

[15] Acartürk TO. Treatment of large ischial ulcers communicating with the hip joint with proximal femoral resection and reconstruction with a combined vastus lateralis, vastus intermedius and rectus femoris musculocutaneous flap. J Plast Reconstr Aesthet Surg. 2009; 62(11):1497–1502

[16] Wolff KD, Grundmann A. The free vastus lateralis flap: an anatomic study with case reports. Plast Reconstr Surg. 1992; 89(3):469–475, discussion 476–477

[17] Cavadas PC, Sanz-Jiménez-Rico JR. Use of the extended-pedicle vastus lateralis free flap for lower extremity reconstruction. Plast Reconstr Surg. 2005; 115(4):1070–1076

[18] Mathes SJ, Nahai F. Classification of the vascular anatomy of muscles: experimental and clinical correlation. Plast Reconstr Surg. 1981; 67(2):177–187

[19] Rozen WM, le Roux CM, Ashton MW, Grinsell D. The unfavorable anatomy of vastus lateralis motor nerves: a cause of donor-site morbidity after anterolateral thigh flap harvest. Plast Reconstr Surg. 2009; 123(5):1505–1509

[20] Taylor GI, Gianoutsos MP, Morris SF. The neurovascular territories of the skin and muscles: anatomic study and clinical implications. Plast Reconstr Surg. 1994; 94(1):1–36

[21] Wong CH, Wei FC, Fu B, Chen YA, Lin JY. Alternative vascular pedicle of the anterolateral thigh flap: the oblique branch of the lateral circumflex femoral artery. Plast Reconstr Surg. 2009; 123(2):571–577

[22] Millican PG, Poole MD. Peripheral neovascularisation of muscle and musculocutaneous flaps. Br J Plast Surg. 1985; 38(3):369–374

15 Basic Local Perforator Flaps of the Lower Extremity

Geoffrey G. Hallock, Mouchammed Agko, Hung-Chi Chen, S. Raja Sabapathy, Hari Venkatramani, and Madhu Periasamy

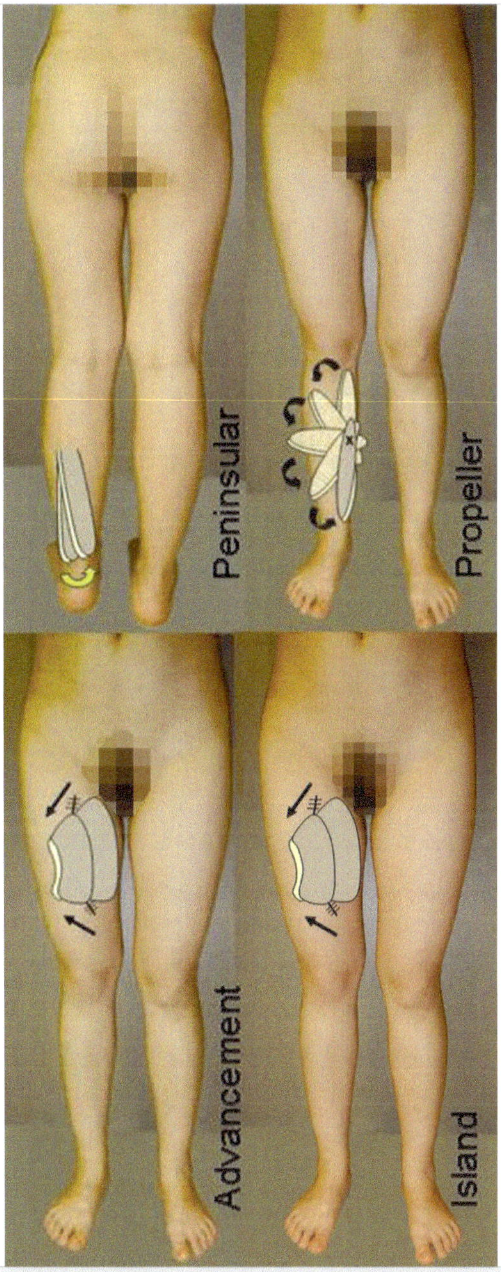

Fig. 15.1 The fundamental subtypes of local perforator flaps.

Summary

Some consider a perforator flap to be a variant of a fasciocutaneous flap that has a specific circulation pattern arising from a known vessel that has perforated the deep fascia. The lower extremity has numerous such perforators that arise in predictable regions or "hot spots," but are individually highly variable. Each supplies a perforasome that can be the basis of a local flap. Local flaps have had increasing popularity as a means to avoid the detriments of free flaps. Yet it must be appreciated that even the harvest of local perforator flaps still requires microsurgical skills, although there need not be a microvascular anastomoses. There are four basic subtypes of local perforator flaps as defined using the traditional nomenclature. These are the peninsular, V-Y or keystone advancement, propeller, or true island flaps that have a lengthy vascular pedicle. Important variants of this theme include the plantar flaps, valuable for solving difficult glabrous sole challenges, and the distal-based sural flap that can similarly be useful without the need for microvascular surgery.

Keywords: perforator flap, peninsular flap, keystone flap, propeller flap, island-pedicled flap, medialis pedis, distal-based sural flap

15.1 Introduction (▶ Fig. 15.1)

Some might say "back to the future." Old-fashioned random flaps survived "randomly" on a subdermal vascular plexus of unknown origin.[1] They could be distinguished from each other only according to their means of transposition (e.g., advancement or rotation)[1] or their geometrical configuration (e.g., as a tubed flap).[2] Strict length-to-width ratios were enforced to ensure reliability, and varied depending on the body region. Methods to delay random flaps for their enlargement or greater reach required multiple time-consuming stages.[3] Milton[4] then abruptly destroyed these concepts demonstrating that the source of circulation was the most important factor for flap survival.

McGregor and Morgan[5] proved Milton right, pointing out that flaps with an intrinsic arteriovenous network would be viable to greater lengths as an axial flap. Even then as shown in their statement regarding the deltopectoral axial flap, they were aware that its network was nourished by "perforating branches of the internal mammary system."[6] Bigger skin flaps without a delay could also be immediately obtained by inclusion of the underlying muscle as a musculocutaneous flap.[7] Then Pontén[8] reintroduced the fasciocutaneous flap that had neither muscle nor an axial pedicle, yet achieved similar results. Although Pontén never specified the source of circulation to his superflaps,[8] Cormack and Lamberty[9] in their classification schema for fasciocutaneous flaps nicknamed them as being random flaps, but they understood well that their circulation relied on fascial feeders with multiple inputs to a fascial plexus. Fasciocutaneous flaps as such became valuable throughout the lower extremity,[10,11] and that of Donski and Fogdestam[12] probably was the precursor to the distal-based sural flap.

But Cormack and Lamberty also knew their other fasciocutaneous flap subtypes differed, since they were nourished by discrete septocutaneous perforators.[9] Song et al[13] published the anterolateral thigh flap also as a septocutaneous perforator perfused flap, although today more often usually this has been found to be via a musculocutaneous perforator. The latter would qualify as a "true" perforator flap,[14] and this genre was soon widely used primarily as a free flap.[15] Wei and Mardini,[16,17] in the search for the perfect donor site, believed that only an adequate perforator needs to be present there, about which could be designed the so-called free-style free flaps. Yet why not use these same perforators in this "free-style" fashion to also be the pedicle to a local flap in the lower extremity in lieu of more complex free flaps?[18,19] So began a gradual transition in that direction with a comparison of the risks and benefits in using local versus free perforator flaps just in the lower extremity.[20,21] No significant difference was found, as long as it was appreciated that from a technical standpoint, a local perforator flap had to be carefully harvested as a microsurgical yet nonmicrovascular tissue transfer.[22] To simplify the technique for the construction and nomenclature for these lower limb local perforator flaps, Lu et al[23] classified them into four subtypes leaning on traditional terminology. Their simplest form was the peninsular flap, which has limited rotation.[24] The V-Y[25,26] or keystone flaps[27] are those most practical for advancement. The propeller flap version that Hyakusoku et al introduced, based on a random subcutaneous pedicle,[28] in the lower limb is more useful if the hub instead is a perforator.[24,29] Finally, a "true" island flap has a pedicle that extends beyond the perforator to allow astounding reach.[30,31]

There can be no question, and for whatever reasons, a paradigm shift has occurred with the preferred selection of local perforator flaps whenever feasible for coverage problems throughout the lower extremity.[32] This is the rationale here for further emphasis on the fundamental subtypes of local perforator flaps pertinent for use in the lower limb, as well as an additional bonus about the role of plantar flaps and the distal-based sural flap for foot and ankle soft-tissue closure. Anatomists have found that the subdermal vascular plexus that nourished the random flaps of past eras in truth intimately relied on deep fascial perforators. No longer just random flaps, these now are actually perforator flaps. The history of flaps has come full circle.

References

[1] Hallock GG. Classification of flaps. In: Wei FC, Mardini S, eds. Flaps and Reconstructive Surgery. Philadelphia, PA: Elsevier; 2009:7–15

[2] Webster JP. The early history of the tubed pedicle flap. Surg Clin North Am. 1959; 39(2):261–275

[3] Bowen J, Meares A. Delayed local leg flaps. Br J Plast Surg. 1974; 27(2):167–170

[4] Milton SH. Pedicled skin-flaps: the fallacy of the length: width ratio. Br J Surg. 1970; 57(7):502–508

[5] McGregor IA, Morgan G. Axial and random pattern flaps. Br J Plast Surg. 1973; 26(3):202–213

[6] McGregor IA, Jackson IT. The groin flap. Br J Plast Surg. 1972; 25(1):3–16

[7] Orticochea M. The musculo-cutaneous flap method: an immediate and heroic substitute for the method of delay. Br J Plast Surg. 1972; 25(2):106–110

[8] Pontén B. The fasciocutaneous flap: its use in soft tissue defects of the lower leg. Br J Plast Surg. 1981; 34(2):215–220

[9] Cormack GC, Lamberty BGH. A classification of fascio-cutaneous flaps according to their patterns of vascularisation. Br J Plast Surg. 1984; 37(1):80–87

[10] Hallock GG. Local fasciocutaneous flaps for cutaneous coverage of lower extremity wounds. J Trauma. 1989; 29(9):1240–1244

[11] Hallock GG. Local knee random fasciocutaneous flaps. Ann Plast Surg. 1989; 23(4):289–296

[12] Donski PK, Fogdestam I. Distally based fasciocutaneous flap from the sural region. Scand J Plast Surg (Oakv). 1983; 17:191–196

[13] Song YG, Chen GZ, Song YL. The free thigh flap: a new free flap concept based on the septocutaneous artery. Br J Plast Surg. 1984; 37(2):149–159

[14] Wei FC, Jain V, Suominen S, Chen HC. Confusion among perforator flaps: what is a true perforator flap? Plast Reconstr Surg. 2001; 107(3):874–876

[15] Hallock GG. Preservation of lower extremity amputation length using muscle perforator free flaps. J Plast Reconstr Aesthet Surg. 2008; 61(6):643–647

[16] Bravo FG, Schwarze HP. Free-style local perforator flaps: concept and classification system. J Plast Reconstr Aesthet Surg. 2009; 62(5):602–608, discussion 609

[17] Wei FC, Mardini S. Free-style free flaps. Plast Reconstr Surg. 2004; 114 (4):910–916

[18] Lee BT, Lin SJ, Bar-Meir ED, Borud LJ, Upton J. Pedicled perforator flaps: a new principle in reconstructive surgery. Plast Reconstr Surg. 2010; 125(1):201–208

[19] Hallock GG. Lower extremity muscle perforator flaps for lower extremity reconstruction. Plast Reconstr Surg. 2004; 114(5):1123–1130

[20] Koh K, Goh TLH, Song CT, Suh HS, Rovito PV, Hong JP, Hallock GG. Free versus pedicled perforator flaps for lower extremity reconstruction: a multicenter comparison of institutional practices and outcomes. J Reconstr Microsurg. 2018; 34(8):572–580

[21] Jakubietz RG, Jakubietz DF, Gruenert JG, Schmidt K, Meffert RH, Jakubietz MG. Reconstruction of soft tissue defects of the Achilles tendon with rotation flaps, pedicled propeller flaps and free perforator flaps. Microsurgery. 2010; 30(8):608–613

[22] Georgescu AV, Matei I, Ardelean F, Capota I. Microsurgical nonmicrovascular flaps in forearm and hand reconstruction. Microsurgery. 2007; 27(5):384–394

[23] Lu TC, Lin CH, Lin CH, Lin YT, Chen RF, Wei FC. Versatility of the pedicled peroneal artery perforator flaps for soft-tissue coverage of the lower leg and foot defects. J Plast Reconstr Aesthet Surg. 2011; 64(3):386–393

[24] Mohan AT, Sur YJ, Zhu L, et al. The concepts of propeller, perforator, keystone, and other local flaps and their role in the evolution of reconstruction. Plast Reconstr Surg. 2016; 138(4):710e–729e

[25] Brunetti B, Tenna S, Aveta A, Segreto F, Persichetti P. Free-style local perforator flaps: versatility of the V-Y design to reconstruct soft-tissue defects in the skin cancer population. Plast Reconstr Surg. 2013; 132(2):451–460

[26] Venkataramakrishnan V, Mohan D, Villafane O. Perforator based V-Y advancement flaps in the leg. Br J Plast Surg. 1998; 51(6):431–435

[27] Behan FC. The keystone design perforator island flap in reconstructive surgery. ANZ J Surg. 2003; 73(3):112–120

[28] Hyakusoku H, Yamamoto T, Fumiiri M. The propeller flap method. Br J Plast Surg. 1991; 44(1):53–54

[29] Hallock GG. The propeller flap version of the adductor muscle perforator flap for coverage of ischial or trochanteric pressure sores. Ann Plast Surg. 2006; 56(5):540–542

[30] Gravvanis AI, Tsoutsos DA, Karakitsos D, et al. Application of the pedicled anterolateral thigh flap to defects from the pelvis to the knee. Microsurgery. 2006; 26(6):432–438

[31] Hallock GG. The proximal pedicled anterolateral thigh flap for lower limb coverage. Ann Plast Surg. 2005; 55(5):466–469

[32] Hallock GG. A paradigm shift in flap selection protocols for zones of the lower extremity using perforator flaps. J Reconstr Microsurg. 2013; 29(4):233–240

15.2 Chapter 15A: The Island Perforator Flap

Geoffrey G. Hallock

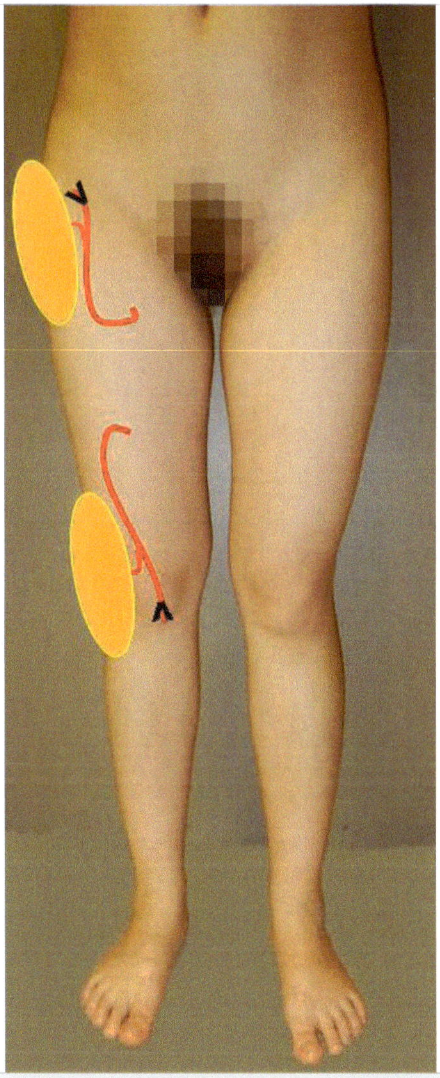

Fig. 15.2 Proximal and distal-based versions of an island flap.

15.2.1 Introduction to the Island Perforator Flap

Just what is a "true" island perforator flap (▶ Fig. 15.2) is a highly controversial idea. Theodore Dunham[1] (1892) is credited with using the term clinically for the first time, and he defined an island flap as one having an axial pedicle that is skeletonized and then tunneled under a cutaneous bridge to allow coverage of a nonadjacent defect. Today the term has become less specific, often applied to any flap whose peripheral boundaries are separated in toto from its donor site,[2,3] remaining attached only by whatever is its source of vascularization. For example, a V-Y or keystone "island" advancement flap remains attached only by a broad base to the underlying deep fascia.[4] A propeller perforator flap is connected only at its hub, that typically being a single perforator that at most has been dissected back to its source vessel to form what is often called an island flap. Rather than an "island" flap, which is somewhat of a misnomer, a better term for the latter two examples might be "islanded" flaps.

Yet Dunham's[1] definition still has merit for describing this subtype of lower limb local perforator flaps. What is a "true" island perforator flap must be approached somewhat differently in order to obtain its somewhat unique attributes. Not only must all skin margins be disconnected at the donor site, but also the axial pedicle providing the flap circulation must be extended beyond just the requisite diminutive perforator to include a major branch if not the source vessel itself. Early examples obeying Dunham's[1] definition in the lower leg were fasciocutaneous flaps that indeed were sustained by perforators from the anterior tibial,[5] posterior tibial,[6] or peroneal[7,8] vessels, but these source vessels themselves were also elevated with the flap over considerable distances. For foot and ankle defects, usually these major vessels would be divided just proximal to the connected perforator-based flap, then the source vessel pedicle dissected distal to the desired point of rotation that allowed appropriate flap insetting. Reverse flow was essential for flap survival, and the source vessel itself was sacrificed irrespective of any risks of long-term sequela. The omnipresence of peripheral vascular disease would make this option unacceptable today, and fortunately many of the other perforator local flap subtypes can now provide the same benefit.

Nevertheless, from a practical standpoint, several possibilities for "true" island flaps still exist in the lower extremity. Zheng et al[9] have described use of a constant perforator of the descending genicular artery (DCA) to sustain a distal anteromedial thigh flap as a propeller flap, but this could also be an island flap for proximal thigh transposition if based instead on the DCA itself. Agko and Chen (Chapter 15E: Medialis Pedis and Other Plantar Flaps) have discussed several local plantar flaps that can similarly be extended on the medial plantar artery as island flaps to allow reach to many sites about the foot and ankle. However, two more pragmatic options in the lower limb are island anterolateral thigh (ALT) and medial sural artery perforator (MSAP) flaps. As is well known, the proximal-pedicled ALT island flap can reach superiorly to the lower abdomen, laterally the greater trochanter, and medially the perineum (▶ Fig. 15.3).[10,11] Both a distal-pedicled ALT island flap (▶ Fig. 15.3)[12] and a proximal-pedicled MSAP island flap[13] (▶ Fig. 15.4) can cover the patella or the proximal lower leg. Because these "true" island flaps rely on inclusion of their source vessel, the descending branch of the lateral circumflex femoral (LCF) or medial sural artery, respectively, reach of these flaps is limited only by the potential length of that pedicle.

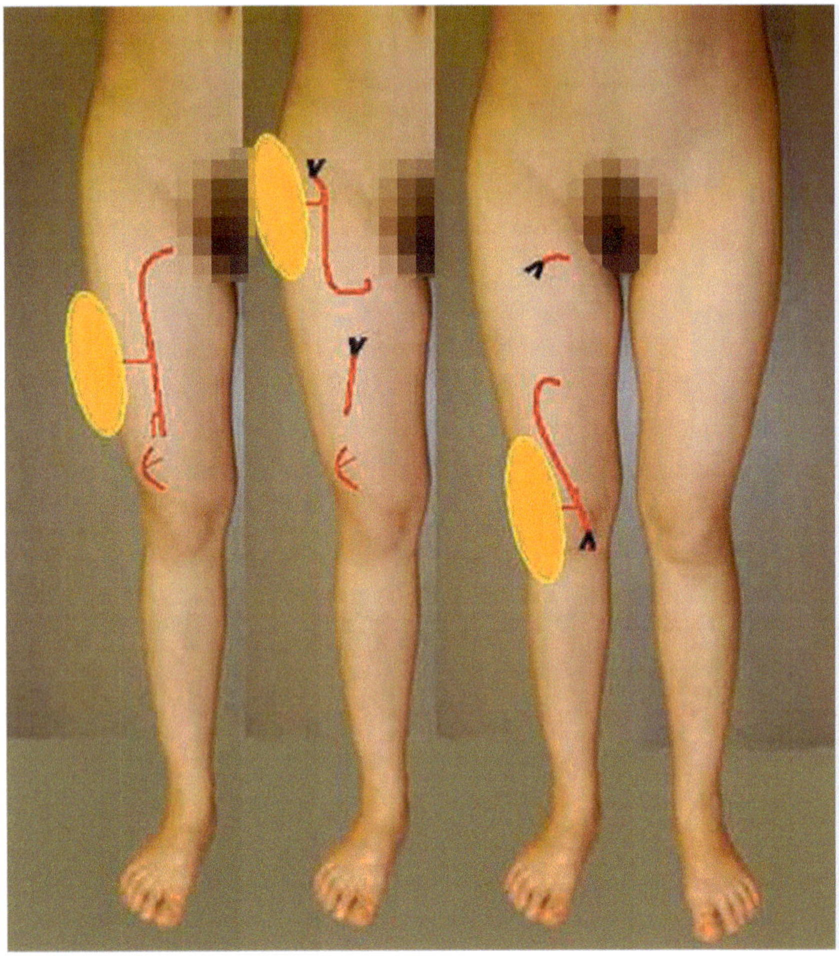

Fig. 15.3 This model of the anterolateral thigh (ALT) flap, based on a perforator of the descending branch of the lateral circumflex femoral, shows that a "true" island flap can have a long proximal pedicle for orthograde perfusion, or instead be based distally to rely on reverse flow. In either scenario, significantly greater reach will be possible than with any other pedicled perforator flap subtype.

15.2.2 Attributes and Detriments

Attributes

- Local flap.
- Normal contour and appearance.
- Long vascular leash with enhanced reach.
- Knee or hip coverage depending on flap selection.
- Function preservation.
- No microsurgery.

Detriments

- Extensive pedicle dissection.
- Sacrifice of source vessel.
- Risk of venous congestion with any distal-based variant.

15.2.3 Anatomical Considerations

To avoid redundancy, the basic anatomy of the ALT and MSAP flaps is no different than as catalogued in Chapter 16. As a local island flap, however, the difference will be the need to extend the source vessel pedicle while always being retained in situ at the point of flap rotation. For example, the pedicle of the MSAP flap can be lengthened to improve reach by dissection back to its origin from the popliteal vessels. The ALT flap pedicle similarly can be freed up back to the LCF vessels. Once this maneuver has been accomplished, passing the island ALT flap under the rectus femoris muscle will further increase reach to the midline or beyond.[14] If the ALT flap is used as a distal-based flap, maintenance of communications of the descending branch of the LCF system, which presumably also services the flap perforator, with collaterals from the lateral superior geniculate vessels for reverse flow will be essential.[12]

15.2.4 Anatomical Variations and Potential Pitfalls

Sural Artery Flaps

Almost always a single major musculocutaneous perforator will be found exiting the medial head of the gastrocnemius muscle.[15] The more distal the perforator, the longer the potential vascular pedicle to allow an MSAP island flap to reach the patella or the proximal tibia. A musculocutaneous perforator of the lateral head is often absent, so another alternative must always be anticipated.[15]

Distal-Based Anterolateral Thigh Flap

The source vessel of the perforator to the ALT flap may not be the descending branch of the LCF, but instead a different LCF branch. In that situation, a distal pedicle leash that will still be attached to the flap to allow this option will not exist. Lin et al[12] in their series using large distal-based ALT flaps for the knee or proximal lower leg found that venous congestion occurred in all flaps except for those that had an intentional venous supercharging for antegrade venous outflow performed at the time of the initial flap surgery. Not only was the source vessel of the flap dissected distally until entering the vastus lateralis muscle to extend reach, but also proximal dissection of the same pedicle was done as far as necessary so that a venous microanastomosis could be made to the greater saphenous vein for orthograde venous outflow.

15.2.5 Flap Design

Design of the ALT or MSAP island flaps will be identical as outlined in Chapter 16 when used as a free flap. Eccentric placement of the skin boundaries as distal to the chosen perforator as possible will allow the longest possible pedicle to extend reach as a local island flap.

15.2.6 Flap Harvest

The elevation of a proximal-pedicled MSAP (▶ Fig. 15.4; see ▶ Video 15.1) or ALT (▶ Fig. 15.5 and also ▶ Fig. 16.5; see ▶ Video 15.2) island flap will be no different than as described if used as a free flap (see Chapter 16) with patient positioning being also the same, except that the pedicle must be dissected as far proximally as necessary to obtain the required reach. Maximally, this would be the popliteal artery for the MSAP

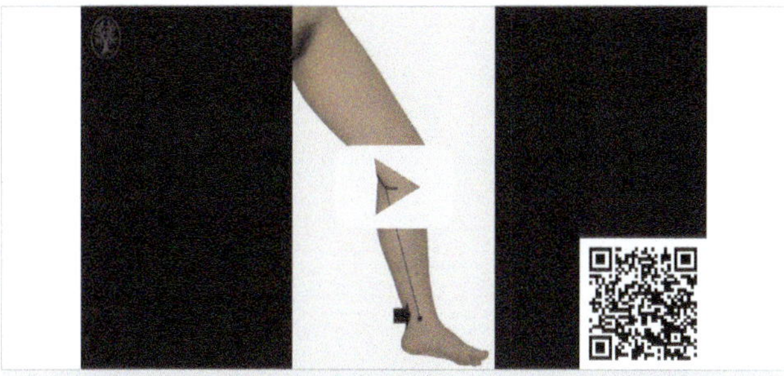

Video 15.1 Island Flap: Medial Sural Artery Perforator Flap. https://www.thieme.de/de/q.htm?p=opn/cs/20/7/12265268-f12f31bb

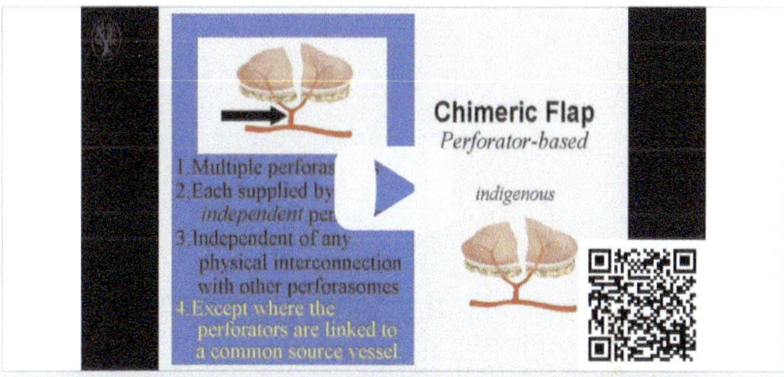

Video 15.2 Island Flap: ALT Chimeric Perforator Flap. https://www.thieme.de/de/q.htm?p=opn/cs/20/7/12265269-459e13e0

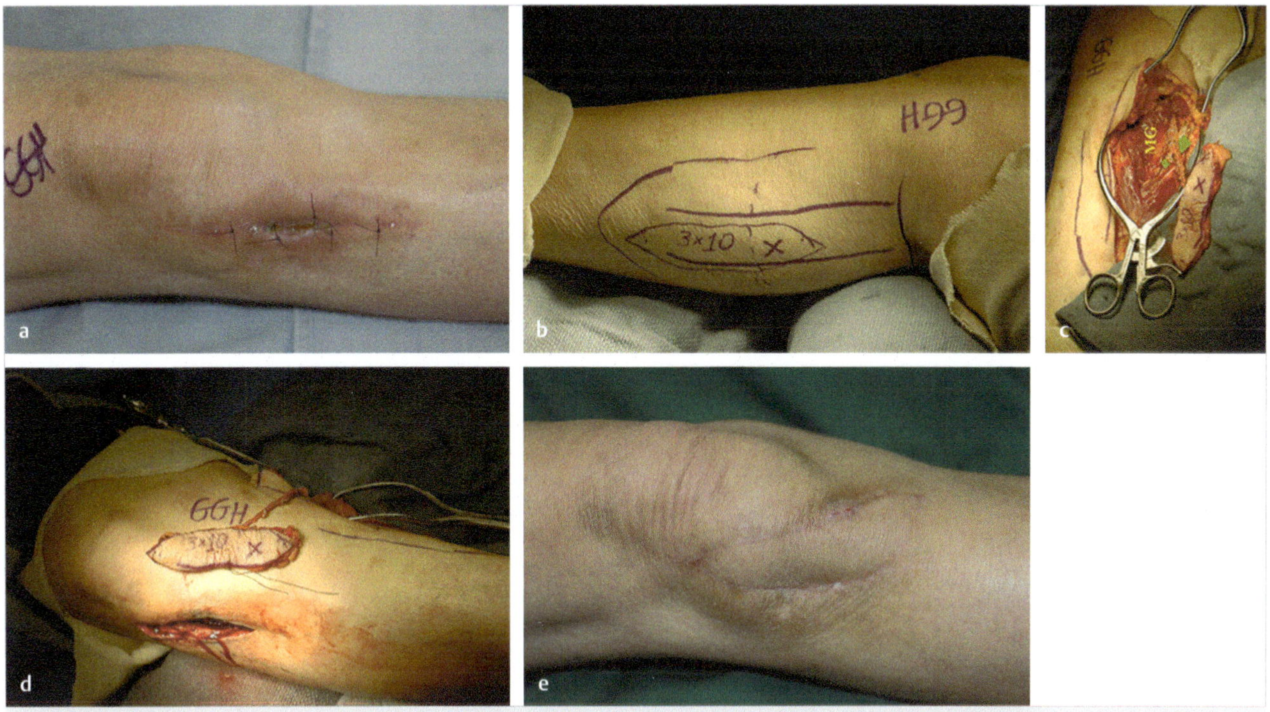

Fig. 15.4 **(a)** Dehisced wound after right total knee replacement with quadriceps tendon exposure. **(b)** Following debridement, a medial sural artery perforator (MSAP) island flap was designed over the outlined medial gastrocnemius (MG) muscle, intentionally eccentric distal to a perforator identified with audible Doppler marked "x." **(c)** Perforator dissected through the MG muscle back to a main medial sural artery branch (*green microgrid*) to extend the flap vascular leash. **(d)** Reach of this island MSAP flap seen before passing through a shorter pathway via a subcutaneous tunnel to the defect, **(e)** allowing tension free healing.

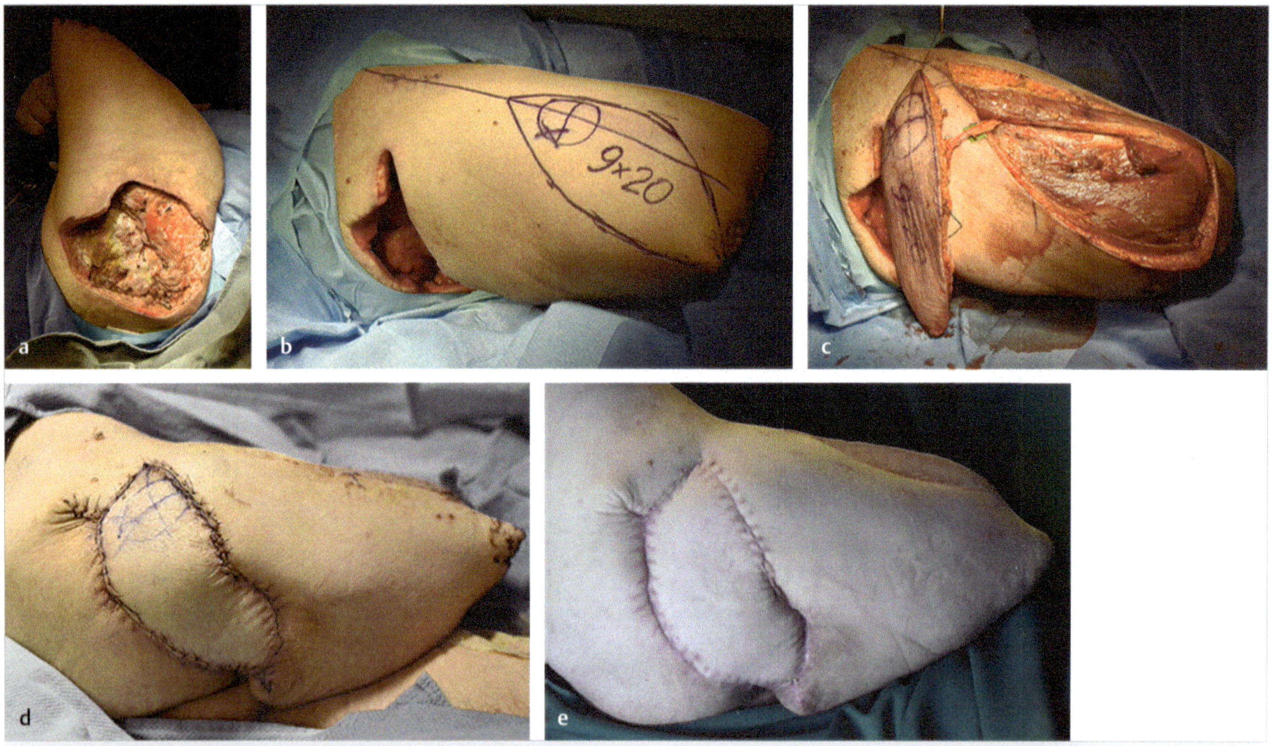

Fig. 15.5 **(a)** Necrotic right hip wound, with right above-knee amputation after frostbite. **(b)** Following serial wound debridement, planned anterolateral thigh (ALT) island flap designed as eccentrically as possible toward stump distal to perforator "x" to maximize flap reach. **(c)** Proximal-pedicled (on microgrid) ALT flap transposed toward right hip. **(d)** Flap inset after it is drawn through the subcutaneous tunnel between the thigh donor site and the right hip. **(e)** Right hip healing after 5 weeks, as is skin graft necessary to close the donor site.

island flap or the LCF artery for the ALT island flap. A distal-pedicled ALT flap should still have the same dissection of its proximal pedicle.[12] This will not only allow potential supercharging whether arterial or venous, but also confirm that the flap perforator arises from a vessel in some way connected to the distal portion of the descending branch of the LCF, which will then still provide reversed flow to sustain the flap. Distal dissection of this pedicle into the vastus lateralis muscle must be enough so that reach to the defect is possible, but at the same time maintaining vessels of reasonable caliber to ensure collateralization with the lateral superior geniculate vessels. After insetting the flap, Lin et al[12] recommend venous supercharging in all cases with an end-to-end microanastomosis of the largest vena comitantes of the proximal ALT pedicle to the greater saphenous vein that can be brought to the flap from the medial leg.

15.2.7 Postoperative Care Protocols

The potential for compression not just of the vascular pedicle to these island flaps that are usually passed through a subcutaneous or submuscular tunnel, but also the diminutive perforators themselves requires that the flaps be observed as carefully as per the usual protocol for a free flap. If the flap crosses a joint, immobilization is essential to prevent movement resulting in stretching of the pedicle, its obstruction or disruption, or even flap dehiscence.

15.2.8 Conclusion

A "true" island perforator flap not only will have all its skin boundaries disconnected from those of its donor site but also will have an elongated pedicle extending beyond just the flap perforator itself, or else would more properly be called an "islanded" flap. This will therefore require inclusion of a major branch or the source vessel of the perforator itself as part of the flap pedicle. Previously, this has been accomplished by sacrificing either the anterior tibial,[5] posterior tibial,[6] or peroneal[7] artery, but this is no longer an acceptable risk under any conditions for fear of eventual devascularization or ischemia of the foot. Other more straightforward local perforator flap alternatives today have become superior options.[16] However, the territories of the ALT or MSAP flaps still represent pragmatic choices for island flaps that as such have far greater reach for coverage of proximal or distal defects of the lower limb than do other local perforator flap subtypes.

References

[1] Fraser JF, Halvorson EG, Mulliken JB. Theodore Dunham's discovery of an Island Flap. Ann Plast Surg. 2014; 72:493–497

[2] Kim JT, Ho SYM, Kim YH. An improved perforator-based island flap: the heart balloon flap. Plast Reconstr Surg. 2015; 135(5):1472–1475

[3] Akita S, Mitsukawa N, Rikihisa N, et al. Descending branch of the perforating branch of the peroneal artery perforator-based island flap for reconstruction of the lateral malleolus with minimal invasion. Plast Reconstr Surg. 2013; 132(2):461–469

[4] Behan FC. The keystone design perforator island flap in reconstructive surgery. ANZ J Surg. 2003; 73(3):112–120

[5] Wee JT. Reconstruction of the lower leg and foot with the reverse-pedicled anterior tibial flap: preliminary report of a new fasciocutaneous flap. Br J Plast Surg. 1986; 39(3):327–337

[6] Liu K, Li Z, Lin Y, Cao Y. The reverse-flow posterior tibial artery island flap: anatomic study and 72 clinical cases. Plast Reconstr Surg. 1990; 86(2):312–316, discussion 317–318

[7] Yoshimura M, Imura S, Shimamura K, Yamauchi S, Nomura S. Peroneal flap for reconstruction in the extremity: preliminary report. Plast Reconstr Surg. 1984; 74(3):402–409

[8] Lu TC, Lin CH, Lin CH, Lin YT, Chen RF, Wei FC. Versatility of the pedicled peroneal artery perforator flaps for soft-tissue coverage of the lower leg and foot defects. J Plast Reconstr Aesthet Surg. 2011; 64(3):386–393

[9] Zheng HP, Zhuang YH, Lin J, et al. Revisit of the anatomy of the distal perforator of the descending genicular artery and clinical application of its perforator "propeller" flap in the reconstruction of soft tissue defects around the knee. Microsurgery. 2015; 35(5):370–379

[10] Gravvanis AI, Tsoutsos DA, Karakitsos D, et al. Application of the pedicled anterolateral thigh flap to defects from the pelvis to the knee. Microsurgery. 2006; 26(6):432–438

[11] Hallock GG. The proximal pedicled anterolateral thigh flap for lower limb coverage. Ann Plast Surg. 2005; 55(5):466–469

[12] Lin CH, Zelken J, Hsu CC, Lin CH, Wei FC. The distally based, venous supercharged anterolateral thigh flap. Microsurgery. 2016; 36(1):20–28

[13] Hallock GG. The medial sural$_{\text{MEDIAL GASTROCNEMIUS}}$ perforator local flap. Ann Plast Surg. 2004; 53(5):501–505

[14] Mohan AT, Sur YJ, Zhu L, et al. The concepts of propeller, perforator, keystone, and other local flaps and their role in the evolution of reconstruction. Plast Reconstr Surg. 2016; 138(4):710e–729e

[15] Hallock GG. Anatomic basis of the gastrocnemius perforator-based flap. Ann Plast Surg. 2001; 47(5):517–522

[16] Koshima I, Moriguchi T, Ohta S, Hamanaka T, Inoue T, Ikeda A. The vasculature and clinical application of the posterior tibial perforator-based flap. Plast Reconstr Surg. 1992; 90(4):643–649

15.3 Chapter 15B: Perforator Advancement Flaps Including the Keystone Flap

Geoffrey G. Hallock

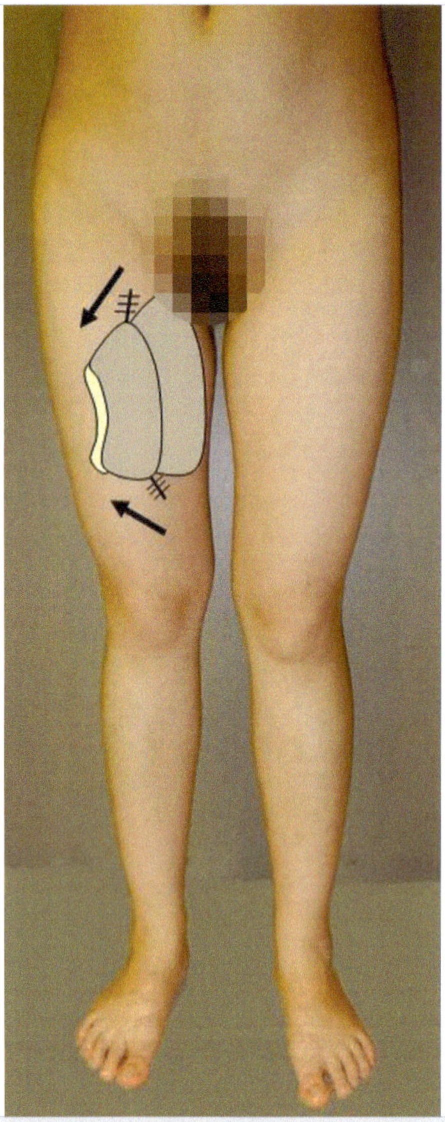

Fig. 15.6 The Keystone Advancement Flap.

15.3.1 Introduction to the Perforator Advancement Flaps Including the Keystone Flap

An advancement flap by definition is always moved in a forward direction into a defect without any rotation or lateral movement.[1] A classic prototype was a unipedicled quadrilateral-shaped random flap sustained by a skin bridge on one side that is now primarily only of historical interest as this geometric arrangement has limited mobility and therefore inadequate reach in the lower extremity.[1] The advent of the perforator flap concept provided an improved means for advancement flap vascularization, but practically has been limited in the lower extremity to V-Y advancement and keystone island flap designs.

According to Niranjan et al,[2] Blasius (1848) should be credited with the idea of the V-Y advancement flap, which for a long time was based on a subcutaneous pedicle[3] with reach dependent on the sliding capability of these triangular shaped skin flaps.[4,5] Since in actuality the fascial plexus alone within the subcutaneous tissues can be quite tenuous, these flaps more likely have always received their circulation from unrecognized perforators of the deep fascia and fascia feeders surrounding it.[2] The same comments also apply to the recent variation introduced by Behan[6] as the "keystone design perforator island flap (▸ Fig. 15.6)." This basically is a trapezoidal islanded flap[7] that consists of two conjoined[7,8] or opposed[9] V-Y advancement flaps. Although usually stated to be islanded, the keystone flap still maintains some connection to the deep fascia directly underneath it. In contradistinction, additional reach no longer relying on skin laxity of a V-Y advancement flap is possible if the flap can be isolated on a distinct perforator,[2,7,10,11] whereas the multiple perforators to a keystone flap are never specifically sought out.[12]

15.3.2 Attributes and Detriments

Attributes

- Local flaps adjacent to defect.
- Similar texture and contour.
- Design simplicity.
- Rapid elevation.
- Nonmicrovascular tissue transfers.
- Minimal donor site morbidity.

Detriments

- Often require adequate soft-tissue laxity for advancement.
- V-Y advancement flap limited to smaller defects.
- Although gigantic keystone flaps are possible, significant scar residue is a sequela.
- If deep fascia cannot be readily separated, these may not easily span space across bone, joint, or prosthesis.
- Lower extremity defects are more likely to require circumferential deep fascia release for keystone flaps.

15.3.3 Anatomical Considerations

Neither a V-Y advancement flap nor a keystone flap absolutely requires identification of a specific perforator. Both can be supplied by perforators of the deep fascia, which could be no more than the ubiquitous capillary perforator,[13] or fascia feeders.[2] As such, these flaps should be oriented to overlie known perforators or areas of high perforator density, that is, "hot spots,"[12] following the longitudinal course of the three source vessels to the foot. If a perforator can be precisely determined preoperatively using available adjunctive techniques, a V-Y advancement flap could instead become an islanded flap connected only to that specific perforator, which would thereby have farther reach, albeit still limited by the length of the perforator itself.

As with any local perforator flap, the condition of local tissues and possible compromise of perforators must always be assessed carefully. In addition, unique to the lower extremity, advancement flaps may be more difficult,[14] as tissue laxity or slipperiness may be nonexistent over the deep fascia although still probably adequate over the muscles of the thigh and calf, if anywhere. As a consequence, transverse oriented V-Y advancement flaps are more mobile,[5,11] as would be longitudinally designed keystone flaps.[9] For keystone flaps, this is an advantage, as this best recruits circulation from multiple captured perforators perhaps from adjacent territories according to the perforasome theory.[15]

15.3.4 Anatomical Variations and Potential Pitfalls

Extended Reach

Salvage of Intrinsic Flap Tissues

Rather than discarding the tissues of the margins of the leading edge of an advancement flap, these can be sewn together, thereby increasing the width of the flap and consequently lessening the amount of advancement needed. For the V-Y advancement flap, this maneuver has been called the PAC-Man technique[2,16,17] (▶ Fig. 15.7) and for the keystone flap, the omega technique[14] (▶ Fig. 15.8).

Deep Fascia Release

Often an incision of the deep fascia as needed about either the V-Y advancement or keystone flap will allow greater movement, as restraints from connections to the underlying tissues are partially released. Usually this begins at the greater curvature border of the keystone flap[9,12] and progresses outward as required to obtain the desired flap mobility. Subfascial extension of this dissection to get even more release should best be away from areas of known high perforator density so they will not be injured.

Suprafascial Flap Release

Instead of incising the deep fascia and violating perforators and perhaps fascial feeders, a suprafascial dissection raising the subcutaneous tissues of either the V-Y advancement or keystone flap from the deep fascia as needed for further advancement can be done. This requires careful preservation of any small vessels encountered, which makes this a more difficult alternative as microdissection will be required.[18] The V-Y advancement flap should be elevated at its apex and base first, whereas for the keystone flap, margins should be explored where perforator density is known to be the least.

Rotation Advancement Flap

If an islanded V-Y advancement flap is intended, but during the subfascial dissection through the exploratory incision via one side of the flap no adequate perforator is found, the flap should be redesigned retaining the contralateral side intact. The base can then be advanced forward with some rotation about its intersection and the retained side to then close the defect[19] (▶ Fig. 15.9). This may require a small back-cut of the retained side starting at the flap apex to allow adequate rotation.

Keystone "Plus" Flap Design

A "V"-shaped extension half of the defect width is designed in the center of the greater curvature of the arc that connected the tangential wings of the standard keystone flap (▶ Fig. 15.10).[20] After flap advancement, this donor site is also closed in a V-Y fashion, which should relieve tension on closure of the greater curvature side of the overall donor defect.

Keystone Flap Skin Bridge Design

The cutaneous central member of the greater arc of the keystone flap is not incised, although the deep fascia is released in its entirety underneath this skin bridge that has been left intact (▶ Fig. 15.11). This should not restrict closure of the donor site. Subdermal lymphatics from the flap are preserved, and Moncrieff et al[21] believe the flap will also have greater vascularity via this connection. However, this contradicts the opinion of Behan[14,22] who believes that the creation of a completely islanded flap causes a sympathectomy effect that results in augmented, not diminished, flap perfusion.

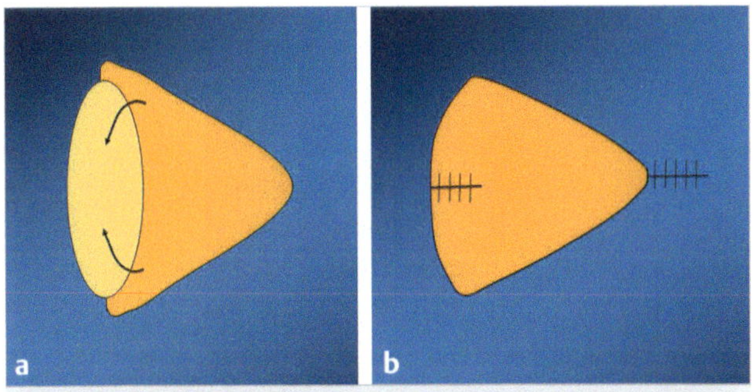

Fig. 15.7 (a) PAC-Man technique: sides of base of V-Y advancement flap (orange) are sewn together in the direction of the *arrows*, **(b)** which lengthens flap, reduces the needed advancement, and otherwise is inset in a V-Y fashion.

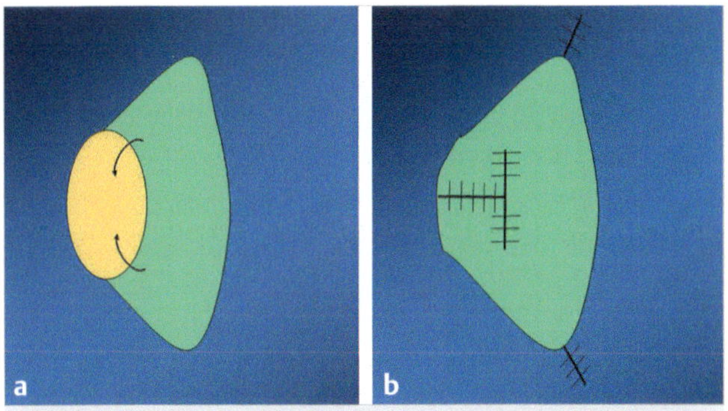

Fig. 15.8 (a) Omega technique: sides of lesser curvature of keystone flap (*green*) are brought together in the direction of the *arrows* and **(b)** then sewn to each other and to the middle of the lesser curvature to form a resemblance of the Greek letter "Ω" that increases the overall width of the flap.

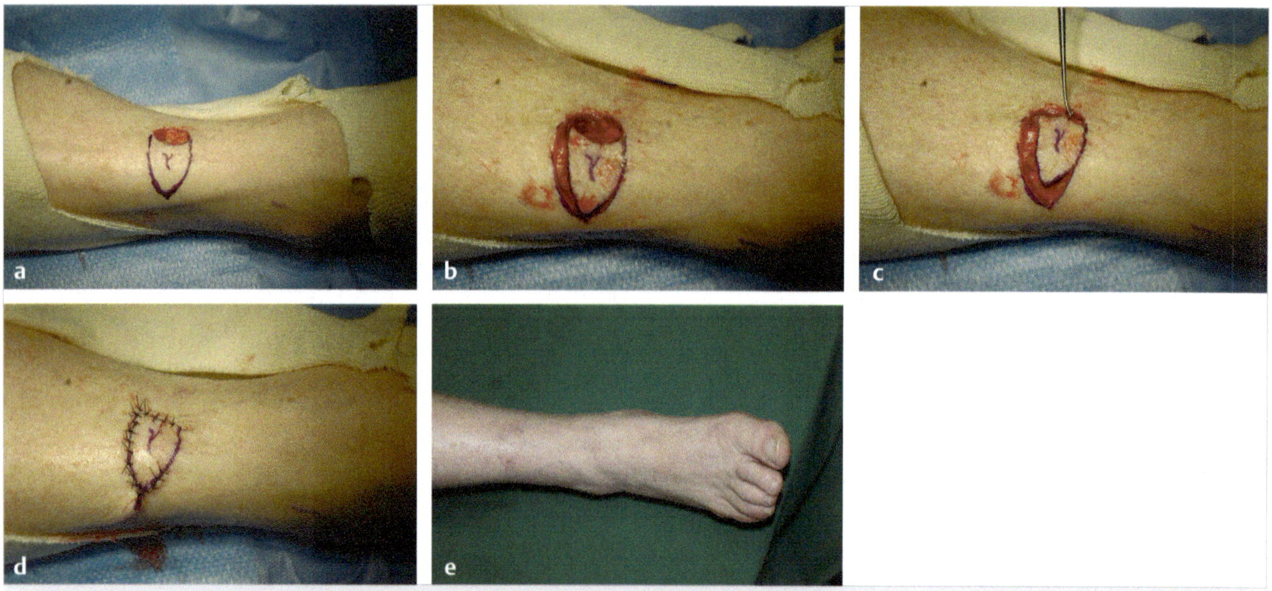

Fig. 15.9 **(a)** Anterior right distal leg skin cancer excision, with proposed transverse oriented V-Y advancement flap for closure about perforator marked "y." **(b)** Subfascial exploratory incision through one side of the triangle did not reveal a perforator, **(c)** so the other side of the flap was left intact except for short back-cut that facilitated flap rotation and advancement to reach the defect. **(d)** Completed flap insetting with direct donor site closure. **(e)** Ultimate superior appearance of the leg without a skin graft.

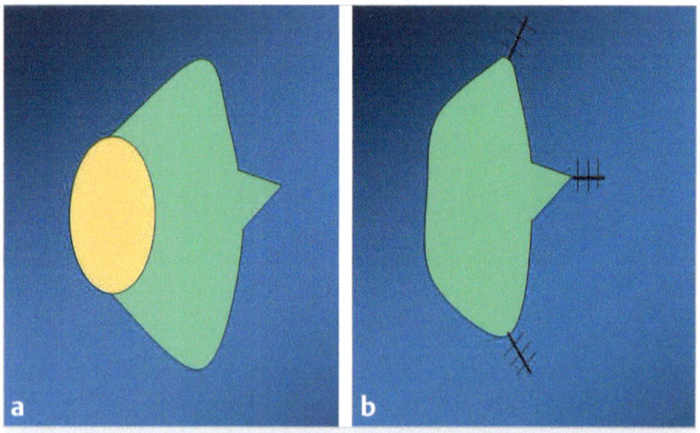

Fig. 15.10 **(a)** Keystone plus flap: "V" extension at the center of the greater curvature of the keystone flap (green) is intended to decrease tension on the latter's closure after advancement, **(b)** as that extension donor site will be closed to gain the same advantage as a V-Y advancement.

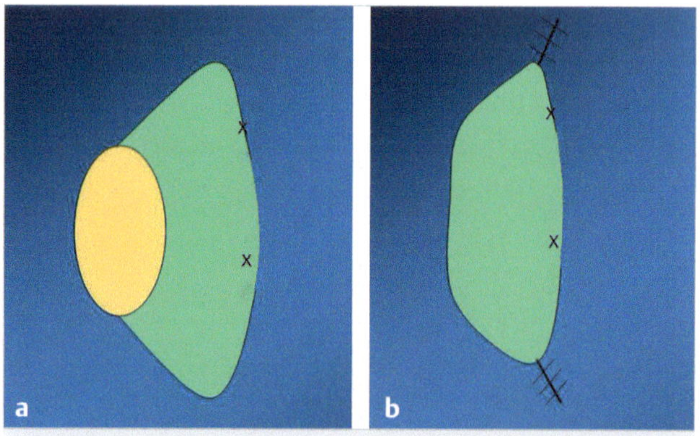

Fig. 15.11 **(a)** Keystone bridge flap: skin of the central portion of the greater curvature (area between "Xs") of the keystone flap (green) is not incised and **(b)** always remains attached to the advanced flap when inset as well as at the original donor site.

15.3.5 Flap Design

V-Y Advancement

The laxity of tissues adjacent to the defect will determine the orientation or even possibility of using this option as a subcutaneous pedicled flap as the keystone flap is typically used. The base of the isosceles triangular shaped flap should slightly exceed the width of the defect (▶ Fig. 15.12). The altitude of the flap will extend perpendicular to the base up to 1.5 to 2.0 times the height of the defect, with a longer flap probably allowing easier closure of the donor site at the apex of the flap that will be in the vicinity of the most pliable donor site tissues.

If subcutaneous tissue elasticity is known to be inadequate for the needed advancement, preoperative search for a nearby perforator should be undertaken. If the perforator is close to the defect, a propeller flap may be a preferred option.[7] If the perforator is further from the defect, it may be more appropriate to design a V-Y advancement flap using the same dimensions as for the subcutaneous pedicled version, although now instead centered over the requisite perforator (▶ Fig. 15.13).

Keystone Flap

Behan classified keystone flaps into four types that varied by the degree of undermining of the deep fascia, number of flaps used, or treatment of the donor site, which rarely required a skin graft.[6] His standard format is a representative model of all his subtypes that will be the focus here (▶ Fig. 15.14). Although in the past many have extended the original defect in an elliptical fashion to coincide with the lesser curvature of the flap,[14] in the lower extremity this can be a waste of precious normal tissues that may instead require alteration of the flap design (▶ Fig. 15.15).[8] Local tissues about the defect should be assessed for the presence of perforators and compared to areas with maximum skin laxity. This can be facilitated by the use of an audible Doppler; however, knowledge of known high-density perforator locations, that is, "hot spots,"[12] or the fact that perforators commonly emanate following the longitudinal course of the source vessels to the foot can be used safely with impunity. Since

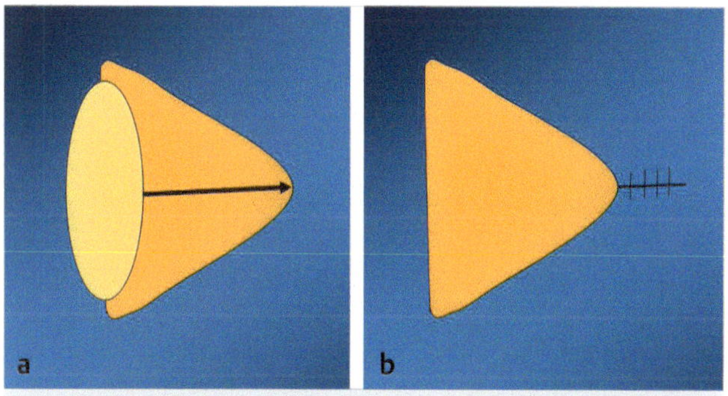

Fig. 15.12 **(a)** Basic design of V-Y advancement flap (orange) as a triangle with the base slightly greater than the width of the defect (*yellow*), and altitude (*perpendicular line* to the apex) 1.5 to 2.0 times the height of the defect itself. **(b)** After advancement to close the defect, the donor area behind the apex is closed primarily to result in the ultimate "Y" appearance of the overall closure.

perforasomes in the lower extremity interconnect in a longitudinal direction,[15] the keystone flap should have a similar axis especially if the most pliable tissues can be simultaneously captured.

Wings starting tangential to the defect on opposite sides should proceed at about a 90-degree angle away for at least as far as the height of the defect. This distance determines the width of the keystone flap. The two tangent lines are joined by an arc to complete the trapezoidal or keystone shape of the flap. If the lesser curvature edge of the flap has already been undermined, its tissues are of poor quality such as irradiated, inelastic, or traumatized, the wings and thus the width of the flap can be increased even up to 5:1 the size of the defect so as to capture adequately perfused and elastic tissues having the desired qualities that can then be advanced as needed.[12]

15.3.6 Flap Harvest

The position of the patient on the operating room table will depend on the location of the defect and the proposed design of the local perforator flap chosen for its correction, so as to most simply allow access to both.

V-Y Advancement

If subcutaneous tissue laxity is readily mobile, the sides of the designed triangle are incised down to at least the equivalent of Scarpa's fascia, or to the deep fascia itself if necessary. Often, the subcutaneous tissues at the base of the flap can be carefully

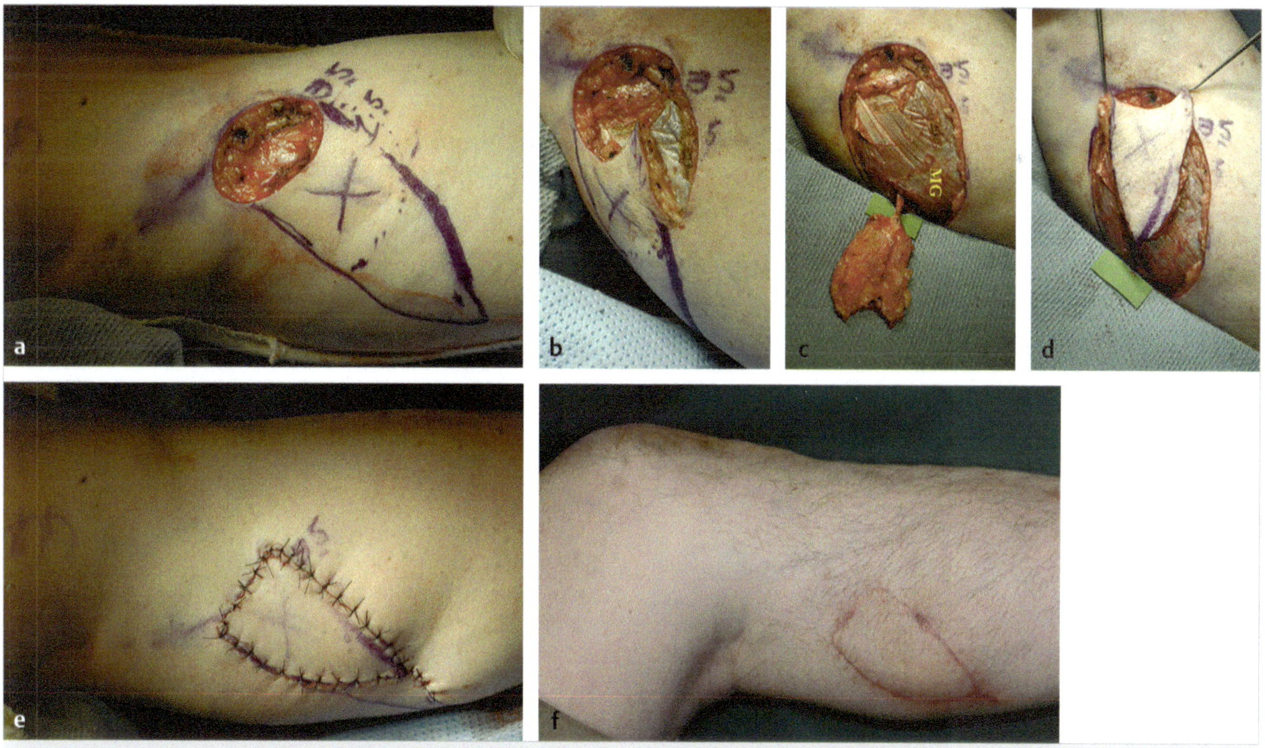

Fig. 15.13 **(a)** Following excision of a basal cell carcinoma from the right calf, a propeller flap was initially planned on a medial sural artery perforator (MSAP) "x" heard with the audible Doppler, **(b)** yet the obligatory exploratory incision revealed that the perforator instead was near the apex of the flap, so a V-Y advancement flap design became a more reasonable alternative. **(c)** Enough reach required some intramuscular dissection of that perforator (microgrid) into the medial gastrocnemius muscle (MG), **(d)** sufficient so that the required tension-free advancement of this MSAP V-Y advancement flap was possible, **(e)** allowing insetting for closure of the defect and donor site in a "Y" fashion, **(f)** with result 3 months later where a skin graft had been avoided.

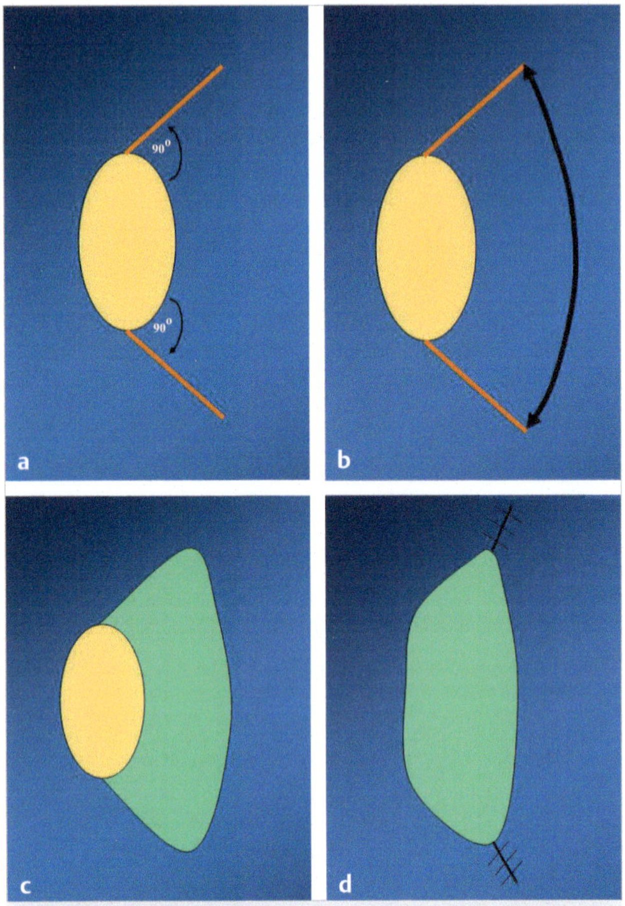

Fig. 15.14 **(a)** Standard keystone flap: tangents on opposite sides of the defect (*yellow*) are drawn at about a 90-degree angle, with length at least equal to the defect width, **(b)** an arc connects the ends of the tangents **(c)** to form a trapezoid- or keystone-shaped flap (*green*) **(d)** that will then be advanced to close the defect, with the small open areas remaining on either side of the greater curvature closed in a V-Y fashion.

raised from the deep fascia as is also done at the apex, as far as required, to then allow additional reach so that the base can be sewn to the farthest edge of the defect. This dissection requires preservation of any small vessels encountered as would be done routinely in the raising of a perforator flap. The triangle's sides are sewn where advanced to the corresponding sides of the defect and donor site. The donor site inferior to the flap apex can then be closed primarily to complete the repair and "Y" appearance of the closure.

If the initial plan is to seek a preoperatively identified subfascial perforator that will better allow advancement of an islanded V-Y advancement flap, only one side of the triangle is incised through the deep fascia as an exploratory incision. The perforator is isolated and lengthened as necessary by coagulation of side branches back to its source vessel or branch. If found adequate, the other flap side is then completely incised, and the flap advanced without tension for insetting just as was done for the subcutaneous pedicled version. However, if no adequate subfascial perforator is confirmed, the backup option of a rotation advancement flap must be considered (▶ Fig. 15.9).[19]

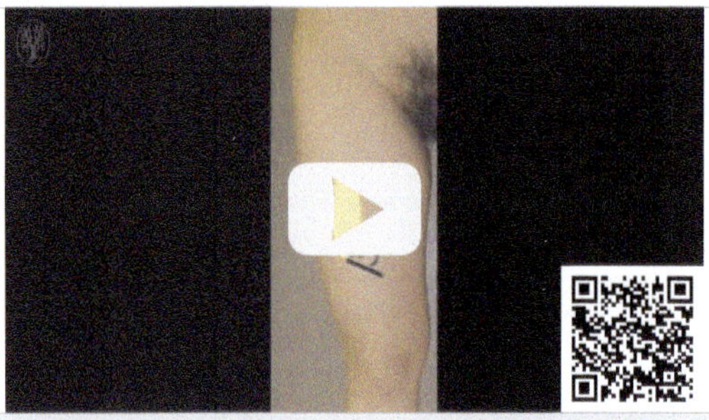

Video 15.3 Keystone Advancement flap. https://www.thieme.de/de/q.htm?p=opn/cs/20/7/12265270-583aca14

Keystone Flap

The wings and greater arc of the standard designed keystone flap are incised (see ▶ Video 15.3). This is carried down to Scarpa's fascia or its equivalent first; if flap advancement is easily possible, some portion of the subcutaneous fascial plexus from tissues adjacent to the flap itself can be preserved for vascular augmentation. However, if necessary, a stepwise release even of the deep fascia starting at the midpoint of the outer curvature incision, then even circumferentially about the flap may have to be done until the flap can be advanced for closure without tension.[9,12] In addition, this could require even some subfascial dissection for further release from underlying tissues, but always away from the known location of flap perforators. Once satisfactory, the center of the flap's inner curvature border is advanced to the middle of the farthest edge of the defect, where subcutaneous sutures are placed to reinforce the attachment. The skin there is next closed as are the sides of the flap, with trimming of any excess tiny remnants at the leading edge of the flap. Only the skin of the outer curvature line is then reclosed in a relatively loose fashion. This will leave a short open area on either side of the arc of the flap, which is closed in the typical V-Y flap fashion to complete the reconstruction.

15.3.7 Postoperative Care Protocols

Both the V-Y and keystone advancement flap versions pedicled by their deep fascial attachments are extremely robust flaps requiring little additional scrutiny as long as pressure is kept off them and adjacent joints relatively immobilized to minimize compression and stretch. On the contrary, an islanded V-Y advancement flap must be carefully protected so that the perforator itself will not be compromised, by appropriate dressings and positioning of the patient, for at least a week or more in most patients until wound healing stability is satisfactory. Sutures, especially in the keystone flap, should never be removed in a hurry, perhaps waiting several weeks or more sometimes so that dehiscence does not occur.

15.3.8 Conclusion

Local perforator advancement flaps basically allow only forward movement of tissues adjacent to a given defect. In the lower extremity, the most pragmatic variations are limited to the V-Y advancement or keystone flap. These on a geometric basis have great similarity in design, and also both can survive on multiple

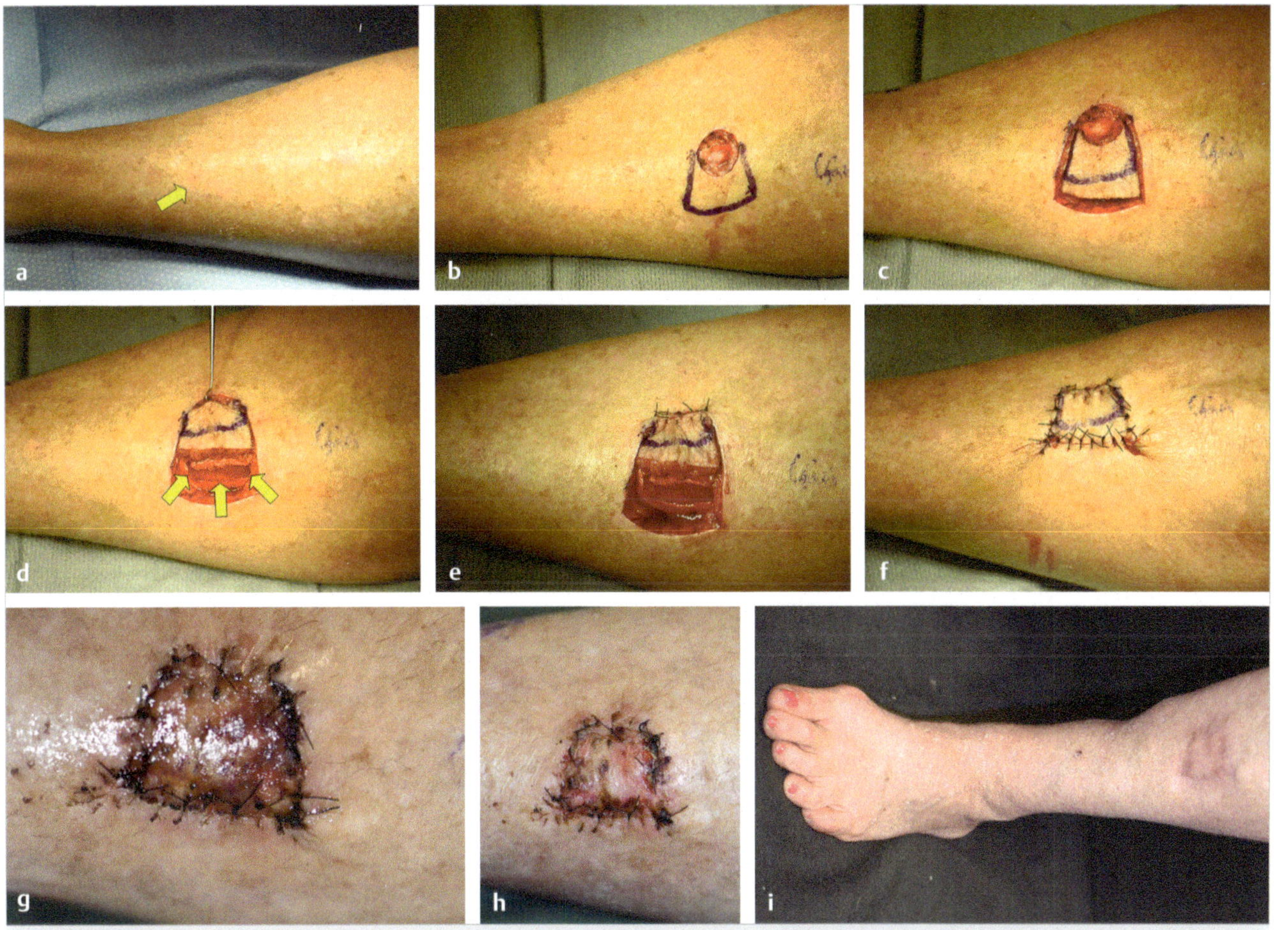

Fig. 15.15 **(a)** Squamous cell carcinoma (*arrow*) of left anterior mid-leg. **(b)** Longitudinally oriented keystone flap designed about excision site over the more mobile posterior leg tissues. **(c)** All sides of the flap were incised to the deep fascia as subcutaneous tissues were extremely thin. **(d)** Necessary lesser curvature advancement required a deep fascia release (*arrows*) along the greater curvature. **(e)** The lesser curvature of the flap is first inset. **(f)** Complete flap insetting. **(g)** Ischemic flap seen 10 days later presumably because the flap was not directly over a lower limb source vessel or tangents were drawn too acutely. **(h)** Marked spontaneous improvement by day 26 postoperative. **(i)** Reasonable contour 3 months later with total keystone flap survival.

perforators through the deep fascia without the need for specific perforator identification. Yet in this form, both rely on tissue laxity to allow the required advancement, with the keystone flap concept necessitating at times even gigantic flaps if need be to obtain this reach. The V-Y advancement flap overall is limited to small or moderate-sized defects, where any additional reach if desired requires instead that a specific perforator be found so that an islanded version tethered only by the length of that as the vascular pedicle will prove to be sufficient.

References

[1] Jankauskas S, Cohen IK, Grabb WC. Basic technique of plastic surgery. In: Smith JW, Aston SJ, eds. Grabb and Smith's Plastic Surgery. 4th ed. Boston, MA: Little Brown; 1991:61–64

[2] Niranjan NS, Price RD, Govilkar P. Fascial feeder and perforator-based V-Y advancement flaps in the reconstruction of lower limb defects. Br J Plast Surg. 2000; 53(8):679–689

[3] Emmett AJJ. The closure of defects by using adjacent triangular flaps with subcutaneous pedicles. Plast Reconstr Surg. 1977; 59(1):45–52

[4] Trevaskis AE, Rempel J, Okunski W, Rea M. Sliding subcutaneous-pedicle flaps to close a circular defect. Plast Reconstr Surg. 1970; 46(2):155–157

[5] Coombs CJ, Ng S, Stewart DA. The use of V-Y advancement flaps for closure of pretibial skin defects after excision of cutaneous lesions. Ann Plast Surg. 2013; 71(4):402–405

[6] Behan FC. The keystone design perforator island flap in reconstructive surgery. ANZ J Surg. 2003; 73(3):112–120

[7] Brunetti B, Tenna S, Aveta A, Segreto F, Persichetti P. Free-style local perforator flaps: versatility of the V-Y design to reconstruct soft-tissue defects in the skin cancer population. Plast Reconstr Surg. 2013; 132(2):451–460

[8] Stone JP, Webb C, McKinnon JG, Dawes JC, McKenzie CD, Temple-Oberle CF. Avoiding skin grafts: the keystone flap in cutaneous defects. Plast Reconstr Surg. 2015; 136(2):404–408

[9] Mohan AT, Rammos CK, Akhavan AA, et al. Evolving concepts of keystone perforator island flaps (KPIF): principles of perforator anatomy, design modifications, and extended clinical applications. Plast Reconstr Surg. 2016; 137 (6):1909–1920

[10] Venkataramakrishnan V, Mohan D, Villafane O. Perforator based V-Y advancement flaps in the leg. Br J Plast Surg. 1998; 51(6):431–435

[11] Brunetti B, Poccia I, Tenna S, Campa S, Persichetti P. Transversally oriented pedicled perforator flaps: a reliable alternative for lower leg reconstruction. Microsurgery. 2015; 35(7):541–545

[12] Mohan AT, Sur YJ, Zhu L, et al. The concepts of propeller, perforator, Keystone, and other local flaps and their role in the evolution of reconstruction. Plast Reconstr Surg. 2016; 138(4):710e–729e

[13] Koshima I, Narushima M, Mihara M, et al. New thoracodorsal artery perforator (TAPcp) flap with capillary perforators for reconstruction of upper limb. J Plast Reconstr Aesthet Surg. 2010; 63(1):140–145

[14] Lanni MA, Van Kouwenberg E, Yan A, Rezak KM, Patel A. Applying the Keystone design perforator island flap concept in a variety of anatomic locations: a review of 60 consecutive cases by a single surgeon. Ann Plast Surg. 2017; 79 (1):60–67

[15] Saint-Cyr M, Wong C, Schaverien M, Mojallal A, Rohrich RJ. The perforasome theory: vascular anatomy and clinical implications. Plast Reconstr Surg. 2009; 124(5):1529–1544

[16] Bonomi S, Sgrò A, Salval A. Avoiding skin grafts: The V-Y Pac-Man perforator flap. Plast Reconstr Surg. 2016; 138(3):561e–562e

[17] Bonomi S, Salval A, Brenta F, Rapisarda V, Settembrini F. The Pacman perforator-based V-Y advancement flap for reconstruction of pressure sores at different locations. Ann Plast Surg. 2016; 77(3):324–331

[18] Chan STS. A technique of undermining a V-Y subcutaneous island flap to maximise advancement. Br J Plast Surg. 1988; 41(1):62–67

[19] Sungur N, Kankaya Y, Gursoy K, Dölen UC, Koçer U. A local flap that never disappoints: V-Y rotation advancement flap. Ann Plast Surg. 2013; 71(5):575–580

[20] Rubino C, Faenza M, Di Pace B, Campitiello N, Brongo S, Zingone G. A new keystone flap "plus" design: case series and analysis of follow-up. J Plast Reconstr Aesthet Surg. 2017; 70(7):976–979

[21] Moncrieff MD, Thompson JF, Stretch JR. Extended experience and modifications in the design and concepts of the keystone design island flap. J Plast Reconstr Aesthet Surg. 2010; 63(8):1359–1363

[22] Lo CH, Menezes H, Behan F. The island perforator flap design augments vascularity. Plast Reconstr Surg. 2013; 132(3):468e–469e

15.4 Chapter 15C: The Peninsular Perforator Flap

Geoffrey G. Hallock

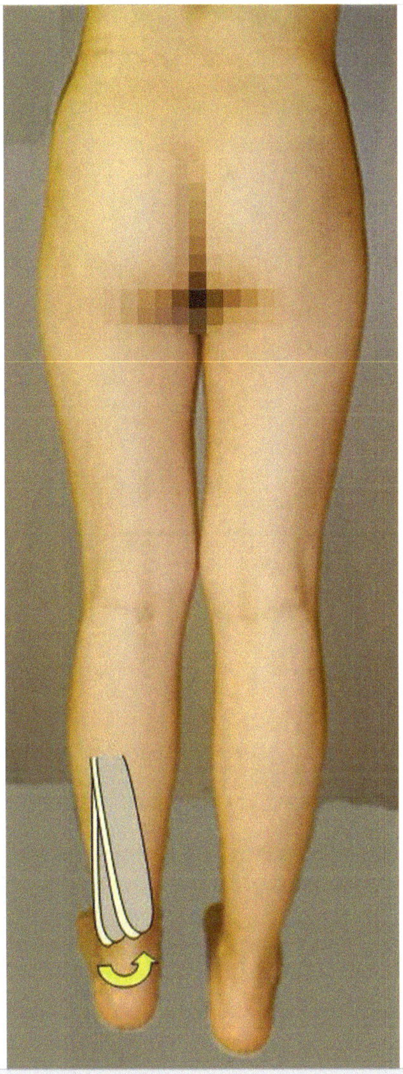

Fig. 15.16 The peninsular flap.

15.4.1 Introduction to the Peninsular Perforator Flap

The traditional dictum for decades stated that skin flaps raised below the knee were destined to failure, as these would be just random flaps expected to survive a length-to-width ratio[1] of no more than 1:1. This was to change in the 1980s when Pontén[1] in a somewhat heretical thrust proved that large skin flaps connected only by a proximal skin bridge to the lower leg integument could survive with a length-to-width ratio up to 4.5:1 if only the deep fascia was included. Thus was born the era of the fasciocutaneous flap in the shape of a peninsula as another means for soft-tissue coverage of the lower extremity (▶ Fig. 15.16).

Yet the vascularity of the deep fascia itself may actually be quite poor,[2] in spite of the known presence of fascial feeder end-arterial branches as espoused by Niranjan et al.[3] Even Gillies was quite aware that inclusion of the deep fascia with a flap was important,[1,4] perhaps based empirically to protect the overlying subcutaneous tissues and what we now term its intrinsic fascial plexus. Pontén[1] never elucidated the actual source of circulation to his "superflaps," but usually oriented them longitudinally overlying one of the three source vessels to the foot, and often included a superficial vein or cutaneous nerve, so that in reality these may have been what we now call neurocutaneous flaps.

In any event, from a geometric standpoint, Pontén's fasciocutaneous flaps were *peninsular* flaps.[5] He was well aware that the fascial plexus nourishing his flaps entered the base above the deep fascia and that the latter could be back-cut to improve rotation as long as care was observed not to injure any direct cutaneous or musculocutaneous perforators that might be encountered.[1] Cormack and Lamberty were cognizant in their type A fasciocutaneous flaps that this peninsular variety in addition could be nourished by yet another distinct source vessel branch, the septocutaneous perforator.[4] Pontén's flaps,[1] as is true with most peninsular flaps today, do not require the precise identification of the source of circulation to the flap as long as his guidelines are followed. Although Pontén's flaps were usually proximal based,[6] peninsular flaps may be transverse based[7,8] or distal based[9,10,11] as long as an adequate perforator system is included nearby. Distal-based flaps, especially valuable near the foot and ankle, will less likely result in bone or tendon exposure at the donor site after flap rotation, an important quality as that donor site will inevitably require a skin graft (▶ Fig. 15.17). Nevertheless, in general some consider the peninsular flap to be their pedicled perforator flap of choice for the lower extremity.[12]

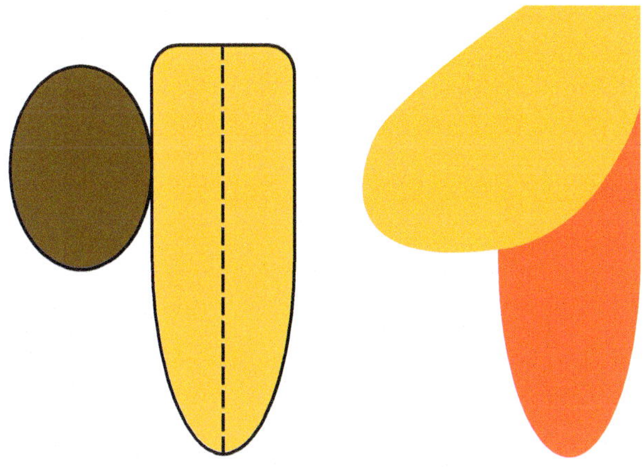

Fig. 15.17 (a) The vertical axis (*dotted line*) of a peninsular flap must have height and width exceeding the dimensions of the defect (*shaded brown*) to compensate for any loss of reach during the rotation.
(b) After clockwise insetting of the flap, the donor site, typically, will be exposed (*shaded red*) and will require a skin graft.

15.4.2 Attributes and Detriments

Attributes

- Local flap.
- Unlimited possibilities.
- Normal contour and appearance.
- Simple to harvest.
- No venous congestion.
- Minimizes risk of lymphedema.
- Function preservation.
- No microsurgery.

Detriments

- Uncertain vascular supply.
- Limited arc of rotation.
- Donor site skin graft.

15.4.3 Anatomical Considerations

There is no need to actually identify a perforator at the base of a peninsular flap, although confirmation of their existence nearby is a practical maneuver. However, if it is uncertain that a specific perforator will be available, the flap design should overlie the course of one of the source vessels of the lower extremity, or the longitudinally oriented superficial veins and often accompanying cutaneous nerves that have their intrinsic vascular system that will simultaneously be captured (▶ Fig. 15.18). Particularly in the latter circumstances, their inclusion alone and without the deep fascia may be all that is necessary to support a peninsular flap. This assures that structures below the deep fascia, especially tendons as the foot and ankle are approached, will not be exposed, and therefore donor site skin grafting will more likely be successful.

15.4.4 Anatomical Variations and Potential Pitfalls

Perforator-Plus Peninsular Flaps

Sometimes a reasonable perforator can be found within the design of a peninsular flap (▶ Fig. 15.19) or by chance alone encountered while the flap is elevated. If this is retained and the base of the flap still connected to the donor area, then this would by definition be a *perforator-plus peninsular flap*.[13] This flap will have a dual blood supply, and unimpeded outflow via the base pedicle so that venous congestion will never be a concern.[14] Now more robust, this subtype can be longer and have a narrower base so that reach and arc of rotation are enhanced.[15,16] To achieve uninhibited transposition, this may require further lengthening of the perforator itself by intramuscular dissection if a musculocutaneous perforator, or source vessel exposure likewise if septocutaneous, as if it is too short, tautness will impede flap movement.[17] Similarly, if the pedicle base proved to be too constrictive, it may be totally divided, and the flap either advanced or rotated as needed, now relying only on the perforator itself for vascularization.

Rotation

The deep fascia will restrain rotation of the peninsular flap about its long axis. Even if the deep fascia is back-cut, to expect rotation more than 90 degrees into the defect would be wishful without creating a significant "dog-ear" at the point of rotation

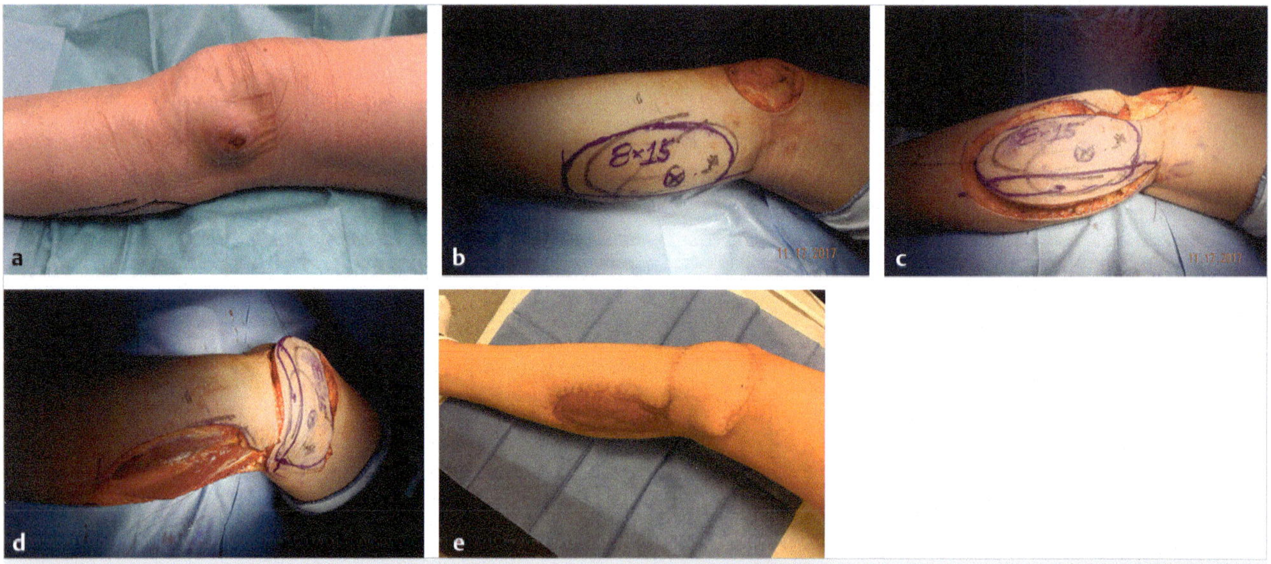

Fig. 15.18 **(a)** Malignant dermatofibroma of the lateral aspect of left knee joint. **(b)** After radical tumor excision, proposed lateral sural artery island perforator flap designed with anticipated perforator "x" heard with audible Doppler. **(c)** No actual perforator was found during exploratory subfascial incision, but the median sural nerve and accompanying vessels were grossly obvious on the flap undersurface, so this was converted to a 8 × 30 cm proximal-based peninsular flap. **(d)** Well-perfused peninsular flap rotated over excision site, with large donor site defect. **(e)** Joint protected by well-healed flap, and skin grafted donor site deformity as seen 2 months later prior to initiation of adjuvant therapy. (This image is provided courtesy of Kariel Claes, MD, Department of Plastic and Reconstructive Surgery, University Hospital, Gent, Belgium.)

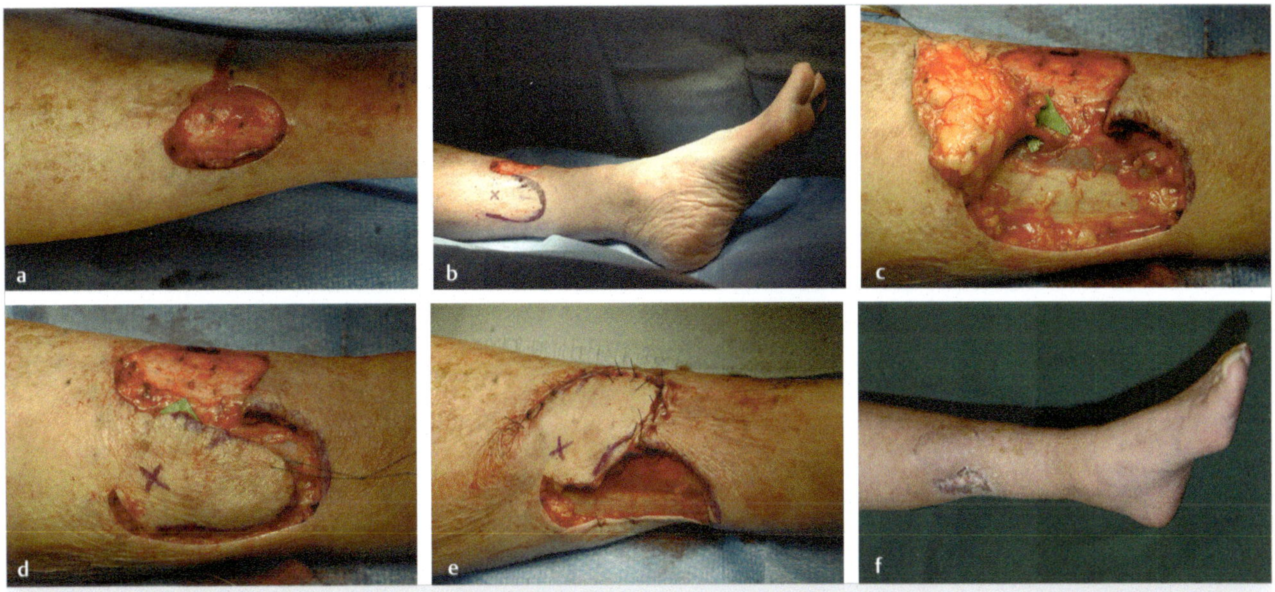

Fig. 15.19 (a) Mohs defect with exposure of left mid-tibia. (b) Proximal-based 4 × 10 cm peninsular flap designed with posterior tibial perforator "x" heard at the base using audible Doppler. (c) Suprafascial flap elevation was possible with dissected perforator seen on microgrid. (d) Back-cut anteriorly at flap base was deemed safe since this was a perforator-plus peninsular flap, as that facilitated tension-free rotation over tibia. (e) Flap inset, with typical donor site defect seen that will require a skin graft. (f) Stable skin coverage of the tibia 2 months later.

or compression impeding circulation. The "dog-ear" should always be retained, as the exact source of circulation to these flaps is never completely known.

Donor Site

If the deep fascia is included with a peninsular flap, great care must be taken to preserve the flimsy soft tissues beneath it. This will better ensure a vascularized base upon which a skin graft of the donor site must be placed. Better yet, if the deep fascia itself can be excluded even if only in part, this will also assure a better chance of skin graft take.

15.4.5 Flap Design

The base of the peninsular flap will depend on the location of the defect. Usually, proximal-based[6] or distal-based flaps[10,11] with the base juxtaposed to one side of the defect are preferable. Knowledge of the ultimate location of the donor site defect is important as this usually must be skin grafted. The more distal the defect, the more likely tendons and/or bone will be exposed, so that a distal-based flap may be preferred as the base of the flap will still provide some donor site coverage.

The axis of the flap preferably should have a longitudinal orientation to ensure maximal length following the perforasome theory for the lower extremity.[18] This should overlie the course of the peroneal, posterior tibial, or anterior tibial vessels so that their perforators will be found at the chosen base of the flap. An alternative would be placement over the greater or lesser saphenous vein or other cutaneous nerves such as the sural or superficial peroneal in the same fashion. Inclusion of these neurovascular structures may even allow elevation of the flap without the need to retain the deep fascia.

One border of the flap will coincide with a side of the defect (▶ Fig. 15.17). The length must exceed the distal extent of the defect as some reach will be lost during flap rotation. Similarly, the width of the flap must exceed that of the defect. If the potential donor site will expose periosteum of the fibula or tibia, another option should be chosen if possible so that a relatively immobile skin graft is not placed upon bone.

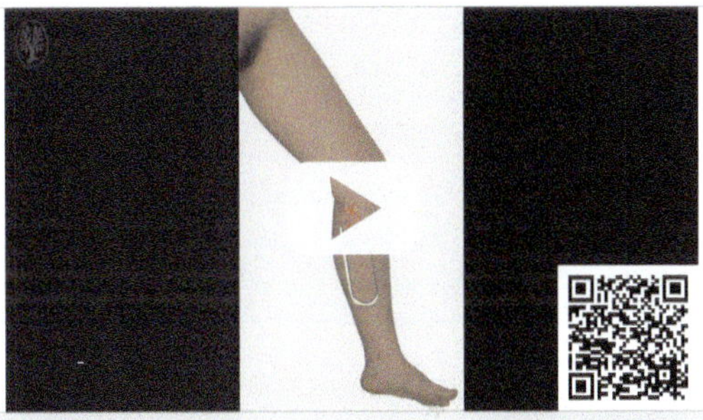

Video 15.4 Peninsular Flap Harvest. https://www.thieme.de/de/q.htm?p=opn/cs/20/7/12265271-d9519f65

15.4.6 Flap Harvest

Positioning of the patient will be dependent on the location of the defect and the chosen donor site for a peninsular flap. Use of a tourniquet if possible will maximize visualization, with or without limb exsanguination. Note the latter approach will facilitate identification especially of perforator veins that could be included optionally. All sides of the peninsular flap are incised leaving the base intact with dissection continuing through the deep fascia (see ▶ Video 15.4). A suture through the free end of the flap including the deep fascia will provide a means to hold up the flap, while the rapid subfascial dissection in a relatively bloodless plane will proceed up to the base. If a dominant perforator is found, this could be retained to make a perforator-plus flap.[13]

Once the base of the flap is reached, if need be, the vertical sides of the flap can be extended to improve reach, or the deep fascia cut horizontally as a back-cut. In both circumstances, destruction of any significant perforators must be avoided. Reach to the defect must be without tension. Tourniquet deflation will allow in situ assessment of perfusion to the flap. If adequate, the flap can then be inset and the donor site skin grafted.

15.4.7 Postoperative Care Protocols

Unless the peninsular flap crosses a joint or is nearby, no specific unusual postoperative care is needed other than to protect inosculation of the skin grafted donor site. Otherwise, some form of immobilization is warranted as long as deemed necessary to prevent stretching of the flap during joint movement that may cause a dehiscence.

15.4.8 Conclusion

The peninsular type of pedicled perforator flap is a valuable ally for skin restoration of many small to medium-sized defects of particularly the lower extremity below the knee. This alternative was the pattern of design for many of the original fasciocutaneous flaps.[6,11,19] No discrete perforator needs to be found during the elevation of most of these flaps, but if one is included to make this a perforator-plus peninsular flap, even more robust flaps having greater reach are possible. Movement of peninsular flaps is limited, and the donor site must usually be skin grafted, the major drawbacks of this choice, which many still consider to have a high priority as a local flap for coverage of the leg.

References

[1] Pontén B. The fasciocutaneous flap: its use in soft tissue defects of the lower leg. Br J Plast Surg. 1981; 34(2):215–220

[2] Gumener R, Montandon D, Marty F, Zbrodowski A. The subcutaneous tissue flap and the misconception of fasciocutaneous flaps. Scand J Plast Reconstr Surg. 1986; 20(1):61–65

[3] Niranjan NS, Price RD, Govilkar P. Fascial feeder and perforator-based V-Y advancement flaps in the reconstruction of lower limb defects. Br J Plast Surg. 2000; 53(8):679–689

[4] Cormack GC, Lamberty BGH. A classification of fascio-cutaneous flaps according to their patterns of vascularisation. Br J Plast Surg. 1984; 37(1):80–87

[5] Bravo FG, Schwarze HP. Free-style local perforator flaps: concept and classification system. J Plast Reconstr Aesthet Surg. 2009; 62(5):602–608, discussion 609

[6] Hallock GG. Local fasciocutaneous flaps for cutaneous coverage of lower extremity wounds. J Trauma. 1989; 29(9):1240–1244

[7] Franchi A, Scaglioni MF. Application of posterior thigh three-dimensional profunda artery perforator perforasomes in refining next-generation flap designs: transverse, vertical, and S-shaped profunda artery perforator flaps. Plast Reconstr Surg. 2017; 140(6):818e–819e

[8] Brunetti B, Poccia I, Tenna S, Campa S, Persichetti P. Transversally oriented pedicled perforator flaps: a reliable alternative for lower leg reconstruction. Microsurgery. 2015; 35(7):541–545

[9] Donski PK, Fogdestam I. Distally based fasciocutaneous flap from the sural region. Scand J Plast Surg (Oakv). 1983; 17:191–196

[10] Hallock GG. The fallacy of presumed superiority of proximally based versus distally based flaps. Plast Reconstr Surg. 1995; 96(6):1372–1377

[11] Hallock GG. Distal lower leg local random fasciocutaneous flaps. Plast Reconstr Surg. 1990; 86(2):304–311

[12] Lu TC, Lin CH, Lin CH, Lin YT, Chen RF, Wei FC. Versatility of the pedicled peroneal artery perforator flaps for soft-tissue coverage of the lower leg and foot defects. J Plast Reconstr Aesthet Surg. 2011; 64(3):386–393

[13] Mehrotra S. Perforator-plus flaps: a new concept in traditional flap design. Plast Reconstr Surg. 2007; 119(2):590–598

[14] Mehrotra S. Perforators in local peninsular and island flaps: are they always useful? Plast Reconstr Surg. 2008; 121:author reply 1866–1867

[15] Sharma RK. Perforators in local peninsular and island flaps: are they always useful? [Reply]. Plast Reconstr Surg. 2008; 121:1867

[16] Mehrotra S. Perforator-plus concept: adding versatility to traditional flaps. Plast Reconstr Surg. 2009; 123(6):219e–220e

[17] Rampazzo A, Gharb BB, Chong MWT, Yao SF, Chen HC. Perforators in local peninsular and island flaps: are they always useful? Plast Reconstr Surg. 2008; 121(5):1864–1865, author reply 1866–1867

[18] Saint-Cyr M, Wong C, Schaverien M, Mojallal A, Rohrich RJ. The perforasome theory: vascular anatomy and clinical implications. Plast Reconstr Surg. 2009; 124(5):1529–1544

[19] Hallock GG. Local fasciocutaneous flap skin coverage for the dorsal foot and ankle. Foot Ankle. 1991; 11(5):274–281

15.5 Chapter 15D: The Perforator Propeller Flap

Geoffrey G. Hallock

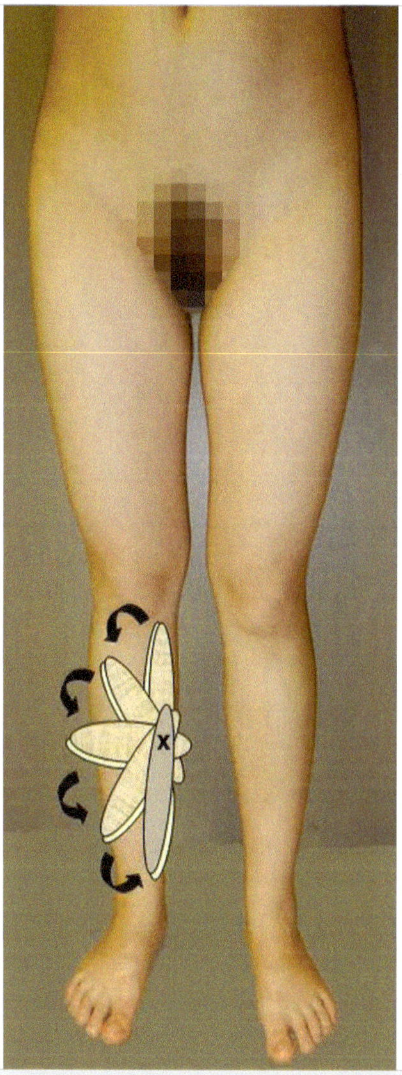

Fig. 15.20 The propeller flap.

15.5.1 Introduction to the Perforator Propeller Flap

The rotation of islanded flaps as a solution for unique coverage problems has long-standing precedents,[1] but Hyakusoku et al[2] deserve full credit for first describing their variant introducing the term "propeller" flap. They used adipocutaneous flaps with two skin extensions that appeared like the blades of a propeller, centered over a random subcutaneous tissue pedicle. The bulkiness of the pedicle itself limited flap rotation to less than 90 degrees. If instead a discrete and identifiable perforator were the pedicle, this perforator-pedicled propeller flap version could be turned up to 180 degrees and thereby be more versatile.[3] The "Tokyo" consensus attempted to strictly define a propeller flap as an islanded flap that reached the recipient site through an axial rotation of its blades about a vascular hub that remained the only physical connection with the donor site (▶ Fig. 15.20).[4]

The intrigue of propeller flaps especially in the lower extremity is that more proximal skin territories that are usually found outside any zone of injury can be transferred to more distal defects where tissue redundancy is sparse, and this can be done as long as an adequate perforator can be found without the need for microvascular surgery, although microsurgical dissection techniques are still required.[5] This concept has allowed "local" perforator propeller flaps to reach not only the foot and ankle,[6] but also the toe.[7] Common donor sites such as for the harvest of the fibula[8] or anterolateral thigh[9] could now be closed directly without the need for skin grafts.

Many believe that comorbidities like diabetes, peripheral vascular disease, a smoking history, or morbid obesity make the risk of propeller flap total failure or partial necrosis unacceptable in the lower extremity,[10,11] although others deny there is any concomitant risk.[12] Free flaps, which would often be the only reasonable alternative, in comparison studies have been found to have a similar rate of complications, but at a greater cost of resources.[13,14,15] Discretion in the process of selection of a propeller flap will still always be the best precaution to minimize unexpected outcomes.

15.5.2 Attributes and Detriments

Attributes

- Local flap.
- Proximal tissues available for distal transport.
- Rapid harvest.
- Nonmicrovascular tissue transfer.
- Function preservation.

Detriments

- Venous congestion common.
- Pedicle torsion or traction unacceptable.
- Potential donor site morbidity and scarring.

15.5.3 Anatomical Considerations

Although the vascular hub of a propeller flap can be a subcutaneous pedicle[2] or even an axial vessel,[16] most often a discrete perforator is selected. In the lower extremity, Geddes et al[17] found a mean of 93 ± 26 perforators that qualify to be so chosen. In the leg, "hot spots" of these perforators are found near articulations or the midportion of the tibia or the fibula,[12] arising from any of the three source vessels to the foot. Perforators from the peroneal[18] or posterior tibial artery[13] have proven to be the most useful, particularly more distally where they tend to be septocutaneous in origin. Since perforasomes in the lower extremity capture those contiguous in a longitudinal direction as is also the direction of the source vessels themselves, the axis of any planned propeller flap should also have as vertical an orientation as possible to minimize any risk of inadequate perfusion.[19]

Any perforator chosen to be the vascular supply to a propeller flap should be close to the defect, so that the size of the major blade and its subsequent donor site residue will be minimized.

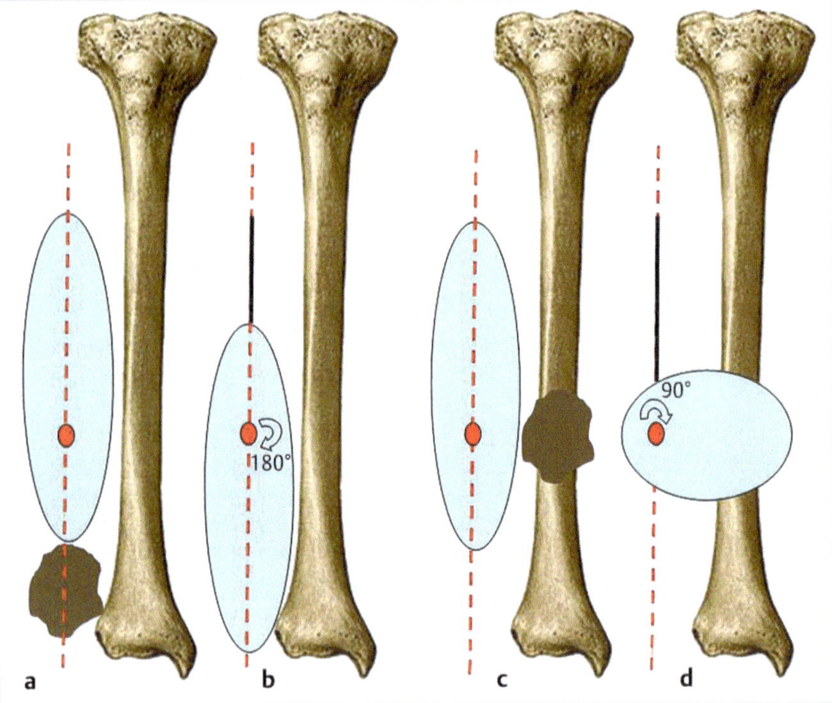

Fig. 15.21 Flap rotation angle. **(a)** For a given defect (*brown*), if the prime perforator (*red dot*) is along the same longitudinal axis of the lower limb, as is the defect, then the designed flap must have the same axis **(b)** and the flap must then be rotated 180 degrees to be inset; **(c)** however, if the given defect is adjacent to the longitudinal axis of this same prime perforator, **(d)** the identically designed flap may only have to be rotated 90 degrees or even less to complete coverage, which is less likely to compromise perforator patency.

Even if sometimes two potential hub perforators are found, retaining the better as a solitary pedicle is usually a superior choice, as that eliminates any risk of the pedicles twisting closed upon each other during the axial rotation.[20] For similar reasons, all fascial strands about the perforator artery and vein should be released perhaps up to the source vessels, as particularly veins will be prone to obstruction from any twisting. Wong et al,[21] in a finite-element simulation model, found that the best perforator would be at least 1 mm in diameter, and, if released up to 30 mm, vessel patency would not be at risk.

15.5.4 Anatomical Variations and Potential Pitfalls

Anterior Tibial Artery Perforator Hubs

Perforators arising from the anterior tibial artery, if adequate, can be used to base a propeller flap, although their selection has been uncommon.[15] Often, these arise near the rigid tibia, which may make perforator release difficult while also generating unrelievable pedicle pressure after rotation. In addition, there is a paucity of tissue redundancy overlying the tibia, so primary donor site closure may be impossible.[20] Even if just encroaching on the edge of the tibia, long term stability of a necessary skin graft may be compromised.

Variable Axis Rotation Angles

In general, the less the angle of rotation of a propeller flap about its hub, the greater the assurance that the perforator vessels will not be compressed. This would be especially true if all fascial strands had not been released. To take advantage of rotation less than the standard 180 degrees, it will require a design where the axis of the defect will lie outside the axis of the proposed flap (▶ Fig. 15.21).

Blade Morphology

Typically, the major and minor blades of a propeller flap look just like that, a propeller. Yet even the existence of a minor blade is not essential. For that matter, the width of each blade can also be variable, primarily designed to ensure direct donor site closure. The axis of the blades can even be curvilinear,[20] yet realize that in the lower extremity adjacent perforasomes interconnect in a longitudinal fashion, so that depending on flap size complete perfusion with such a design may be risky.

Short Pedicles

The further that the pedicle to a propeller flap can be freed of any restraining strands, the greater will be the freedom of rotation without risk of vascular compression. Note that the more distal the source vessel perforators to the lower leg arise, the less subcutaneous tissues that have to be traversed to reach the subdermal plexus. As a corollary, these distal perforators tend to arise more perpendicular to the source vessels and have a shorter course,[22] so that their complete release if chosen to be a vascular hub to a propeller flap may require dissection back to include even the source vessel itself to ensure sufficient release.

Delay Procedures

Venous congestion is a common problem in propeller flaps. If further pedicle inspection and release of obstructing bands does not resolve the concern, the flap should be returned in situ for rotation 2 to 3 days later. If it is longer than that, inflammatory changes and edema may make it impossible to move. In fragile or high-risk patients, the "venous perforasome" is sometimes not immediately obvious,[23] so that a multistaged plan including a delay procedure from the outset may avoid the risk of retaining a portion of a congested territory that would then become a partially nonviable flap.

Supercharge

Sometimes venous congestion or arterial pallor of a propeller flap cannot be resolved with conventional tactics. It may still be possible after flap rotation to perform a microvenous or microarterial anastomosis, especially if multiple perforators had been found initially servicing the flap.[24,25] A leg with prior signs of skin injury may be at obvious risk for considering this option or may be an indication to not hesitate to choose instead a different method for wound salvage.

Composite Flaps

An adipofascial extension of the major blade will provide upon flap rotation tissue for fill of a three-dimensional void.[26] Since the overlying skin remains at the donor site, primary donor site closure will not be inhibited. Sometimes the deep fascia component can be separated partially from the subcutaneous tissues like the hands of a clock to also increase surface area coverage.[27] Teo has included muscle left intact to the deep fascia of the major blade for the same purposes.[20]

15.5.5 Flap Design

An adequate perforator closest to the defect should always be selected as the proposed propeller flap hub. If adjunctive methodologies such as color Duplex ultrasound or CT angiography are not available to localize this perforator, an audible Doppler may still be valuable. Since most problems where a propeller flap will be beneficial involve the distal leg or foot and ankle, the posterior tibial or peroneal artery perforators are best to consider.[28] The latter will be found along a line corresponding to the posterior border of the fibula. The posterior tibial artery and its perforators will be in the septum between the deep and superficial posterior compartments found a few fingers' breadth posterior to the medial border of the tibia.

If considering a planned 180-degree rotation, the minor blade will extend from the hub to the most proximal margin of the defect (▶ Fig. 15.22). The major blade must be longer than the sum of the lengths of the defect and the minor blade, as some reach will be lost upon flap rotation. In the lower extremity, the axis of each blade should parallel the source vessels as well as possible in a vertical direction while still capturing any donor site skin excess that would then best assure its primary closure (▶ Fig. 15.22). The width of the major blade must be appropriate so that the defect will be filled, and again usually somewhat wider so that there will be no tension on insetting that could impede pedicle flow.

15.5.6 Flap Harvest

Patient positioning on the operating table depends on the location of the defect and the proposed propeller flap. A sterile tourniquet is always used after partial exsanguination by limb elevation. This ensures that especially the veins remain visible to minimize risk of injury. Working from anterior to posterior for elevation of the flap is usually easiest (see ▶ Video 15.5). An exploratory incision along the skin border anterior to where the perforator is considered to be is first made (▶ Fig. 15.23). Dissection toward it can be suprafascial or subfascial,[29] but the latter is the easiest and safest. Once confirmed, the design of the flap is altered as necessary (▶ Fig. 15.23).

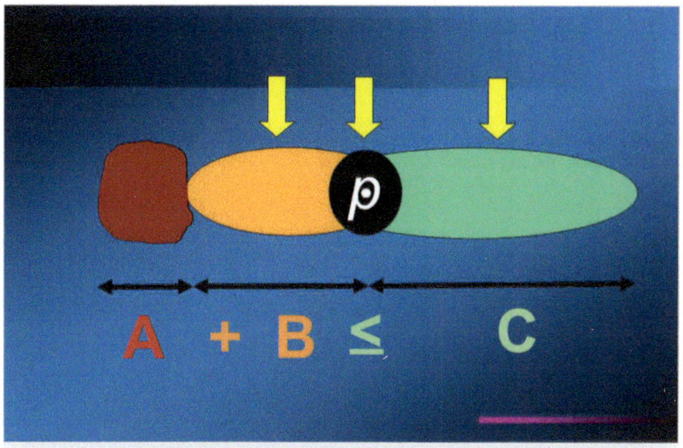

Fig. 15.22 Propeller flap design. Given that the length of a defect (*brown*) is "A," the closest margin of the defect to the perforator hub (*p*) of the propeller flap will be the length "B" of the minor blade (*orange*). The major blade (*green*) must have length "C" slightly exceeding the sum of "A + B" to compensate for the minor loss of reach during flap rotation, with a width adequate to fill the width of the defect.

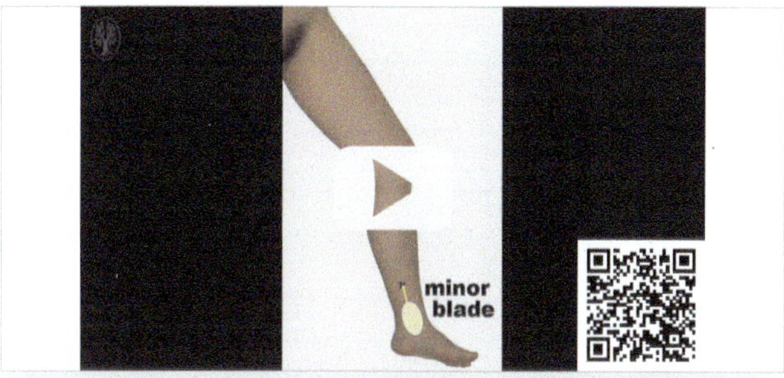

Video 15.5 Propeller Flap Harvest. https://www.thieme.de/de/q.htm?p=opn/cs/20/7/12265272-1bca58c5

Sufficient skeletonization of the perforator pedicle with release of any fascial constraints as well as coagulation of muscle or other side branches should be performed going back to the source vessel itself if necessary to minimize the risk of later kinking.[30] If done adequately without injury, and if more than one adequate perforator is found, the best with regard to caliber and appearance is usually kept to prevent them from twisting about each other later. The remaining boundaries of the flap are next incised and the paddles are raised in a superficial or subfascial plane. Rotation of the flap in a clockwise or counterclockwise direction is done to see the effect on the pedicle. Once unrestrained, the flap is replaced in situ, and the tourniquet is deflated to allow reperfusion, resolution of any vascular spasm, and overall reevaluation.

Once flap circulation is reasonable, the flap is rotated again into the defect. Sutures placed on either side of the hub will ensure that this point remains static and pedicle traction will be avoided. Tension-free insetting of the major lobe is accomplished. The minor lobe will facilitate closure of the major lobe donor site. If primary closure is not possible without tension, a

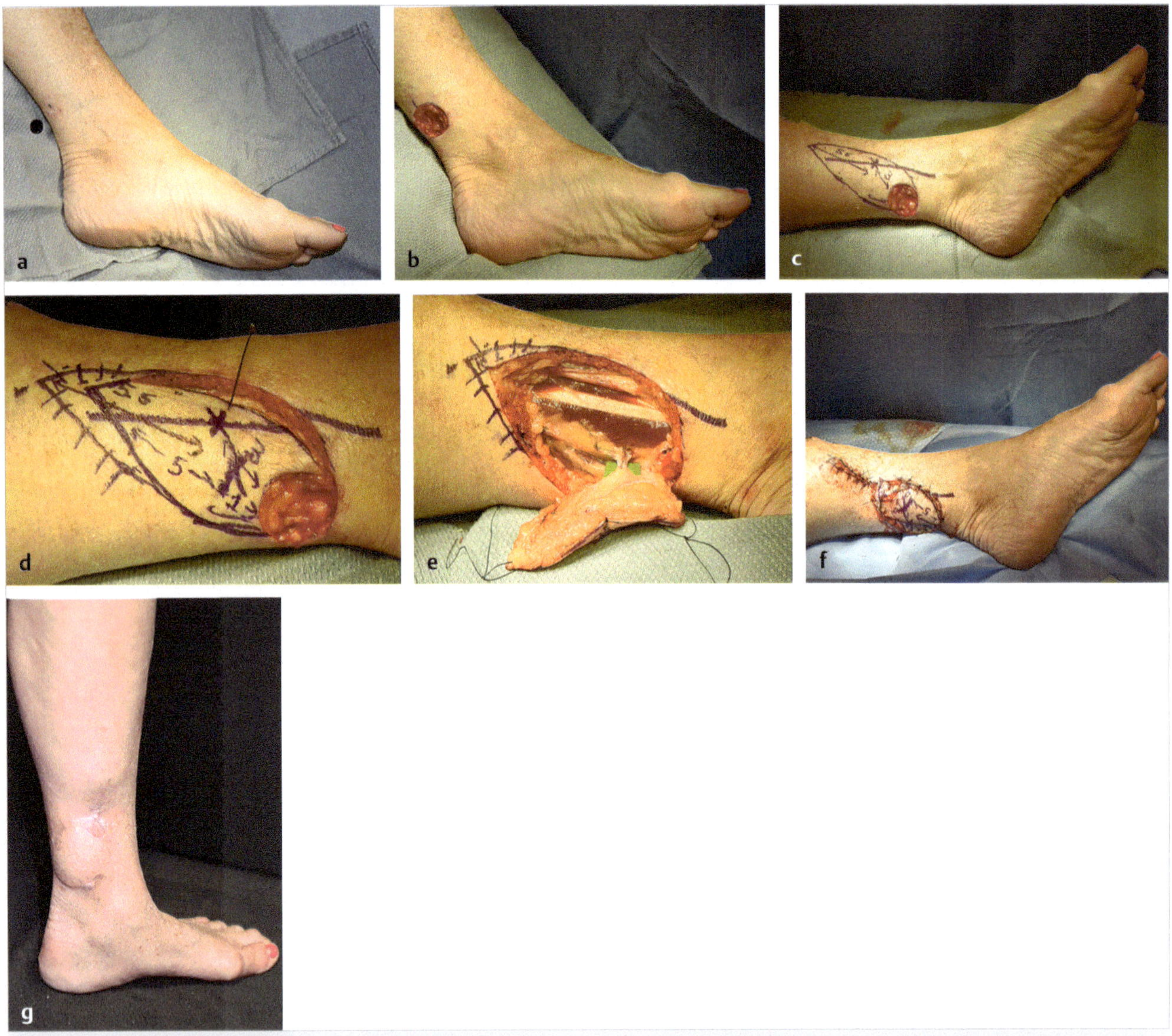

Fig. 15.23 (a) Basal cell carcinoma near the anterior border of the left Achilles tendon (*black dot*). **(b)** After a wide excision leaving a 2.5-cm circular defect barely exposing the tendon. **(c)** Initial design of the propeller flap oriented to capture the presumed posterior tibial artery perforator "x." **(d)** Anterior border exploratory incision revealed the actual perforator (large "X") to be closer to the defect, so flap boundaries were redrawn to minimize major lobe donor site residue. **(e)** Completion of flap elevation in the subfascial plane with release of restricting fascial strands about perforator (microgrid). **(f)** Flap inset after clockwise rotation into the defect with near total primary donor site closure. **(g)** Reasonable appearance 4 months later.

skin graft will always be preferable to embarrassment of circulation in the flap hub.

15.5.7 Postoperative Care Protocols

Any means to minimize lower limb edema, such as elevation, should be utilized to prevent stretch on the hub perforator even by edema. Use of compressive dressings and stockings should be avoided as flap circulation will always be disturbed. Careful monitoring much like a free flap will still be necessary. Signs of venous congestion are not unusual, but, if progressive, release of some sutures perhaps causing excessive tension by the closure will be necessary. If inadequate, a return to the operating room for reinspection of the vascular pedicle may be mandatory. Leeches represent another unwelcome alternative. Leg dangling and ambulation will have to await the elimination of these concerns.

15.5.8 Conclusion

The perforator-pedicled propeller flap is probably the most versatile of local perforator flaps, as this technique will allow the transfer of uninjured or uninvolved skin territories from the proximal lower limb to the more distal regions of the leg or foot and ankle where skin reserves are sparse and usually inadequate. As with any flap of the lower extremity, there are risks, with venous congestion being the most common. However, the risks of catastrophic loss of the flap do not exceed that of free flaps in this region[13,14,15] and since no microvascular surgery is required, even patients with significant comorbidities may be candidates for a propeller flap, while the stress on the surgeon is perhaps also reduced. The propeller flap represents a recognized alternative for restoration of small or medium-sized defects of the lower extremity, but overzealous use of propeller flaps with large major blades can sometimes result in unacceptable donor site morbidity.

References

[1] Hallock GG. Evaluation of fasciocutaneous perforators using color duplex imaging. Plast Reconstr Surg. 1994; 94(5):644–651

[2] Hyakusoku H, Yamamoto T, Fumiiri M. The propeller flap method. Br J Plast Surg. 1991; 44(1):53–54

[3] Hallock GG. The propeller flap version of the adductor muscle perforator flap for coverage of ischial or trochanteric pressure sores. Ann Plast Surg. 2006; 56(5):540–542

[4] Pignatti M, Ogawa R, Hallock GG, et al. The "Tokyo" consensus on propeller flaps. Plast Reconstr Surg. 2011; 127(2):716–722

[5] Georgescu AV, Matei I, Ardelean F, Capota I. Microsurgical nonmicrovascular flaps in forearm and hand reconstruction. Microsurgery. 2007; 27(5):384–394

[6] Chang SM, Wang X, Huang YG, Zhu XZ, Tao YL, Zhang YQ. Distally based perforator propeller sural flap for foot and ankle reconstruction: a modified flap dissection technique. Ann Plast Surg. 2014; 72(3):340–345

[7] Hallock GG. The first dorsal metatarsal artery perforator propeller flap. Ann Plast Surg. 2016; 76(6):684–687

[8] Sharma M, Balasubramanian D, Thankappan K, et al. Propeller flaps in the closure of free fibula flap donor site skin defects. Ann Plast Surg. 2013; 71 (1):76–79

[9] Iida T, Yoshimatsu H, Koshima I. Reconstruction of anterolateral thigh defects using perforator-based propeller flaps. Ann Plast Surg. 2017; 79(4):385–389

[10] Chaput B, Bertheuil N, Carloni R, Bekara F, Laloze J, Herlin C. Propeller perforator flaps of extremities seem less reliable. J Reconstr Microsurg. 2017; 33 (8):603–604

[11] Jakubietz RG, Jakubietz DF, Gruenert JG, Schmidt K, Meffert RH, Jakubietz MG. Reconstruction of soft tissue defects of the Achilles tendon with rotation flaps, pedicled propeller flaps and free perforator flaps. Microsurgery. 2010; 30(8):608–613

[12] Mohan AT, Sur YJ, Zhu L, et al. The concepts of propeller, perforator, keystone, and other local flaps and their role in the evolution of reconstruction. Plast Reconstr Surg. 2016; 138(4):710e–729e

[13] Nelson JA, Fischer JP, Brazio PS, Kovach SJ, Rosson GD, Rad AN. A review of propeller flaps for distal lower extremity soft tissue reconstruction: Is flap loss too high? Microsurgery. 2013; 33(7):578–586

[14] Cajozzo M, Toia F, Innocenti A, et al. Retrospective analysis in lower limb reconstruction: propeller perforator flaps versus free flaps. J Reconstr Microsurg. 2017; 33 S 01:S34–S39

[15] Bekara F, Herlin C, Somda S, de Runz A, Grolleau JL, Chaput B. Free versus perforator-pedicled propeller flaps in lower extremity reconstruction: what is the safest coverage? A meta-analysis. Microsurgery. 2018; 38(1):109–119

[16] Toia F, D'Arpa S, Pignatti M, Noel W, Cordova A. Axial propeller flaps: a proposal for update of the "Tokyo consensus on propeller flaps.". J Plast Reconstr Aesthet Surg. 2017; 70(6):857–860

[17] Geddes CR, Tang M, Yang D, Morris SF. Anatomy of the integument of the lower extremity. In: Blondeel PN, Morris SF, Hallock GG, Neligan PC, eds. Perforator Flaps: Anatomy, Technique, & Clinical Applications. 2nd ed. St. Louis, MO: Quality Medical Publishing; 2013:667–703

[18] Lu TC, Lin CH, Lin CH, Lin YT, Chen RF, Wei FC. Versatility of the pedicled peroneal artery perforator flaps for soft-tissue coverage of the lower leg and foot defects. J Plast Reconstr Aesthet Surg. 2011; 64(3):386–393

[19] Saint-Cyr M, Wong C, Schaverien M, Mojallal A, Rohrich RJ. The perforasome theory: vascular anatomy and clinical implications. Plast Reconstr Surg. 2009; 124(5):1529–1544

[20] Teo TC. Propeller flaps of the lower extremity. In: Blondeel PN, Morris SF, Hallock GG, Neligan PC. eds. Perforator Flaps: Anatomy, Technique, & Clinical Applications. 2nd ed. St. Louis, MO: Quality Medical Publishing; 2013:1223–1241

[21] Wong CH, Cui F, Tan BK, et al. Nonlinear finite element simulations to elucidate the determinants of perforator patency in propeller flaps. Ann Plast Surg. 2007; 59(6):672–678

[22] Jakubietz RG, Schmidt K, Zahn RK, et al. Subfascial directionality of perforators of the distal lower extremity: an anatomic study regarding selection of perforators for 180-degree propeller flaps. Ann Plast Surg. 2012; 69(3):307–311

[23] Chaput B, Grolleau JL, Garrido I, et al. Delayed procedure in propeller perforator flap: defining the venous perforasome. J Plast Reconstr Aesthet Surg. 2017; 70(2):286–289

[24] Yildiz K, Ozeren M, Kelahmetoglu O, Guneren E. The increasing of pedicled propeller perforator flap survival by an extra vein anastomosis. Microsurgery. 2017; 37(5):451–452

[25] Chaput B, Bertheuil N, Grolleau JL, Bekara F, Carloni R, Laloze J, Herlin C. Comparison of propeller perforator flap and venous supercharged propeller perforator flap in reconstruction of lower limb soft tissue defect: a prospective study. Microsurg. 2018; 38 2:177–184

[26] Zhou ZB, Pan D, Tang JY. Adipofascial extension of the propeller perforator flap: achieve two things at one stroke. J Plast Reconstr Aesthet Surg. 2017; 70(4):542–543

[27] Antonini A, Rossello C, Salomone C, Carrega G, Felli L, Burastero G. The propeller concept applied to free flaps and the proposal of a "clock flap" nomenclature. J Reconstr Microsurg. 2017; 33 S 01:S48–S52

[28] Gir P, Cheng A, Oni G, Mojallal A, Saint-Cyr M. Pedicled-perforator (propeller) flaps in lower extremity defects: a systematic review. J Reconstr Microsurg. 2012; 28(9):595–601

[29] Brunetti B, Tenna S, Poccia I, Persichetti P. Propeller flaps with reduced rotational angles: clinical experience on 40 consecutive reconstructions performed at different anatomical sites. Ann Plast Surg. 2017; 78(2):202–207

[30] John JR. Subfascial directionality of perforators of the distal lower extremity: an anatomic study regarding selection of perforators for 180-degree propeller flaps. Ann Plast Surg. 2014; 72(2):261–262

15.6 Chapter 15E: Medialis Pedis and Other Plantar Flaps

Mouchammed Agko and Hung-Chi Chen

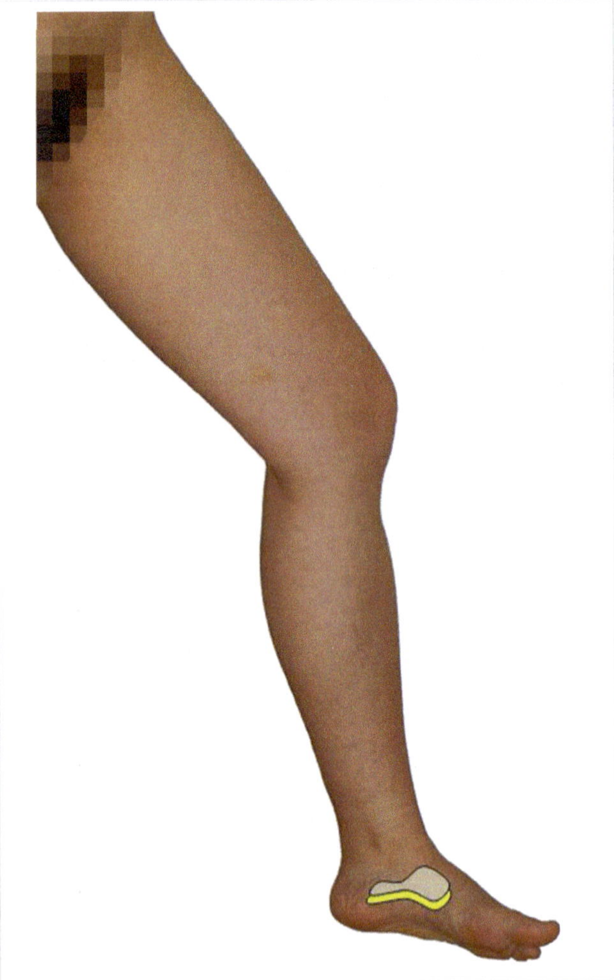

Fig. 15.24 The medialis pedis flap.

15.6.1 Introduction to the Medialis Pedis and Other Plantar Flaps

The plantar aspect of the foot can serve as a source for several muscle, musculocutaneous, fasciocutaneous, or purely cutaneous flaps that can be transposed, rotated, or transferred as a free tissue flap. In terms of ankle and foot reconstruction, these flaps, due to their sizes and special features of the skin, are mainly used to cover small to moderate-size defects involving the plantar surface and hind foot (▶ Fig. 15.30).

Mir y Mir (1954)[1] first used a random, cross-leg plantar arch flap transferred in three stages to cover heel defects on the contralateral foot. Later, Shanahan and Gingrass first described the pedicled medial plantar artery sensory flap from the ipsilateral foot based on the homonymous artery and nerve.[2] Reiffel and McCarthy further refined the flap by narrowing its pedicle and suggesting a subfascial dissection.[3] Harrison and Morgan reported the harvest of an island "instep flap" from the same area but including the underlying abductor hallucis muscle.[4] Morrison et al transferred this instep flap in a fasciocutaneous form (i.e., without the muscle) both as a pedicled island flap and as a free flap, extending its application to forefoot defects.[5] Finally, in 2001, Koshima et al introduced the free medial plantar artery perforator flap wherein a purely cutaneous instep flap is elevated based on a single perforator emanating through the intermuscular septum between the abductor hallucis and flexor digitorum brevis muscles.[6] This is where the superficial branch of the medial plantar artery, the pedicle of all the aforementioned flaps, is located. More recently, the medial plantar artery perforator flap has been successfully applied to defects involving all three weight-bearing regions of the sole: forefoot, midfoot, and heel.[7,8]

Alternatively, the medial aspect of the midfoot can serve as a donor site for the distinct medialis pedis flap. In 1990, Masquelet and Romana demonstrated, both in cadaveric specimens and in clinical cases, the feasibility and reliability of this fasciocutaneous flap based on the medial (cutaneous) branch(es) that arise(s) from the deep branch of the medial plantar artery.[9] Due to the thin and thus pliable nature of the skin and size of this flap, it is particularly suitable for coverage for distal medial malleolus, distal Achilles tendon, and heel. Other less commonly used plantar flaps are the lateral plantar artery flap and various intrinsic muscle flaps that can be used to cover exposed structures and provide a reliable bed for skin grafting.[10]

15.6.2 Medialis Pedis Flap

Attributes and Detriments

Attributes

- Thin, glabrous skin that can allow good recovery of protective sensation even if a cutaneous nerve is not included.
- No major artery sacrificed.
- Pedicled or free flap.
- Donor site primary closure possible with small-sized flaps.

Detriments

- Careful dissection of the short and delicate pedicle is required.
- Previous trauma and peripheral vascular disease may endanger the vascular supply of the flap.
- At times, skin graft take may be a problem at the donor site.
- Skin graft required for flaps wider than 2 to 3 cm.

Anatomical Considerations

Despite numerous publications on the subject, there is considerable confusion in the literature as to the surgical anatomy of the medial plantar vessels.[11] While the division of the posterior tibial artery into the medial and lateral plantar vessels is not contested, the terminology for the subsequent branching of the medial plantar artery is much less uniform presumably reflecting the considerable anatomical variation. However, this should not dampen interest in these flaps, as irrespective of the specific branching pattern, there always is a reliable vessel that can nourish both the medialis pedis and the medial plantar artery flaps.

For the sake of simplicity, the predominant pattern will first be described and then the clinically relevant variations will be explored as appropriate. The posterior tibial artery divides into the medial and lateral plantar arteries at the posterior edge of the sustentaculum tali that corresponds to the lower edge of the flexor retinaculum. After coursing for 2.5 to 3.5 cm, the medial plantar artery further divides into its superficial and deep branches at the level of the talonavicular joint deep to the abductor hallucis muscle (▶ Fig. 15.25a). The superficial branch, which is the vascular source for the medial plantar (instep) flaps, proceeds distally in the intermuscular septum between the abductor hallucis and flexor digitorum brevis muscles (▶ Fig. 15.25b).

The deep branch remains deep to the abductor hallucis muscle and then divides into medial and lateral branches. The lateral branch dives deep in the foot to connect to the deep plantar arch. The medial branch courses over the tibialis posterior tendon (close to its insertion into the tubercle of the navicular bone) and wraps around the medial osseous arch. The cutaneous vessels from the medial branch (of the deep branch of the medial plantar artery) supply the medialis pedis flap (▶ Fig. 15.25b).

The tibial nerve is closely associated with the posterior tibial artery and in a similar fashion divides into medial and lateral plantar nerves. The medial plantar nerve accompanies the superficial branch of the medial plantar artery and provides sensation for the medial plantar flap. The sensory innervation of the medialis pedis flap on the contrary is provided by the saphenous nerve, which reaches the area as a continuation of the femoral nerve. The saphenous nerve can be included in the medialis pedis flap, yet reasonable protective sensation and moving two-point discrimination can be achieved even without coaptation of the nerve.[12]

A network of venae comitantes accompanies the medial plantar artery and its branches, and maintains the venous drainage of these flaps. Nevertheless, the superficial venous system should be included in the medialis pedis flap in case the deep venous system accompanying the arterial pedicle is diminutive and, therefore, inadequate.

Anatomical Variants and Potential Pitfalls

The distal pedal pulses should be examined by palpation and audible Doppler auscultation to confirm patency of all inflow vessels prior to committing to this flap. The cutaneous arterial branches supplying the medialis pedis flap sometimes arise directly from the trunk of the medial plantar artery instead of originating from the deep branch. Regardless, this does not preclude safe harvest of the flap, as in either situation the pedicle can be traced proximally to a suitable sized vessel if necessary.

Another important consideration is to avoid exsanguination of the limb before tourniquet inflation to more readily enable

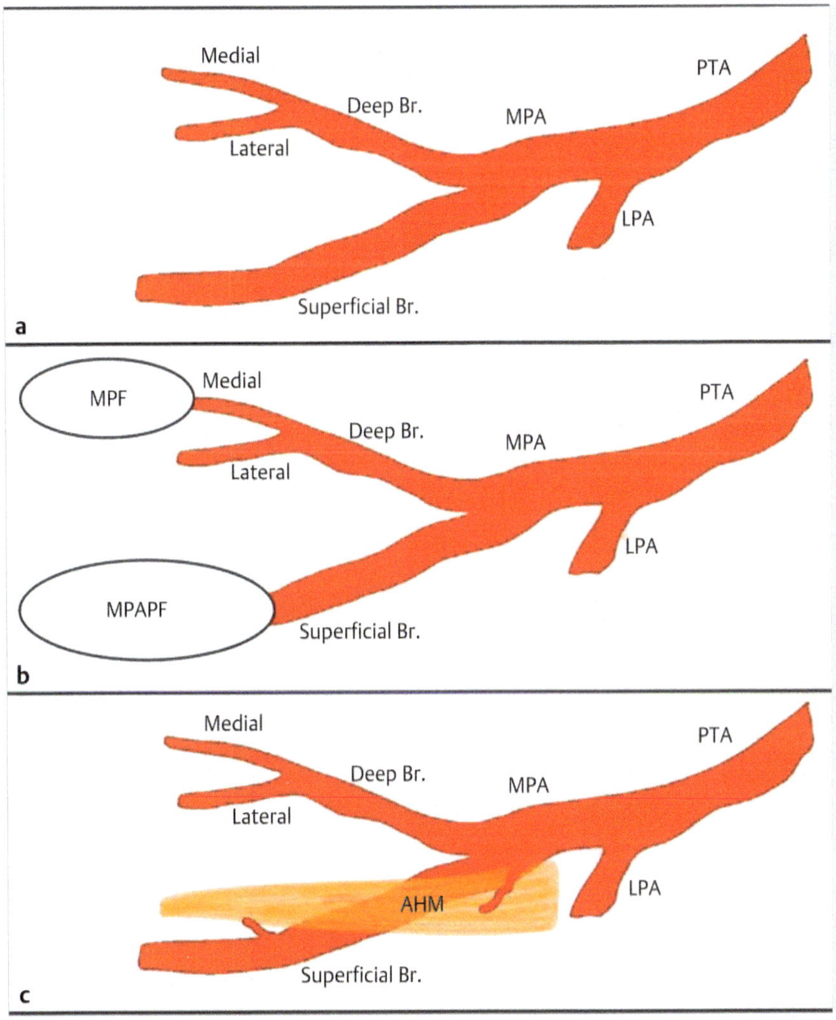

Fig. 15.25 **(a)** The posterior tibial artery (PTA) typically terminates into the medial plantar artery (MPA) and lateral plantar artery (LPA). The MPA then divides into a superficial and a deep branch. **(b)** The medial branch of the deep branch of the MPA provides the vascular supply for the medialis pedis flap (MPF). The superficial branch of the MPA gives off several usually septocutaneous perforators that nourish the medial plantar artery perforator flap (MPAPF), which would be the perforator form of the medial plantar (instep) flap. **(c)** The MPA and its superficial branch also send branches to the abductor hallucis muscle (AHM).

the identification and preservation of all small nourishing vessels. Finally, since the medialis pedis flap is raised at the supraperiosteal layer, alternative donor sites should be contemplated if skin grafting would be required and the tubercle of the navicular bone is unusually prominent. Failing to do so might result in delayed donor site wound healing and repeated ulcerations.

Flap Design

The four surface landmarks that can aid in designing the medialis pedis flap include the medial malleolus, posterior tibial artery, tubercle of the navicular bone, and abductor hallucis muscle. The long axis of the flap over the medial aspect of the foot parallels the medial plantar arch and is centered over the tubercle of the navicular bone. This is where the cutaneous branches consistently cross over the tibialis posterior tendon insertion and then proceed distally into the skin. The flap can extend from the medial inframalleolar area to the metaphysis of the first metatarsal bone. It is quite helpful to locate the skin perforators with a Doppler preoperatively around the tubercle and draw the perimeter of the flap accordingly. Flap size can be up to 5 cm in width and 10 cm in length, but a width greater than 2 to 3 cm will prevent primary donor site closure.

Flap Harvest

After preoperative markings are made, a more proximal tourniquet is inflated without limb exsanguination. Initially, the superior border of the flap is incised down to, but not including, the periosteum of the underlying bone. Dissection continues in a plantar direction immediately above the periosteum of the navicular bone and above the paratenon of the tibialis posterior tendon until the cutaneous branches are visualized on the undersurface of the flap. Once it is confirmed that a reliable skin perforator(s) can be included, the distal end of the flap is incised in a similar manner, as is the proximal curvilinear mark extending from the proximal end of the flap toward the medial inframalleolar area.

With retraction of the abductor hallucis muscle away from the osseous arch, the junction of the medial cutaneous branches with the lateral branch of the deep branch of the medial plantar artery is visualized. Next, the plantar border of the flap is incised down to abductor hallucis muscle. Further dissection proceeds in a superior direction over the muscle in a subfascial plane toward the vascular pedicle until the junction of the lateral and medial branches is encountered. At this time, utmost attention is required to avoid a traction injury to the lateral branch. To allow safe dissection proximally along the deep branch of the medial plantar artery, the lateral branch is preemptively ligated distal to the medial cutaneous branches. If a longer pedicle is desired, the medial plantar artery or even the posterior tibial artery can be exposed. In the latter case, the superficial branch of the medial plantar artery also needs to be ligated to enable proximal mobilization of the pedicle. Flap reach will then be sufficient for transposition to a mid or hind foot defect (▶ Fig. 15.26).[13] An alternative flap elevation technique involves exposure of the posterior tibial vessels first, and then tracing all the named branches distally in an orthograde fashion (see ▶ Video 15.6).

If tension-free primary closure of the donor site is not possible, a nonmeshed split-thickness skin graft should always be used to cover the donor defect to minimize the risk of further wound healing issues.

15.6.3 Medial Plantar (Artery Perforator) Flap

Attributes and Detriments

Attributes

- Like-with-like reconstruction for plantar defects (color, glabrous nature, thickness)
- No major artery sacrificed.
- Donor site in a concealed area
- Flap dissection relatively straightforward.
- No loss of function.
- A sensate flap is possible.
- Constant anatomy.

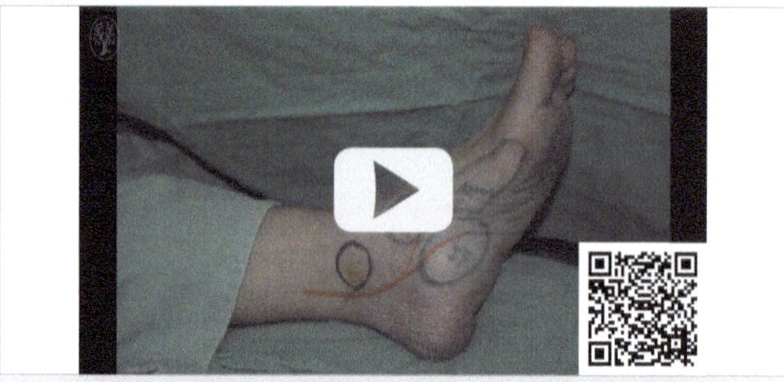

Video 15.6 Pedicled Medialis Pedis Flap. https://www.thieme.de/de/q.htm?p=opn/cs/20/7/12265273-a2dfac4e

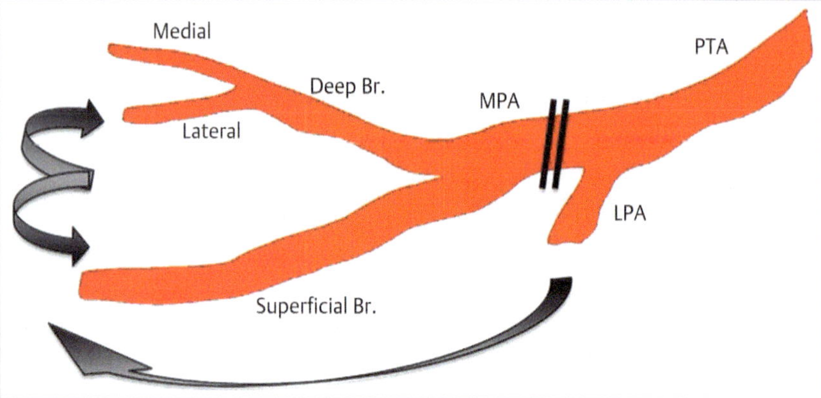

Fig. 15.26 Due to distal interconnections between the branches of the medial plantar artery and the dorsalis pedis (*double arrow*) and/or deep plantar arch (LPA, lateral plantar artery; *single arrow*) vascular networks, viability of the medialis pedis or medial plantar flaps, and abductor hallucis muscle can be maintained by reverse flow. After proximal division of the respective vascular pedicle (*double-cross hatch*), the flap can then be transposed to cover a defect in the distal aspect of the foot.

- Coverage of all hind, mid, or forefoot defects.
- Wide arc of rotation.

Detriments

- Large size defects may require alternative flaps.
- Primary closure usually not possible.
- Foot deformity with alteration of the weight-bearing area on the plantar surface could be a contraindication for this flap.
- Meticulous dissection of the cutaneous fascicles from the trunk of the medial plantar nerve is necessary so as to prevent sensory deficit at the donor site.

Anatomical Considerations

The predominant pattern of the posterior tibial artery is to divide into the medial and lateral plantar arteries at the posterior edge of the sustentaculum tali that correspond to the lower edge of the flexor retinaculum. After coursing for 2.5 to 3.5 cm, the medial plantar artery further divides into its superficial and deep branches at the level of the talonavicular joint deep to the abductor hallucis muscle (▶ Fig. 15.25a). The superficial branch, along with the medial plantar nerve, proceeds distally in the intermuscular septum between the abductor hallucis and flexor digitorum brevis muscles (▶ Fig. 15.25b). At the midsole, this neurovascular bundle becomes more superficial, and always in the intermuscular septum. Both the artery and nerve send cutaneous branches through this septum and around the medial border of the plantar fascia to supply the non-weight-bearing area of the sole. At least two (up to four) septocutaneous branches or perforators arise from the superficial branch in this manner. More distally, the superficial branch divides into two branches that communicate with tributaries of the dorsalis pedis and lateral plantar arteries. These connections are the anatomical basis for the distal-based (reverse) medial plantar (artery perforator) flaps.

Anatomical Variants and Potential Pitfalls

The distal branching pattern of the superficial branch may vary considerably. While this is inconsequential for proximal-based (antegrade) flaps, the reliability of the distal-based flaps ultimately will depend on the nature of the interconnections of these branches with the dorsal and lateral plantar vascular networks. Thus, temporary clamping proximally of the superficial branch in order to test whether these distal vascular anastomoses can reliably sustain the flap is crucial (▶ Fig. 15.27).

Flap Design

As with the medialis pedis flap, audible Doppler examination aids both to confirm patency of major pedal vessels and to identify the septocutaneous perforators on which the flap should be designed. The maximum skin surface that can be elevated depends on the boundaries of the individual's non-weight-bearing sole, with reports ranging from 4 to 6 cm possible for width and 10 to 12 cm for length. With smaller sized flaps, the design template can be shifted in both directions (anteroposterior and mediolateral) based on the spatial relationship with the defect. However, at least one perforator should be included within the circumference of the marked flap, and the boundaries of the flap should always be confined within the non-weight-bearing area.

The flap can be elevated in a subfascial (fasciocutaneous) or suprafascial (purely cutaneous) plane. The latter is preferred if a more pliable flap is desired. Additionally, preservation of the muscle fascia might improve the outcome of skin grafting of the donor area.

Flap Harvest

A proximal tourniquet is inflated after elevation of the limb only for exsanguination. A medial incision is made over the abductor hallucis muscle, followed by dissection in a suprafascial level over that muscle toward the intermuscular septum. Once the septocutaneous perforators are identified, the lateral incision is made over the flexor digitorum brevis muscle with a similar dissection continuing toward the septum. After isolation of the septum from the muscles on both sides, the perforators are followed toward the superficial branch of the medial plantar artery by retracting the two muscles apart from each other.

The decision to proceed more proximally for exposure of the main medial plantar artery or even the posterior tibial artery depends on the position of the defect that must be reached. A more posteriorly located heel defect will, of course, require a longer pedicle (▶ Fig. 15.28). A midfoot defect adjacent to the donor site will only necessitate enough dissection of the chosen perforator to allow rotation even as a propeller flap, as long as there is no kinking of the vessels.

A medial or lateral location of a forefoot defect will determine the type of flap needed. If possible, a medial forefoot defect can be covered with a proximally based flap in a propeller flap fashion. If this variation would fall short of reaching the defect, then a distal-based flap would be selected taking the aforementioned precautions. A pedicled flap often will fail to reach a lateral foot defect. A free medial artery perforator flap can then be transferred with microsurgical anastomosis to the lateral plantar artery or a branch thereof.

Standard microsurgical acumen should be exercised when deciding which or how many perforators to include in the medial plantar flap. If the first identified perforator is small, a second one preferably should be included whether it is a pedicled or a free flap. Tension on the pedicle should be avoided requiring

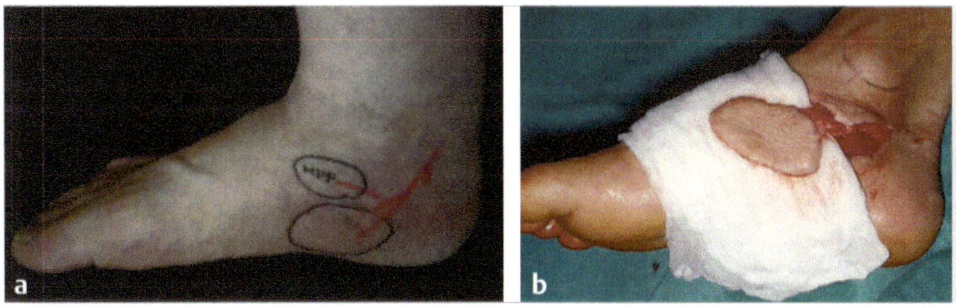

Fig. 15.27 (a) The skin territories of the medialis pedis flap (MPF) superiorly and medial plantar artery perforator flap inferiorly are demonstrated on the medial aspect of the foot. **(b)** The skin island of the MPF here has been harvested and its pedicle skeletonized.

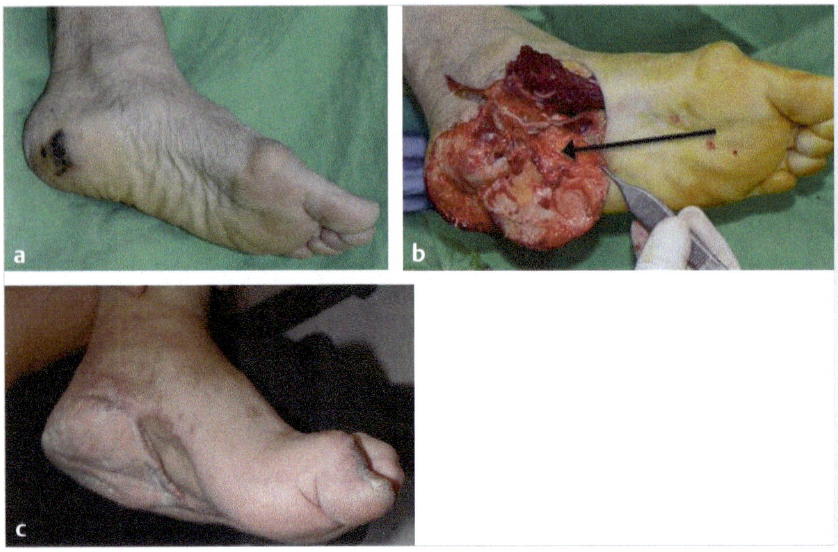

Fig. 15.28 **(a)** A 63 year old patient with melanoma of the heel pad underwent a wide local excision **(b)** with immediate reconstruction using a pedicled medial plantar artery perforator flap (MPAPF). The *black arrow* points to one of the perforators on the undersurface of the flap. The origin of the abductor hallucis muscle was divided to allow unimpeded transposition of the flap. **(c)** The MPAPF flap provided a durable plantar heel surface as seen at 3-year follow-up, without recurrence of the melanoma, but the donor site required a split-thickness skin graft.

more extensive dissection and release of any tethering. The cutaneous sensory branches should be identified and separated from the main trunk of the medial plantar nerve with a nerve-splitting technique to preserve distal sensation. A nonmeshed split-thickness skin graft is routinely used to cover the donor site, as any attempt at primary closure is ill advised since at high risk for dehiscence or skin necrosis if tension is excessive.

15.6.4 Other Plantar Flaps

Lateral Plantar Artery Perforator Flap

The lateral plantar artery passes deep to the flexor digitorum brevis muscle in a lateral and distal direction to reach the intermuscular septum between this muscle and the abductor digiti minimi. Not unlike the medial plantar vessels, septocutaneous perforators supply the lateral sole. Due to the weight-bearing nature of this region, which would poorly tolerate skin grafting, this flap should only be used as a second-tier flap to cover perhaps a small defect along the lateral aspect of the sole in a V-Y fashion along a longitudinal axis so that there would be primary closure of the wound and all incisions.

Intrinsic Muscle Flaps

As the medialis pedis and medial plantar artery perforator flaps have gained greater popularity in recent years, the enthusiasm for intrinsic foot muscle flaps has weaned. Yet, they continue to be a perfectly viable option for small defects. Even though good working knowledge of the foot anatomy is a prerequisite, their dissection is relatively easy and quick compared to other flaps and will cause a minimal functional and aesthetic deficit. Primary closure of all wounds is often possible. Preexisting denervation of the foot renders these muscles atrophic and therefore unusable as a flap. Therefore, be very careful in considering the use of these intrinsic muscle flaps for patients who have diabetes mellitus, peripheral vascular occlusive disease, or denervation of the foot as after trauma.

Abductor Hallucis Muscle

The abductor hallucis muscle originates from the medial aspect of the calcaneus and adjacent plantar aponeurosis to insert into the medial surface of the proximal phalanx of the great toe. For harvest, the muscle is first palpated along the medial foot and an incision made along the medial border of the foot. After exposure of the muscle, its tendon is divided just proximal to its insertion site, followed by division of minor vascular branches entering the muscle distally. The dominant blood supply, a proximal branch from the medial plantar artery, must be preserved. If necessary, the muscle can be further mobilized by separation of the origin from the calcaneus. The muscle flap can then be transposed much like an island flap to cover any reasonable nearby defect. The muscle can also be advanced anteriorly for coverage of medial forefoot defects by complete mobilization of the muscle, basing its vascular supply on reverse flow from the connections of the distal branches of the medial plantar artery with the dorsal vascular system and deep plantar arch (▶ Fig. 15.29).

Abductor Digiti Minimi Muscle

On the opposite side of the sole, the abductor digiti minimi muscle is the lateral counterpart of the abductor hallucis muscle. It originates broadly from the calcaneus and adjacent plantar aponeurosis to insert into the lateral aspect of the proximal phalanx of the little toe. A lateral foot incision lateral to the weight-bearing surface is used to expose the muscle. After disinsertion of the distal tendon, the distal minor branches from the lateral plantar artery are divided. With careful proximal dissection, the muscle is separated from the adjacent flexor digiti minimi brevis muscle up to the level of the cuboid bone where the dominant pedicle, a proximal branch from the lateral plantar artery, is identified and preserved. It should be remembered that the lateral plantar neurovascular bundle is situated between the abductor digiti minimi and the flexor digitorum brevis muscle. Depending on the amount of mobilization required to cover the

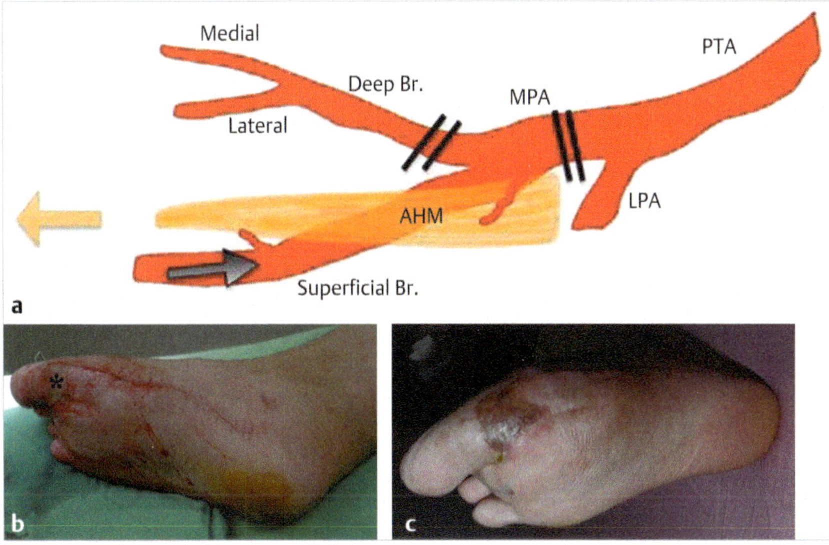

Fig. 15.29 A 56-year-old farmer had an injury to the right foot with tissue loss at the first metatarsophalangeal joint with tendon and bone exposure. **(a)** As seen schematically, an abductor hallucis muscle (AHM) was advanced distally for coverage (*orange arrow*). The AHM was based on retrograde flow (*black arrow*) to the superficial branch of the medial plantar artery (MPA) from the dorsalis pedis arterial system and deep plantar arch. Both the proximal MPA and its deep branch had to be divided (double-cross hatches) to permit this transposition. **(b)** A split-thickness skin graft (*star*) was used to cover the advanced muscle flap. Note the closure of the medial plantar incision necessary to harvest the AHM. **(c)** By 3 months of follow-up, the wound had healed well.

lateral heel or ankle defect, the muscle may be left attached to its origin or partially, and if necessary, completely detached.

Flexor Digitorum Brevis Muscle

The flexor digitorum brevis muscle occupies the space between the two abductor muscles just deep to the plantar aponeurosis. The proximal plantar aponeurosis and a narrow area of the adjacent calcaneus constitute the origin of this muscle that separates distally into four tendons, which themselves split into two before attaching to the sides of the middle phalanges. The lateral plantar neurovascular bundle supplies the muscle as it crosses deep to the muscle on its way to the lateral aspect of the foot. Through a midline skin incision on the sole, the plantar aponeurosis can be divided to allow reach to the muscle. All four tendons are divided near their insertion from the muscle, while utmost attention must be observed to avoid injury to the digital neurovascular bundles that run between them. The muscle is then reflected posteriorly to reach a heel defect.[14]

Alternatively, a musculocutaneous flap can be used to avoid a skin graft over the heel. This flap is planned to include the sole overlying the second and third metatarsals, encompassing the area between the intermuscular septa of the flexor digitorum brevis, that is, medial to the abductor digiti minimi, and lateral to the abductor hallucis muscles. The plantar aponeurosis immediately under the skin paddle is included with the flap, with the rest dissected away to expose the flexor digitorum brevis. The remaining elevation will be just as for a muscle-only flap, with the exception that the lateral plantar artery and venae comitantes must be divided in the midfoot and kept with the flap. If a sensate flap is desired, sensory branches from the medial plantar nerve entering the skin must be dissected from the main nerve trunk to be included.[15]

15.6.5 Postoperative Care Protocols

A protective splint is always applied to avoid compression of any plantar flap, and the limb is elevated to 30 degrees to minimize swelling. With pedicle flaps, the patient is kept in bed for 3 days. With free flaps, the bed rest period is prolonged to 1 week. This is followed by a cautious dangling protocol and then careful ambulation.

15.6.6 Conclusion

Reconstruction of the plantar foot poses a formidable challenge to the plastic surgeon. The outcome has far-reaching implications on the functional capacity and overall well-being of the patient. The medialis pedis and medial plantar artery perforator flaps are two workhorse flaps from the non–weight-bearing aspect of the foot that can safely and reliably resurface small and medium-size defects of the foot and ankle. Their glabrous skin provides an ideal form of coverage. Alternatively, the intrinsic muscles of the foot offer a time-tested option for small-sized defects of the mid and hind foot, and serve as a reliable bed for skin grafts. Their presence should not be forgotten.

References

[1] Mir y Mir, L, Functional Graft of the Heel, Plast Reconstr Surg, 1954;14(6): 444–450
[2] Shanahan RE, Gingrass RP. Medial plantar sensory flap for coverage of heel defects. Plast Reconstr Surg. 1979; 64(3):295–298
[3] Reiffel RS, McCarthy JG. Coverage of heel and sole defects: a new subfascial arterialized flap. Plast Reconstr Surg. 1980; 66(2):250–260
[4] Harrison DH, Morgan BD. The instep island flap to resurface plantar defects. Br J Plast Surg. 1981; 34(3):315–318
[5] Morrison WA, Crabb DM, O'Brien BM, Jenkins A. The instep of the foot as a fasciocutaneous island and as a free flap for heel defects. Plast Reconstr Surg. 1983; 72(1):56–65
[6] Koshima I, Urushibara K, Inagawa K, Hamasaki T, Moriguchi T. Free medial plantar perforator flaps for the resurfacing of finger and foot defects. Plast Reconstr Surg. 2001; 107(7):1753–1758
[7] Zelken JA, Lin CH. An algorithm for forefoot reconstruction with the innervated free medial plantar flap. Ann Plast Surg. 2016; 76(2):221–226
[8] Scaglioni MF, Rittirsch D, Giovanoli P. Reconstruction of the heel, middle foot sole, and plantar forefoot with the medial plantar artery perforator flap: clinical experience with 28 cases. Plast Reconstr Surg. 2018; 141(1):200–208
[9] Masquelet AC, Romana MC. The medialis pedis flap: a new fasciocutaneous flap. Plast Reconstr Surg. 1990; 85(5):765–772
[10] Attinger CE, Ducic I, Cooper P, Zelen CM. The role of intrinsic muscle flaps of the foot for bone coverage in foot and ankle defects in diabetic and nondiabetic patients. Plast Reconstr Surg. 2002; 110(4):1047–1054, discussion 1055–1057

[11] Rodriguez-Vegas M. Medialis pedis flap in the reconstruction of palmar skin defects of the digits: clarifying the anatomy of the medial plantar artery. Ann Plast Surg. 2014; 72(5):542–552
[12] Chen HC, Mardini S, Liu YT. Medial plantar artery perforator flaps with emphasis on the medialis pedis flap. In: Blondeel PN, Hallock GG, Morris SF, Neligan PC, eds. Perforator flaps. Anatomy, technique and clinical applications. St Louis, MO: Quality Medical Publishing; 2006:741–753
[13] Park JS, Lee JH, Lee JS, Baek JH. Medialis pedis flap for reconstruction of weight bearing heel. Microsurgery. 2017; 37(7):780–785
[14] Zenn MR, Jones G. Flexor Digitorum Brevis Flap, Reconstructive Surgery: Anatomy, Technique, and Clinical Applications. St. Louis, MO: Quality Medical Publishing; 2012:1762–1763
[15] Ikuta Y, Murakami T, Yoshioka K, Tsuge K. Reconstruction of the heel pad by flexor digitorum brevis musculocutaneous flap transfer. Plast Reconstr Surg. 1984; 74(1):86–96

15.7 Chapter 15F: The Distally Based Sural Flap

S. Raja Sabapathy, Hari Venkatramani, and Madhu Periasamy

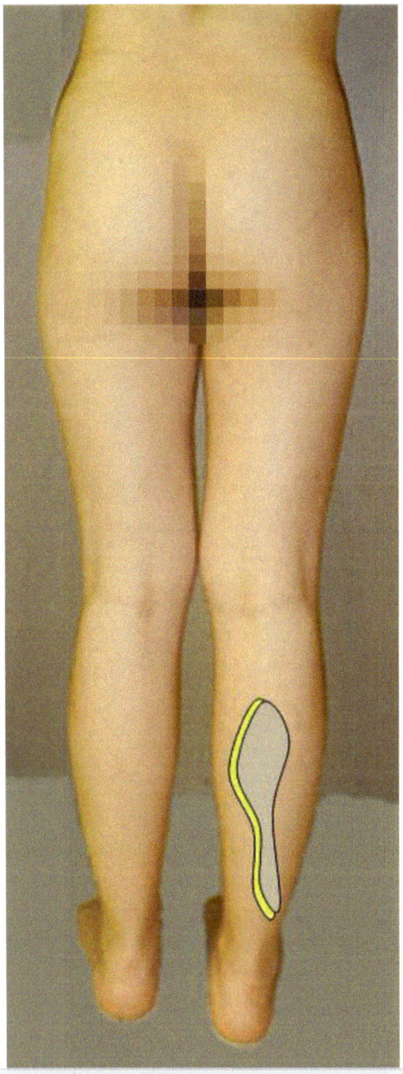

Fig. 15.30 The distal-based sural flap.

15.7.1 Introduction to the Distally Based Sural Flap

Coverage of soft-tissue defects in the lower third of the leg, ankle, and heel poses an extreme challenge for the reconstructive surgeon. The introduction of free flaps solved most of the problems and is the favored choice in current practice. In situations where free flaps are not possible, or when a microsurgical facility is not available, the distally based sural artery flap is an excellent alternative to cover defects in these areas (▶ Fig. 15.24).

The distally based sural artery flap is based on the vascular network around the sural nerve in the distal two-thirds of its course in the leg. Masquelet et al[1] in anatomical studies found that the median superficial sural artery that accompanies the sural nerve also delivers numerous branches to the skin. These cutaneous branches are present in the suprafascial portion of the course of the nerve. The median superficial sural artery and the interlacing network of branches are connected to the perforators of the peroneal artery, which are constantly found between 5 and 7 cm proximal to the lateral malleolus. This anatomical fact allows the design of a distally based flap based on those peroneal perforators with a pivot point often up to 5 cm above the lateral malleolus.

15.7.2 Attributes and Detriments

Attributes

- The blood supply is reliable, and major arteries are not sacrificed.
- Flap elevation is easy and quickly performed.
- No microsurgical skills or infrastructure is required.
- Useful even in elderly and diabetics since it is based on the perforators of the peroneal vessels, which are usually patent even in people with these comorbidities.
- The flap can comfortably cover defects in the lower third of the leg (▶ Fig. 15.31), lateral and medial malleoli (▶ Fig. 15.32), ankle, tendo-Achilles region, heel (▶ Fig. 15.33), and up to the proximal two-thirds of the dorsum of the foot (▶ Fig. 15.34).
- Can be raised as a fasciocutaneous, adiposofascial, or with a small cuff of gastrocnemius muscle as a musculocutaneous flap.

Detriments

- Has to be used with caution in patients who have fractures in the lower third of the leg, which could have injured the perforators arising from the peroneal artery.
- The donor area, if skin grafted, leaves an aesthetically unacceptable scar.
- The flap, if extended beyond the junction between the upper and the middle third of the leg, is not dependable.

15.7.3 Anatomical Considerations

The distally based sural flap is supplied by the median superficial sural artery that accompanies the sural nerve. As per Masquelet et al,[1] this artery descends to the ankle 65% of the time, and in the other 35% it is reduced to an interlacing suprafascial network of vessels that anastomose with the usually septocutaneous perforators arising from the peroneal artery. These peroneal artery perforators are situated between 5 and 7 cm proximal to the lateral malleolus. Thus, by keeping a width of about 3 cm at the flap base, this would include the sural nerve and pertinent vessels so it will be possible to raise a distally based flap incorporating the skin of the posterior aspect of the leg, with the sural nerve defining the axis of the flap. The safe proximal extent of the flap is the junction between the proximal and middle third of the leg, as at that level the sural nerve and its accompanying vessels pass subfascially.

15.7.4 Anatomical Variants and Potential Pitfalls

- The distally based sural flap is based on structures that have a fairly consistent anatomy, so reliable flap planning can almost always be done.[2,3]

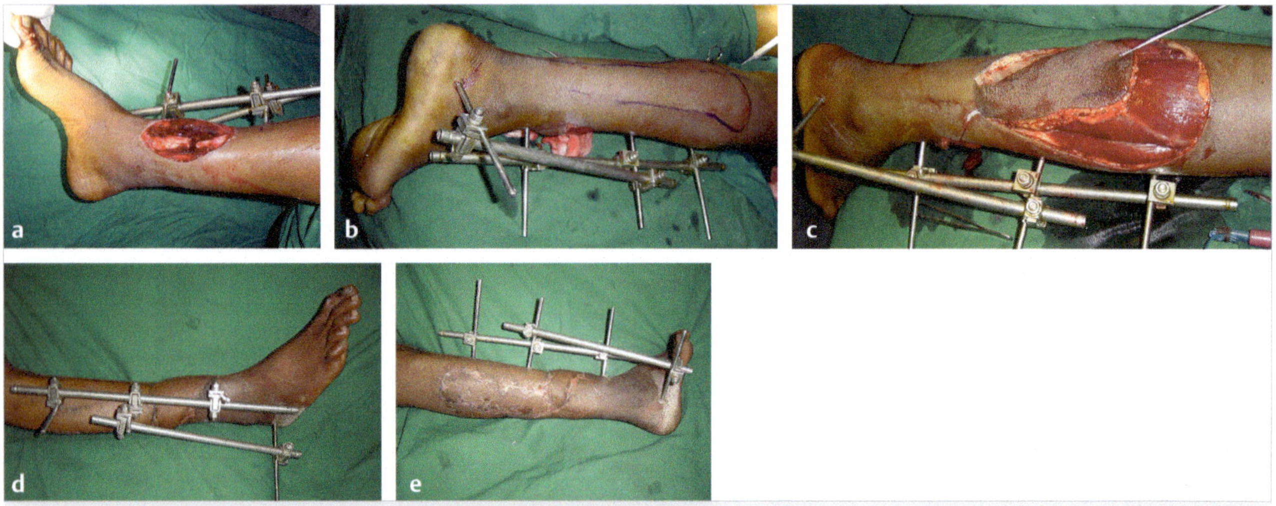

Fig. 15.31 **(a)** Lower third leg open tibia fracture requiring flap coverage. **(b)** Outline of chosen distally based sural flap. **(c)** Subfascial flap elevation. **(d)** Subsequent flap healing. **(e)** Appearance of skin grafted donor site.

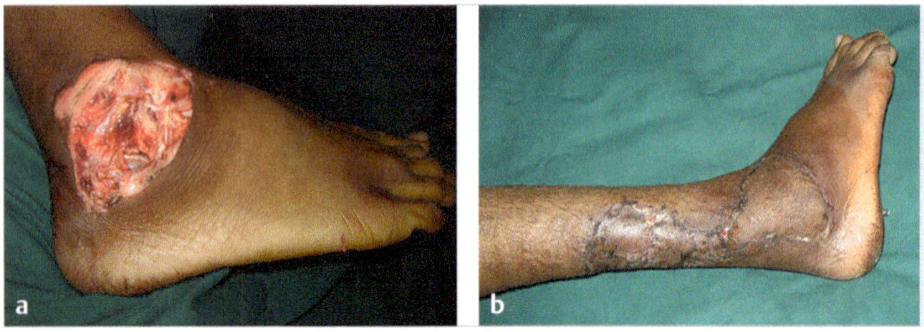

Fig. 15.32 **(a)** Soft-tissue defect over the lateral malleolus, **(b)** easily covered by distally based sural flap.

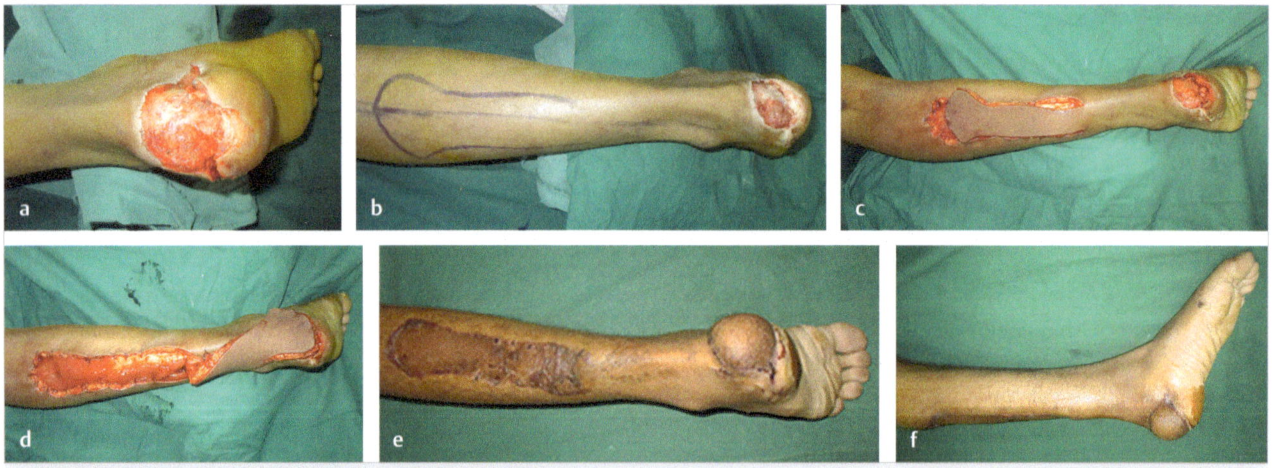

Fig. 15.33 **(a)** Posterior heel defect. **(b)** Proposed distally based sural flap markings. **(c)** The flap raised. **(d)** The flap turned over as in interpolation flap, to be inset. **(e)** Long-term outcome after flap pedicle division at 3 weeks, with expected result after skin grafting of the donor site. **(f)** Medial view showing flap contour over the heel.

- In closed degloving injuries of the lower third of the leg, and in some cases with fractures of both bones of the leg where the fracture site is situated around 5 cm proximal to the lateral malleolus, there is risk of disruption of the interconnections between the perforators of the peroneal artery and the vascular network around the sural nerve, thereby rendering potential distally based sural flap viability questionable.
- If the upper boundary of the distally based sural flap is designed proximal to the junction of the proximal and the middle third of the leg, the sural nerve at that level is subfascial and lies between the two heads of the gastrocnemius muscle. If care is not taken to include the nerve by deeper dissection and to sometimes include a portion of the gastrocnemius muscle as a vascular mesentery, that portion of the flap may be devascularized.

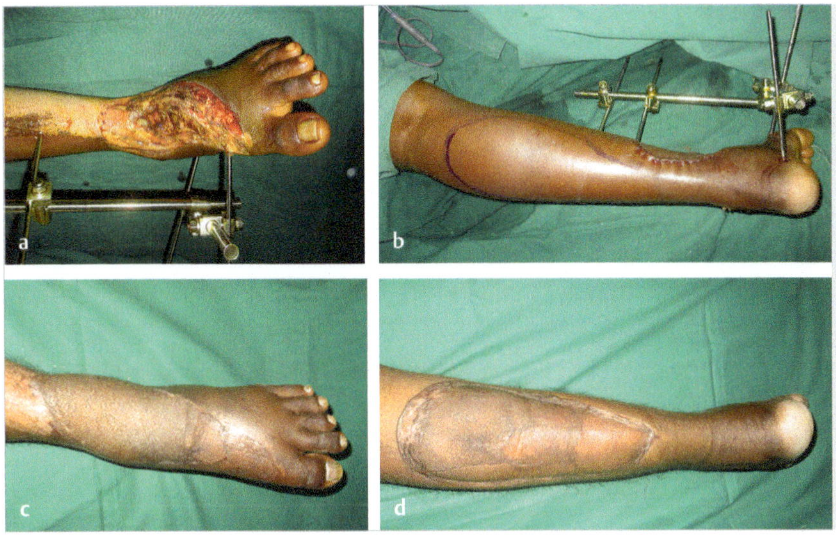

Fig. 15.34 **(a)** Large dorsal foot defect prior to definitive debridement. **(b)** Distally based sural flap marked. **(c)** The flap covered the critical area in the proximal two-thirds of the defect, and the rest was skin grafted. **(d)** Typical skin grafted donor site.

- The sural nerve can be spared from inclusion in the distally based sural flap, or even harvested as a nerve graft. This requires a careful dissection of the nerve from the fascia while preserving the accompanying vascular network. Though sometimes successful, many consider this maneuver risky and to be attempted only in exceptional circumstances.

15.7.5 Flap Design

The defect size is marked on a template and the outline of the distally based sural flap is marked on the line corresponding to the sural nerve, which extends from posterior to the lateral malleolus to the junction of the two heads of the gastrocnemius muscle, and then to the midpoint of the popliteal fossa. Sufficient pedicle length must be included to allow turnover at the location of the chosen peroneal artery perforator. Some would place this pivot point 7 to 10 cm above the lateral malleolus to ensure inclusion of several perforators to better provide flap perfusion.[4]

The flap can be designed to be entirely fasciocutaneous, or adiposofascial by sparing the skin in its entirety or just along the pedicle alone (▶ Fig. 15.35). The pedicle could be planned in such a way that it is tunneled to reach the recipient destination or could be used as a turnover interpolation flap, and the pedicle disconnected 3 weeks later. The former choice allows a single-staged transposition, but risks pedicle compression and flap devascularization. The maximum safe size of the flap in general practice is about 10-cm wide and 12-cm long. A skin graft will be necessary if primary donor site closure is not possible.

15.7.6 Flap Marking

The patient is usually placed in the prone position, and will then need to have general anesthesia. In our unit, we sometimes use regional anesthesia so the patient can lie in a lateral position on the side of the involved leg. The affected leg is kept straight, while the contralateral leg is draped with the hip and the knee flexed 90 degrees. This has been found to be a very comfortable position. A tourniquet is applied high up in the thigh, and the lower limb prepped and draped from the lower thigh to the heel. This simultaneously allows access to harvest a split skin graft from either thigh if needed to cover the flap donor area.

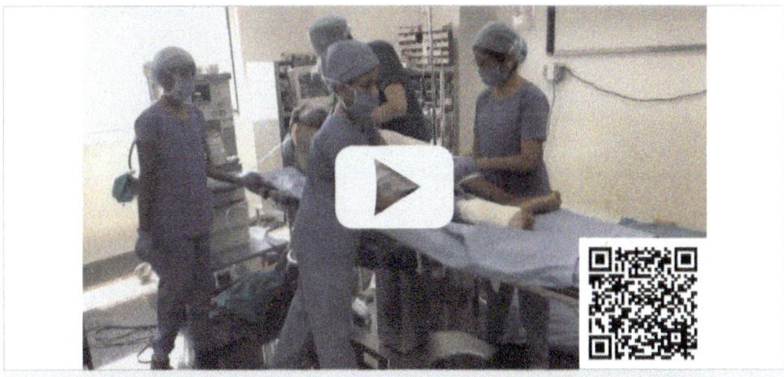

Video 15.7 Reverse Sural Neurocutaneous Flap. https://www.thieme.de/de/q.htm?p=opn/cs/20/7/12265274-30ce9dc7

The posterior midline of the leg is marked first following the course of the sural nerve and neighboring short saphenous vein. This line extends from a point between the lateral malleolus and the tendo-Achilles, should reach the midline between the heads of the gastrocnemius muscle at the junction of the middle and the lower third of the leg, to then pass proximally to the midpoint of the popliteal space.

The distally based sural flap is centered on the line as drawn with a pedicle length determined that is sufficient to reach the defect, with a point 5 to 7 cm proximal to the lateral malleolus as the pivot point. If a large flap must be taken, the flap can extend for 2 to 3 cm medial to the line of the sural nerve and laterally it can just cross the line of the lateral intermuscular septum where the perforators arise from the peroneal artery.

We keep a 2- to 3-cm strip as the width of the pedicle base centered on the axis of the sural nerve. This pedicle can contain skin, subcutaneous tissue, and fascia, or be without the integument. In the latter case, the skin is raised from the flap at the subdermal level, leaving a wide strip of adipose tissue with fascia containing the sural nerve and the short saphenous vein. These thin skin flaps can then be used to partially close the donor site.

15.7.7 Flap Harvest

After the distally based sural flap is marked, the proximal boundary is incised first down through the underlying deep fascia (see ▶ Video 15.7). The short saphenous vein, median superficial

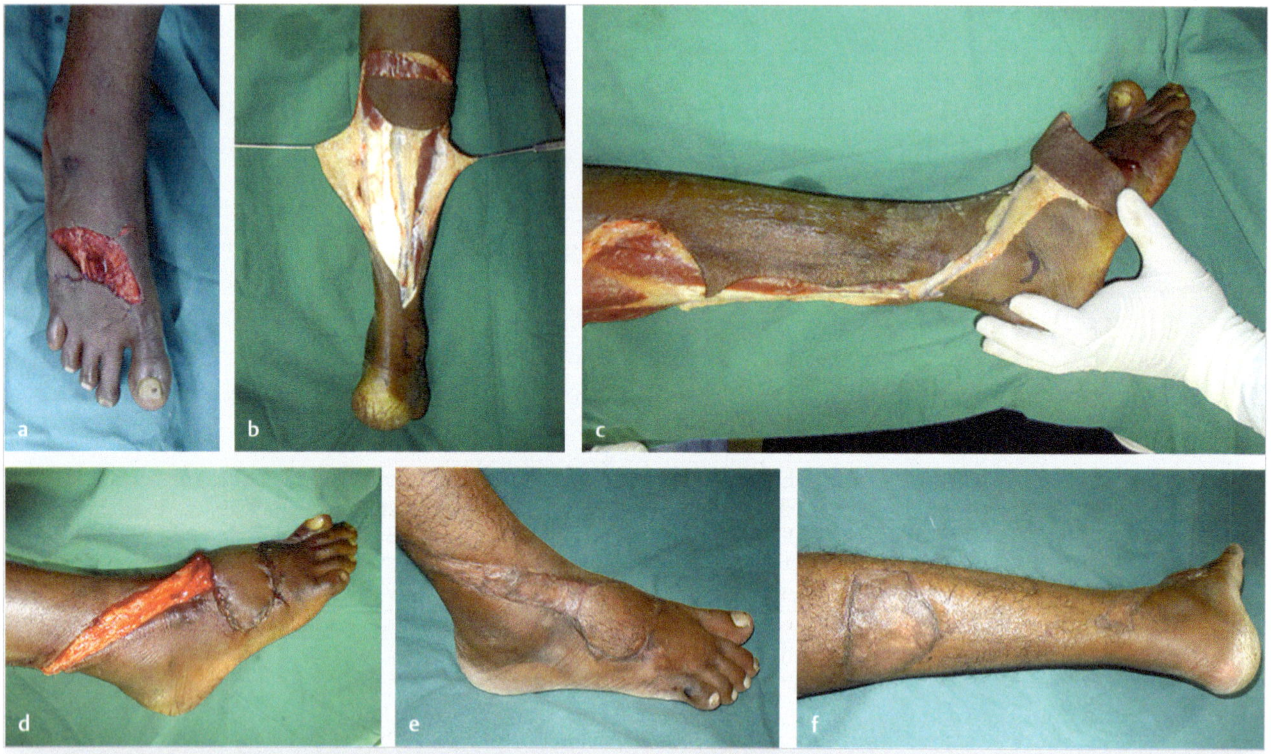

Fig. 15.35 **(a)** Distal dorsal foot defect. **(b)** Distally based sural flap raised with adiposofascial pedicle. **(c)** Turned over to anticipate reach to the defect. **(d)** Dorsal foot skin was incised and undermined to allow passage of the flap pedicle. **(e)** Flap was inset, and the pedicle covered with a skin graft. **(f)** This approach minimized but did not eliminate the need for donor site skin grafting.

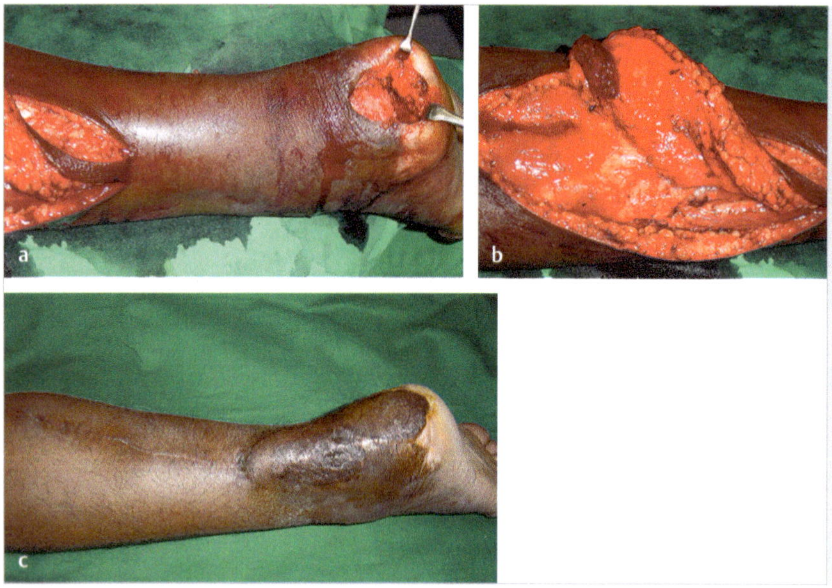

Fig. 15.36 **(a)** Deep cavity in calcaneus with simultaneous skin defect. **(b)** Extending the distally based sural flap proximally required that the proximal end of the flap be raised with a cuff of gastrocnemius muscle surrounding the sural nerve as a vascular mesentery to ensure viability. **(c)** The muscle here was also used to fill the defect in the calcaneus, while the skin flap simultaneously provided soft-tissue coverage.

sural artery, and the sural nerve will be found in that order from medial to lateral. The short saphenous vein is ligated. The sural nerve is pulled distally and divided after coagulating the end with diathermy. The proximal cut end of the nerve is allowed to retract to prevent a symptomatic neuroma at the scar line. Sutures are placed to retain the deep fascia and nerve with the skin to prevent shearing away of any vascular connections.

If the flap extends beyond the level of the junction of the proximal and middle third of the leg, the sural nerve must be identified in its subfascial location. A cuff of gastrocnemius muscle still attached to the deep fascia should be taken alongside the nerve, as this provides a vascular mesentery. This muscle can also be used to fill gaps in bone or dead spaces after flap transposition[5,6] (▶ Fig. 15.36).

Next, the medial boundary is incised a few centimeters to the medial side of the sural nerve. The lateral incision is finally completed, also incising the deep fascia. If a large flap is raised, this lateral limit can be 2 cm beyond the line of the lateral intermuscular system.

After the flap proper has been elevated, the next step is to raise the pedicle. If it is fasciocutaneous, a 3-cm-wide strip of skin centering on the course of the sural nerve is raised. If the flap is to be adiposofascial, subdermal skin flaps are first raised for 2 cm on either side of the line of the sural nerve, so that the encompassed adipofascial tissues will serve as the pedicle (▶ Fig. 15.35). Distal pedicle dissection is continued until the pivot point at the desired peroneal artery perforator is reached, often 5 cm proximal to the lateral malleolus.

Once the pedicle dissection reaches the pivot point, the flap can be turned over to the defect and inset. The pedicle can be tunneled to the defect or the intervening skin incised, and that sutured to the flap margins. The skin flap can also be turned over as an interpolation flap, and the pedicle divided 3 weeks later after adequate neovascularization has occurred. The last option will not leave any scar or bulkiness in the tendo-Achilles region. Advancement of skin at the margins of the donor site can narrow the defect, but if primary closure is not possible, the open area must be covered by split skin graft.

15.7.8 Postoperative Course and Protocols

A below-knee plaster slab is applied with padding about the distally based sural flap area with a window for monitoring the flap. If the flap is on the heel area, a special offloading technique must be used to prevent compression.[7]

Since the flap is used most commonly to cover fracture sites, weight bearing will depend upon restrictions imposed by fracture healing. When the flap is on the plantar heel, weight bearing is usually not started until after 6 weeks, and always with special soft footwear.

15.7.9 Conclusion

The distally based sural flap is a reliable, easy-to-raise flap that could be used to cover open areas in the lower third of the leg, ankle, or for heel defects. It does not require microsurgical techniques or capabilities, and does not sacrifice any major vessel. Detriments include sensory loss of the lateral foot if the sural nerve is included with the flap. Also, skin grafts if needed for the donor area will leave a conspicuous scar on the leg.

References

[1] Masquelet AC, Romana MC, Wolf G. Skin island flaps supplied by the vascular axis of the sensitive superficial nerves: anatomic study and clinical experience in the leg. Plast Reconstr Surg. 1992; 89(6):1115–1121

[2] Hasegawa M, Torii S, Katoh H, Esaki S. The distally based superficial sural artery flap. Plast Reconstr Surg. 1994; 93(5):1012–1020

[3] Rajacic N, Darweesh M, Jayakrishnan K, Gang RK, Jojic S. The distally based superficial sural flap for reconstruction of the lower leg and foot. Br J Plast Surg. 1996; 49(6):383–389

[4] Al-Qattan MM. Distally based sural artery flap. In: Blondeel PN, Morris SF, Hallock GG, Neligan PC, eds. Perforator Flaps: Anatomy, Technique, & Clinical Applications. St. Louis, MO: Quality Medical Publishing; 2013:847–854

[5] Al-Qattan MM. A modified technique for harvesting the reverse sural artery flap from the upper part of the leg: inclusion of a gastrocnemius muscle "cuff" around the sural pedicle. Ann Plast Surg. 2001; 47(3):269–274, discussion 274–278

[6] Hallock GG. Invited discussion: a modified technique for harvesting the reverse sural artery flap from the upper part of the leg: inclusion of a gastrocnemius muscle cuff around the sural pedicle. Ann Plast Surg. 2001; 47:274–278

[7] Venkataramani H, Jain DK, Sabapathy SR. Comments: a useful modification of the plaster backslab to off-load pressure from reconstructions of the heel and elbow. Indian J Plast Surg. 2012; 45(3):588–589

16 Common Versatile Free Flaps for the Lower Extremity

Geoffrey G. Hallock, Waleed Gibreel, Karim Bakri, and Samir Mardini

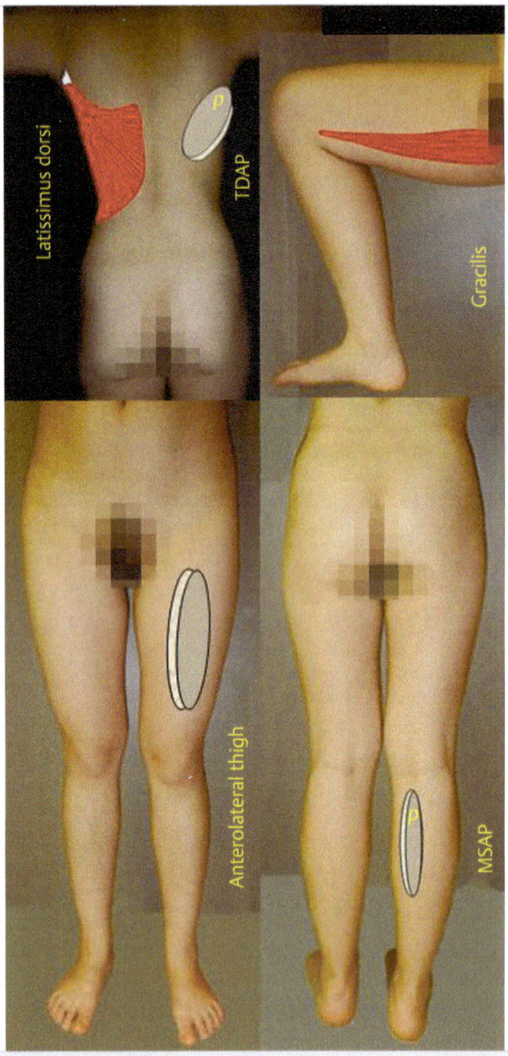

Fig. 16.1 "Workhorse" lower extremity free flaps.

Summary

Few would argue that the lower extremity might be the most difficult body region to resurface not just due to the paucity of skin redundancy but also due to not uncommon vascular deficiencies as it is so distant from the heart itself. A surge in interest lately for the use of local flaps as the solution when a vascularized flap is indicated for lower extremity reconstruction, presumably to avoid the risks of microanastomotic failure or technical challenges, should not obscure the fact that free flaps will still always sometimes be needed. Local tissue damage or vascular embarrassment will instead require the selection of a free flap. Some have called the anterolateral thigh flap the "ideal" soft-tissue flap for all purposes in this regard. Other "workhorse" donor sites are the relatively thin medial sural artery perforator flap, the thoracodorsal artery perforator flap that can capture the large dorsal thoracic fascial territory, or the more malleable and versatile gracilis and latissimus dorsi muscle flaps. Many other options do exist such as the superficial circumflex iliac perforator flap, but competency at least in using the aforementioned flaps should be expected, as they each have almost universal applications.

Keywords: anterolateral thigh flap, gracilis muscle, latissimus dorsi muscle, medial sural artery perforator flap, thoracodorsal artery perforator flap, free flap, microsurgical tissue transfer

16.1 Introduction (▶ Fig. 16.1)

What exactly is reconstructive surgery? An exact answer easily eludes us, but Tagliacozzi was on the right tract when he stated that it is rebuilding missing parts so as to restore the function that has been lost.[1,2] So how do reconstructive surgeons stand out from the wound center crowds who also claim this capability? Can it be because of our ability to solve more complex problems that require vascularized tissues in the form of what we call flaps? If simpler local options were inadequate, how could then a flap be moved from point A to point B? Hamilton (1854) answered that question by attaching one leg to another as a cross-leg flap.[3] Even a staged toe-to-hand transfer was similarly possible using the Nicoladoni method.[4] Filatov[5] (1917) and Gillies[6] (1920) independently developed the tubed pedicle as another means for distant tissue movement. Yet evolution was imperative as the immobilization necessary for success of these now-considered primitive maneuvers was lengthy, could lead to joint stiffness, and required multiple surgical interventions, while risking pressure sores, incompletely surviving flaps, or thromboembolic events. And most important, the outcome was suboptimal compared to today's high expectations.

The beginning of this new beginning relied on animal experiments in the early 1900s by Carrel[7] and Guthrie[8] who perfected anastomoses of blood vessels permitting replantations and organ transfers in the laboratory. Many others followed, developing fundamental reliable and consistent operative techniques, the discovery of anticoagulation essential to decrease the risk of thrombosis, and obtained intraoperative magnification for better visualization.[8] Jacobson and Tamai,[8] then latter Acland,[9,10,11] fabricated new designs in instrumentation and suture material that would facilitate what now is called the microvascular anastomoses. O'Brien set up a microsurgical research unit specifically to find answers to previously unrecognized physiological and clinical challenges at the microvascular level.[12]

Then a tsunami began. McLean and Bunke[13] used the omentum as an autotransplant to the scalp. Harii et al,[14] in 1972, performed the first successful free skin transfer using the temporal scalp for hair transplantation. Credit for the first composite tissue transfer, however, usually is given to Daniel and Taylor[15] for their iliofemoral island flap placed in a single stage on a distal lower limb defect. The "Introduction" of that paper is preceded by some provocative and prophetic words by Harry J. Buncke, Jr., himself that cannot be overlooked: "The successful transplantation of a block of composite tissue by reanastomosing the microvascular pedicle has untold experimental and clinical possibilities."[15]

And so it would be, and it was good. Soon muscle,[16] bone,[17] nerve,[18] viscera,[19] and every imaginable microsurgical tissue transfer as a "free" flap would be used anywhere in the body. Innovators willing to risk criticism and resistance instead flourished. Godina showed superior results for lower extremity trauma by the immediate use of free flaps.[20,21] Hong honed technical expertise with supermicrosurgery.[22] Millennials even proved a true value of the cell phone by obtaining thermographic images for perforator localization equal to that possible with CT angiography.[23] The Chang Gung group obtained better outcomes using an intensive care "free flap" unit with well-trained nurses for monitoring that could detect earlier microanastomotic catastrophes that could then be more easily rectified, as the sooner the better.[24]

In this day of perforator flaps where a paradigm shift is being seen prioritizing local flaps for lower extremity soft-tissue coverage,[25] is there still a role for free flaps? The answer even for the most casual observer should be "yes." There can be no argument if local tissues have been too compromised or even absent as in a limb amputation where a joint or limb length must nevertheless be preserved.[26] Almost all large wounds and even some small to moderate-sized wounds might still be better served by a free flap. Today, donor site morbidity also must be considered, as oftentimes just the aesthetics would be superior with a small free flap as opposed to a local flap where donor site closure had required a skin graft. Perusal of the process of flap selection in Chapter 13 recites all reasonably available free flap options, but those chosen here have been carefully selected for emphasis. The anterolateral thigh flap, some say, is the "ideal" soft-tissue flap.[27] The thinness of the medial sural flap for many has supplanted use of the radial forearm flap as it avoids sacrifice of the radial artery.[28] The thoracodorsal artery perforator flap can capture the same dorsal thoracic fascial territory as does the scapular/parascapular flap,[29,30] but it has a potentially much longer vascular pedicle that could reach beyond a zone of injury. If a perforator flap is not an option or has failed, more malleable muscle flaps such as the gracilis and latissimus dorsi are also available, which are not only important for the lower extremity, but also are truly "workhorse" flaps for throughout the body.[31] Finally, the groin flap has been reborn as the superficial circumflex iliac perforator flap and is better explained in Chapter 22.

References

[1] Tagliacozzi G. De Curtorum Chirurgica per Insitionem Libri Duo. Venice: G Bindonus; 1597

[2] Park JE, Chang DW. Advances and innovations in microsurgery. Plast Reconstr Surg. 2016; 138(5):915e–924e

[3] Stark RB, Kaplan JM. Cross-leg flaps in patients over 50 years of age. Br J Plast Surg. 1972; 25(1):20–21

[4] Huemer GM. Carl Nicoladoni and the concept of toe-to-hand transfer at the turn of the nineteenth century. Plast Reconstr Surg. 2005; 115(5):1432–1433

[5] Barsky AJ. Filatov and the tubed pedicle. Plast Reconstr Surg Transplant Bull. 1959; 24:456–462

[6] Bingham HG, Moore CE. Farewell to Queen's Hospital, Sidcup. Br J Plast Surg. 1976; 29(4):297–301

[7] Carrel A. La Technique Operatoire des Anastomoses Vasculaires et de la Transplantation des Visceres. Lyon Med. 1902; 98:859–863

[8] Tamai S. History of microsurgery. Plast Reconstr Surg. 2009; 124(6) Suppl: e282–e294

[9] McGrouther DA. Robert Acland (1941–2016) innovator, microsurgeon, anatomist and teacher. J Plast Reconstr Aesthet Surg. 2018; 71(2):126–131

[10] Acland R. A new needle for microvascular surgery. Surgery. 1972; 71(1): 130–131

[11] Acland RD. Microvascular anastomosis: a device for holding stay sutures and a new vascular clamp. Surgery. 1974; 75(2):185–187

[12] Morrison WA. Bernard McCarthy O'Brien. Br J Plast Surg. 1994; 47:204–205

[13] McLean DH, Buncke HJ, Jr. Autotransplant of omentum to a large scalp defect, with microsurgical revascularization. Plast Reconstr Surg. 1972; 49(3):268–274

[14] Harii K, Omori K, Omori S. Successful clinical transfer of ten free flaps by microvascular anastomoses. Plast Reconstr Surg. 1974; 53(3):259–270

[15] Daniel RK, Taylor GI. Distant transfer of an island flap by microvascular anastomoses. A clinical technique. Plast Reconstr Surg. 1973; 52(2):111–117

[16] Research Laboratory for Replantation of Severed Limb. Free muscle transplantation by microsurgical neurovascular anastomoses. Report of a case. Chin Med J (Engl). 1976; 2(1):47–50

[17] Taylor GI, Miller GD, Ham FJ. The free vascularized bone graft. A clinical extension of microvascular techniques. Plast Reconstr Surg. 1975; 55(5): 533–544

[18] Taylor GI, Ham FJ. The free vascularized nerve graft. A further experimental and clinical application of microvascular techniques. Plast Reconstr Surg. 1976; 57(4):413–426

[19] Hallock GG, Koch TJ. External monitoring of vascularized jejunum transfers using laser Doppler flowmetry. Ann Plast Surg. 1990; 24(3):213–215

[20] Hong JPJ, Colen LB. How has Dr. Marko Godina influenced us? Plast Reconstr Surg. 2017; 140(3):641–642

[21] Godina M. Early microsurgical reconstruction of complex trauma of the extremities. Plast Reconstr Surg. 1986; 78(3):285–292

[22] Hong JP. The use of supermicrosurgery in lower extremity reconstruction: the next step in evolution. Plast Reconstr Surg. 2009; 123(1):230–235

[23] Pereira N, Valenzuela D, Mangelsdorff G, Kufeke M, Roa R. Detection of perforators for free flap planning using smartphone thermal imaging: a concordance study with computed tomographic angiography in 120 perforators. Plast Reconstr Surg. 2018; 141(3):787–792

[24] Chen KT, Mardini S, Chuang DCC, et al. Timing of presentation of the first signs of vascular compromise dictates the salvage outcome of free flap transfers. Plast Reconstr Surg. 2007; 120(1):187–195

[25] Hallock GG. A paradigm shift in flap selection protocols for zones of the lower extremity using perforator flaps. J Reconstr Microsurg. 2013; 29(4): 233–240

[26] Hallock GG. Preservation of lower extremity amputation length using muscle perforator free flaps. J Plast Reconstr Aesthet Surg. 2008; 61(6):643–647

[27] Wei FC, Jain V, Celik N, Chen HC, Chuang DCC, Lin CH. Have we found an ideal soft-tissue flap? An experience with 672 anterolateral thigh flaps. Plast Reconstr Surg. 2002; 109(7):2219–2226, discussion 2227–2230

[28] Kao HK, Chang KP, Wei FC, Cheng MH. Comparison of the medial sural artery perforator flap with the radial forearm flap for head and neck reconstructions. Plast Reconstr Surg. 2009; 124(4):1125–1132

[29] Stokes R, Whetzel TP, Stevenson TR. Three-dimensional reconstruction of the below-knee amputation stump: use of the combined scapular/parascapular flap. Plast Reconstr Surg. 1994; 94(5):732–736

[30] Rautio J, Asko-Seljavaara S, Laasonen L, Härmä M. Suitability of the scapular flap for reconstructions of the foot. Plast Reconstr Surg. 1990; 85(6):922–928

[31] Hallock GG. The role of muscle flaps for salvage of failed perforator free flaps. Plast Reconstr Surg Glob Open. 2015; 3(11):e564

16.2 Chapter 16A: The Anterolateral Thigh Flap for Lower Extremity

Waleed Gibreel, Karim Bakri, and Samir Mardini

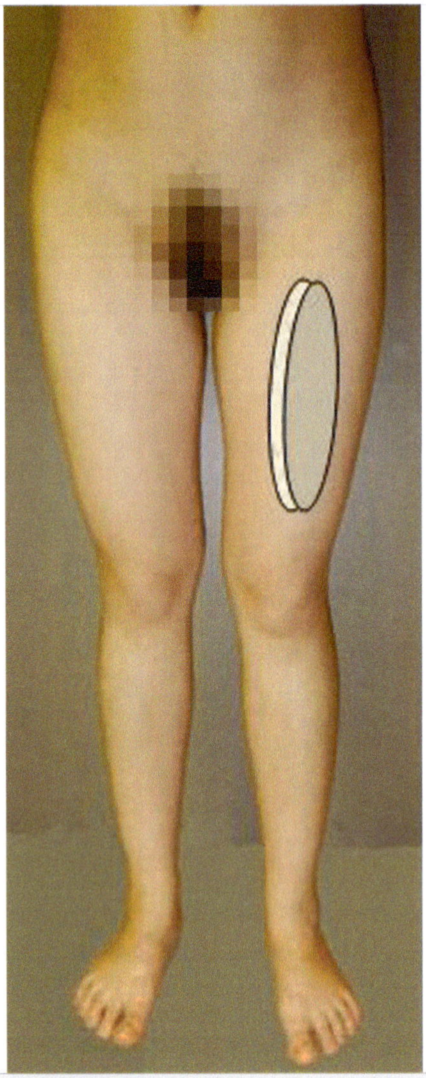

Fig. 16.2 The anterolateral thigh flap.

16.2.1 Introduction to the Anterolateral Thigh Flap for Lower Extremity

Following the initial description by Song et al,[1] the utility of the anterolateral thigh (ALT) flap (▶ Fig. 16.2) by reconstructive surgeons has increased tremendously. It is now considered the workhorse soft-tissue flap for reconstructive surgeries in various regions of the body.[2,3,4,5,6,7,8] The relatively consistent anatomy, minimum donor site morbidity, ability to reconstruct simple and composite soft-tissue defects, versatility, long pedicle, and satisfactory caliber of vessels are among the attributes that have led to the popularity of this flap and expanded its utility for both locoregional and free tissue transfer in different body regions including lower extremity reconstruction.

16.2.2 Attributes and Detriments

Attributes

- Relatively constant anatomy with slight anatomic variations.
- Ease of harvest when anatomic variation is understood.
- Ability to reconstruct complex soft-tissue defects.
- Minimum donor site morbidity when used as a perforator flap.
- Ability to harvest the flap in the supine and lateral positions.
- Allows a two-team approach when used for contralateral lower extremity reconstruction.
- Adequate pedicle length that maximizes reach when used for locoregional reconstruction.
- Adequate caliber of vessels suitable for free tissue transfer.
- Pliable flap that can be thinned without compromising flap vascularity.
- Ability to be used as a sensate flap especially for weight-bearing areas such as heel reconstruction.

Detriments

- Skin graft may be required for donor site coverage when the flap width exceeds 8 or 9 cm at the mid-thigh.
- Even if direct donor site closure is possible, the mid-thigh scar may be considered nonaesthetic.
- Rare inconsistency of the perforator anatomy.

16.2.3 Flap Components

The ALT flap can be harvested as a cutaneous, fasciocutaneous, or musculocutaneous flap. It can also be harvested as a chimeric flap to include other tissues such as the rectus femoris, tensor fascia lata, or vastus lateralis muscles or even femoral bone, where the ALT flap itself is supplied by a separate perforator or even independent source vessel. The missing tissues at the recipient site will dictate the necessary size, thickness, and components of the ALT flap.

16.2.4 Anatomic Consideration

Vascular Anatomy

The blood supply of the ALT flap is primarily derived from the descending branch of the lateral circumflex femoral artery (LCFA). Clinical and anatomic studies have demonstrated that about 86% of the perforators follow a musculocutaneous course, while 14% follow a septocutaneous course.

Following its origin from the lateral aspect of the deep femoral artery, the LCFA courses posterior to the sartorius and rectus femoris muscles and divides into the ascending, transverse, and descending branches. The transverse branch passes laterally to pierce the vastus lateralis muscle, while the descending branch passes down in the septum between the rectus femoris and vastus lateralis muscles, giving off numerous muscular branches before anastomosing with the lateral superior genicular artery about the knee joint.

The flap pedicle length can be up to 10 to 13 cm with an arterial diameter of 2.0 to 2.5 mm at its origin, and a pair of accompanying veins of diameter from 1.8 to 3.0 mm.

Sensory Innervation

The skin of the ALT is supplied by branches of the lateral cutaneous nerve of the thigh and branches of the anterior cutaneous nerve of the thigh. The predominant nerve supplying the ALT skin territory is the anterior division of the lateral cutaneous nerve of the thigh. The lateral cutaneous nerve of the thigh (L2–L3) passes about 1 cm medial to the anterosuperior iliac spine (ASIS) and behind the inguinal ligament. It passes anterior to the sartorius muscle into the thigh. There its larger anterior branch then pierces the fascial lata about 10 cm below the ASIS to supply the skin of the ALT, while the posterior branch pierces the fascia higher to supply the skin of the lateral thigh.

Motor Innervation

The vastus lateralis muscle is supplied by a motor branch from the posterior division of the femoral nerve. This branch runs with the descending branch of the LCFA and can be included with the flap for coaptation with a motor branch at the recipient site when the vastus lateralis muscle is used for functional muscle transfer.

16.2.5 Anatomic Variations

The pattern and distribution of the vessels supplying the ALT cutaneous territory is variable and failure to understand these anatomic variations can lead to flap vascular compromise. The descending branch of the LCFA commonly arises from the LCFA but can originate from the deep femoral or common femoral arteries. A large-scale systematic review revealed that the majority of perforators to the ALT skin originate from the descending branch of the LCFA in 75 to 100% of cases. Origin from the transverse, ascending, and oblique branches has also been described with wide range of reported frequency. The same study revealed that septocutaneous perforators were present in about 20% of cases and ALT perforators were absent about 2% of the time.[9]

16.2.6 Patient Positioning

The flap is usually harvested with the patient in a supine position, but can also be harvested with the patient in a semilateral or true lateral position. The lower extremity is circumferentially prepped. Harvesting the flap from the contralateral thigh allows for a two-team approach.

16.2.7 Flap Design

Routinely examine the patient in the preoperative area or in the operating room while awake to determine the location of the septum between the rectus femoris and vastus lateralis muscles. With a straight leg raise test, this septum may be palpated or even potentially visualized in patients with a thin body habitus. Otherwise, a line joining the ASIS and the superolateral border of the patella is marked and will represent the location of the septum, and potential location of septocutaneous perforators. Note that the septum is neither a straight line nor a fixed point, and its location could shift medially or laterally depending on the patient position on the table or if the lower extremity has undergone medial or lateral rotation. All markings will be more reliable with the patient supine and the lower extremity kept in neutral rotation.

A handheld audible Doppler is commonly used next to identify perforator signals, which are concentrated within a 3-cm-diameter circle centered over the midpoint of the septal line. The perforators themselves are most frequently found within the inferolateral quadrant of this circle. Musculocutaneous perforators, of course, will pierce the vastus lateralis muscle posterior to this line. When designing the chosen skin island, it is advisable to encompass more than one perforator, and to preferably shift the flap boundaries slightly posterior to the line joining the ASIS and superolateral patella so as to be able to capture both septocutaneous and musculocutaneous perforators, if present.

In patients with thicker thighs, identification of perforators with the audible Doppler examination can be misleading. Yu's group proposed a very reliable, simple, and accurate model (ABC model) to guide perforator location.[10] That is, there are usually one to three perforators in the ALT flap territory in predictable locations (A, B, or C). In an average person, perforator B is located near the midpoint, whereas perforators A and C are approximately 5 cm proximal or distal to perforator B. All three perforators are located approximately 1.4 cm lateral to the line joining the ASIS and superolateral patella, but again this can be highly variable.

A longitudinally oriented skin island is designed to incorporate the marked perforators. A skin island up to 35-cm long and 25-cm wide can be harvested on a single dominant perforator, but inclusion of more than one perforator is advisable. This will provide the surgeon the option of using more than one skin island, each based on a separate perforator, or just as a safety factor to prevent inadvertent flap twisting or devascularization.

Variations of the skin island design can place the perforator at centric or eccentric locations. Designing the skin island distally places the chosen perforator at an eccentric position proximally, and thereby increases the effective pedicle length when the flap is based on a proximal pedicle. When using the ALT as a distal-based pedicled flap for coverage of soft-tissue defects about the knee, the perfusion of the flap will be retrograde through communications with the superior lateral genicular system. In these circumstances, designing the skin island proximally on the ALT increases the effective distal pedicle length and enhances the arc of rotation and reach.

16.2.8 Flap Harvest

Suprafascial Approach

The medial flap boundary incision is made first and dissection is carried down to the level of the deep fascia (▸ Fig. 16.3 and ▸ Video 16.1). If additional soft-tissue bulk is necessary, the

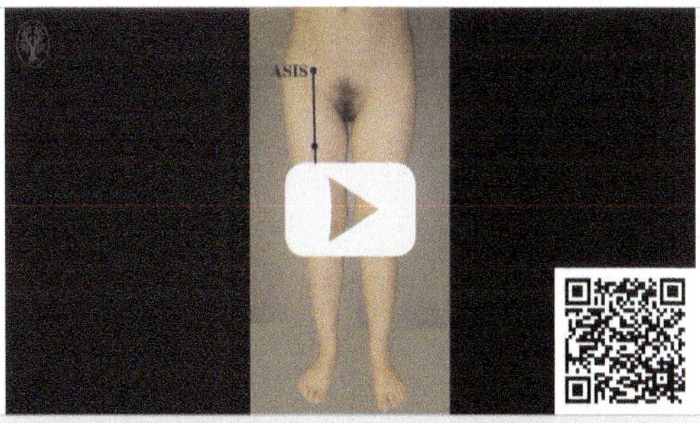

Video 16.1 ALT Flap for Lower Extremity Reconstruction. https://www.thieme.de/de/q.htm?p=opn/cs/20/7/12265275-1a6625fc

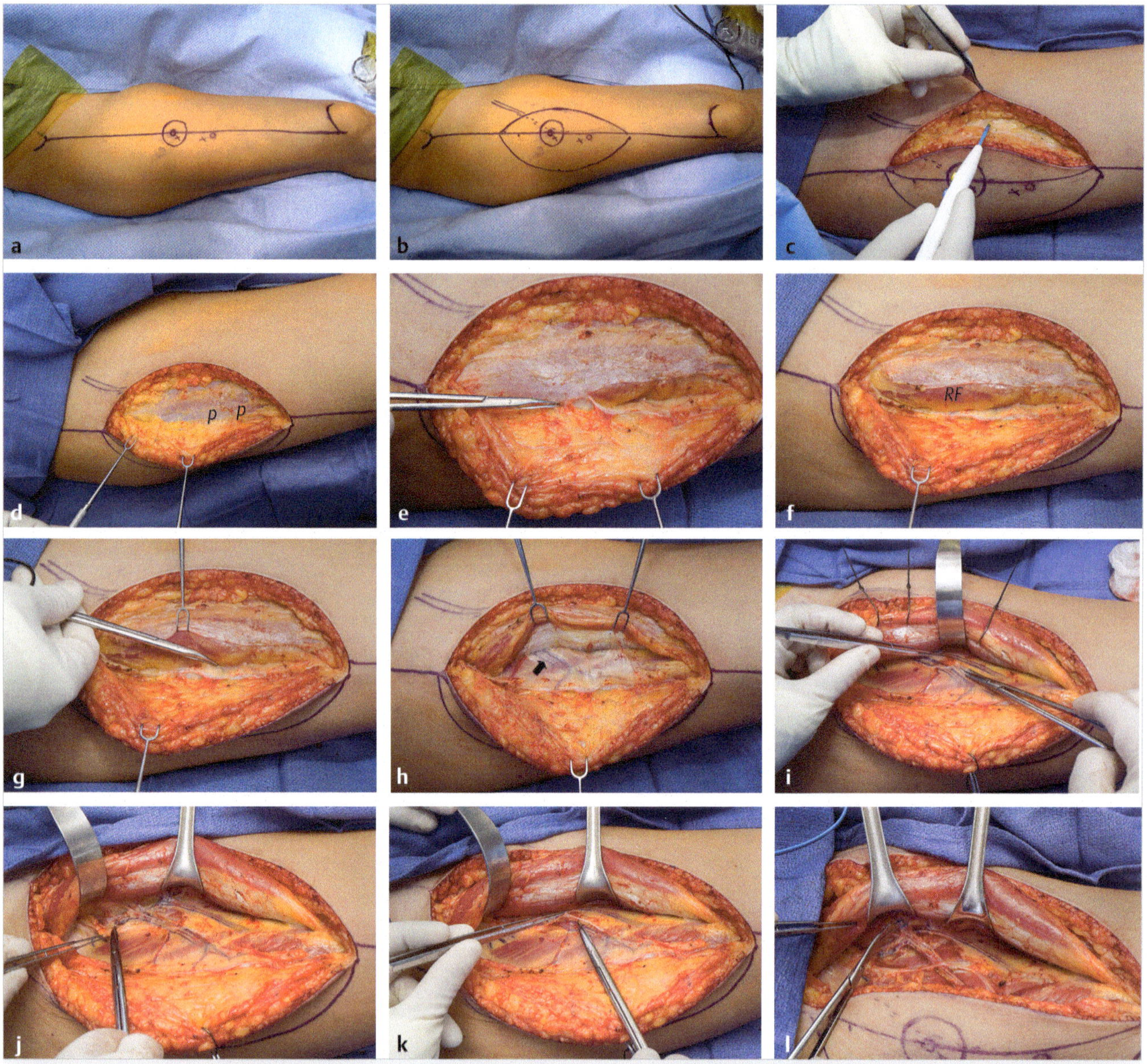

Fig. 16.3 Suprafascial anterolateral thigh (ALT) flap harvest. **(a)** A line is drawn from the anterosuperior iliac spine (ASIS) to the superolateral border of the patella. This represents the location of the septum between the vastus lateralis and rectus femoris muscles. At the midpoint of this line, a circle of 3-cm. diameter is drawn. Usually in the inferolateral quadrant of this circle a perforator can be found, here marked "x." In addition, in this case a second perforator "x" was identified 5 cm more inferiorly. **(b)** Design of the skin island is best made to include at least two major perforators, and if placed eccentric to the perforators distally, it ensures not only a longer pedicle length, but also often a thinner flap at least in its distal portion. **(c)** The medial flap border incision is made first, and dissection carried down to the level of the deep fascia. Additional subcutaneous fat/fascia can be obtained while doing this by beveling the dissection in a more medial direction. **(d)** Next, dissection is performed in a medial to lateral direction directly above the deep fascia until the perforators (*p*) are visualized. **(e)** The fascia medial to the perforators is sharply incised and the septum between the rectus femoris and vastus lateralis muscles is visualized. **(f)** The remainder of the fascia is opened to completely expose the septum and the lateral border of the rectus femoris (RF) muscle. 8**(g)** One of the perforators (tip scissors) is seen emanating along the septum before entering the flap. **(h)** The rectus femoris muscle is retracted medially to expose the descending branch of the lateral circumflex femoral vessel (LCFV) pedicle (*arrow*) to the perforators. **(i)** Retrograde dissection of the pedicle commences from distal to proximal toward the descending branch of the LCFV proper. **(j)** Proximal pedicle dissection continues until the required length is obtained. **(k)** The motor branch to the vastus lateralis muscle (forceps) must be carefully separated from the vascular pedicle and preserved. **(l)** Here the vascular branch to the rectus femoris muscle has been clipped and is about to be divided, as will be any other distal branches if additional pedicle length is needed.

(*Continued*)

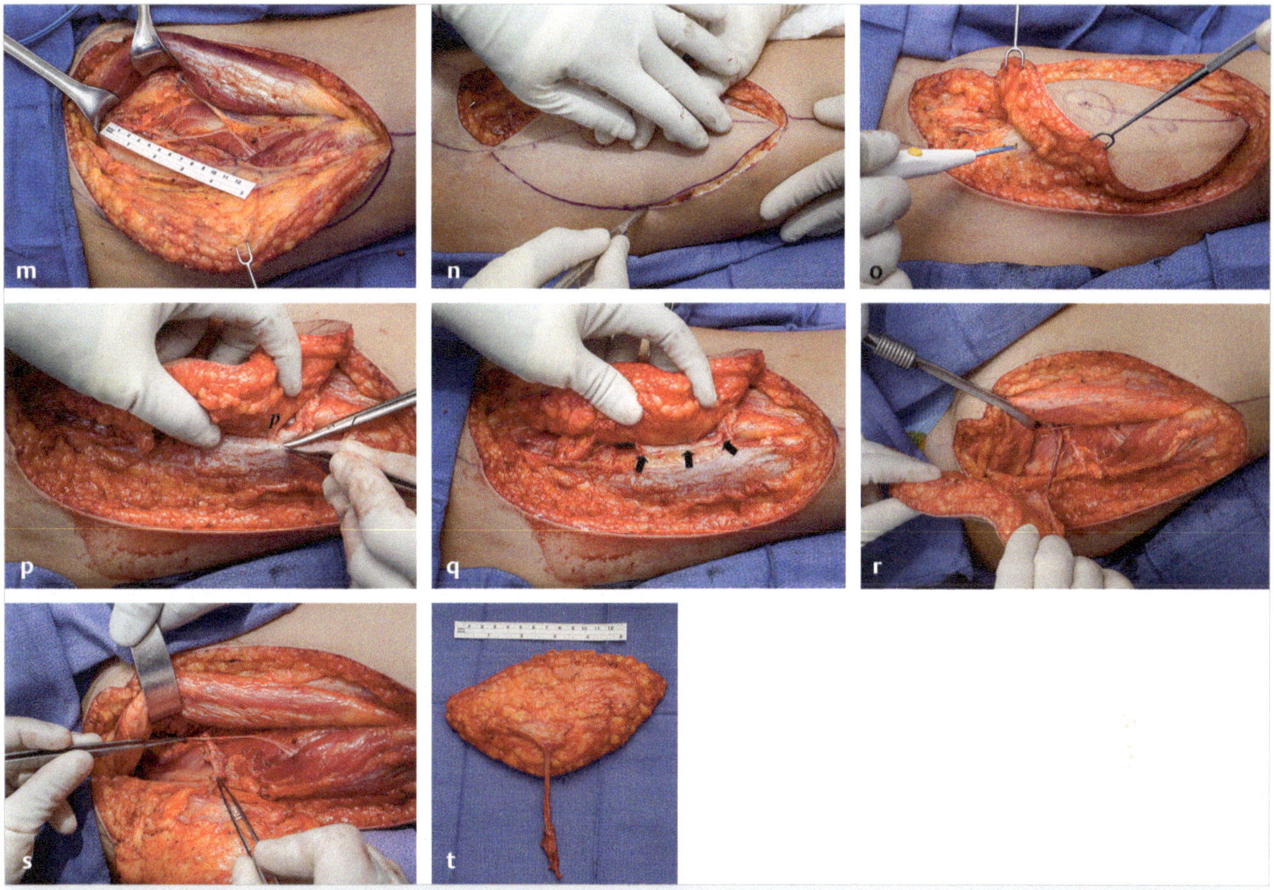

Fig. 16.3 (*Continued*) **(m)** By following these steps, a 13-cm-long pedicle has been obtained. **(n)** Now the lateral flap border incision can be made. **(o)** Dissection will proceed from lateral to medial in the suprafascial plane. **(p)** This dissection stops when the previously selected perforators (*p*) are identified on their lateral side. The fascia is incised just lateral to them, preserving a small cuff of fascia with the flap. **(q)** Final narrow fascial cuff (*arrows*) seen around and protecting the two perforators as their intramuscular dissection is completed back to the source pedicle. **(r)** All dissection has been completed, making this an island flap connected to the thigh only by the source pedicle. **(s)** For a free flap, the pedicle is divided as far proximally as required, then as seen here passed underneath the motor nerve while being removed from the thigh. **(t)** The ALT free flap ready for transfer to the recipient site.

dissection could be beveled away from the flap to include more subcutaneous fat. The flap is then raised from medial to lateral in a suprafascial plane directly above the fascia lata, using cautery or tenotomy scissor until a skin perforator is identified piercing the fascia. Once perforators of adequate caliber are identified, the fascia is incised and opened medial to the perforators, and the remainder of the septum is opened to expose the descending branch of the LCFA. Dissection is then continued proximally toward the latter's origin itself from the LCFA. While doing this, multiple motor branches will need to be carefully dissected away from the vascular pedicle and protected to avoid iatrogenic denervation of the thigh musculature, especially when the flap is used as a perforator flap without including part of the vastus lateralis muscle.

The extent of proximal pedicle dissection will be determined by the length and caliber of vessels required. When the ALT is used for locoregional reconstruction, a long pedicle is frequently needed to maximize reach. In these circumstances, the branch to the rectus femoris muscle can be safely divided to obtain an additional effective pedicle length.[11,12] When the rectus femoris branch is divided, care should be taken to avoid extensive dissection around the rectus femoris muscle distally so the blood supply from minor distal pedicles can be maintained. The rectus femoris branch can also be divided if additional pedicle length is needed when using the ALT for free tissue transfer.

The lateral boundary incision is then made, and suprafascial dissection is continued from lateral to medial till the same perforators identified earlier are visualized. If the course of the perforator(s) is purely septocutaneous, they can easily be dissected down to the source vessel. If the perforators follow an intramuscular course, the usual tedious intramuscular dissection is performed with all muscular branches carefully ligated (muscle branches usually arise from the lateral and posterior surfaces of the perforators). A small cuff of fascia left around the perforator helps prevent pedicle twisting or avulsion, while also being something that can be held safely and maneuvered with forceps. Intramuscular dissection is usually carried out in a retrograde fashion back to the source vessel, but antegrade dissection is also possible.

When the flap is used as a sensate flap, the lateral cutaneous nerve of the thigh is included with the flap. The nerve is identified proximally below the fascial lata and additional length can be obtained by extending the dissection proximally toward the ASIS.

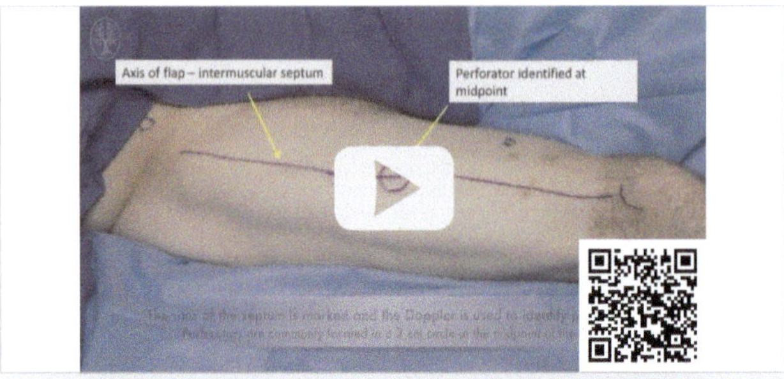

Video 16.2 Subfascial Harvest of the ALT Free Flap. https://www.thieme.de/de/q.htm?p=opn/cs/20/7/12265276-d0a33d54

Suprafascial dissection is preferred when a thin flap is required. This allows also for preservation of sensory nerves in the thigh that traverse over the fascia. In addition, preserving the fascia may minimize donor site morbidity such as by preventing muscle herniation.

Subfascial Approach

The medial flap boundary incision is made first and dissection is carried down to the level of the deep fascia (See ▶ Video 16.2). When bulk or deeper fascia is needed, dissection is beveled away from the flap to incorporate more subcutaneous fat or an extension of the fascia. The fascia is sharply incised directly exposing the underlying rectus femoris muscle. Subfascial dissection is then carried from medial to lateral, until the septum between the rectus femoris and vastus lateralis muscles is identified. If septocutaneous perforators are identified, the remainder of the dissection is straightforward. If no septocutaneous perforators are present (as in the majority of cases), careful dissection is then continued over the vastus lateralis muscle to identify musculocutaneous perforators. Once perforators of adequate caliber are identified, intramuscular perforator dissection back to the descending branch, further pedicle dissection, and nerve preservation continues in a fashion similar to the suprafascial approach. After completion of perforator and pedicle dissection, the lateral boundary incision is made, and subfascial dissection is carried from lateral to medial, back to the first deep fascial incision.

16.2.9 Pitfalls, Flap Modification, and Tips to Optimize Outcomes

Perforator Dissection and Flap Handing

Adequate hemostasis is of paramount importance as in all perforator flap surgery to allow unimpeded visualization of the perforator at all times. All side branches must be carefully clipped, then divided, or gently cauterized with bipolar cautery. Care should be taken to avoid placing excessive traction on the perforators, as an iatrogenic traction injury to the perforators can occur even with slight traction.

Absent or Inadequate Lateral Thigh Skin Perforators

The surgeon should be prepared for the possibility of absent or inadequate caliber lateral thigh skin perforators, as this has been reported to occur in about 2 to 4.3% of cases.[9,13,14,15,16,17,18] The presence of adequate skin perforators should be confirmed first before making the lateral incision. If the vessels supplying the skin island are too small to perform safe intramuscular dissection, the flap can be raised as a musculocutaneous flap to include the vastus lateralis muscle with the skin island.

In the rare situation that a perforator is absent or injured, the surgeon has the following options:

- Perform audible Doppler mapping of the medial thigh skin. Dissection is then carried in a medial direction to identify those skin perforators. This is based on the knowledge that there is an inverse relationship between the number and caliber of vessels in the lateral and medial thigh regions. Almost always a perforator can be found in the medial thigh, and a flap harvested through the same medial incision without creating another donor site defect.[13,19]
- A freestyle approach is followed to look for vessels supplying the region of the thigh.[15]
- The lateral circumflex femoral vessel is exposed and the vessel branch supplying the tensor facial lata muscle is identified. A tensor fascia lata perforator flap is then harvested based on this vessel.
- Closure of the initial donor site and selection of an alternative flap.

Use of the Anterolateral Thigh as a Pedicled Flap

The ALT flap can be used as a pedicled or island flap for groin, medial thigh, perineum, trochanter, posterior thigh, contralateral inguinal, and knee coverage (see Chapter 15A: The Island Perforator Flap). Multiple techniques have been described to maximize reach when used as a locoregional flap, such as passage through a subcutaneous tunnel, placement below the rectus femoris muscle, and transmuscular transfer to the posterior thigh.[11] The vascular branch to the rectus femoris muscle can be safely divided to maximize effective pedicle length.[12]

When the ALT flap is used for knee coverage, it must be based distally on retrograde blood flow through the communication between the superior lateral genicular system and the descending branch of the LCFA or, less commonly, the profunda femoris artery. The pivot point is usually 3 to 10 cm above the patella. A higher incidence of venous congestion has been reported when the flap is based distally. To mitigate against this unfavorable outcome, the pedicle should routinely be dissected proximally to obtain extra length so that supercharging the flap will be facilitated if venous congestion occurs.[20]

The adequacy of distal retrograde blood inflow must also be confirmed before dividing the proximal pedicle. A vascular clamp applied temporarily to occlude the proximal pedicle will allow assessment of flap perfusion via the retrograde flow. If inadequate, the ALT flap can still be transferred as a free flap.

Use as a Flow-Through Flap

The ALT flap can be used as a flow-through flap in various situations. For example, when a vascular segment in the lower extremity is missing due to trauma or surgical resection, the ALT pedicle can be used to bridge the missing vascular gap. In addition, the distal end of the pedicle can be used to provide

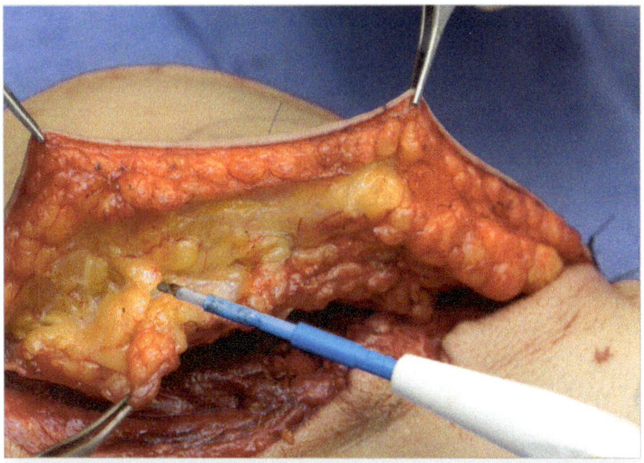

Fig. 16.4 Primary anterolateral thigh (ALT) flap thinning. Note the difference in shape and size of fat lobules between the superficial and deep subcutaneous layers. The larger deep layer fat lobules are being removed along the thin, white fascial layer that is retained, which serves to separate them from the superficial layer.

inflow/outflow to another free flap, serving as the recipient site for the latter.

Flap Thinning

When the ALT flap is used for pretibial, dorsum of the foot, ankle, or heel coverage, primary thinning of the flap can be considered especially in patients with excess subcutaneous fat. Thin flaps may have the ability to regain sensation quicker even when transferred as insensate flaps.

Flap thinning is performed while the flap is still being perfused before division of the pedicle to enable continuous monitoring of flap perfusion as well as obtaining adequate hemostasis. Preservation of a 2- to 3-cm soft-tissue cuff around the pedicle entrance into the flap is advised to maintain perfusion. To best accomplish this, the plane between the superficial and deep fat layers is first identified (▶ Fig. 16.4). The deep fat layer has larger fat lobules, while the superficial layer has smaller and more round lobules, the two usually separated by a thin fascial layer. Flap thinning requires removing the deep fat layer lobules until the superficial layer is reached. Further thinning can actually be performed up to the level of the subdermal plexus; however, flap survival after transfer may be more likely affected by how the flap is inset. Caution must then be observed if tension is excessive, or if a complex defect requires folding of the flap, as viability will be less reliable. Secondary flap thinning is a much easier and safer procedure, and should be a consideration until experience with primary flap thinning is reasonable.

Harvest as an Adipofascial Flap

This is particularly helpful when a thin flap is required (such as coverage of exposed tendons on the foot dorsum) in patients with excess subcutaneous fat. Raising an adipofascial flap follows the same technique as for subfascial ALT flap harvest. The dissection should be performed with a subfascial approach to preserve the vascular network that runs on the surface of the fascia. A minimum of 3 mm of fat should be preserved over the fascia to avoid damage to this fine vascular network.[21]

Adding Bulk to the Flap

Flap bulk can be increased by inclusion of the vastus lateralis, rectus femoris, or tensor fascia lata muscles, or by including more subcutaneous fat as by beveling away from the incisions of the flap boundaries themselves as needed.

Use for Tendon Reconstruction

The fascia lata component of the ALT flap has been described for primary tendon reconstruction.[2] This is best done by keeping the more lateral and thicker fascia lata with the cutaneous paddle as a composite flap, then rolling it up as a tube to serve much like a vascularized tendon graft.

16.2.10 Donor Site Management

Primary closure of the donor site is preferable, but obtaining a flap of adequate size always takes precedence. A skin island with width exceeding 8 to 9 cm at the mid-thigh level may preclude direct donor site closure, which otherwise could result in a thigh compartment syndrome. The donor site may still then be closed primarily at the superior and inferior aspects, but the middle portion may require split-thickness skin grafting. Using a dermal regeneration template prior to skin grafting or tissue stretching devices will allow time for swelling to subside, which could permit even further or complete closure of the middle portion of the donor site. This may then avoid the risk of skin graft failure, particularly common after a suprafascial flap harvest, and definitely provide a better aesthetic outcome.

Alternatively, synchronous local advancement flaps based on other perforators (e.g., keystone or V-Y flaps) may facilitate complete primary donor site closure, but at the price of additional scarring of the thigh. Preoperative and postoperative thigh tissue expansion has also been described to avoid the need for a skin graft.[22,23]

Another option, if a wider skin island is needed, is to select a long but narrow longitudinal design. This will require the preoperative identification of at least two major perforators within that design based on that same source vessel, so that the skin paddle can be split into two islands, each based on an individual perforator. The skin islands can then be inset side by side at the recipient site using the "kiss" principle to provide the necessary coverage width, while still allowing primary closure of the donor site.[24]

16.2.11 Case Examples

Case 1: Locoregional ALT flap

A 19-year-old woman had a right groin mass excised that proved to be a synovial sarcoma (▶ Fig. 16.5). Following neoadjuvant radiation, radical sarcoma excision resulted in a right groin defect requiring soft-tissue coverage. This was achieved by transposition of an ipsilateral island ALT flap.

Case 2: ALT Free Tissue Transfer

Following a motorcycle accident, this young man sustained a comminuted right tibia/fibula fracture with extensive soft-tissue degloving. Single vessel runoff remained, making this a Gustilo grade IIIC tibial fracture. Following plate and intramedullary rod

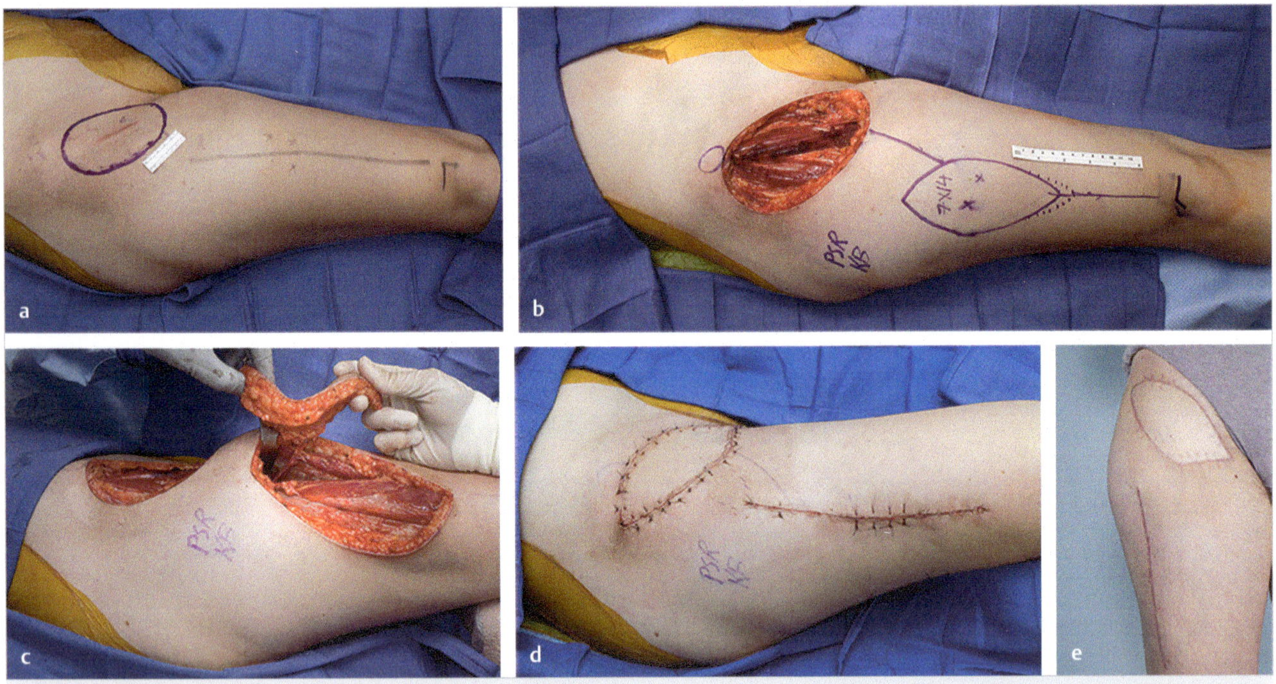

Fig. 16.5 Locoregional anterolateral thigh (ALT) flap transfer. **(a)** Planned radical excision of right groin synovial sarcoma, with preoperative location (x) of ALT perforators. **(b)** Resultant soft-tissue defect in irradiated wound. An ipsilateral ALT flap was designed about the previously marked perforators (x). **(c)** Following a suprafascial dissection, an island ALT flap was raised based on a single perforator. The retractor permitted visualization for enough pedicle lengthening that allowed sufficient reach to the defect and also creation of a subcutaneous tunnel through which the flap would be passed. **(d)** Island ALT flap inset with simultaneous primary donor site closure. **(e)** Excellent contour at 4-month follow-up. Vertical linear scar typical of mid-thigh donor site residue.

fixation, the large defect was covered elsewhere with a latissimus dorsi free muscle flap that was unsuccessful. As a backup option for this now chronic wound, a contralateral ALT free flap was planned (▶ Fig. 16.6), not only to obtain another huge soft-tissue flap that was needed, but also to have a long pedicle with large caliber vessels that would reach the popliteal vessels outside the zone of injury and permit facile end-to-side microanastomoses. That proved to be successful, allowing limb salvage.

16.2.12 Postoperative Care Protocols

Extreme vigilance and attention to details are required to identify early flap compromise. Studies have shown that the most important factor in salvage of the failing free flap is early identification of any vascular compromise. Even pedicled flaps should undergo serial clinical examination by the surgical/nursing team (every 2–4 hours) starting in the recovery area for the first 24 hours. After the first 24 hours, the frequency of clinical examination varies based on individual cases.

Free flap monitoring typically follows a specified protocol of hourly clinical and, if nothing else is available, audible Doppler examination by a nursing staff specifically trained to care for free flap patients. Familiarity and experience of the nursing staff with the management of free flap patients has enabled care for this subset of patients on a general plastic surgery hospital floor. Admission to an intensive care unit is then rarely needed following lower extremity reconstructions with free flaps unless the general health of the patient and associated medical comorbidities require a higher level of care. Patients are maintained on strict bed rest for 5 days, followed by gradual resumption of lower extremity dangling.

16.2.13 Conclusion

The ALT perforator flap is a versatile flap often used in lower extremity reconstruction. The relatively constant anatomy, adequate pedicle length and caliber of vessels, ability to modify flap components based on the recipient site needs, minimal donor site morbidity, and excellent reported outcomes are among the reasons that have led to widespread adoption and utilization as both a pedicled and as a free flap, for challenges that so commonly present in the lower extremity.

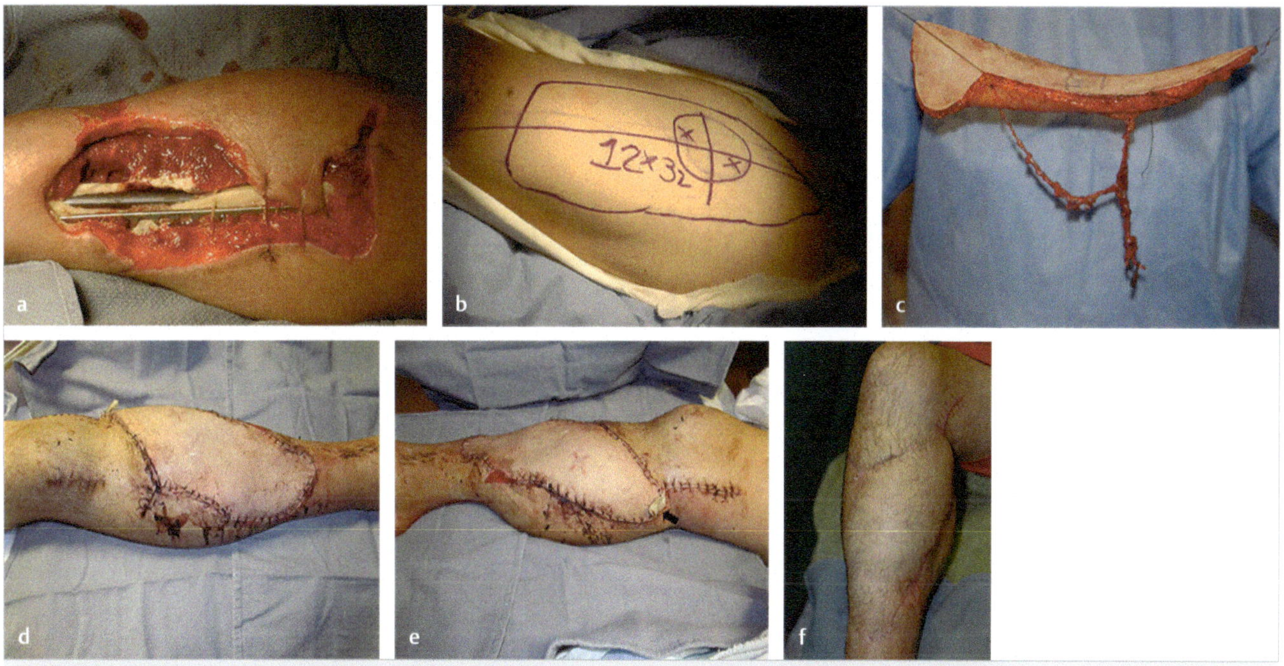

Fig. 16.6 Anterolateral thigh (ALT) free flap. (a) Motorcycle accident with chronic open right tibia fracture after failed latissimus dorsi free muscle flap done elsewhere. (b) Huge contralateral ALT free flap designed about two perforators (x) identified using audible Doppler. (c) ALT free flap after subfascial harvest, supplied by two perforators connected to the descending branch of lateral circumflex femoral vessel (LCFV) pedicle. (d) Anterior view of inset ALT free flap and (e) medial view demonstrating the near circumferential extent of coverage following wound preparation. In addition, a corner of the flap was inset into the incision needed to expose the popliteal vessels that were used as the new recipient site (arrow), so as to minimize the risk of compression of its long pedicle that was needed to reach the latter. (f) Early successful coverage of this extensive right leg defect.

References

[1] Song YG, Chen GZ, Song YL. The free thigh flap: a new free flap concept based on the septocutaneous artery. Br J Plast Surg. 1984; 37(2):149–159

[2] Dayan JH, Lin CH, Wei FC. The versatility of the anterolateral thigh flap in lower extremity reconstruction. Handchir Mikrochir Plast Chir. 2009; 41(4): 193–202

[3] Gedebou TM, Wei FC, Lin CH. Clinical experience of 1284 free anterolateral thigh flaps. Handchir Mikrochir Plast Chir. 2002; 34(4):239–244

[4] Hong JP, Kim EK. Sole reconstruction using anterolateral thigh perforator free flaps. Plast Reconstr Surg. 2007; 119(1):186–193

[5] Hong JP, Shin HW, Kim JJ, Wei FC, Chung YK. The use of anterolateral thigh perforator flaps in chronic osteomyelitis of the lower extremity. Plast Reconstr Surg. 2005; 115(1):142–147

[6] Kuo YR, Jeng SF, Kuo MH, et al. Free anterolateral thigh flap for extremity reconstruction: clinical experience and functional assessment of donor site. Plast Reconstr Surg. 2001; 107(7):1766–1771

[7] Nosrati N, Chao AH, Chang DW, Yu P. Lower extremity reconstruction with the anterolateral thigh flap. J Reconstr Microsurg. 2012; 28(4):227–234

[8] Hallock GG. The proximal pedicled anterolateral thigh flap for lower limb coverage. Ann Plast Surg. 2005; 55(5):466–469

[9] Lakhiani C, Lee MR, Saint-Cyr M. Vascular anatomy of the anterolateral thigh flap: a systematic review. Plast Reconstr Surg. 2012; 130(6):1254–1268

[10] Lin SJ, Rabie A, Yu P. Designing the anterolateral thigh flap without preoperative Doppler or imaging. J Reconstr Microsurg. 2010; 26(1):67–72

[11] Vijayasekaran A, Gibreel W, Carlsen BT, et al. Maximizing the utility of the pedicled anterolateral thigh flap for locoregional reconstruction: technical pearls and pitfalls. Clin Plast Surg. 2017; 44(2):371–384

[12] Wong CH, Ong YS, Wei FC. Revisiting vascular supply of the rectus femoris and its relevance in the harvest of the anterolateral thigh flap. Ann Plast Surg. 2013; 71(5):586–590

[13] Yu P. Inverse relationship of the anterolateral and anteromedial thigh flap perforator anatomy. J Reconstr Microsurg. 2014; 30(7):463–468

[14] Yu P, Selber J, Liu J. Reciprocal dominance of the anterolateral and anteromedial thigh flap perforator anatomy. Ann Plast Surg. 2013; 70(6):714–716

[15] Chang CC, Shen JH, Chan KK, Wei FC. Selection of ideal perforators and the use of a free-style free flap during dissection of an anterolateral thigh flap for reconstruction in the head and neck. Br J Oral Maxillofac Surg. 2016; 54(7): 830–832

[16] Hong JP, Kim EK, Kim H, Shin HW, Hwang CH, Lee MY. Alternative regional flaps when anterolateral thigh flap perforator is not feasible. J Hand Microsurg. 2010; 2(2):51–57

[17] Lin YT, Lin CH, Wei FC. More degrees of freedom by using chimeric concept in the applications of anterolateral thigh flap. J Plast Reconstr Aesthet Surg. 2006; 59(6):622–627

[18] Lu JC, Zelken J, Hsu CC, et al. Algorithmic approach to anterolateral thigh flaps lacking suitable perforators in lower extremity reconstruction. Plast Reconstr Surg. 2015; 135(5):1476–1485

[19] Wong CH, Wei FC, Fu B, Chen YA, Lin JY. Alternative vascular pedicle of the anterolateral thigh flap: the oblique branch of the lateral circumflex femoral artery. Plast Reconstr Surg. 2009; 123(2):571–577

[20] Lin CH, Zelken J, Hsu CC, Lin CH, Wei FC. The distally based, venous supercharged anterolateral thigh flap. Microsurgery. 2016; 36(1):20–28

[21] Hsieh CH, Yang CC, Kuo YR, Tsai HH, Jeng SF. Free anterolateral thigh adipofascial perforator flap. Plast Reconstr Surg. 2003; 112(4):976–982

[22] Hallock GG. The preexpanded anterolateral thigh free flap. Ann Plast Surg. 2004; 53(2):170–173

[23] Hallock GG. Tissue expansion techniques to minimize morbidity of the anterolateral thigh perforator flap donor site. J Reconstr Microsurg. 2013; 29(9): 565–570

[24] Tsai FC, Yang JY, Mardini S, Chuang SS, Wei FC. Free split-cutaneous perforator flaps procured using a three-dimensional harvest technique for the reconstruction of postburn contracture defects. Plast Reconstr Surg. 2004; 113 (1):185–193, discussion 194–195

16.3 Chapter 16B: The Gracilis Muscle Free Flap

Geoffrey G. Hallock

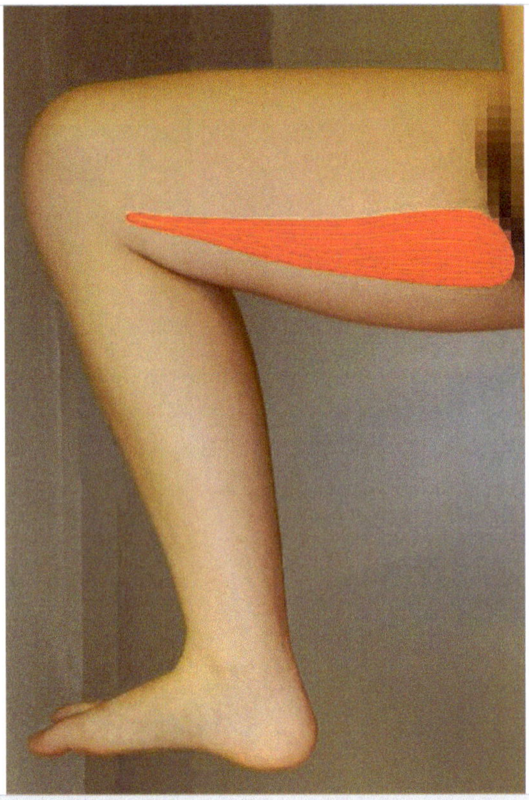

Fig. 16.7 The gracilis muscle.

16.3.1 Introduction to the Gracilis Muscle Free Flap

The advent of the realization of the clinical value of microvascular tissue transfers soon followed McLean and Buncke's[1] use of the omentum to cover a scalp defect, and Daniel and Taylor's[2] first successful composite tissue transfer. But imperfections of the latter's groin flap such as anatomical inconsistencies rapidly led to the investigation for more pragmatic donor sites. The rebirth of muscle flaps around the same time frame as an important entity can be traced to Orticochea,[3] who raised large peninsular flaps from the thigh safely without delay maneuvers, with reliability ensured by inclusion of the underlying gracilis muscle. However, without microsurgical capabilities, this had to be a multistaged regional flap for coverage of an exposed ankle bone.[3] Quickly thereafter, the gracilis muscle (▶ Fig. 16.7) alone proved to be a reliable free flap donor site when Harii et al[4] showed its utility for functional restoration of facial paralysis. Musculocutaneous free flap versions that followed were not always completely viable if the skin paddle had a vertical axis, but Yousif et al[5] in cadaver studies proved this was because the "true" perforasome of the perforators from the dominant pedicle of the gracilis muscle had a transverse orientation in the upper thigh.

The gracilis muscle indeed deserves the appellation as a "workhorse flap," as it has been found to solve all conceivable problems within the "skin and its contents," the realm of the "true" reconstructive surgeon. Often preferable about the upper portion of the lower extremity as a local flap (see Chapter 14B: The Gracilis Local Muscle Flap), the gracilis muscle is extremely versatile also as a free flap. As a musculocutaneous version, the transverse myocutaneous gracilis (TMG)[6] or transverse upper gracilis (TUG)[5,7,8] free flap in the appropriate candidate is a secondary option for breast reconstruction. The gracilis muscle can be a dynamic transfer apropos for facial reanimation[4,8,9] or restoration of a myriad of upper extremity functions.[10] Although its small cross-sectional area limits potential power, ankle dorsiflexion has been achieved.[11] More conventional roles in the lower extremity have been dictated when malleable fill is essential or coverage of small to moderate-sized defects needed.[12] In the ubiquitous obese patient, this may be the best available thin flap that will not interfere with shoe wear and ambulation.

The gracilis muscle functions as a thigh adductor, knee and hip flexor, and medial hip rotator,[8] but only a minimal deficit is noted if absent, so it is considered expendable.[13] Potential donor site morbidity is minimal, and the resultant scarring on the medial thigh usually can be well hidden.[13,14,15] It should be reiterated that all these attributes and unlimited roles demand that a complete knowledge of this donor site be mastered by all who use it!

16.3.2 Attributes and Detriments

Attributes

- Versatile "workhorse flap."
- Expendable.
- Consistent anatomy.
- Expeditious harvest.
- Harvest possible in supine, lithotomy, or prone positions.
- Coverage of small and medium-sized defects.
- Thin contour.
- Autologous tendon reconstruction.
- Dynamic restoration.
- Virtually nonexistent donor site morbidity.
- Hidden donor site scar.
- Reliable to approach even in the morbidly obese.

Detriments

- Often found far more posterior in the medial thigh than believed possible.
- Not suited for large defects.
- Hyperesthesia of the medial distal thigh if the cutaneous branch of the obturator nerve is injured.
- Inconsistent reliability of vertical cutaneous paddle if composite flap.
- Significant arterial orifice atherosclerosis may make this unusable in end-stage peripheral vascular disease patient.

16.3.3 Anatomical Considerations

The gracilis muscle is found in the more posterior aspect of the medial thigh. It is the most superficial of the muscles of the adductor compartment, extending longitudinally for some

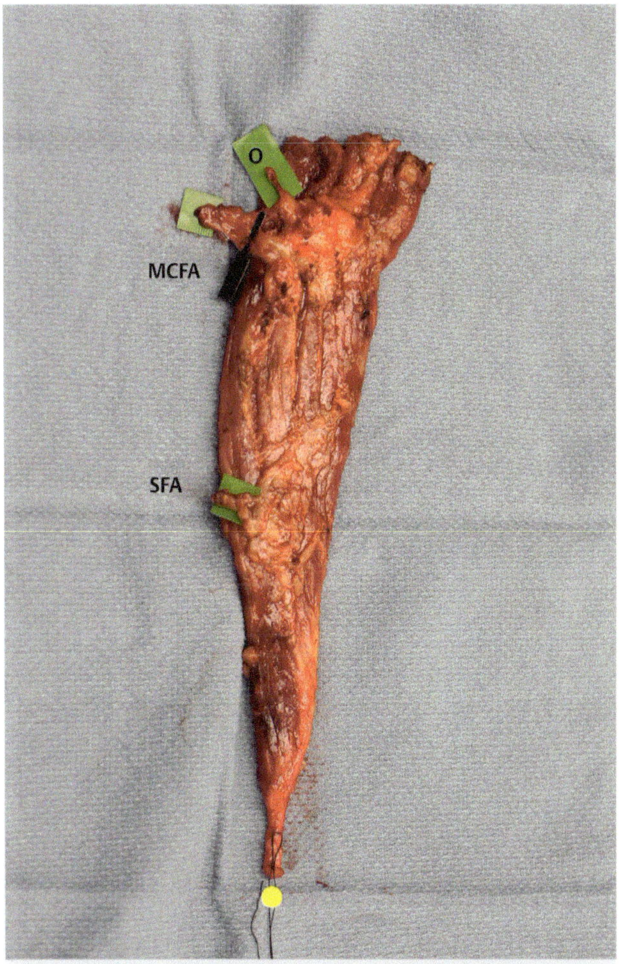

Fig. 16.8 The gracilis muscle has a triangular shape extending from a wide base at its origin until narrowing around its tendon distally (*yellow dot*). Here the medial circumflex femoral artery (MCFA) was the source of the dominant vascular pedicle, entering on the undersurface of the anterior border of the muscle. The anterior branch of the obturator nerve (O) entered obliquely just superior to the vascular hilum. A single distal secondary or minor pedicle originated from the superficial femoral artery (SFA).

30 cm from its aponeurotic origin at the symphysis pubis and pubic arch to where its tendon inserts as part of the pes anserinus on the medial tibial condyle, where found inferior to the tendon of sartorius and above that of semitendinosus.[7,8] The width of the muscle may be up to about 7 cm at the level of the major vascular hilum,[16] then tapers distally toward its long tendon, thereby overall forming a somewhat triangular shape (▶ Fig. 16.8).

The dominant vascular supply most commonly is considered to be the medial circumflex femoral artery (MCFA),[7] although others state it may be the adductor branch or even the first profunda perforator[16,17]; however, regardless of what it is, it always ultimately arises from the profunda femoris.[16,18] The MCFA then courses medially between the adductor longus and magnus muscles before entering the anterolateral undersurface of the gracilis at a point about 10 cm (range: 5–14 cm[16]) inferior to the pubic tubercle.[5] The artery caliber varies from 1.5 to 3 mm,[8] and venae comitantes that are usually larger are always present. The potential pedicle length is about 7 cm.[8] As with most muscles, minor pedicles may be found near the origin and insertion. For example, Tremp et al[19] describe a more proximal pedicle that was a deep branch of the MCFA. Cavadas et al[17] found a mean of 2.2 distal secondary pedicles that arose from the superficial femoral or descending genicular arteries, with the most proximal of these commonly entering near the midportion of the muscle. Since circulation to the entire muscle is routinely satisfactory via just its dominant pedicle in spite of these minor pedicles, this would be considered a type II muscle using the classification of Mathes and Nahai.[20]

Motor innervation of the gracilis muscle is via the anterior branch of the obturator nerve.[8] That takes an oblique course between the adductor longus and the magnus muscle before entering the gracilis muscle just superior to its dominant vascular hilum. Following the nerve proximally as far as the obturator foramen will allow harvest up to 13 cm in length.[8] After entry into the gracilis muscle, the nerve splits into branches, allowing segmental functional muscle transfers, making this a type I muscle according to the mode of innervation following the schema of Taylor et al.[21]

16.3.4 Anatomical Variations and Potential Pitfalls

Extending Pedicle Length

Many consider the vascular pedicle length of the gracilis muscle to be very short, making it difficult to manipulate as well as reach outside a zone of injury to a chosen recipient site. However, a few centimeters' extension as well as increased vessel caliber can be obtained if the vascular origin at the profunda femoris vessels themselves can be reached during pedicle dissection. Exposure to allow this is best achieved following the advice of Hasen et al,[22] where after a subfascial dissection above the adductor longus muscle at the level of the gracilis pedicle, the sartorius and vastus medialis muscles are retracted laterally to expose the desired origin at the profunda femoris vessels.

Reliable Musculocutaneous Version

Both septocutaneous and musculocutaneous perforators to the skin overlying the gracilis muscle exist, and are found predominantly about the dominant vascular hilum.[23] A single and then usually large musculocutaneous perforator will often arise from the muscle that coincides with the entry point of the dominant pedicle,[5,7,24] and is a good clue as to its whereabouts. Unfortunately, more typically multiple perforators are present and of smaller caliber that are difficult to individually dissect.[23] It is far better to include all the fascia between the adductor longus and gracilis muscle to ensure inclusion of even septocutaneous perforators with the gracilis muscle if a musculocutaneous free flap is considered. Historically, long vertical skin paddles have been taken with the gracilis muscle with inevitable necrosis of their distal portion.[24,25] However, if this described fascial preservation is carefully observed, a vertically oriented flap at least to the mid-thigh level is usually reliable. Remember also that Yousif et al[5] showed in cadaver and then clinical studies that the true perforasome of the gracilis skin perforators had a transverse orientation extending anteriorly from the sartorius and adductor longus muscles to the posterior mid-thigh in its upper third. This more reliable skin orientation is the rationale for the TUG[5,7,8] or identical TMG[6] free flap, often acceptable as a secondary option for breast reconstruction.

Multiple Segmental Free Flaps

The gracilis muscle can be split into multiple segmental muscle free flaps simultaneously, each depending on a secondary pedicle or in combination with the dominant pedicle.[17,26] If the proximal secondary pedicle alone is used to supply a segmental portion of the gracilis muscle as a free flap, the rest of the muscle and its unviolated dominant pedicle can be reserved for later use if needed.[19]

Autogenous Tendon Graft

If the gracilis tendon needs to be used, for example, to replace the Achilles tendon,[13] the distal harvest incision should be made in a longitudinal fashion over the tendon insertion at the medial proximal aspect of the lower leg where it will be divided so as to maximize length. The gracilis tendon will be found in the middle of the pes anserinus, and the more posterior semitendinosus tendon can also be removed to provide more autologous tendon tissue as needed.

Option for Large Extremity Wound

After completion of the microanastomoses, careful scoring of the superficial epimysium under magnification with removal of excessive connective tissue while preserving the intrinsic vasculature, followed by distraction perpendicular to the muscle fibers will modify the tubular shape of the gracilis into more like a sheet.[27] The muscle thereby becomes thinner, but now can be suitable to cover a larger defect.[27]

16.3.5 Flap Design

When possible, depending on the lower extremity defect, the patient most easily will be kept in a supine position, with the hip and knee flexed and thigh abducted for the easiest approach to the gracilis muscle. Except in the most obese patient, the course of the adductor longus muscle can be palpated from the pubic tubercle to the medial condyle of the femur. The gracilis muscle will be found posterior to a vertical line drawn between these two points.[28] Since the vascular pedicle to the gracilis muscle enters on the anterolateral border of the muscle, the thigh chosen as the donor site must be determined by the location of the defect and recipient site so that a direct path to the latter without twisting is possible.

If a vertical oriented composite flap is required, the skin paddle should be planned in the upper two-thirds of the thigh below the aforementioned line, centered over the gracilis muscle, and of a width that allows primary donor site closure. For the lower extremity, a transverse elliptical design from the proximal thigh will rarely be necessary. However, if preferred, this should extend no more anteriorly than the hollow overlying the profunda femoris vessels, found just lateral to the anterior border of the adductor longus muscle.[6] The upper border of this ellipse should be a few centimeters below the groin crease so as not to distort it, continuing posteriorly to the gluteal crease to almost the ischial tuberosity. The lower border of this flap will correspond to the amount of skin that can be pinched together to also permit direct donor site closure.[6]

16.3.6 Flap Harvest

For problems confined to the lower extremity, the supine position with the hip and knee flexed and thigh abducted is adequate for harvest and use of the gracilis muscle as a free flap. A bump under the knee will hold the leg steady. Since the gracilis muscle lies almost immediately posterior to the adductor longus muscle, which corresponds to a line drawn from the pubic tubercle to the medial condyle of the femur, a lengthy longitudinal incision just inferior to this line along the medial thigh, or instead a transverse incision paralleling the groin crease as if performing an upper thigh lift, will allow adequate exposure of almost the entire muscle.[19] However, the scar length can be better minimized by first making a short vertical incision just proximal to the knee joint in the more posterior aspect of the medial thigh (▶ Fig. 16.9[29]; see ▶ Video 16.3). This approach is extended down through the deep fascia to expose the sartorius muscle fibers that can be seen to run

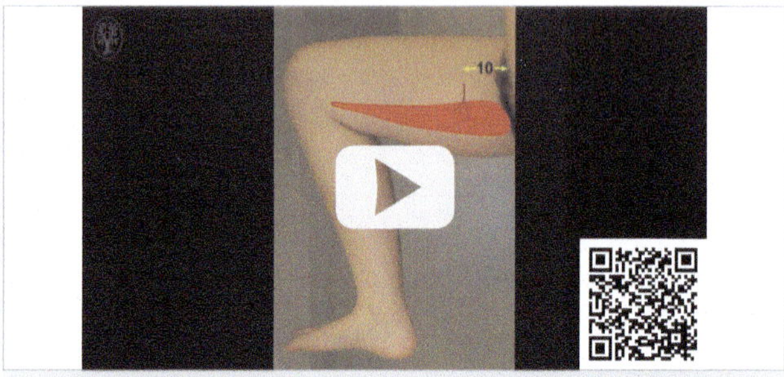

Video 16.3 The Gracilis Muscle Free Flap. https://www.thieme.de/de/q.htm?p=opn/cs/20/7/12265277-20e3ba8e

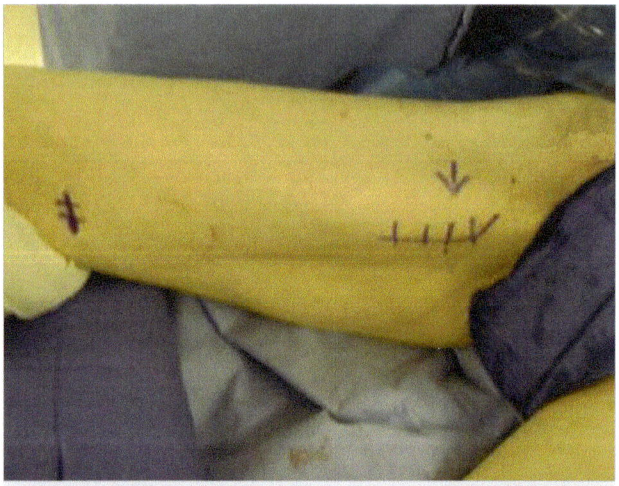

Fig. 16.9 Planned incisions for a customary approach to the gracilis muscle as marked on the posteromedial thigh. The distal vertical incision just proximal to the knee joint facilitates exposure of the gracilis tendon upon which traction will more accurately identify the site of the muscle belly near the proximal markings. The *arrow* is about 10 cm below the pubic tubercle, and is an estimate of the anticipated region to find the vascular hilum.

parallel to the femur. If the greater saphenous vein is first seen in the subcutaneous tissues, the dissection should proceed more inferiorly, remembering that the gracilis muscle will be more posterior and just below the sartorius at this level. A circumferential finger dissection below the sartorius muscle permits retrieval of the gracilis tendon much like when grabbing the vas deferens during an inguinal herniorrhaphy.

A Penrose drain wrapped around the gracilis tendon when distracted medially and distally causes movement of the gracilis muscle that can be observed in the proximal thigh. This location is marked on the skin, as well as an arrow above it at about 10 cm distal to the pubic tubercle as a good estimate of where to anticipate the location of the medial circumflex femoral vessels (MCFV), the usual dominant pedicle. If a vertical musculocutaneous flap is planned, the skin paddle should be centered over the muscle now outlined. For the more typical situation just as a muscle flap, only a short longitudinal incision centered about this arrow, once through the deep fascia, allows access to the anterior border of the muscle. With medial muscle retraction, by careful dissection the exact location of the vascular hilum must be identified. The incision can then be extended proximally in a curvilinear fashion upward toward the groin crease to better expose the adductor longus muscle and aponeurotic origin of the gracilis muscle.

The gracilis muscle proximal and distal to the hilum of its vascular pedicle is carefully freed circumferentially from any fascial connections. A Penrose drain distally around the muscle will allow medial retraction for better exposure during lengthening of the vascular pedicle. Likewise, a vessel loop around the pedicle lateral to the hilum facilitates exposure of side branches. The anterior branch of the obturator nerve will be identified just above this point and preserved only if a dynamic muscle transfer is desired. The fascial adhesions of the adductor longus to the adductor magnus are released for several centimeters above and below where the pedicle is seen to go under the former. This allows gentle lateral retraction of the adductor longus muscle, thereby exposing branches to it arising vertically from the MCFV. These are carefully ligated individually, which upon doing so better defines the further course of the MCFV. More lateral dissection ceases when the pedicle is considered long enough. If an extended pedicle is required, the adductor longus muscle is freed by a lateral subfascial approach and retracted medially to expose the MCFV origin from the profunda femoris (see sections on "Anatomical Variations" for details).

Once pedicle dissection is completed, the proximal incision is extended distally only until blunt finger dissection around the more distal unexposed muscle is completely possible via the two incisions that have been made. Often this will expose a prominent secondary pedicle that will have to be ligated. A long silk suture is sewn to the tendon with its free ends then brought with a long gooseneck clamp through the distal subfascial tunnel so created into the proximal incision. The tendon is divided distally, and traction on the suture will bring the tendon and distal muscle into the proximal wound. Next, the aponeurotic origin at a level just below the symphysis pubis is taken down to create an island flap, only attached to the thigh by its vascular pedicle. When ready, the vascular pedicle is divided, and the flap transferred to whatever is the recipient site.

16.3.7 Postoperative Care Protocols

The gracilis muscle free flap requires no unique protocols for management. Institutional policies for monitoring, dressings, and subsequent ambulation should be followed as is the routine.

16.3.8 Conclusion

The gracilis muscle as a free flap for the lower extremity is adequate for small to moderately sized defects (▶ Fig. 16.10). Minimal bulk allows coverage of the foot and ankle (▶ Fig. 16.11),

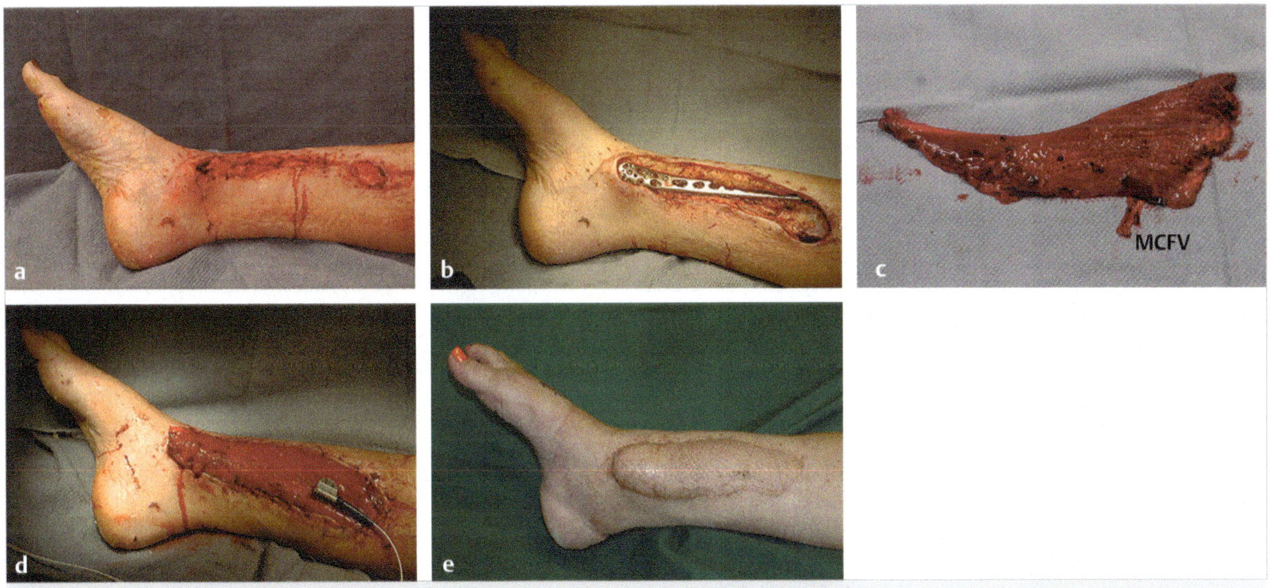

Fig. 16.10 **(a)** Wound breakdown following internal fixation of a right distal tibial fracture. **(b)** Following adequate debridement, the entire fixation plate is exposed creating a long narrow defect. **(c)** Here apropos, a long narrow left gracilis muscle free flap was selected as the donor muscle, as the medial circumflex femoral vessel (MCFV) pedicle is anatomically directed posteriorly toward the planned posterior tibial recipient site. **(d)** Muscle flap once revascularized and inset. **(e)** Reasonable contour of the right leg after skin grafted gracilis muscle free flap.

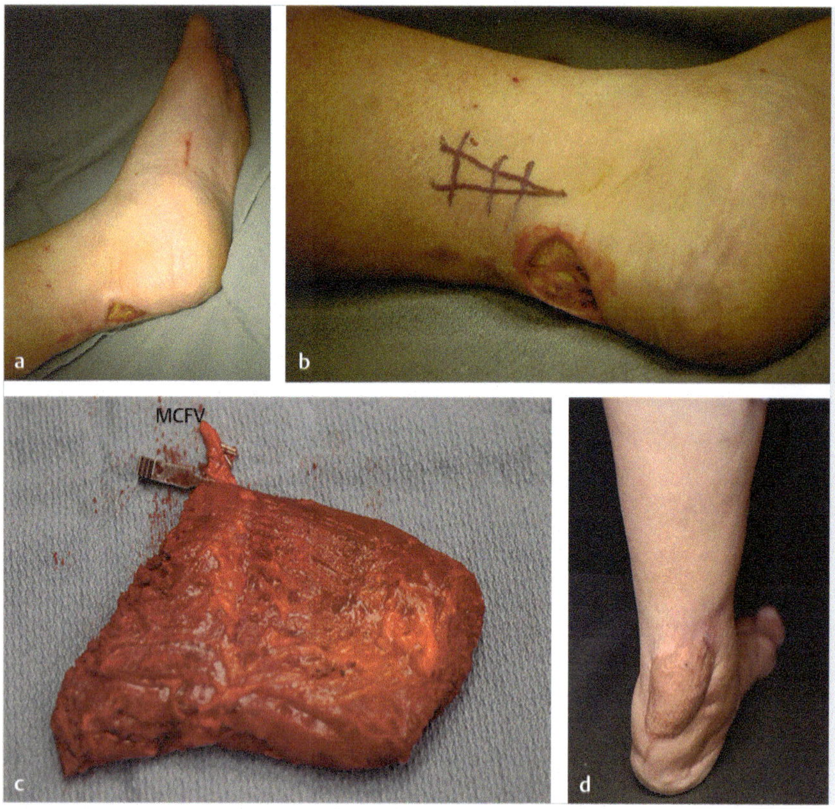

Fig. 16.11 (a) Obese diabetic with infected, exposed left Achilles tendon after tenorrhaphy wound breakdown. **(b)** Small wound after adequate debridement. **(c)** Small segmental ipsilateral gracilis muscle free flap chosen with vascular pedicle (medial circumflex femoral vessel) oriented toward the posterior tibial recipient site. **(d)** Reasonable thin skin grafted gracilis muscle free flap covering Achilles tendon preserved function and did not interfere with use of conventional shoe wear.

where especially after muscle atrophy use of shoe wear and subsequently ambulation will not be impeded. Since extremely malleable, fill or three-dimensional insetting is an asset. There is a limited role as a dynamic flap for the lower extremity. The anatomy and vascular supply of this muscle is consistent to allow an expeditious harvest. However, in the presence of severe atherosclerotic peripheral vascular disease, the arterial orifice may be extremely difficult to visualize or allow passage of sutures, so an alternative donor site should be considered for this subset of patients.

References

[1] McLean DH, Buncke HJ, Jr. Autotransplant of omentum to a large scalp defect, with microsurgical revascularization. Plast Reconstr Surg. 1972; 49(3):268–274

[2] Daniel RK, Taylor GI. Distant transfer of an island flap by microvascular anastomosis. A clinical technique. Plast Reconstr Surg. 1973; 52:111–117

[3] Orticochea M. The musculo-cutaneous flap method: an immediate and heroic substitute for the method of delay. Br J Plast Surg. 1972; 25(2):106–110

[4] Harii K, Ohmori K, Torii S. Free gracilis muscle transplantation, with microneurovascular anastomoses for the treatment of facial paralysis. A preliminary report. Plast Reconstr Surg. 1976; 57(2):133–143

[5] Yousif NJ, Matloub HS, Kolachalam R, Grunert BK, Sanger JR. The transverse gracilis musculocutaneous flap. Ann Plast Surg. 1992; 29(6):482–490

[6] Fattah A, Figus A, Mathur B, Ramakrishnan VV. The transverse myocutaneous gracilis flap: technical refinements. J Plast Reconstr Aesthet Surg. 2010; 63(2):305–313

[7] Zenn MR, Jones G. Gracilis and TUG/TMG flaps. In: Reconstructive Surgery: Anatomy, Technique, and Clinical Applications. St. Louis, MO: Quality Medical Publishing; 2012:1418–1465

[8] Zuker RM, Bains RD. Gracilis flap. In: Wei FC, Mardini S, eds. Flaps and Reconstructive Surgery. Edinburgh: Elsevier; 2017:559–569

[9] Fattah A, Borschel GH, Manktelow RT, Bezuhly M, Zuker RM. Facial palsy and reconstruction. Plast Reconstr Surg. 2012; 129(2):340e–352e

[10] Zuker RM, Bezuhly M, Manktelow RT. Selective fascicular coaptation of free functioning gracilis transfer for restoration of independent thumb and finger flexion following Volkmann ischemic contracture. J Reconstr Microsurg. 2011; 27(7):439–444

[11] Lin CH, Lin YT, Yeh JT, Chen CT. Free functioning muscle transfer for lower extremity posttraumatic composite structure and functional defect. Plast Reconstr Surg. 2007; 119(7):2118–2126

[12] Redett RJ, Robertson BC, Chang B, Girotto J, Vaughan T. Limb salvage of lower-extremity wounds using free gracilis muscle reconstruction. Plast Reconstr Surg. 2000; 106(7):1507–1513

[13] Huemer GM, Larcher L, Schoeller T, Bauer T. The free gracilis muscle flap in Achilles tendon coverage and reconstruction. Plast Reconstr Surg. 2012; 129(4):910–919

[14] Carr MM, Manktelow RT, Zuker RM. Gracilis donor site morbidity. Microsurgery. 1995; 16(9):598–600

[15] Deutinger M, Kuzbari R, Paternostro-Sluga T, et al. Donor-site morbidity of the gracilis flap. Plast Reconstr Surg. 1995; 95:1240–1244

[16] Hussey AJ, Laing AJ, Regan PJ. An anatomical study of the gracilis muscle and its application in groin wounds. Ann Plast Surg. 2007; 59(4):404–409

[17] Cavadas PC, Sanz-Giménez-Rico JR, Landín L, Martínez-Soriano F. Segmental gracilis free flap based on secondary pedicles: anatomical study and clinical series. Plast Reconstr Surg. 2004; 114(3):684–691

[18] King ICC, Obeid N, Woollard AC, Jones ME. Maximizing length and safety in gracilis free flap dissection. J Plast Reconstr Aesthet Surg. 2016; 69(10):1452–1453

[19] Tremp M, Oranges CM, Wang WJ, et al. The "nugget design": a modified segmental gracilis free flap for small-sized defect reconstruction on the lower extremity. J Plast Reconstr Aesthet Surg. 2017; 70(9):1261–1266

[20] Mathes SJ, Nahai F. Classification of the vascular anatomy of muscles: experimental and clinical correlation. Plast Reconstr Surg. 1981; 67(2):177–187

[21] Taylor GI, Gianoutsos MP, Morris SF. The neurovascular territories of the skin and muscles: anatomic study and clinical implications. Plast Reconstr Surg. 1994; 94(1):1–36

[22] Hasen KV, Gallegos ML, Dumanian GA. Extended approach to the vascular pedicle of the gracilis muscle flap: anatomical and clinical study. Plast Reconstr Surg. 2003; 111(7):2203–2208

[23] Hallock GG. The gracilis (medial circumflex femoral) perforator flap: a medial groin free flap? Ann Plast Surg. 2003; 51(6):623–626

[24] Serafin D. The gracilis muscle: musculocutaneous flap. In: Atlas of Microsurgical Composite Tissue Transplantation. Philadelphia, PA: W.B. Saunders; 1996:293–299

[25] Persichetti P, Cogliandro A, Marangi GF, et al. Pelvic and perineal reconstruction following abdominoperineal resection: the role of gracilis flap. Ann Plast Surg. 2007; 59(2):168–172

[26] Temmen TM, Perez J, Smith DJ. Transverse splitting of the gracilis muscle free flap: Maximal use of a single muscle. Microsurgery. 2011; 31(6):479–483

[27] Calotta NA, Pedreira R, Deune EG. The gracilis free flap is a viable option for large extremity wounds. Ann Plast Surg. 2018; 81(3):322–326

[28] Hallock GG, Morris SF. Skin grafts and local flaps. [CME]. Plast Reconstr Surg. 2011; 127(1):5e–22e

[29] Hallock GG. Minimally invasive harvest of the gracilis muscle. Plast Reconstr Surg. 1999; 104(3):801–805

16.4 Chapter 16C: The Versatile Latissimus Dorsi Muscle Free Flap

Geoffrey G. Hallock

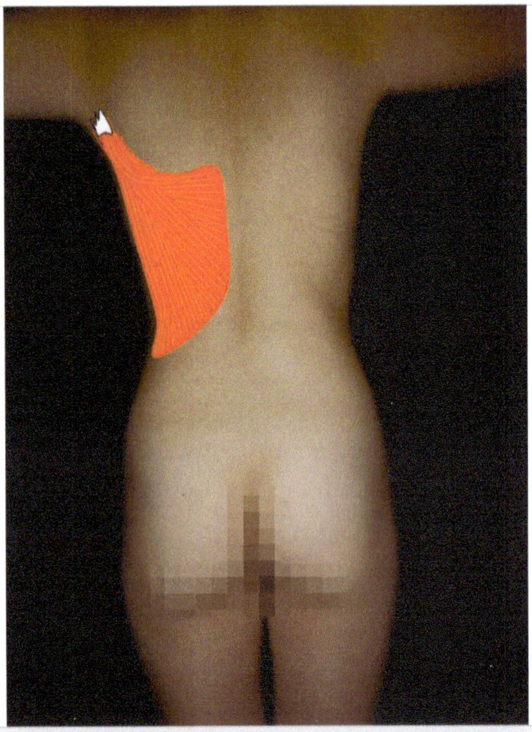

Fig. 16.12 The latissimus dorsi muscle.

16.4.1 Introduction to the Versatile Latissimus Dorsi Muscle Free Flap

In the search for a more reliable method to ensure viability of a random-patterned axillary skin flap used for replacement of the chest skin after mastectomy, Tansini[1] resorted to his own cadaver dissections to conclude that keeping the underlying latissimus dorsi (LD) muscle (▸ Fig. 16.12) attached would be the answer. And so a "new procedure,"[1] was born, the LD musculocutaneous flap as a local flap. But not until Olivari[2] some seven decades later was this rediscovered. The near synchronous introduction of microvascular surgery led to the quest for more reliable donor sites, so as a logical progression, Maxwell et al[3] realized that this quite robust island flap with its large caliber and lengthy pedicle would also make an ideal free flap.

The function of the LD muscle is to extend, medially rotate, and adduct the humerus,[4,5,6] as well as stabilize the pelvis during locomotion and hold the inferior angle of the scapula against the chest wall.[4] The synergistic action of some six other muscles in the shoulder girdle does not replace all these functions, as Lee and Mun[7] in a systematic review have shown that there is an overall impairment such as weakness in 40% of patients. However, most have little difficulties in daily life or work activities,[7,8] a finding that explains why this muscle is even considered by Zenn and Jones[9] to be "the most expendable muscle in the body." The numerous attributes of this large muscle explain its longstanding and widespread use as a local flap for the head and neck, breast, thorax, and upper arm.[6,9] The very same characteristics have made it an ideal free flap for use throughout the lower extremity as well. The fact that Bartlett et al[5] in their cadaver dissections found no pedicle occlusive atherosclerosis makes the LD muscle a first consideration instead of using lower extremity free flap donor sites especially in the elderly or those with peripheral vascular disease, even though a different body region must be violated. To quote Serafin,[4] for all patients needing a free flap, the LD muscle is the "gold standard of donor composite tissue because of its dependability and applicability." And so it is.

16.4.2 Attributes and Detriments

Attributes

- Muscle with largest available surface area in the body.
- Versatile local or free flap donor site.
- Flat.
- Expendable.
- Consistent anatomy.
- Superficial, allowing a rapid harvest.
- Reliable viability.
- Macrosurgical caliber vessels.
- Long vascular pedicle.
- Cornucopia of chimeric and composite flap combinations.
- Potential for vascular flow-throughs.
- Segmental splitting for multiple flaps.
- Restoration of function elsewhere.

Detriments

- Bulkiness of musculocutaneous flap.
- Potential weakness limits crutch bearing in general, and transfer abilities for paraplegics.
- Function disturbance in locomotion in various neuromuscular disorders.
- Possible winging of scapula.
- High incidence of seroma after harvest.

16.4.3 Anatomical Considerations

The LD is a flat, triangular-shaped muscle found most superficial on the posterior thorax except on its superior and medial borders where it is overladen by the trapezius muscle.[10] A broad aponeurosis that joins the thoracolumbar fascia and attaches to the spine of the lower six thoracic, lumbar, and sacral vertebrae, as well as the supraspinatus ligament and outer lip of the posterior iliac crest, serves as its origin.[4,5,6] Commonly, some fibers interdigitate with those of the external oblique and serratus anterior muscles to arise from the 10th to 12th ribs.[4] Also, not unusual is a sometimes distinct small slip that takes origin from the tip of the scapula. All these muscle fibers converge proximally to contribute to the posterior fold of the axilla, then spiral around the teres major muscle and insert into the intertubercular groove of the humerus.[5,6] The muscle length ranges from 21 to 42 cm[11] and has a mean surface area of 25 × 35 cm.[9]

The vascular supply to the LD muscle is highly consistent as a branch of the subscapular artery. The thoracodorsal artery, and

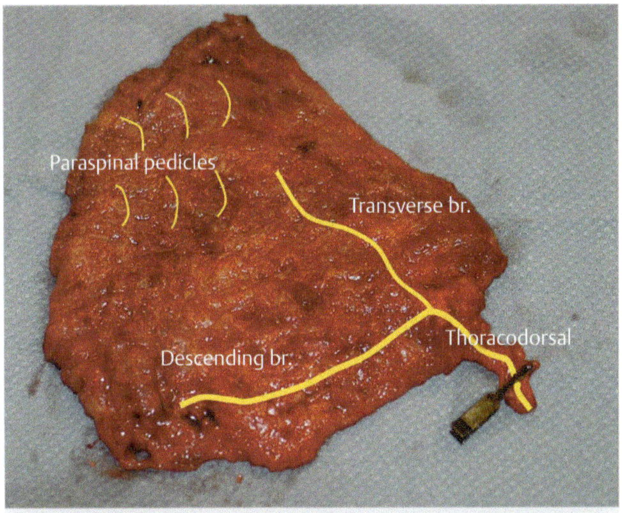

Fig. 16.13 Arterial anatomy of the latissimus dorsi muscle. The dominant thoracodorsal artery soon after entering its vascular hilum bifurcates into transverse and descending branches. Posterior intercostal and lumbar branches are secondary paraspinal minor pedicles.

usually a single venae comitantes, 99% of the time according to Tobin et al[12] enter on the medial undersurface of the muscle. This vascular hilum is usually about 10 cm inferior to its muscular insertion in the posterior axilla, and near the tip of the angle of the scapula.[9,11] The latter is found about 2.5 cm medial to the lateral border of the muscle that is often palpable.[4,12] The artery has a mean pedicle length of 9 cm, and caliber at its origin of 2.7 mm, with the vein averaging 3.4 cm.[5] Shortly after entering the muscle, this solitary dominant pedicle divides into a transverse (medial) and descending (lateral) branch (▶ Fig. 16.13).[4] These run at a 45-degree angle to each other to parallel the medial and lateral borders of the muscle, respectively, with numerous interconnecting collaterals. More caudally and medially will be found secondary segmental pedicles that have a lateral row arising from the posterior intercostals and a medial row from the lumbar vessels. This vascular pattern makes this a type V muscle according to Mathes and Nahai.[13] Venous outflow parallels the dominant arterial supply except in the region of the secondary pedicles where valves direct outflow via the intercostal and lumbar veins, which may explain why sometimes the muscle expected to survive on either source of arterial supply does not in the most inferior portion that can become congested.[11,14]

The thoracodorsal nerve courses with the dominant vascular pedicle to also enter the muscle at what would be its neurovascular hilum. Although some sensory fibers may be present, this nerve primarily serves as the source of motor innervation for the entire muscle.[3] Taylor et al[15] classify the LD muscle as having a type I mode of innervation with a single nerve that does not branch before entering the muscle, although Tobin et al[12] in their anatomical studies found that the thoracodorsal nerve bifurcated at a mean of 1.3 cm prior to this entry, which would make this a type II muscle.[15] Numerous intercostal nerves penetrate the LD muscle to provide sensation to the skin, but these are usually divided during muscle elevation, so a musculocutaneous version would be essentially insensate.

16.4.4 Anatomical Variants and Potential Pitfalls

Vascular Supply

The subscapular artery arises from the third portion of the axillary artery, and soon thereafter branches into the circumflex scapular and thoracodorsal arteries, which is the typical anatomy 94% of the time.[4] Otherwise, the thoracodorsal artery may directly originate from the axillary artery itself (5%) or the lateral thoracic artery (1%),[4] presumably because the circumflex scapular artery itself sometimes arises directly from the axillary artery. The subscapular artery and vein 92% of the time are found together where they enter the axillary artery or vein. If not, the artery arises a mean distance of 4.2 cm proximal to the vein and may not rejoin it until reaching the serratus artery branch.[5] Note on rare occasion a double thoracodorsal vein will be found and should be preserved, especially if they later join together upstream.[5]

Once intramuscular, the thoracodorsal artery does not always bifurcate into transverse and descending branches, as about 14% of the time the transverse branch is diminutive or nonexistent or has multiple branches,[16] which would mitigate against traditional splitting of the muscle or require use of some other muscle preservation techniques.[4,16] Although the thoracodorsal artery can capture the territory of the secondary pedicles, the same is not true for the venous outflow. Valves in the veins of the latter direct outflow via the intercostal and lumbar veins, and away from the dominant vascular hilum. This may explain why sometimes the harvested muscle initially seems to have adequate inflow, but becomes dark and congested over time in the most inferior and medial portions that ultimately will not survive.[11]

Vascular Flow-Throughs

A segment of the circumflex scapular or serratus anterior artery can be kept intact with the thoracodorsal artery. Either that branch or the thoracodorsal artery that is also the pedicle to the flap is anastomosed in an end-to-end fashion to the proximal recipient artery, with the other then connected to the distal recipient artery in an orthograde end-to-end fashion. This can in similar fashion be done for the venous side. This avoids the need for an end-to-side microanastomosis if the operator is uncomfortable with that. If the flow-through is long enough, a gap in the recipient vessel can be overcome without resorting to using a vein graft. Miyamoto et al[17] believe that depending on the caliber of branches and connections, this technique can stabilize flow into the flap so that if either the donor or recipient veins are relatively small, they will not then be overcome by excessive inflow.

Musculocutaneous Version

Although the muscle is relatively thin, the usual overlying skin and subcutaneous tissues that are used as a musculocutaneous flap can be bulky,[18] especially if foot and ankle reconstruction is done where shoe wear would then be impeded. Exceptions do exist. Most musculocutaneous perforators are found near the dominant vascular hilum, so this region must be part of any planned skin paddle. A design transversely across the muscle (which would appear to have an oblique orientation) captures the looser skin in this region leading to a more aesthetic scar that can be better hidden, such as by a bra on a woman.[9] Yet a vertical design allows a larger skin flap. The size can be maximized by including the circumflex scapular vessels as a conjoined parascapular/LD flap, where not only can the skin portion extend from the triangular space to near the pelvic origin of the muscle with total viability, but the distal muscle also probably survives more than expected via retrograde inflow from the musculocutaneous perforators emanating from the skin or from improved venous outflow in the opposite direction.[19]

Muscle Splitting/Function Preservation

The conventional description of splitting of the LD muscle would be between its transverse and descending branches to thereby make multiple flaps possible, but usually with the intent to keep one segment intact at the donor site for function preservation.[12] However, if the transverse branch is inadequate, which occurs about 14% of the time,[4] this would not be a viable possibility. Another approach would be to plan a thoracodorsal artery perforator (TDAP) flap as a chimeric flap, usually using the descending branch as the perforator source vessel with its continuation to a lateral portion of the muscle itself that would be tailored to the desired size.[20,21] If dissection of the perforators needs to be avoided, a composite flap retaining a small portion of the muscle with the skin paddle is an alternative as a muscle-sparing LD flap.[22] In actuality, when the LD muscle alone is taken as a free flap, only a lateral segment is typically used, keeping the medial muscle still perfused by the secondary pedicles. Of course, in this scenario the dominant vascular hilum is taken with the free flap, so the rest of the muscle segment would be denervated if the thoracodorsal nerve is not independently preserved.

Dynamic Transfer

The LD muscle is not considered the first choice for most applications if restoration of function elsewhere is desired. Motor function for the entire muscle is via the solitary thoracodorsal nerve,[3,9] which can be reanastomosed to a motor nerve in the lower extremity that remains at the site where function has been lost. The LD muscle should be marked to length prior to release of its origin and insertion so that the exact tension is reestablished at the given recipient site. This has been used to replace absent quadriceps muscle to provide knee extension,[23] posterior compartment muscles for ankle plantar flexion,[24] and anterior compartment muscles for ankle dorsiflexion.[25]

Chimeric Flaps

The subscapular axis with its numerous branches to cutaneous flaps (e.g., scapular, parascapular, TDAP), muscles (e.g., LD, serratus anterior), and bone (e.g., scapula via angular or descending branch of the circumflex scapular), allows the creation of over five dozen combinations and permutations of these flaps that each have their own independent branch for independent insetting, but remain attached together only to the same source vessel—the subscapular vessels.[26] This not only allows simultaneous three-dimensional fill, but provides multiple tissues each with different functions, as well as the potential for coverage of multiple sites.[27] In addition, especially if recipient sites are limited as is frequently the case in the lower extremity, the multiple flaps require only a single recipient site as they are all connected ultimately to the same source vessel. Some examples include LD muscle–serratus anterior muscle (muscle–muscle chimera),[28] LD muscle–serratus anterior fascia (muscle–fascia chimera),[25] LD muscle–TDAP flap (muscle–skin chimera),[20,21] LD muscle–scapula (muscle–bone chimera),[29] LD muscle–TDAP flap–scapula (muscle–skin–bone chimera),[30] and LD muscle–serratus anterior/rib (muscle–muscle/bone chimera).[31] Chimeric flaps are somewhat more difficult to harvest, and certainly make monitoring of the combination as a free flap more challenging (▶ Fig. 16.14).

Donor Site Morbidity

Methods to preserve muscle function, if important such as to preserve the contour of the posterior axillary fold, have been described previously in this section. Another major concern common to this flap harvest is seroma. An 80% seroma rate has been reported, and usually with the use of drains.[32] Incorporating quilting sutures to reattach the subcutaneous layer to the remaining muscle bed is helpful. Care must be observed as sutures placed too deeply can cause a pneumothorax. The combination of quilting sutures with a fibrin sealant has reduced the incidence of seroma to 9.4%.[32]

Most often the amount of muscle needed as a free flap can be reached by an 8- to 10-cm vertical scar extending from the cupola of the axilla along the posterior axillary fold. Kiiski et al[33] have reduced this to 3 to 5 cm using standard endoscopic techniques with CO_2 insufflation. This does not count scars left from necessary access portals. Of course, if a musculocutaneous flap is used, this approach would be unnecessary. If the width of the flap then exceeded typically 8 to 10 cm, primary skin closure would not be possible, and skin grafts that are sometimes difficult to heal, potentially later unstable, and certainly aesthetically displeasing would be required. A larger skin surface area is possible by designing multiple small skin paddles on independent perforators over the latissimus muscle that can after transfer be rearranged at the recipient site to close a big defect using the "kiss" principle.[34,35,36] Primary closure using this alternative still leaves just a scar on the back, but the lower extremity skin flaps themselves will have more scarring where approximated together than just around their perimeter if there had been only a solitary skin paddle.

16.4.5 Flap Design

With the patient erect and hands on their hips, forceful contraction implies an innervated muscle with usually an intact thoracodorsal blood supply that can be searched for.[11] In the thin individual, contraction also allows identification of the most anterior border of the muscle. The angle of the scapula should also be marked, as the superior border of the muscle adjacent to the teres major will be found there. Usually, only a muscle free flap will be necessary for the lower extremity. However, if for some reason a musculocutaneous variant is needed, the skin paddle should not exceed in width 8 to 10 cm or what can be pinched together, as primary closure would not be possible and

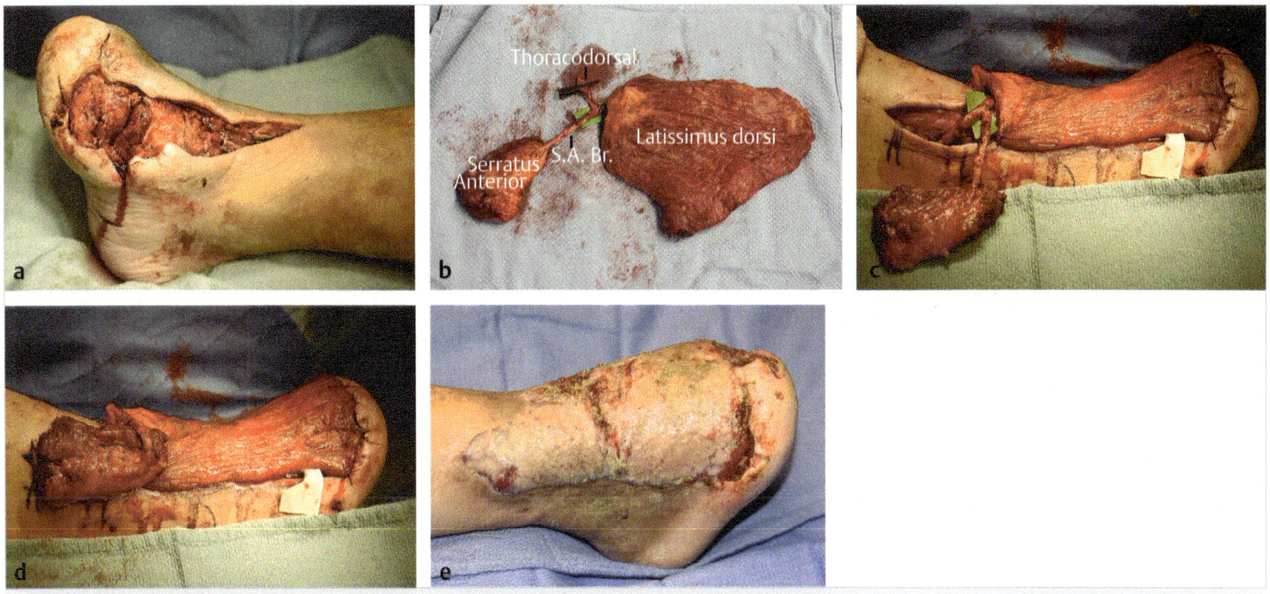

Fig. 16.14 **(a)** This hemodialysis patient had exposed joints in an open right transmetatarsal amputation (TMA) stump. **(b)** A chimeric latissimus dorsi (LD) and serratus anterior muscle free flap was raised with the serratus anterior branch (SA Br.) joining the thoracodorsal branch that is then common to both muscles. **(c)** The LD muscle could just reach for insetting over the TMA stump, with the still exposed vascular pedicle seen entering to the peroneal vessels in this single vessel extremity. **(d)** The serratus anterior muscle could then be independently inset specifically for coverage of the recipient site. **(e)** Slow healing at 2 months, but chimeric muscle free flap has sustained joint coverage and so far preserved his right TMA.

a skin graft or some other local flap must be utilized. The design of the chosen skin paddle must include the musculocutaneous perforators arising from the thoracodorsal vessels, which are near its hilum. This can be transverse to the muscle to capture the loose skin in the mid-back region, allowing a scar easily hidden by a bra in women.[9] A longer skin paddle is possible with a vertical ellipse with its axis parallel to the anterior border of the muscle, which must be included to ensure capture of the descending branch of the thoracodorsal. Greater amounts of skin can be transferred, but the design will have to be unique for each case, using the "kiss" principle as Zhang et al have proposed.[36]

16.4.6 Flap Harvest

The position of the patient on the operating table depends on the defect and the goals of reconstruction. A posterior lower limb defect may best have both the donor site and the recipient site reached with the patient in a prone position. If bilateral LD muscles need to be harvested simultaneously, again the prone position to start may be best. Usually, the lower limb defect is anterior, and many use a supine position.[31,37] However, most often the lateral decubitus position is used even though it is somewhat more awkward, and this will be discussed further here in detail (▶ Fig. 16.15). If the anterior tibial or peroneal vessels will be the recipient site, the contralateral side will be positioned down on the table. If the posterior tibial vessels are the recipient site, the ipsilateral side will be placed downward.

Important landmarks should be marked to provide orientation with the patient in the lateral decubitus position (see ▶ Video 16.4). The lateral border of the muscle sometimes can be grasped while grabbing the external skin and fat. This often surprisingly can be as anterior as the anterior axillary fold.[10] The angle of the scapula is always palpable and corresponds to the superior border of the muscle that must be separated from

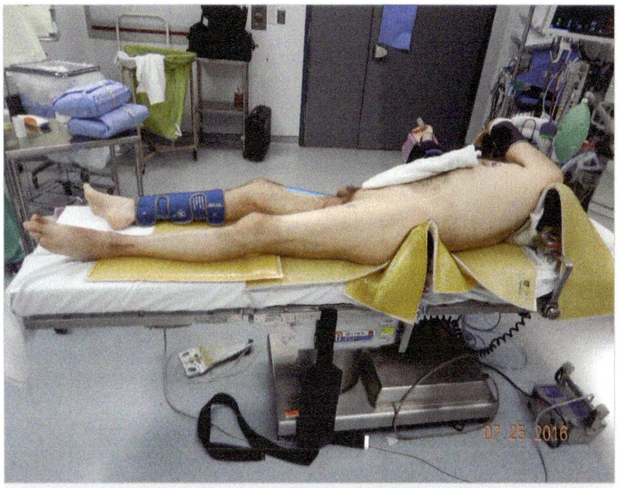

Fig. 16.15 Positioning on the operating table for harvest of the latissimus dorsi (LD) muscle can be variable depending on the location of the defect. In this case, a not quite full lateral position allowed access to the ipsilateral LD muscle and proposed recipient site above the defect at the medial left ankle.

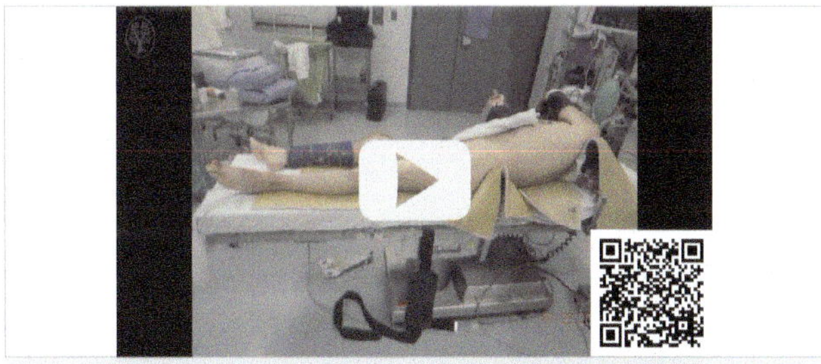

Video 16.4 Latissimus Dorsi Muscle Free Flap. https://www.thieme.de/de/q.htm?p=opn/cs/20/7/12265278-b8fddfff

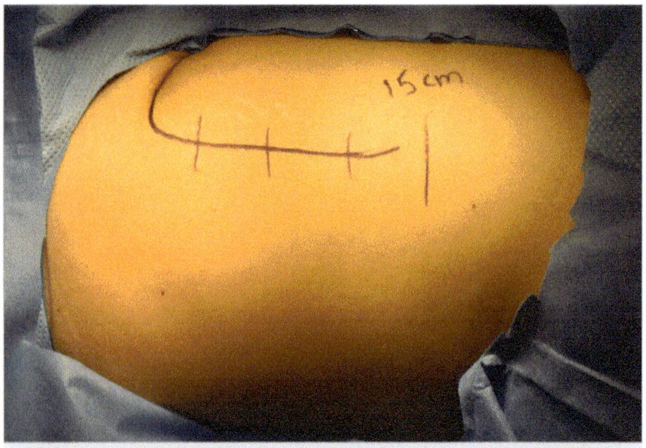

Fig. 16.16 Planned incision to harvest a latissimus dorsi muscle free flap only, here curving from the cupola of the axilla (which facilitates exposure of the tendinous insertion) to a vertical line dropping down along the posterior axillary fold as needed. In this case, the designed scar will be hidden by adduction of the arm upon the thorax.

the adjacent and more cephalad teres major muscle. At the highest point of the posterior axillary fold, a vertical line is dropped from the cupola of the axilla for about 10 cm where the location of the neurovascular hilum of the LD muscle must be carefully sought.

When a musculocutaneous flap is planned, the design of the skin paddle will determine the skin incision. Most commonly for the lower extremity, however, only a muscle flap is required. This is approached via a curved line from the cupola of the axilla to the border of the posterior axillary fold, proceeding then vertically as far caudally as needed (▶ Fig. 16.16). If the entire muscle must be used, this line is then distally curved back medially so that wide exposure is possible, fully realizing that the resulting scar now cannot be hidden when the arm is adducted to the thorax.

After the skin incision, the subcutaneous tissues are divided down to expose the muscle. Usually there will be a somewhat loose areolar layer found, which with retractor traction upward on the skin and fat will expose this plane that can be swept away from the muscle. First, proceed anteriorly to identify the LD lateral border throughout the incision. Then starting above the angle of the scapula, dissect posteriorly until it is reached. LD muscle fibers here are oriented obliquely toward the axilla, as are the fibers of the teres major above them, both originating to some degree from the scapula. Usually a thin layer of fat will separate the two so that the superior border of the latissimus is readily discernible. More inferior and medial separation of the posterior side of the muscle from the subcutaneous fat continues to establish the flap dimensions as planned. If a very wide flap is needed, during medial dissection the trapezius muscle will be encountered, which must be expected and elevated above the LD muscle that courses below it toward the spinous processes.

Once the dimensions of the standard muscle free flap have been completely exposed, beginning at the most inferior aspect of the lateral border, division of the origin starts to proceed medially in a perpendicular direction. As the lateral muscle is raised, the underlying serratus posterior inferiorly and serratus anterior muscles superiorly must not also be included inadvertently. Once the designated medial border has been reached, this is divided vertically as the undersurface of the muscle is freed caudal to cephalad up to the tip of the scapula to join the superior border. Numerous paraspinal secondary pedicles in this region must be carefully ligated, as these can bleed profusely. The thick fat pad encountered during this elevation, if left behind, best allows visualization of the deep surface of the latissimus and its vascular arborization. This maneuver also ensures that the serratus anterior muscle underneath the fat pad has been separated away properly.

At the angle of the scapula, a search for the crow's foot of the serratus branch on the serratus anterior muscle is initiated, then using bipolar cautery only until the thoracodorsal vessels are found nearby entering the undersurface of the LD muscle. More proximally, these diverge away from the muscle to pass under a fascial septum. Toward its insertion near the axilla, on the posterior LD surface, tendinous fibers start to appear. If the muscle insertion is completely divided here and retracted, better exposure of this fascial septum is possible to facilitate seeing and lengthening the vascular pedicle underneath it as desired. Normally, skeletonization of the vascular pedicle only back to the circumflex scapular vessels is necessary, as a long pedicle with not excessively large caliber vessels is available, and the latter will remain as a backup donor site. Further dissection back to the subscapular vessels will lengthen the pedicle, but is more difficult and will result in having very large caliber vessels. The serratus branch is protected until adequate flow through the thoracodorsal vessels is assured, as this by itself can supply the muscle enough as a backup option.[9] The thoracodorsal pedicle to the now island flap is not divided for transfer, until the lower extremity recipient site is prepared. The donor site then is closed primarily, following the usual protocols of the operator.

16.4.7 Postoperative Care Protocols

Positioning the patient on the back donor site is never a major concern. However, if a joint is crossed or any risk of pressure on the flap itself by the patient's position exists, this must be avoided by proper use of splints or traction devices. Monitoring of any free flap must follow the unit's protocols.

16.4.8 Conclusion

The LD muscle is the largest muscle in the body that is considered expendable, and therefore useful not only as a pedicled flap, but also as a free flap for transfer anywhere to any region of the body. Small as well as large flaps, multiple intrinsic flaps, and a possible combination with a multitude of other donor sites as chimeric flaps based on the subscapular axis increase the reconstructive options. The large caliber vessels with long vascular pedicle make this an ideal free flap donor site. The LD muscle is a dependable, reliable, and versatile "workhorse" flap that has a long-proven history that always deserves consideration when a microsurgical tissue transfer has been declared the solution for a lower extremity defect (▶ Fig. 16.17).

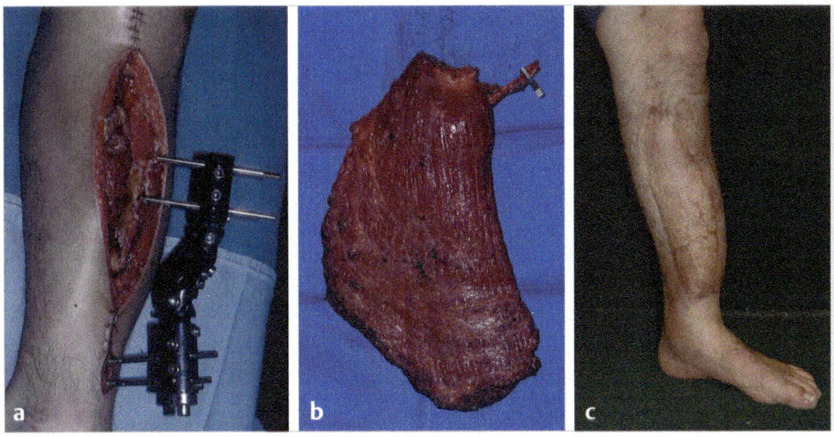

Fig. 16.17 (a) Open Gustilo IIIB fracture of the left mid-tibia with extensive soft-tissue loss precluding use of local tissues. **(b)** Latissimus dorsi (LD) muscle free flap with thoracodorsal vessels in microclamp. **(c)** Final appearance of the skin grafted LD muscle.

References

[1] Maxwell GP. Iginio Tansini and the origin of the latissimus dorsi musculocutaneous flap. Plast Reconstr Surg. 1980; 65(5):686–692

[2] Olivari N. The latissimus flap. Br J Plast Surg. 1976; 29(2):126–128

[3] Maxwell GP, Stueber K, Hoopes JE. A free latissimus dorsi myocutaneous flap: case report. Plast Reconstr Surg. 1978; 62(3):462–466

[4] Serafin D. The latissimus dorsi muscle-musculocutaneous flap. In: Atlas of Microsurgical Composite Tissue Transplantation. Philadelphia, PA: W.B. Saunders; 1996:205–216

[5] Bartlett SP, May JW, Jr, Yaremchuk MJ. The latissimus dorsi muscle: a fresh cadaver study of the primary neurovascular pedicle. Plast Reconstr Surg. 1981; 67(5):631–636

[6] Mathes SJ, Nahai F. Latissimus dorsi. In: Clinical Atlas of Muscle and Musculocutaneous Flaps. St. Louis, MO: C.V. Mosby; 1979:369–391

[7] Lee KT, Mun GH. A systematic review of functional donor-site morbidity after latissimus dorsi muscle transfer. Plast Reconstr Surg. 2014; 134(2):303–314

[8] Repo JP, Barner-Rasmussen I, Roine RP, Sintonen H, Tukiainen EJ. Treatment of compound tibia fracture with microvascular latissimus dorsi flap and the Ilizarov technique: a cross-sectional study of long-term outcomes. J Plast Reconstr Aesthet Surg. 2016; 69(4):524–532

[9] Zenn MR, Jones G. Latissimus dorsi flap. In: Reconstructive Surgery: Anatomy, Technique, and Clinical Applications. St. Louis, MO: Quality Medical Publishing; 2012:726–757

[10] Hallock GG, Morris SF. Skin grafts and local flaps. [CME]. Plast Reconstr Surg. 2011; 127(1):5e–22e

[11] Germann G, Reichenberger M. Latissimus dorsi flap. In: Wei FC, Mardini S, eds. Flaps and Reconstructive Surgery. Edinburgh: Elsevier; 2017:446–463

[12] Tobin GR, Schusterman M, Peterson GH, Nichols G, Bland KI. The intramuscular neurovascular anatomy of the latissimus dorsi muscle: the basis for splitting the flap. Plast Reconstr Surg. 1981; 67(5):637–641

[13] Mathes SJ, Nahai F. Classification of the vascular anatomy of muscles: experimental and clinical correlation. Plast Reconstr Surg. 1981; 67(2):177–187

[14] Levin LS. The latissimus dorsi muscle-musculocutaneous flap. (Discussion). In: Serafin D, ed. Atlas of Microsurgical Composite Tissue Transplantation. Philadelphia, PA: W.B. Saunders; 1996:218–219

[15] Taylor GI, Gianoutsos MP, Morris SF. The neurovascular territories of the skin and muscles: anatomic study and clinical implications. Plast Reconstr Surg. 1994; 94(1):1–36

[16] Elzawawy EM, Kelada MN, Al Karmouty AF. Design of mini latissimus dorsi flap based on thoracodorsal vascular patterns. Ann Plast Surg. 2018; 80(6): 607–615

[17] Miyamoto S, Fujiki M, Sakuraba M. Clinical analysis of 33 flow-through latissimus dorsi flaps. J Plast Reconstr Aesthet Surg. 2015; 68(10):1425–1431

[18] Barton RM, Vasconez LO. Microvascular free transfer of a latissimus dorsi muscle and musculocutaneous flap. In: Strauch B, Vasconez LO, Herman CK, Lee BT, eds. Grabb's Encyclopedia of Flaps. 4th ed. Philadelphia, PA: Wolters Kluwer; 2016:1397–1400

[19] Hallock GG. The combined parascapular fasciocutaneous and latissimus dorsi muscle conjoined free flap. Plast Reconstr Surg. 2008; 121(1):101–107

[20] Lee KT, Wiraatmadja ES, Mun GH. Free latissimus dorsi muscle-chimeric thoracodorsal artery perforator flaps for reconstruction of complicated defects: does muscle still have a place in the domain of perforator flaps? Ann Plast Surg. 2015; 74(5):565–572

[21] Kim SW, Youn DG, Kim JT, Kim YH. A thoracodorsal artery perforator chimeric free flap for prevention of microvascular pedicle compression in lower extremity reconstruction. Microsurgery. 2018; 38(1):46–50

[22] Schwabegger AH, Harpf C, Rainer C. Muscle-sparing latissimus dorsi myocutaneous flap with maintenance of muscle innervation, function, and aesthetic appearance of the donor site. Plast Reconstr Surg. 2003; 111(4):1407–1411

[23] Hallock GG. Restoration of quadriceps femoris function with a dynamic microsurgical free latissimus dorsi muscle transfer. Ann Plast Surg. 2004; 52(1):89–92

[24] Rednam RS, Rinker BD. Reconstruction of posterior compartment of lower extremity using a functional latissimus dorsi free flap: a case report. Microsurgery. 2016; 36(1):77–80

[25] Patel KM, Mantell M, Sosin M, Ramineni P. Chimeric functional latissimus flap transfer to restore ankle dorsiflexion following a traumatic defect of the lower leg: a case report. J Reconstr Microsurg. 2014; 30(4):279–282

[26] Hallock GG. Permutations of combined free flaps using the subscapular system. J Reconstr Microsurg. 1997; 13(1):47–54

[27] Hallock GG. The chimera flap: a quarter century odyssey. Ann Plast Surg. 2017; 78(2):223–229

[28] Kim SW, Jeon SB, Hwang KT, Kim YH. Coverage of amputation stumps using a latissimus dorsi flap with a serratus anterior muscle flap: a comparative study. Ann Plast Surg. 2016; 76(1):88–93

[29] Junnila J, Repo JP, Mustonen A, Tukiainen EJ. Treatment of compound tibial fracture with free osteomuscular latissimus dorsi scapula flap. J Reconstr Microsurg. 2015; 31(3):217–224

[30] Ozcan Akcal A, Ünal K, Gorgulu T, Akif Akcal M, Bigat Z. Reconstruction of midfoot bone and soft tissue loss with chimeric partial scapula and latissimus dorsi muscle flap and short perforator-based skin flap following gunshot injuries: report of two cases. Microsurgery. 2016; 36(7):598–603

[31] Trignano E, Fallico N, Nitto A, Chen HC. The treatment of composite defect of bone and soft tissues with a combined latissimus dorsi and serratus anterior and rib free flap. Microsurgery. 2013; 33(3):173–183

[32] Al-Ani SA, Soumian S, Zapantioti P, Sterne GD. Latissimus dorsi donor-site morbidity: the combination of quilting and fibrin sealant reduce length of drain placement and seroma rate. Ann Plast Surg. 2014; 72(6):729–730

[33] Kiiski J, Kaartinen I, Kotaluoto S, Kuokkanen H. Modified approach for endoscopic harvest of the latissimus dorsi free flap with CO2 insufflation and standard laparoscopic equipment. Microsurgery. 2017; 37(5):383–387

[34] Zhang YX, Messmer C, Pang FK, et al. A novel design of the multilobed latissimus dorsi myocutaneous flap to achieve primary donor-site closure in the reconstruction of large defects. Plast Reconstr Surg. 2013; 131(5):752e–758e

[35] Miyamoto S, Kayano S, Fujiki M, Kamizono K, Fukunaga Y, Sakuraba M. Flow-through divided latissimus dorsi musculocutaneous flap for large extremity defects. Ann Plast Surg. 2015; 74(2):199–203

[36] Zhang YX, Hayakawa TJ, Levin LS, Hallock GG, Lazzeri D. The economy in autologous tissue transfer: part 1. The kiss flap technique. Plast Reconstr Surg. 2016; 137(3):1018–1030

[37] Hwang KT, Kim SW, Sung IH, Kim JT, Kim YH. Is delayed reconstruction using the latissimus dorsi free flap a worthy option in the management of open IIIB tibial fractures? Microsurgery. 2016; 36(6):453–459

16.5 Chapter 16D: The Medial Sural Artery Perforator Flap

Geoffrey G. Hallock

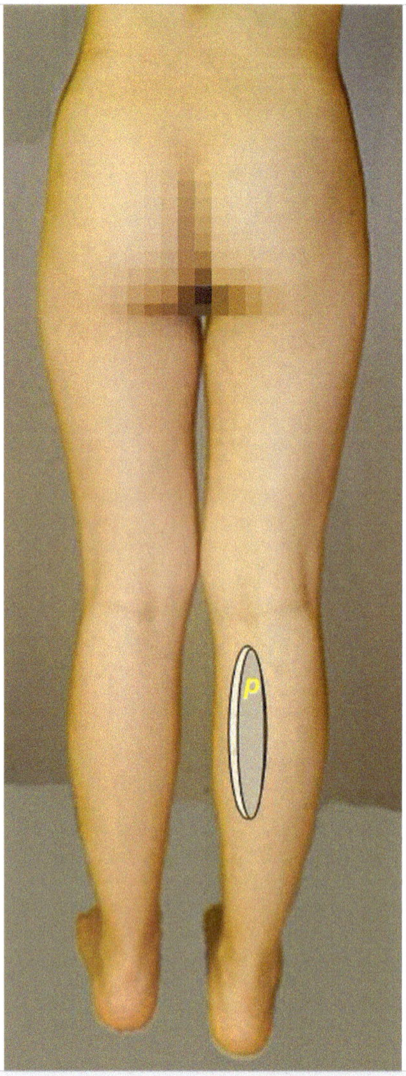

Fig. 16.18 The medial sural artery perforator flap.

16.5.1 Introduction to the Medial Sural Artery Perforator Flap

The medial sural artery perforator (MSAP) flap (▶ Fig. 16.18) essentially captures the skin territory of the more traditional medial gastrocnemius musculocutaneous flap. In their quest for donor site alternatives to the groin flap during the nascent era of microvascular tissue transfers, Taylor and Daniel[1] demonstrated in cadavers that the calf skin theoretically could be nourished by a musculocutaneous perforator of the medial gastrocnemius muscle. Montegut and Allen[2] presented the topographic anatomy of this region, but not until Hallock[3] specifically outlined the anatomy for its use as a potential perforator flap, followed by a clinical series by Cavadas et al[4] would the MSAP flap prove to have valuable clinical applications.

One of only a few lower extremity flap donor site options that have a potentially long vascular pedicle, allowing an island flap configuration, the MSAP flap can possibly reach even as far proximal as the patella (see Chapter 15A: The Island Perforator Flap).[4] However, more often its role has been as a free flap for the head and neck,[5,6] hand,[7] upper extremity,[8] or elsewhere in the lower limb.[9] It is one of few reliable skin flaps possible to harvest with the patient in a prone position.[10] The flap is relatively thin even in the obese individual,[11,12] with many selecting its use in preference to a radial forearm flap as no major source artery needs to be sacrificed.[5] If the reconstruction is limited to the lower extremity, epidural anesthesia alone is possible, which avoids the risks of general anesthesia.[11]

Some consider the residual calf donor site scar even after a primary closure to be a contraindication for selection of the MSAP flap, especially in the female patient (▶ Fig. 16.19). A legitimate exception to this rule might be its use for an ipsilateral distal lower extremity defect, as this untoward donor site morbidity would be limited to the same body region that already has been compromised (▶ Fig. 16.20).[13]

16.5.2 Attributes and Detriments

Attributes

- Function preservation.
- Supine or prone position skin flap donor site.
- Local flap for knee region.
- Thin free flap, substitute for radial forearm flap.
- Long vascular pedicle of large caliber.
- Superb choice for ipsilateral lower extremity defect requiring a free flap.
- Chimeric flap possibilities as when combined with the medial gastrocnemius muscle.

Detriments

- Significant donor site scar residue.
- Small surface area size.
- Relatively small perforators.

16.5.3 Anatomical Considerations

The medial sural artery is a branch of the popliteal artery, originating at or about the knee joint, which then passes for a few centimeters before entering the undersurface of the medial gastrocnemius muscle. Unfortunately, there is no consensus as to the ultimate distribution of the major medial sural artery musculocutaneous perforators,[3,9,11,14,15,16,17] but this may be best summarized by a classification schema devised by Dusseldorp et al.[17] They described three intramuscular branching patterns of the medial sural artery, with dual branches being the most common that can run superficial (posterior) or deep to the muscle surface. A clinically usable major perforator arising from these branches was found in 92% of cadaver dissections,[17] whereas Hallock found at least one in every specimen.[3] These perforators were found on average to be 13 ± 2 cm below the popliteal crease, and 2.5 ± 1 cm from the posterior midline,[17] although this can be highly variable.[10,14,16] Depending on the location of the perforator, the MSAP flap pedicle could range in

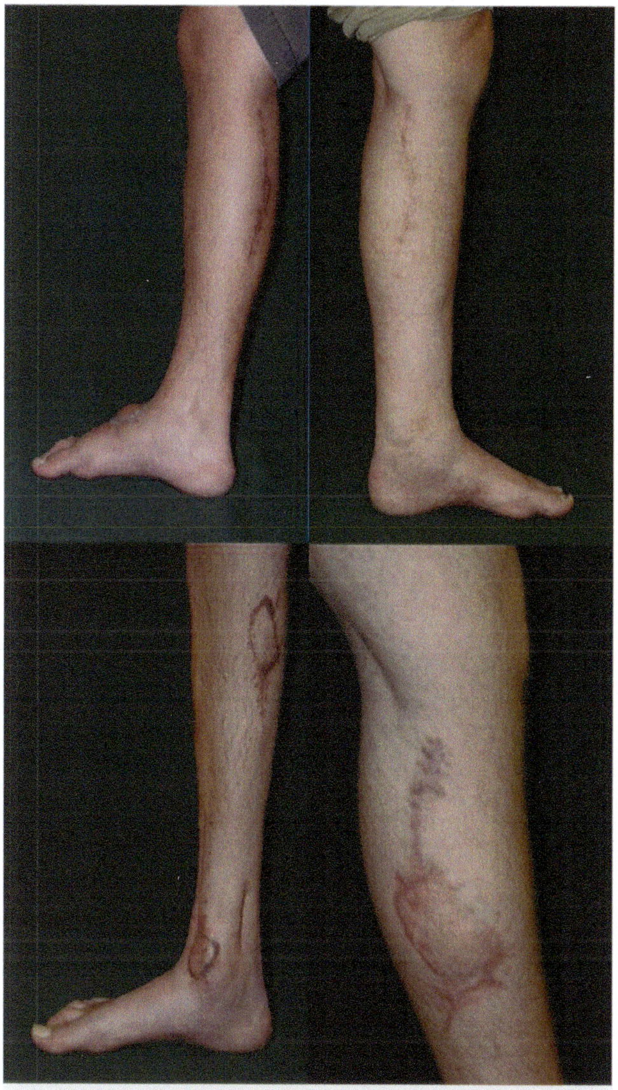

Fig. 16.19 Even a linear scar of the calf (upper two images) after closure of the medial sural artery perforator flap may be unacceptable. This is even worse if a skin graft were necessary (lower two images), but is not much better than the appearance of the flap on the dorsum of the right foot (lower left), suggesting that at least for the ipsilateral defect the overall residue may be not so unreasonable.

length from 9 to 16 cm. Venous outflow follows the course of the perforators. The flap is usually an insensate flap.

16.5.4 Anatomical Variations and Potential Pitfalls

Perforator Anomalies

Variations in the anatomical location of major medial sural artery musculocutaneous perforators are the norm to be expected. Unlike the better known anterolateral thigh flap where preoperative coordinates where most perforators can be expected are very reliable, no similar diagram is consistent for the MSAP flap.[18] For that matter, Dusseldorp et al[17] found that in those specimens without any major MSAP at all there was always a substantial median sural artery or sometimes a lateral sural artery perforator that would suffice instead.

Subfascial Approach

Unlike most perforator flaps where a suprafascial dissection may be preferable, a subfascial dissection of the MSAP flap is safer. Probably to compensate for muscle contraction during ambulation with concomitant perforator stretching, the course of the perforator after it leaves the external muscle border until it pierces the deep fascia may ramble in a coiled fashion for several centimeters like a spring that will recoil without harm. Thus, preoperative imaging studies such as CT angiography, MRA, color duplex ultrasound, and even the ubiquitous handheld audible Doppler may incorrectly target the course of the perforator and its actual perforasome. This confusion can best be overcome by direct visualization of the perforator using endoscopic assistance,[19] most easily done in the subfascial plane (▶ Fig. 16.21). However, of course, this must be at the time of the surgery.

Perforator Selection

Another concern, as is always true with perforator flaps, is how to choose a proper MSAP even once visualized. This would be easy if there were but a solitary perforator, thereby not allowing any choice, or if the visualized venae comitantes were 1.0 mm or larger. However, more often than not there are multiple perforators, which if threadlike are inconsequential and should be discarded. In general, even what is considered an adequate MSAP will be smaller than those of the more conventional perforator flaps, and the dissection therefore more difficult. If a large perforator artery, for example, greater than 0.5 mm caliber, is not found, it would be best to include at least two smaller perforators that line up along the same sagittal line and spread as far apart as possible to nourish disparate ends of the desired flap territory. Inclusion of two perforators is also a reasonable safety factor in case one were injured during the subsequent dissection, and better ensures that twist of the pedicle does not later occur —especially a problem if the flap were to be moved elsewhere as a free flap! Dissection of these multiple perforators will require spreading of the muscle fibers between them, which, again unlike the muscle underlying other major perforator flaps, usually separate easily since that is also the normal vertical direction of the medial gastrocnemius muscle fibers and as such rarely requires any direct cutting of the muscle.

Flap Orientation

Since interconnections between perforasomes in the lower extremity are oriented in a longitudinal direction as Saint-Cyr et al[20] have shown, the major axis of any MSAP flap should also parallel that pattern. If obliquely oriented, the distal portion of the flap, which may cross into a neighboring angiosome, may then otherwise not survive.

16.5.5 Flap Design

The design of the desired MSAP flap must follow a template made of the defect. Next, a rough estimate of the site of the perforator that will service the flap is determined. Although color duplex ultrasound may be better,[15] the handheld audible Doppler is more likely available and sometimes adequate for this purpose. Kim et al,[14] Wang et al,[9] and Wong et al[16] have suggested a series of lines that intersect to facilitate a

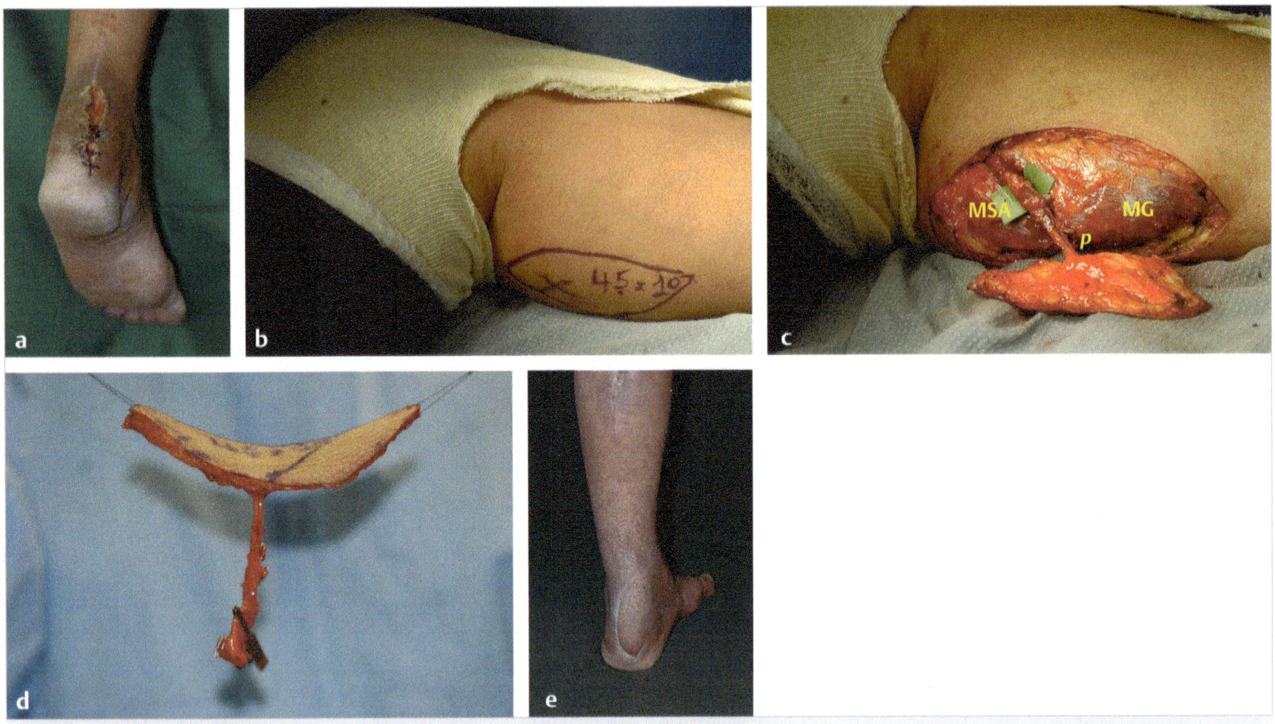

Fig. 16.20 **(a)** Truck door injury with subsequent disruption of left Achilles tendon repair seen weeks later. **(b)** Design of medial sural artery perforator (MSAP) flap on the ipsilateral calf, eccentric to perforator "x" to obtain longer vascular pedicle. **(c)** In situ island MSAP flap based on single perforator (*p*) branching from the MSA unroofed through the medial gastrocnemius (MG) muscle. **(d)** MSAP free flap. **(e)** Thin contour of healed MSAP flap padding posterior hindfoot, with conspicuous wide scar of donor site partially seen above.

beginning point for the identification of the requisite perforator, but are not as pragmatic an idea as those Kao et al[5] have proposed. The latter draw three lines, that is, transversely along the popliteal crease, from the midpoint of that line to bisect the calcaneus, and finally a curved line along the distal border of the belly of the medial gastrocnemius muscle (▶ Fig. 16.22). This, of course, outlines where that latter muscle is, and the perforator of choice will also be within those lines, which in reality is anywhere the muscle is. Usually, fortunately, the perforator will be in the upper 8 cm of the medial gastrocnemius muscle, which should serve as the starting point for its identification.

The actual design of the flap cannot be determined until the precise location where the perforator pierces the deep fascia is known. Through an exploratory aperture along the most anterior border of the flap, if the patient is supine, a subfascially placed endoscope will allow its actual visualization (▶ Fig. 16.21). If a long pedicle is necessary, the template is placed eccentrically distal to that point to form an ellipse with a vertical axis (▶ Fig. 16.20). If two reasonable and spread-out perforators are found, an independent narrow flap can be designed about each, keeping the perforators joined later only by a common branch of the medial sural artery pedicle. When transferred as free flaps, they can then be joined side by side at the recipient defect to cover a larger surface area; yet this maneuver allows primary donor site closure following the "kiss" principle of Zhang et al.[21] Depending on the skin elasticity of the calf, if the width of the flap otherwise exceeds 5 cm, a skin graft will inevitably be required to avoid the risk of a compartment syndrome.[5]

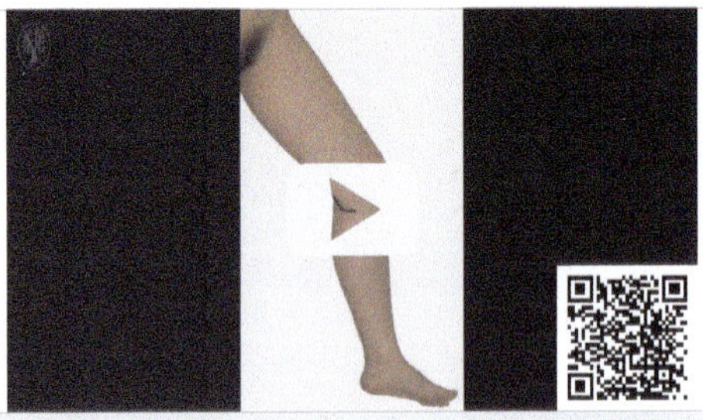

Video 16.5 Medial Sural Artery Perforator Flap Harvest. https://www.thieme.de/de/q.htm?p=opn/cs/20/7/12265279-6546c2f5

Note that the largest MSAP flap as reported by Wang et al[9] was 9 cm wide and 14 cm long.

16.5.6 Flap Harvest

Most commonly, the patient will be in the supine position with the thigh abducted, lower extremity externally rotated, and knee flexed, but the lower limb will maintain a neutral posture if in the prone position. The limb is exsanguinated only by elevation to maintain fill of venae comitantes for their better visualization after inflation of a mid-thigh tourniquet, and to also ensure a bloodless field that will not obscure perforators during their dissection. A small exploratory opening is made along the more medial border of the estimated flap design, directly anterior to where the presumed flap perforator was found using an audible Doppler. The subcutaneous tissues and deep fascia are incised directly downward to expose the medial gastrocnemius muscle (see ▶ Video 16.5). If in the prone position, this

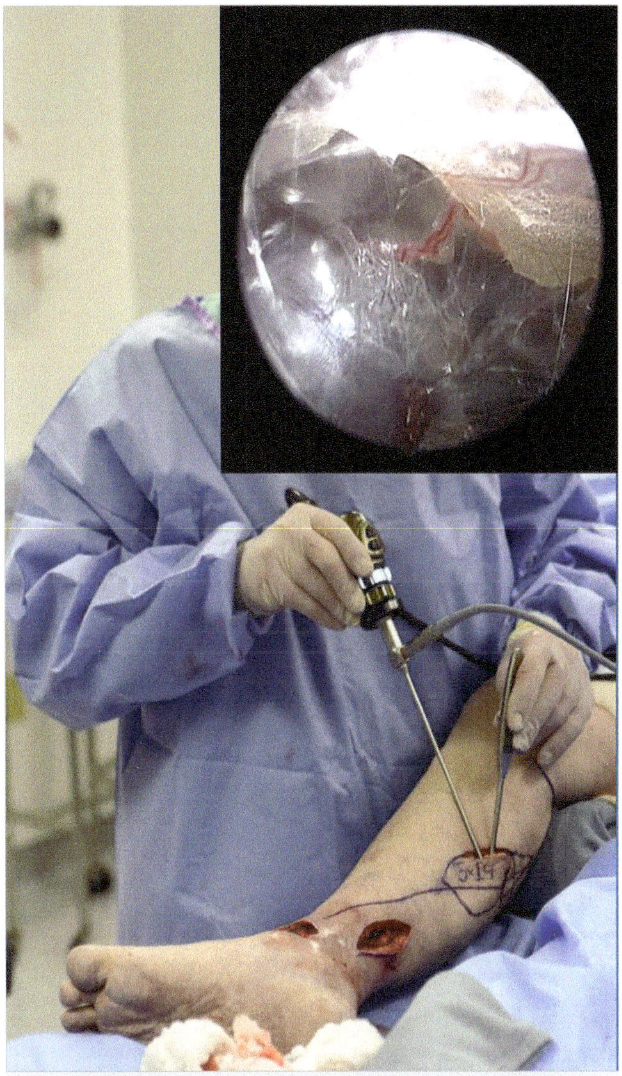

Fig. 16.21 Subfascial endoscopic approach through an exploratory incision anterior to presumed perforator site found with audible Doppler, with monitor view showing perforator seen exiting the muscle (upper right) to enter deep fascia (lower left).

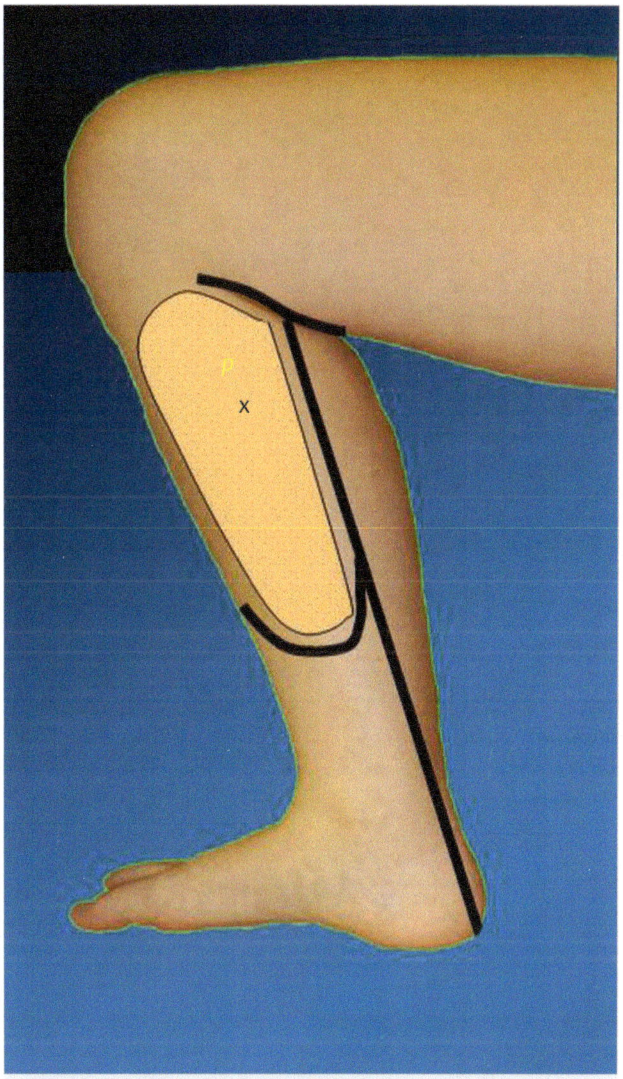

Fig. 16.22 A realistic schematic for finding a dominant medial sural artery perforator (MSAP) using a handheld audible Doppler as proposed by Kao et al.[5] A line is drawn in the popliteal crease.
From its midpoint, a vertical line descends to bisect the calcaneus.
A third line curves along the inferior border of the belly of the medial gastrocnemius muscle. Note that this shaded area essentially encompasses the entire medial head of the gastrocnemius muscle, apropos as anomalies of the location of an MSAP are to be anticipated, but usually found within 8 cm of the popliteal crease as suggested by the "x" site.

approach will be easier instead starting via the lateral border of the proposed flap near the posterior midline. The exploratory incision used must be large enough to allow introduction of a short 5-mm, 30-degree endoscope and a narrow rigid retractor that can press down on the muscle while the endoscope is advanced to locate the perforator (▶ Fig. 16.21).

Once the desired perforator location has been verified by transillumination, the boundaries of the flap are redrawn as necessary. To complete the supine position approach, the exploratory incision is extended to include the entire medial flap boundary. Rapid subfascial exploration in this bloodless plane by pushing away the medial gastrocnemius muscle should confirm the dimensions of the perforator seen by the endoscope plus any others that may be reasonable to retain. Only the most proximal and distal portions of the lateral border of the flap are next incised to allow the flap to fall posteriorly with unimpeded exposure of the perforator(s) as they exit the muscle. Retention of a central portion of the lateral border of the flap while supporting it on a stack of towels will prevent the flap from falling totally upon the operating table and thereby irreversibly stretching the perforator(s).

The tedious intramuscular dissection of the perforator(s) down to its medial sural artery branch then begins per routine. Fortunately, gently spreading apart of the medial gastrocnemius muscle fibers above and below the entry point of the perforator (s) will easily unroof their path to the deeper course of the branch of the MSAP source vessel. A vessel loop around this vascular branch allows traction for then complete circumferential pedicle dissection. Anything that does not separate easily by blunt dissection probably is a vascular branch and should be coagulated with bipolar cautery, or a motor nerve that must be identified and preserved. This dissection of the source pedicle continues proximally until the desired pedicle length or vessel caliber (if a free flap) is reached. If a chimeric flap including a portion of the medial gastrocnemius muscle as a combined flap is desired,[22] the distal end of the medial sural branch is not ligated, but followed distally as long as needed to where it nourishes a portion of muscle of the desired dimensions that will be harvested separately. If used as a local MSAP flap, pedicle length must be sufficient so that advancement is possible without tension.

At this point, the MSAP flap is an in situ island flap. The tourniquet is deflated, and flap perfusion is assessed. Application of vasodilators may be helpful. Bleeding points should be controlled. Once adequate, a local flap can be inset. If chosen as a free flap, the pedicle is divided as is customary. The medial gastrocnemius muscle rent is closed with a running absorbable suture. No attempt is made to close the deep fascia. Primary skin approximation is completed; or, if not possible, a skin graft is placed on the muscle.

16.5.7 Postoperative Care Protocols

As with any perforator flap, pressure on the flap and its vascular pedicle or tension during insetting should be avoided so that compression on the narrow lumens of the perforators, especially veins, leading to thrombosis is prevented. If an island MSAP flap crosses the knee joint, a knee immobilizer may be prudent to avoid movement and stretching of the flap pedicle. For how long this must be worn is unknown, but caution for a few weeks until neovascularization is sufficient to make the flap pedicle independent is probably wise. If used as a microvascular tissue transfer, this flap should be treated as per the institutional protocols for any other free flap.

16.5.8 Conclusion

The MSAP flap has some distinctive attributes that deserve consideration. As a local flap, function preservation is possible as an alternative to the medial gastrocnemius muscle for coverage of the proximal one-third of the lower leg. As a free flap, this is a relatively thin flap even in the more obese patient, and could supplant use of the radial forearm flap, which sacrifices a hand source artery.[5] The MSAP flap vascular pedicle can be long to reach most recipient sites outside a zone of injury, and has a large caliber that does not require supramicrosurgery. The same vascular pedicle can be used as a simpler recipient site for the knee region![23] Unfortunately, the exact location of acceptable perforators is variable, but this shortcoming is best overcome by using endoscopic visualization.[19] The major detriment is the obvious donor site closure residue even if just a scar, which would understandably be unacceptable for a woman (▶ Fig. 16.19). Nevertheless, indications for selecting the MSAP free flap may best be justifiable for the ipsilateral lower extremity defect requiring a microsurgical tissue transfer, as all disfigurement including that of the donor site would be restricted to the same extremity.[13] Some even believe its potential versatility has now made this a workhorse flap that always deserves consideration.[24]

References

[1] Taylor GI, Daniel RK. The anatomy of several free flap donor sites. Plast Reconstr Surg. 1975; 56(3):243–253

[2] Montegut WJ, Allen RJ. Sural Artery Perforator Flap as an Alternative for the Gastrocnemius Myocutaneous Flap. 90th Annual Scientific Assembly of the Southern Medical Association. Baltimore, MD: November 20–24, 1996

[3] Hallock GG. Anatomic basis of the gastrocnemius perforator-based flap. Ann Plast Surg. 2001; 47(5):517–522

[4] Cavadas PC, Sanz-Giménez-Rico JR, Gutierrez-de la Cámara A, Navarro-Monzonís A, Soler-Nomdedeu S, Martínez-Soriano F. The medial sural artery perforator free flap. Plast Reconstr Surg. 2001; 108(6):1609–1615, discussion 1616–1617

[5] Kao HK, Chang KP, Wei FC, Cheng MH. Comparison of the medial sural artery perforator flap with the radial forearm flap for head and neck reconstructions. Plast Reconstr Surg. 2009; 124(4):1125–1132

[6] Shen H, Shen XQ, Lv Y, Xu JH, Lu H. Pharyngoesophageal reconstruction with the medial sural artery perforator flap after total laryngopharyngectomy: a new method. Ann Plast Surg. 2017; 78(2):191–194

[7] Lin CH, Lin CH, Lin YT, Hsu CC, Ng TW, Wei FC. The medial sural artery perforator flap: a versatile donor site for hand reconstruction. J Trauma. 2011; 70(3): 736–743

[8] Ives M, Mathur B. Varied uses of the medial sural artery perforator flap. J Plast Reconstr Aesthet Surg. 2015; 68(6):853–858

[9] Wang X, Mei J, Pan J, Chen H, Zhang W, Tang M. Reconstruction of distal limb defects with the free medial sural artery perforator flap. Plast Reconstr Surg. 2013; 131(1):95–105

[10] Hallock GG, Sano K. The medial sural$_{\text{MEDIAL GASTROCNEMIUS}}$ perforator free flap: an "ideal" prone position skin flap. Ann Plast Surg. 2004; 52(2):184–187

[11] Xie XT, Chai YM. Medial sural artery perforator flap. Ann Plast Surg. 2012; 68(1):105–110

[12] Akdeniz Doğan ZD, Çavuş Özkan M, Tuncer FB, Saçak B, Çelebiler Ö. A comparative clinical study of flap thickness: medial sural artery perforator flap versus anterolateral thigh flap. Ann Plast Surg. 2018; 81(4):472–474

[13] Hallock GG. Medial sural artery perforator free flap: legitimate use as a solution for the ipsilateral distal lower extremity defect. J Reconstr Microsurg. 2014; 30(3):187–192

[14] Kim HH, Jeong JH, Seul JH, Cho BC. New design and identification of the medial sural perforator flap: an anatomical study and its clinical applications. Plast Reconstr Surg. 2006; 117(5):1609–1618

[15] Kosutic D, Pejkovic B, Anderhuber F, et al. Complete mapping of lateral and medial sural artery perforators: anatomical study with Duplex-Doppler ultrasound correlation. J Plast Reconstr Aesthet Surg. 2012; 65(11):1530–1536

[16] Wong MZ, Wong CH, Tan BK, Chew KY, Tay SC. Surgical anatomy of the medial sural artery perforator flap. J Reconstr Microsurg. 2012; 28(8):555–560

[17] Dusseldorp JR, Pham QJ, Ngo Q, Gianoutsos M, Moradi P. Vascular anatomy of the medial sural artery perforator flap: a new classification system of intramuscular branching patterns. J Plast Reconstr Aesthet Surg. 2014; 67(9): 1267–1275

[18] Hallock GG. A primer of schematics to facilitate the design of the preferred muscle perforator flaps. Plast Reconstr Surg. 2009; 123(3):1107–1115

[19] Shen XQ, Lv Y, Shen H, Lu H, Wu SC, Lin XJ. Endoscope-assisted medial sural artery perforator flap for head and neck reconstruction. J Plast Reconstr Aesthet Surg. 2016; 69(8):1059–1065

[20] Saint-Cyr M, Wong C, Schaverien M, Mojallal A, Rohrich RJ. The perforasome theory: vascular anatomy and clinical implications. Plast Reconstr Surg. 2009; 124(5):1529–1544

[21] Zhang YX, Hayakawa TJ, Levin LS, Hallock GG, Lazzeri D. The economy in autologous tissue transfer: part 1. The kiss flap technique. Plast Reconstr Surg. 2016; 137(3):1018–1030

[22] Han SE, Lee KT, Mun GH. Muscle-chimaeric medial sural artery perforator flap: a new design for complex three-dimensional knee defect. J Plast Reconstr Aesthet Surg. 2014; 67(4):571–574

[23] Smith ML, Molina BJ, Dayan E, Kim JN, Kagen A, Dayan JH. Use of distal medial sural vessels as recipient vessels in free tissue transfer. J Reconstr Microsurg. 2017; 33(1):59–62

[24] Daar DA, Abdou SA, Cohen JM, Wilson SC, Levine JP. Is the medial sural artery perforator flap a new workhorse flap? A systematic review and meta-analysis. Plast Reconstr Surg. 2019; 143(2):393e–403e

16.6 Chapter 16E: The Thoracodorsal Artery Perforator Free Flap

Geoffrey G. Hallock

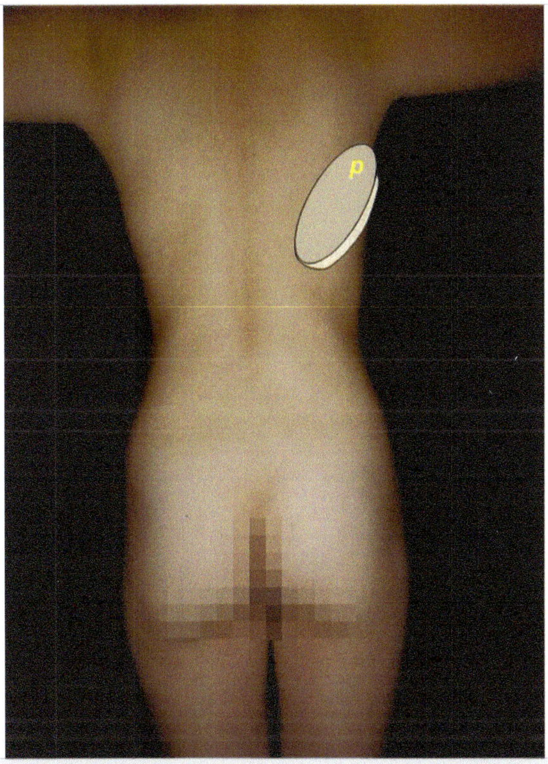

Fig. 16.23 The thoracodorsal artery perforator flap.

16.6.1 Introduction to the Thoracodorsal Artery Perforator Free Flap

Only a century ago, random skin flaps raised in the axilla were notorious for inconsistent distal necrosis. This prompted Tansini[1] (1906) to include the latissimus dorsi (LD) muscle with the overlying skin as a local musculocutaneous flap. He thought the more reliable blood supply so obtained was because he always kept a perforator from the circumflex scapular artery, but did not recognize the importance of the musculocutaneous perforators from the LD muscle itself. Taylor and Daniel,[2] after their first successful free composite tissue transfer,[3] sought other donor site alternatives in cadavers including inspection of the axilla. There they found musculocutaneous perforators to the overlying skin that could be dissected through the LD muscle to the thoracodorsal source pedicle just as done in routine perforator flap surgery today, as well as sometimes direct cutaneous branches from the same source vessel that skirted around the lateral muscle border that may now be considered paramuscular perforators.[4] Baudet et al[5] then clinically transferred successfully what they called "free thoracodorsal axillary flaps," based on either these same LD musculocutaneous perforators or what they called a direct cutaneous branch from the thoracodorsal, exactly as Taylor and Daniel had found.[2] Yet the credit for demonstrating a true perforator dissection through the LD muscle to create the thoracodorsal artery perforator (TDAP) flap (▶ Fig. 16.23) belongs to Angrigiani et al[6,7] who were seeking a way to reduce the bulk of the LD musculocutaneous flap by totally eliminating the muscle. The now-accepted nomenclature of this flap as the "TDAP flap" follows the Ghent consensus that was devised by the faculty of the International Course for Perforator Flaps.[8]

Many have accepted the TDAP flap even in place of the LD muscle flap itself not just because there is reduced bulk; but also because there is function preservation, which is the sine qua non of perforator flaps in general, donor site complications like seroma are much less,[9] and the aesthetic result is superior to a skin grafted muscle flap.[10] Much of the dorsal thoracic fascia can also be served by the cutaneous branches of the circumflex scapular system as an alternative; but the TDAP flap has a much longer pedicle, the dissection of the former through the triangular space is more difficult, and with a preferable transverse-oriented design hypertrophic or wide scars are less frequent, while the TDAP flap itself thereby may be even thinner.[11]

The TDAP flap as a pedicled flap can resurface the axilla, upper arm and elbow, lateral chest, shoulder area, and breast.[12,13] As a free flap, it has been used for all body regions including partial or total breast reconstruction,[14,15] tubed for the esophagus,[16] throughout the lower extremity,[10,17,18,19,20] and even to preserve toes[21] and fingers.[22] This is all possible with almost no donor site morbidity as there is minimal impairment of shoulder function and a scar well hidden by clothing.[11]

16.6.2 Attributes and Detriments

Attributes

- Skin territory as large as the LD musculocutaneous flap.
- Function preservation.
- Regional pedicled flap.
- Versatile free flap.
- Long vascular pedicle of large caliber.
- Possible thin contour.
- Potentially sensate.
- Vascular flow-through possibility.
- Chimeric flaps as part of the subscapular axis.
- Minimal donor site morbidity.
- Hidden scar.

Detriments

- Arterial anomalies commonplace in the axilla.
- Musculocutaneous perforators may be diminutive.
- Sensitive to congestion.
- Vertical flap design can lead to lateral displacement of the nipple–areola complex.
- Perforator verification difficult in obese patients.
- Hypertrophic donor site scarring.

16.6.3 Anatomical Considerations

The TDAP flap as a "true" perforator flap[23] is nourished by musculocutaneous perforators of the underlying LD muscle. Most major LD perforators arise from the descending branch of the thoracodorsal artery. In the original cadaver study by Angrigiani et al,[7] the mean position of the proximal and usually dominant perforator of the descending branch was found 8 cm below the posterior axillary fold and 2 cm posterior to the lateral free border of the muscle. That border is an important landmark to discern preoperatively, facilitated by forceful contraction of the muscle while the patient is erect with hands on their hips, as often then it is easily palpable. However, note that Mun et al[24] based on intraoperative topography found the most proximal perforator to be always present but highly variable in location, being a mean of 10.1 cm from the posterior axillary fold (range: 5.0–15.7), and 1.6 cm (range: 0.5–2.9) inward from the lateral LD muscle border. These findings were corroborated by Schaverien et al[25] in their microanatomical studies in fresh cadavers. Venous outflow was found to have a polygonal patterned network within the subdermal plexus that then fed into the deep system to join the venae comitantes that accompanied the perforator arteries.[25]

Once an acceptable perforator is identified, retrograde dissection to the descending branch can continue to the bifurcation of the thoracodorsal artery at the vascular hilum, or even to the latter's origin, which usually is the subscapular artery, if additional pedicle length or greater vessel caliber is required.[26] Thus, a pedicle length of 14 to 18 cm is possible,[12,27,28] with mean caliber of the artery 2.7 mm and vein 3.4 cm.[29]

16.6.4 Anatomical Variations and Potential Pitfalls

Vascular Supply

Kim,[16,30] in an extensive study, showed that the actual vascular supply to the skin of the lateral thoracic region between the lateral borders of the LD and pectoralis major (PM) muscles can be quite confusing. He found that there are at least three distinct columns of potential perforator patterns that are all interconnected, with consequently a high variation of dominance. The most posterior column is from musculocutaneous perforators usually from the descending branch of the thoracodorsal artery that traverse the LD muscle. More anterior to this is what he calls a septocutaneous perforator that originates from the thoracodorsal artery or serratus branch from 2 to 5 cm proximal to the LD muscle vascular hilum.[31] Some might call this a paramuscular perforator[16] as it travels between the serratus anterior and LD muscle before skirting around the lateral border of the latter to reach the skin, and occurs as often as 40% of the time or more.[16,25] Next is the lateral thoracic artery that has a variable origin and follows the lateral border of the PM muscle on the serratus anterior fascia before giving off a direct cutaneous branch. Of the three variations, this has the most diverse pattern of origin and can be quite diminutive with no associated vein.[32] Shin et al[32] even found, while raising a TDAP flap based on a second perforator of the LD muscle, that it was actually a direct cutaneous perforator from the lateral thoracic artery!

To make things even more complicated, Kim[16] found that 70% of the time there could be an accessory lateral thoracic artery that was a direct branch between the lateral thoracic artery origin and the subscapular artery that would run in the midaxillary line. He solves this anatomical dilemma by always making a vertical midaxillary incision for exploration to find an acceptable perforator first before designing any flap that is required.

Sensate Flaps

A sensate TDAP flap is only possible with a transverse design. Such a flap theoretically will regain tactile discrimination earlier than an insensate flap. The design must include the posterior divisions of the lateral cutaneous branches of intercostal nerves that course medially over the LD muscle to terminate in the subcutaneous tissues either separate or unrelated to the musculocutaneous perforators or joined with them.[22,33] Lin and Chen[22] in color Duplex ultrasound studies found that since the intercostal nerve branches accompany the intercostal arteries, if the latter were found not to accompany the course of the perforator, they would have a separate pattern, making finding and including them more difficult. In addition, they found that a quarter of the time there was no nerve available around the most proximal perforator, so a sensate TDAP flap would be impossible.[22]

Muscle Sparing

If an adequate LD musculocutaneous perforator is not present, but clusters of capillary perforators exist along the lateral border of the muscle as found using color Duplex ultrasound, that is, those with a caliber of 0.3 to 0.5 mm, then a cuff of muscle about them and the descending branch of the thoracodorsal will serve what Tashiro et al[34] call a $TDAP_{cp}$ flap (cp = capillary perforator). Sometimes keeping a small cuff of muscle even around larger perforators can be a safer method to preserve them during their harvest, which in no way would interfere with LD muscle function.[35,36]

Chimeric Thoracodorsal Artery Perforator Flaps

The TDAP flap, based on musculocutaneous or paramuscular perforators, would have access to the subscapular axis with its numerous branches to cutaneous flaps (e.g., scapular or parascapular), muscles (e.g., LD or serratus anterior), and bone (e.g., scapula via angular or descending branch of the circumflex scapular). This would allow the creation of over five dozen combinations and permutations of these flaps that each would have their own independent branch for independent insetting, but remain attached together only by the same source vessel: the subscapular vessels.[20] As such, if recipient sites are limited, as is frequently the case in the lower extremity, these multiple combinations of flaps would require only a single recipient site. The tremendous variability in options allows simultaneously three-dimensional fill, provision of multiple tissues each with different functions, as well as the potential for coverage of multiple sites.[32,37] Some examples include the LD muscle–TDAP flap (muscle–skin chimera),[18,38] serratus anterior muscle–TDAP flap (muscle–skin chimera),[10] scapula–TDAP flap (bone–skin chimera),[39] and LD muscle–TDAP flap–scapula (muscle–skin–bone chimera).[19] Caution must be observed as chimeric flaps are somewhat more difficult to harvest, and certainly monitoring of each component as a free flap is more challenging.

16.6.5 Flap Design

The perforasome captured by the dominant TDAP coincides with the dorsal thoracic fascia covering the LD muscle.[12] The TDAP flap can be designed in this region in any direction about the dominant LD musculocutaneous perforator that is found best by CT angiography[11] or color Duplex ultrasound.[22,34] Use of the handheld audible Doppler can be misleading due to the posterior course of these perforators once exiting the muscle[12] and from background noise from the descending branch itself.[40]

Anatomic landmarks to guide elevation of this flap are inconsistent (▶ Fig. 16.24), but two important landmarks are the tip of the scapula near the upper LD muscle border and often the lateral border of the LD muscle that can be grasped through the subcutaneous tissues or seen during forceful contraction with the patient erect with hands on their hips. With the patient in the position that will be used during the surgery, a line dropped 8 to 10 cm from the posterior axillary fold along this lateral muscle border, then 1.5 cm inward, would be a good starting point to find this perforator.

A transverse flap orientation that captures the looser skin of the mid-flank will permit the easiest closure and least scarring.[18] It matters not that the flap has an eccentric or centrally located perforator,[41] but it is best to be somewhat anterior to the LD muscle lateral border with any design to ensure capture of not only the requisite musculocutaneous perforator, but also any visualization of other vascular pattern variations known to occur in this region.[16] The width of the flap should be that which can be pinched together, and usually less than 10 cm, as otherwise a skin graft or second flap would be necessary to close the donor site. A flap as long as 25 cm can safely survive on a single musculocutaneous perforator;[12] but if larger, either muscle would have to be included with the flap or more than one perforator.[30] In the latter case, the flap orientation would then have to be vertical to parallel the course of the descending branch where those perforators would be found (▶ Fig. 16.25).

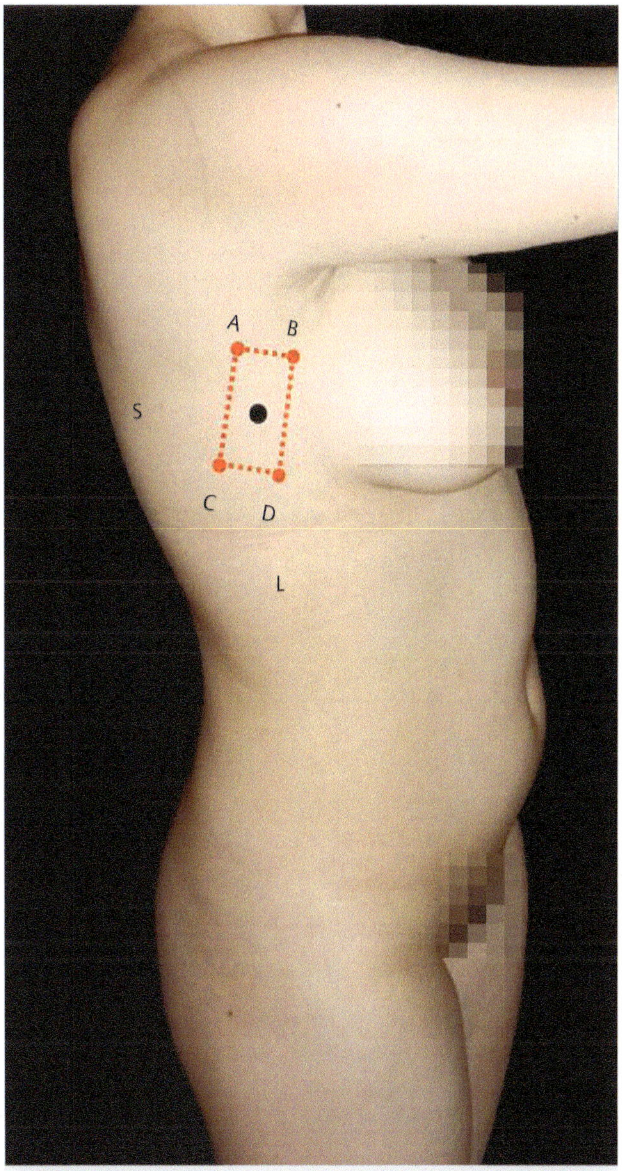

Fig. 16.24 Schematic to assist in finding the most proximal and usually dominant perforator (*black dot*) arising from the descending branch of the thoracodorsal artery, which will be the basis for a thoracodorsal artery perforator (TDAP) flap. Invariably, it will be located within a rectangle ABCD of height 11 cm and width 2.5 cm, centered 10 cm below the posterior axillary fold and 1.6 cm medial to the lateral free border (L) of the latissimus dorsi muscle (S, tip of the scapula).

16.6.6 Flap Harvest

The position on the operating table mainly depends on how readily the perforator supplying the flap will be identified (see ▶ Video 16.6). Kim et al[42] use the convenient supine position if the posterior tibial vessels will be the recipient site, or a semilateral position when instead the anterior tibial vessels are used, to facilitate their access and subsequent microvascular surgery. However, in the Western world where obesity is endemic, the lateral decubitus position that also allows access to both the defect and the recipient site, with the arm abducted 90 degrees at the shoulder and elbow flexed 90 degrees, is preferred.[12] The lateral border of the LD muscle is marked as is the site of the perforator determined by whatever preoperative method. The flap is temporarily designed about that site in whatever direction will satisfy both coverage of the defect and primary donor site closure. In all cases, the most lateral extension of that design should be anterior to the lateral border of the LD muscle.

In general, the incision and dissection should begin at the anteroinferior border of the flap proceeding through the subcutaneous tissues to identify the LD lateral border. With the flap

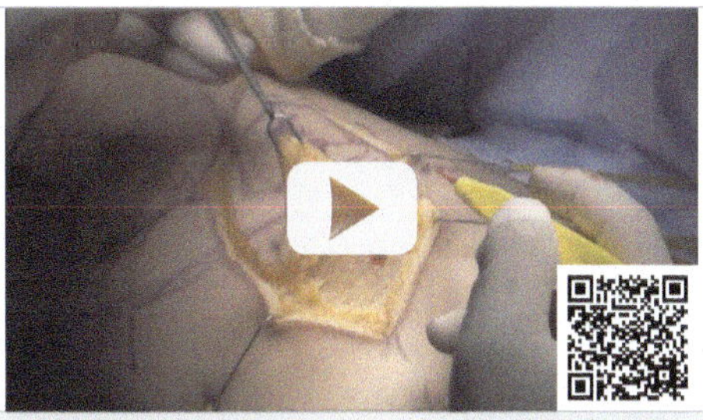

Video 16.6 TDAP Flap Harvest. https://www.thieme.de/de/q.htm?p=opn/cs/20/7/12265280-56208354

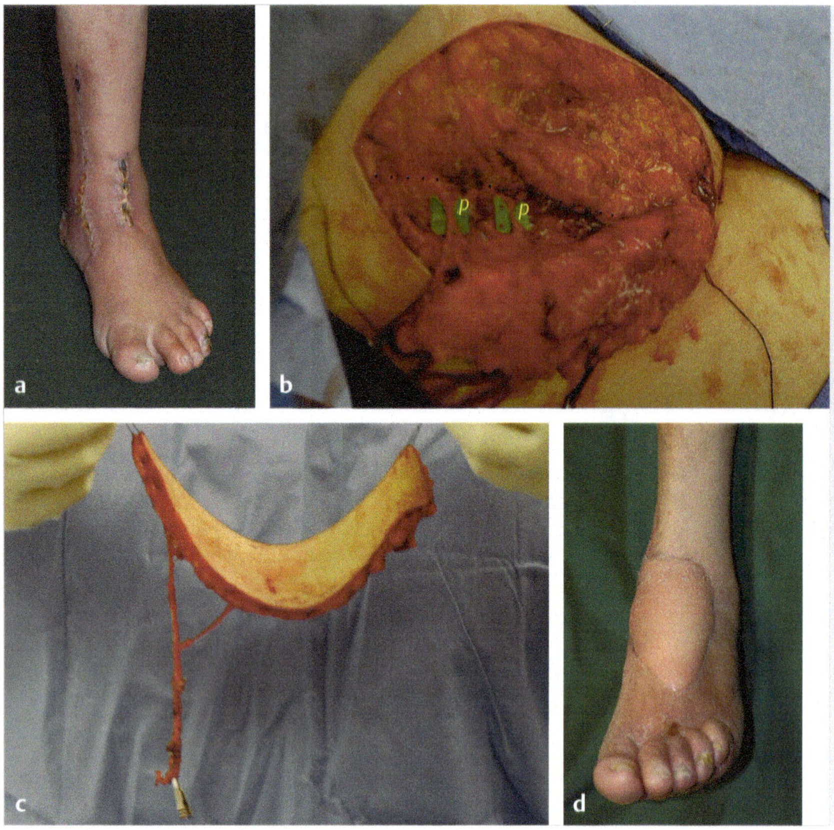

Fig. 16.25 (a) Exposed in situ bypass to the dorsalis pedis artery on the dorsum of the left foot after wound breakdown also involving the greater saphenous vein donor site. (b) in situ vertical orientated thoracodorsal artery perforator (TDAP) flap retracted posteriorly to demonstrate two musculocutaneous perforators (*p*) from the descending branch of the thoracodorsal artery, emanating just medial to the lateral border of the LD muscle (*dotted line*). (c) TDAP free flap based eccentrically on these two perforators to create a long vascular leash needed to reach the more proximal in situ bypass graft for end-to-side microanastomosis. (d) Satisfactory healing of both wounds on the dorsum of the left foot.

retracted posteriorly, dissection over the LD muscle continues cephalad carefully until the requisite perforator is identified and deemed adequate. If not, a more vertical dissection along the LD lateral border to seek out other perforators or even a muscle-sparing flap may have to be considered, usually with the flap boundaries then having to be redrawn. Once an adequate perforator is found, the remaining boundaries of the flap may be incised. Some will proceed in a superficial fascial plane as the flap is raised toward the perforator if immediate thinning is the goal.[16,20,42]

Next, the dissection of the perforator itself proceeds as with any perforator flap with its unroofing and intramuscular dissection back to the descending branch of the thoracodorsal vessels. Muscular branches are then cauterized with a bipolar, and the descending branch ligated distal to the takeoff of the perforator, while being careful to preserve any motor nerve branches. The descending branch is further unroofed and circumferentially raised back to the LD vascular hilum. Once external to the LD muscle, the extent of further pedicle lengthening will be determined by the reach needed to the recipient site[28] and desired vessel caliber. This can continue even back to the subscapular vessels from which the thoracodorsal vessels usually originate.[26] Now temporarily an island TDAP flap, once the defect and recipient site are ready, the vascular pedicle may be disconnected for transfer as a free flap.

16.6.7 Postoperative Care Protocols

Some believe that venous outflow from perforators in general is troublesome and flap congestion common, which often can be relieved by just elevation of the lower extremity until resolved.[16] This will also minimize swelling of the flap, where any tension or compression can compromise fragile perforator patency. Otherwise, precautions and monitoring as for any free flap should be observed.

16.6.8 Conclusion

As with any perforator flap, their major attribute is function preservation. For the TDAP flap, this would be the function of the LD muscle. The TDAP flap even based on a single perforator can be extremely large, and if thinned intraoperatively or in a delayed fashion, it is highly useful for almost any coverage problem in the lower extremity. The vascular pedicle length that is determined by the amount of intramuscular dissection done can be excessively long, to easily reach beyond any zone of injury, a distinct advantage over the circumflex scapular perforator flap that can similarly capture the dorsal thoracic fascia (▶ Fig. 16.26). Since usually dependent on the thoracodorsal artery, multiple flap combinations utilizing branches of the subscapular axis allow creation of chimeric or conjoined flaps

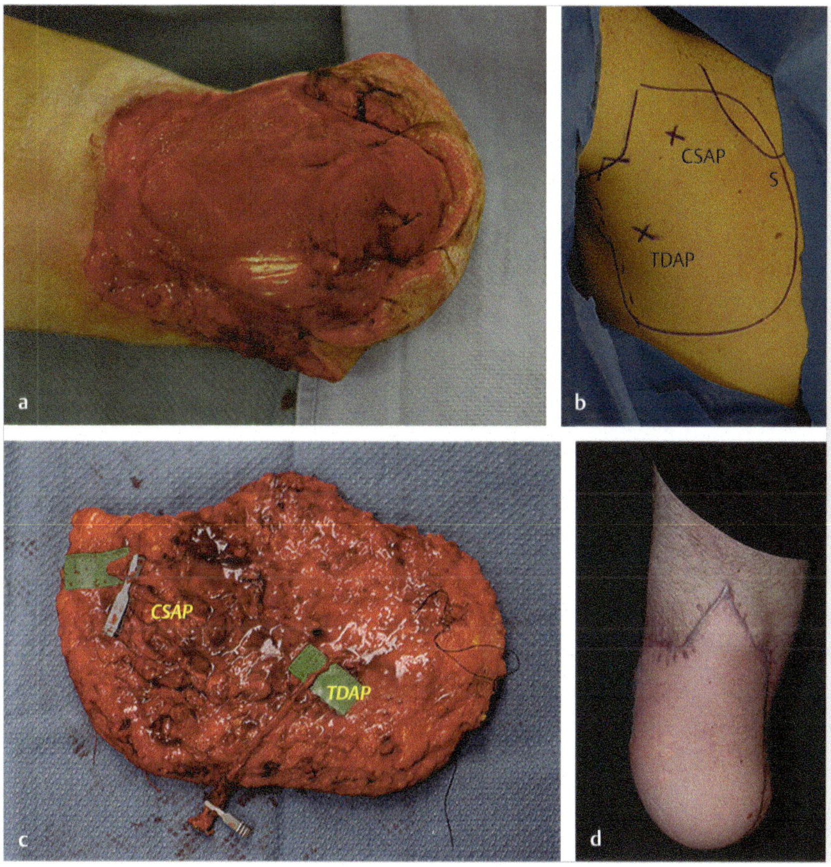

Fig. 16.26 (a) Huge skin deficiency of the posterior aspect of traumatic left below-knee amputation stump. **(b)** A 30 cm × 40 cm conjoined thoracodorsal artery perforator (TDAP) and circumflex scapular artery (CSAP) flap designed to ensure adequate circulation to this large flap by including both a TDAP and the cutaneous branch or perforator of the CSAP that would be found in the triangular space lateral to the scapula (S). **(c)** TDAP–CSAP conjoined free flap. The circumflex scapular vessels, as is the case infrequently, originated directly from the axillary artery, so a second set of microanastomoses to each branch had to be done in an end-to-side fashion to the popliteal vessels. Note the longer pedicle length potential with the TDAP. **(d)** Salvaged knee joint by free flap coverage of the left below-knee amputation stump.

(▶ Fig. 16.26) with a cornucopia of potential simultaneous reconstructive options available including concomitant vascularized bone transfer or malleable muscle that is valuable for filling three-dimensional voids. All these attributes are possible with minimal donor site morbidity, and a scar easily hidden by clothing.

References

[1] Maxwell GP. Iginio Tansini and the origin of the latissimus dorsi musculocutaneous flap. Plast Reconstr Surg. 1980; 65(5):686–692

[2] Taylor GI, Daniel RK. The anatomy of several free flap donor sites. Plast Reconstr Surg. 1975; 56(3):243–253

[3] Daniel RK, Taylor GI. Distant transfer of an island flap by microvascular anastomosis. Plast Reconstr Surg. 1973; 52(2):111–117

[4] Hallock GG. Paramuscular perforators in DIEAP flap for breast reconstruction: an important variation in perforator flap nomenclature. [Letter]. Ann Plast Surg. 2015; 74(6):745–746

[5] Baudet J, Guimberteau JC, Nascimento E. Successful clinical transfer of two free thoraco-dorsal axillary flaps. Plast Reconstr Surg. 1976; 58(6):680–688

[6] Angrigiani C. Thoracodorsal artery perforator (TDAP) flap. In: Strauch B, Vasconez LO, Herman CK, Lee BT, eds. Grabb's Encyclopedia of Flaps. 4th ed. Philadelphia, PA: Wolters Kluwer; 2016:367–369

[7] Angrigiani C, Grilli D, Siebert J. Latissimus dorsi musculocutaneous flap without muscle. Plast Reconstr Surg. 1995; 96(7):1608–1614

[8] Blondeel PN, Van Landuyt KH, Monstrey SJ, et al. The "Gent" consensus on perforator flap terminology: preliminary definitions. Plast Reconstr Surg. 2003; 112(5):1378–1383, quiz 1383, 1516, discussion 1384–1387

[9] Arikawa M, Miyamoto S, Fujiki M, Higashino T, Oshima A, Sakuraba M. Comparison of donor site drainage duration and seroma rate between latissimus dorsi musculocutaneous flaps and thoracodorsal artery perforator flaps. Ann Plast Surg. 2017; 79(2):183–185

[10] Rausky J, Binder JP, Mazouz-Dorval S, Hamou C, Revol M. Perforator-based chimaeric thoracodorsal flap for foot reconstruction. J Plast Reconstr Aesthet Surg. 2013; 66(12):1798–1800

[11] Lee KT, Kim A, Mun GH. Comprehensive analysis of donor-site morbidity following free thoracodorsal artery perforator flap harvest. Plast Reconstr Surg. 2016; 138(4):899–909

[12] van Landuyt K, Morrison CM. Thoracodorsal artery perforator flap. In: Blondeel PN, Morris SF, Hallock GG, Neligan PC, eds. Perforator Flaps: Anatomy, Technique, & Clinical Applications. 2nd ed. Vol. 2. St. Louis, MO: Quality Medical Publishing; 591–604

[13] Park BY, Seo SW, Mun GH. Microsurgical pedicle lengthening for pedicled thoracodorsal artery perforator flap transfer. Ann Plast Surg. 2014; 73(2): 174–176

[14] Angrigiani C, Rancati A, Artero G, Khouri RK, Jr, Walocko FM. Stacked thoracodorsal artery perforator flaps for unilateral breast reconstruction. Plast Reconstr Surg. 2016; 138(6):969e–972e

[15] Santanelli F, Longo B, Germano S, Rubino C, Laporta R, Hamdi M. Total breast reconstruction using the thoracodorsal artery perforator flap without implant. Plast Reconstr Surg. 2014; 133(2):251–254

[16] Kim JT. Perforator flaps in the lateral thoracic region. In: Wei FC, Mardini S, eds. Flaps and Reconstructive Surgery. Edinburgh: Elsevier; 2017:648–667

[17] Fortin AJ, Skoracki RJ. Thoracodorsal artery perforator (TAP) flap reconstruction of a soft-tissue defect of the knee following below-knee amputation. J Reconstr Microsurg. 2004; 20(8):605–609

[18] Lee KT, Wiraatmadja ES, Mun GH. Free latissimus dorsi muscle-chimeric thoracodorsal artery perforator flaps for reconstruction of complicated

defects: does muscle still have a place in the domain of perforator flaps? Ann Plast Surg. 2015; 74(5):565–572
[19] Ozcan Akcal A, Ünal K, Gorgulu T, Akif Akcal M, Bigat Z. Reconstruction of midfoot bone and soft tissue loss with chimeric partial scapula and latissimus dorsi muscle flap and short perforator-based skin flap following gunshot injuries: report of two cases. Microsurgery. 2016; 36(7):598–603
[20] Kim SW, Youn DH, Hwang KT, Sung IH, Kim JT, Kim YH. Reconstruction of the lateral malleolus and calcaneus region using free thoracodorsal artery perforator flaps. Microsurgery. 2016; 36(3):198–205
[21] Kim YH, Kim KH, Sung KY, Kim JT, Kim SW. Toe resurfacing with a thin thoracodorsal artery perforator flap. Microsurgery. 2017; 37(4):312–318
[22] Lin CT, Chen LW. Surgical refinements and sensory recovery of using transverse sensate thoracodorsal artery perforator flaps to resurface ring-avulsed fingers. Ann Plast Surg. 2014; 72(3):299–306
[23] Wei FC, Jain V, Suominen S, Chen HC. Confusion among perforator flaps: what is a true perforator flap? Plast Reconstr Surg. 2001; 107(3):874–876
[24] Mun GH, Lee SJ, Jeon BJ. Perforator topography of the thoracodorsal artery perforator flap. Plast Reconstr Surg. 2008; 121(2):497–504
[25] Schaverien M, Saint-Cyr M, Arbique G, Brown SA, Rohrich RJ. Three- and four-dimensional arterial and venous anatomies of the thoracodorsal artery perforator flap. Plast Reconstr Surg. 2008; 121(5):1578–1587
[26] Serafin D. The latissimus dorsi muscle-musculocutaneous flap. In: Atlas of Microsurgical Composite Tissue Transplantation. Philadelphia, PA: W.B. Saunders; 1996:205–216
[27] Zenn MR, Jones G. Latissimus dorsi flap. In: Reconstructive Surgery: Anatomy, Technique, and Clinical Applications. St. Louis, MO: Quality Medical Publishing; 2012:738
[28] Kim SW, Sung IH, Kim YH. Reconstruction of severe atherosclerotic and obstructive diabetic feet using thoracodorsal artery perforator flaps with long vascular pedicles. Microsurg. 2018; 38(3):287–294
[29] Bartlett SP, May JW, Jr, Yaremchuk MJ. The latissimus dorsi muscle: a fresh cadaver study of the primary neurovascular pedicle. Plast Reconstr Surg. 1981; 67(5):631–636
[30] Kim JT. Two options for perforator flaps in the flank donor site: latissimus dorsi and thoracodorsal perforator flaps. Plast Reconstr Surg. 2005; 115(3): 755–763
[31] Miyamoto S, Arikawa M, Kagaya Y, Fukunaga Y. Septocutaneous thoracodorsal artery perforator flaps: a retrospective cohort study. J Plast Reconstr Aesthet Surg. 2019; 72(1):78–84
[32] Shin JY, Roh SG, Lee NH, Yang KM. Direct cutaneous lateral thoracic artery perforator misdiagnosed as second thoracodorsal artery perforator. Microsurgery. 2017; 37(6):724–725
[33] Lin CT, Yang KC, Hsu KC, Liu WC, Chen JS, Chen LW. Sensate thoracodorsal artery perforator flap: a focus on its preoperative design and harvesting technique. Plast Reconstr Surg. 2009; 123(1):163–174
[34] Tashiro K, Yamashita S, Araki J, Narushima M, Iida T, Koshima I. Preoperative color Doppler ultrasonographic examination in the planning of thoracodorsal artery perforator flap with capillary perforators. J Plast Reconstr Aesthet Surg. 2016; 69(3):346–350
[35] Schwabegger AH, Harpf C, Rainer C. Muscle-sparing latissimus dorsi myocutaneous flap with maintenance of muscle innervation, function, and aesthetic appearance of the donor site. Plast Reconstr Surg. 2003; 111(4):1407–1411
[36] Kim SW, Youn S, Kim JT, Kim YH. A modified method for harvesting thoracodorsal artery perforator flaps in a simple and time-saving approach. Microsurgery. 2016; 36(8):642–646
[37] Hallock GG. The chimera flap: a quarter century odyssey. Ann Plast Surg. 2017; 78(2):223–229
[38] Kim SW, Youn DG, Kim JT, Kim YH. A thoracodorsal artery perforator chimeric free flap for prevention of microvascular pedicle compression in lower extremity reconstruction. Microsurgery. 2018; 38(1):46–50
[39] Momeni A, Krischak S, Bannasch H. The thoracodorsal artery perforator flap with a vascularized scapular segment for reconstruction of a composite lower extremity defect. Microsurgery. 2006; 26(7):515–518
[40] Hallock GG. Attributes and shortcomings of acoustic Doppler sonography in identifying perforators for flaps from the lower extremity. J Reconstr Microsurg. 2009; 25(6):377–381
[41] Kim SW, Kim SY, Kim YH. Eccentric instead of central position of a thoracodorsal artery perforator: is it reliable? Plast Reconstr Surg. 2015; 136(4S): 157–158
[42] Kim KN, Hong JP, Park CR, Yoon CS. Modification of the elevation plane and defatting technique to create a thin thoracodorsal artery perforator flap. J Reconstr Microsurg. 2016; 32(2):142–146

17 Supermicrosurgery Approach to the Lower Limb

Joon Pio Hong

Summary

Supermicrosurgery is manipulating vessels with diameters less than 0.8 mm. In flap surgery, this approach will allow an increase in the selection of recipient pedicles by using a perforator-to-perforator anastomosis approach. Decreased time of surgery, elevation of the flap by taking just a short segment of the perforator pedicle, minimization of any risk for major vessel injury, and utilizing collateral circulation in ischemic diabetic foot are some of the apparent advantages.

Keywords: supermicrosurgery, perforator-to-perforator microsurgery, diabetic foot reconstruction, freestyle reconstruction

17.1 Introduction

Reconstruction of the lower extremity using free flaps remains a difficult procedure. Although limb salvage rates have greatly improved over the past 20 to 30 years, major hurdles regarding single artery limb, atherosclerosis, involvement of hardware, frequent spasm, chronic infections, edema, complexity of lower limb trauma, and diabetes still make it very challenging even for experienced surgeons.[1] In this age of reconstruction, we are faced with the challenge of achieving not only successful soft-tissue coverage but also functional recovery, infection control, and cosmetic improvement. Evolutions in microsurgery have been noted from the days of experimental surgery, finger replantation, and now to perforator flaps and supermicrosurgery, and it has allowed achieving complex goals. These evolutions aim for better results and to minimize complications despite the innate risks of lower extremity soft-tissue reconstruction. The use of perforator-to-perforator supermicrosurgery has reduced complications in high-risk lower extremity reconstructions.

Lower extremity can be extremely difficult to reconstruct with poor outcome. Frequently the lower extremity reconstruction involves major vessel injury leaving only one major vessel to the leg, requires long pedicle length to reach the recipient vessel, may have severe arthrosclerosis in diabetic or elderly patients limiting the choices for recipient vessels, has lower perfusion, being furthest from the heart, and is very difficult to isolate the recipient vessels in the mid and upper leg as it is lying very deep to the skin. How can we overcome these difficult situations without compromising the outcome of reconstruction while maintaining a robust distal flow? This is the key challenge.

The supermicrosurgery technique is defined as microsurgical anastomosis of vessels, with a diameter less than 0.8 mm.[2,3,4,5] This technique, although reported frequently on lymphaticovenous shunting to treat lymphedema, fingertip replantation, finger/toe reconstruction, and sporadically in soft-tissue reconstruction with specific indications, is a relatively new concept for lower extremity reconstruction.[3,6,7,8,9,10,11,12,13] As lymphedema supermicrosurgery will be covered in another chapter, this chapter will focus on soft-tissue reconstruction. For the lower extremity soft-tissue reconstruction, one of the applications can be seen in the perforator-to-perforator anastomosis approach or using small-diameter pedicles of perforator flaps to anastomose on a lager vessel end to side.[4,5,14,15] This concept deserves to be recognized as a new paradigm in microsurgery as it has been mentioned that vessel size less than 1 mm may significantly increase the risk of flap failure.[16] However, with advances in technology and skills, the overall success rate for using supermicrosurgery technique for lower extremity reconstruction compares similar to other reports using vessels larger than 1 mm.[2,16,17,18]

The evolution into this new concept and paradigm shift came naturally as the understanding of single perforasome (perforator angiosome) unfolded as well as the establishment of free styling of perforator flap elevation.[19,20,21,22,23,24] The successful survival of the skin flap based on a single perforator led the hypothesis of using a single perforator artery and veins as a recipient pedicle.[4,5,14] Thus, using the perforator as a recipient vessel may overcome the difficult challenges that the surgeons face during lower extremity reconstruction. Introduction of supermicrosurgery, especially perforator to perforator, also led to true free style free flaps as any perforator-based skin flaps even the one with short pedicles now can be used to reconstruct the defect.[4,10,14,25,26,27]

Another possibility that perforator-to-perforator supermicrosurgery showed was in treating ischemic diabetic foot patients. Patient with ischemic diabetic limb develop multiple collaterals as atherosclerosis develops. It is these collateral vessels that can supply the skin perforators to maintain the vascular flow despite of major artery obstruction. Using these collateral arteries and perforators supplied from these collaterals is essential for the application of supermicrosurgery in ischemic diabetic limb.[15,28,29] The details of this approach is described in the chapter for diabetic foot reconstruction.

In this chapter, we will focus on how the perforator-to-perforator supermicrosurgery can help surgeons to overcome some of the challenges seen in lower extremity reconstruction.

17.2 Attributes and Detriments

17.2.1 Attributes

- Perforators or small end vessels can be used as recipient vessels.
- Perforator-to-perforator supermicrosurgery alleviates the use of major vessels and maintains the distal flow to the leg without disruption.
- Pulsatile perforator or an end vessel is a good indication for use.
- This approach can be minimally invasive, thus minimizing the need for extensive dissection to isolate the recipient.

17.2.2 Detriments

- Special instruments may be required for supermicrosurgery.
- There is a steep learning curve.
- Perforator as a recipient has a limit in providing perfusion to the tissue.
- Volume depletion must be avoided during post-op care.

17.3 Anatomical Consideration

There are more than 420 perforators that are over 0.5 mm in diameter throughout our body.[30] While these perforators can be seen as potential sites for perforator-based flaps, they can be considered as recipient vessels as well. In the lower extremity, there are on average 184 perforators from gluteal, hip, thigh, knee, leg, and foot.[30] The abundance of these potential recipient sites truly allows us to approach in free style in not only elevating the flaps, but also selecting the recipient source.[4,5] The perforator is an end vessel that is the sum of all supplies not only from major vessels but also from all the branches and collaterals heading toward the end vessel perforator.[15,28] Thus, using these perforator or end vessels becomes possible despite the major artery being insufficient from atherosclerosis, trauma, or other relevant causes.[4] Even in legs with single artery, the risk of steal phenomenon or distal flow reduction can be avoided as using perforators will not disturb the flow of this major vessel.

Preoperative CT scans will allow us to view the vascular details of the lower extremity. In the cases where foreign body effect deters from obtaining appropriate images, conventional angiograms can be obtained as well. These images can also show the possible recipient sites as well as give information on potential donor flap sites. Preoperative duplex can be used to enforce the findings from Doppler as this can give you objective measurement such as velocity of flow and the diameter of the vessel as well as more detailed anatomical findings.

In the lower extremity, there are relatively constant and large perforators coming out from the three major vessels. The findings of the study by Schaverien and Saint-Cyr are shown in ▶ Fig. 17.1, which depicts the relatively constant regions where the perforator emerges from the three major arteries.[31] The

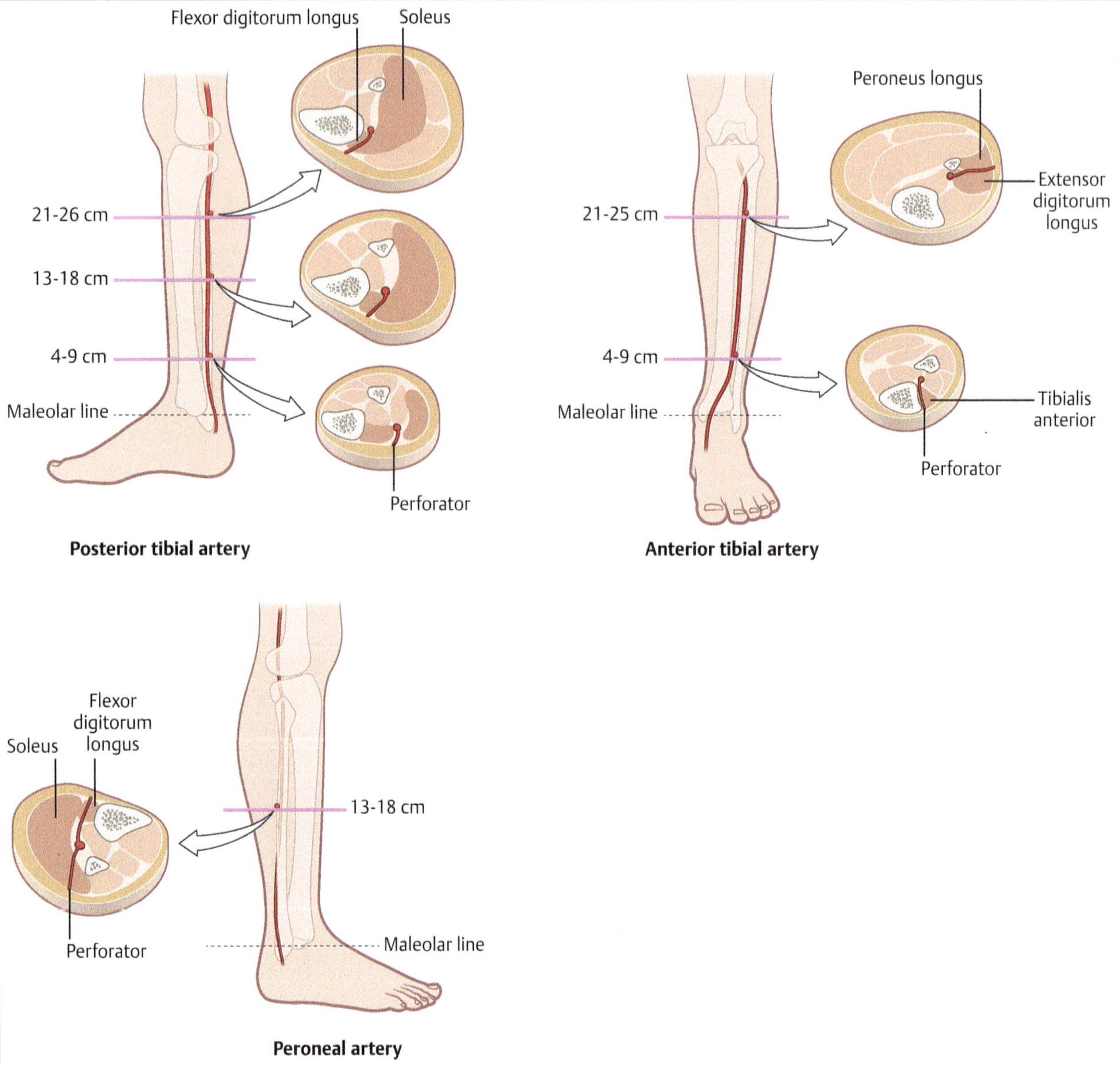

Fig. 17.1 This illustration depicts the relatively constant perforators originating from the three major arteries. If the defect is near these perforators, these are relatively easier to find and use as a recipient.

perforators from the posterior tibial artery are found between the flexor digitorum longus and soleus in all three intervals, with the largest perforators found in the middle cluster. The constant perforators from the anterior tibial artery are located within two clusters. The proximal perforators, 21 to 25 cm from the intermalleolar line, are in the anterior peroneal septum between the extensor digitorum longus and the peroneus longus, and the distal perforators, 4 to 9 cm from the intermalleolar line, are found between the tibia and the tendon of the tibialis anterior muscle. The constant perforator for the peroneal artery is found 13 and 18 cm from the intermalleolar line emerging from various muscles.[31] Using these relatively constantly located perforators will allow the surgeon to approach with some degree of reliability when considering the perforator as a recipient.

17.4 Anatomical Variants and Pitfalls

The first and foremost important factor in using a perforator as a recipient is a visual pulse. With an evident pulse on the perforating artery, it can be successfully used as a recipient vessel to supply a sizable flap. A perforator can be located during the debridement or resection as a projectile bleeding from the artery is encountered at this time. One can dissect these small vessels further toward the source vessel and clamp it temporarily after obtaining a comfortable length for anastomosis. However, as mentioned earlier, there are relatively constant perforators from the three major arteries and can start by examining these clusters using Doppler or duplex examination. Nevertheless, any perforator with a visible pulse and a pulsatile flow can be chosen as a recipient source. This free style of searching perforators as recipient vessels embraces any variants possible.

The biggest pitfall of this approach is the flow of the recipient perforator, as manipulation of the perforator during dissection may cause constriction and vasospasm that may not be irreversible. Meticulous dissection is an absolute prerequisite to maximize the chance for success. Finer instruments and better microscope will help but is not an absolute requirement. In most of the cases, the constriction or vessel spasm will recover. Therefore, before ligating the pedicle of the flap, it is prudent to check the flow (pulsation) of the recipient perforator first. If the recipient perforator has not recovered from the spasm, one can search for a different nearby perforator or dissect the original perforator toward the source vessel. Once the recipient is confirmed with pulsatile flow, the pedicle flap should be ligated accordingly with the length required.

17.5 Surgical Approach

Any reconstructive procedure involves debridement or resection of unwanted tissue. During this time, one can come across bleeders that have strong pulsatile flow. This small bleeding artery can also be considered a potential recipient perforator or end vessel and saved for later use. If the wound is chronic, often the small vessels in the zone of injury will be difficult to use due to scarring of the tissue, which makes the dissection difficult, hence the concept of avoiding the zone of injury. However, with better microscope and equipment, one can dissect the recipient perforator with care and will be able to use it as such.

After complete debridement, recipient vessels should be explored while the second team starts elevating the flap. Then the recipient perforator or end vessel can be located within the defect or adjacent to the defect. Preoperative search using duplex, Doppler, and CT angiogram can help you identify potential recipient sites (▶ Fig. 17.2, ▶ Fig. 17.3). The search for such perforators can begin by examining at high-clustered sites from the three major arteries.[31] During the operation, the exploration begins by searching the marked region. Usually recipient perforators can be easily identified by dissecting the plane between the fascia and subcutaneous fat like the suprafascial elevation of a DIEP (deep inferior epigastric artery perforator) flap under loupe magnification. Once the perforating vessels are noted, further dissection using the microscope makes it easier to prepare the vessels and confirm the flow of the recipient perforator. A firm pulse from the artery of the perforator is a sign of good perfusion despite the location being within or near the zone of injury. Accompanying veins are used for primary venous drainage, but if superficial veins are found while exploring the recipient pedicle, it is prudent to save and isolate it. In fingers or toes, digital arteries can be used to connect the artery in an end-to-side manner to maintain the flow distal to the anastomosis. In regions where major vessels are lying shallow

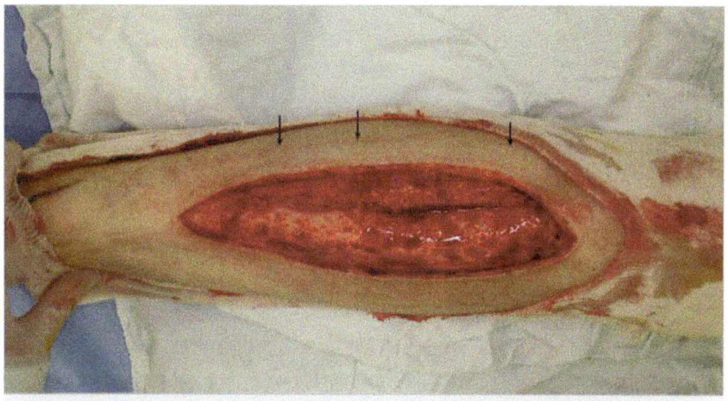

Fig. 17.2 Doppler can be used to mark the potential perforators around or within the defect. The selection of recipient can be started from these potential sites. However, definitive selection of the recipient vessel must rely on the actual pulsation of the perforator.

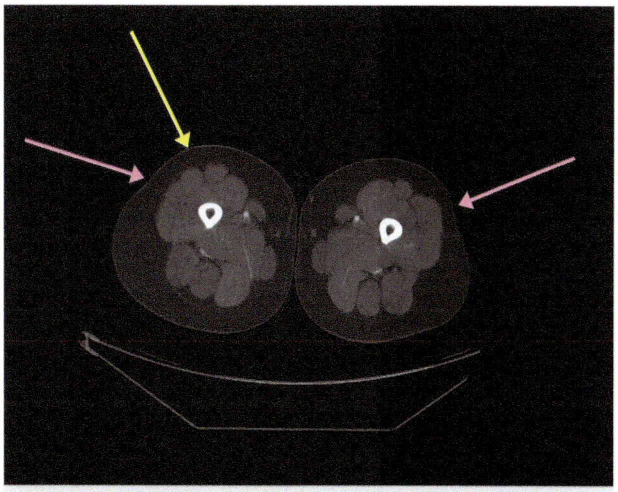

Fig. 17.3 CT angiogram also provides images to locate potential recipient perforators.

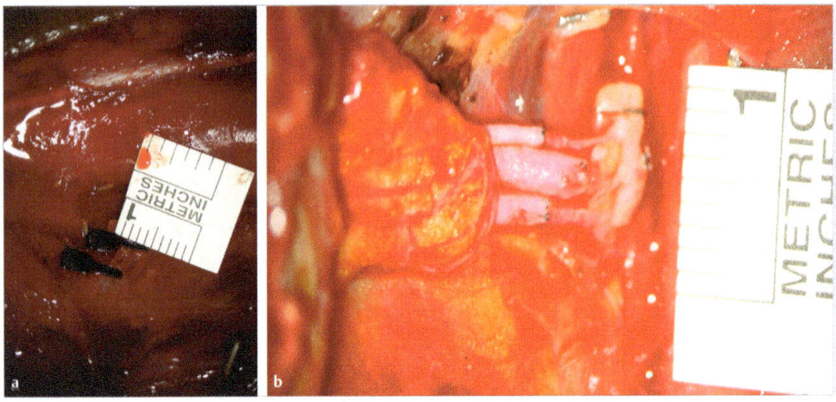

Fig. 17.4 One of the most important procedures in using perforators as recipient vessel is to dilate the recipient and the flap perforators to expand to a comfortable diameter to work with. A dilator is used to expand the vessels. Note the difference **(a)** before dilation and **(b)** after dilation.

from the skin, one can use the branch from the major vessel or connect the artery or vein in an end-to-side manner. However, one must consider the inflow volume when doing an end-to-side inflow to a major vessel as the increased volume of inflow overwhelming the small flap may cause congestion of the flap. There have been reports considering the metabolic demand of the flap, but further research is needed in regard to supermicrosurgery and flap physiology.[4]

Upon securing an adequate recipient vessel, various factors should be considered in relationship to the harvesting flap especially the length of the pedicle. If the intended recipient perforator has poor flow, one can look for a different perforator or trace the initial perforator toward the source vessel until an adequate flow is noted.

Once the flap is ready for final ligation of the pedicle, one should recheck the status of the recipient perforator. Usually, the vasoconstriction recovers by the time flap elevation is finished. If there is no adequate pulse or if the recipient does not recover from the spasm, one can ask the anesthesiologist to increase the perfusion pressure by increasing the blood pressure. If this does not work, one should look for an alternative recipient as mentioned earlier. The ligation of the flap pedicle should be performed only after the adequate recipient vessel has been obtained.

The anastomosis begins by the surgeon's preference. The author usually prefers to do the vein first or whatever recipient vessel is located deeper as it is more difficult to anastomose. Once the artery or vein is aligned for anastomosis, the critical step is dilating the vessel to a sufficient diameter, which makes microanastomosis easier. The vessels are dilated using dilators (▶ Fig. 17.4). After dilation, for diameters less than 0.8 mm but greater than 0.5 mm, an 11–0 or 12–0 nylon with a 50- to 30-µm needle can be used. If the diameter is less than 0.5 mm, a 12–0 nylon with a 50- to 30-µm needle is used. The anastomosis is the same as any microsurgery anastomosis. A minimum of six stitches and average of nine stitches were performed.[4] After anastomosis, brisk bleeding from the margin of the flap is confirmed and the flap is set over the defect.

A video is shown going over the overall approach to this technique (▶ Video 17.1).

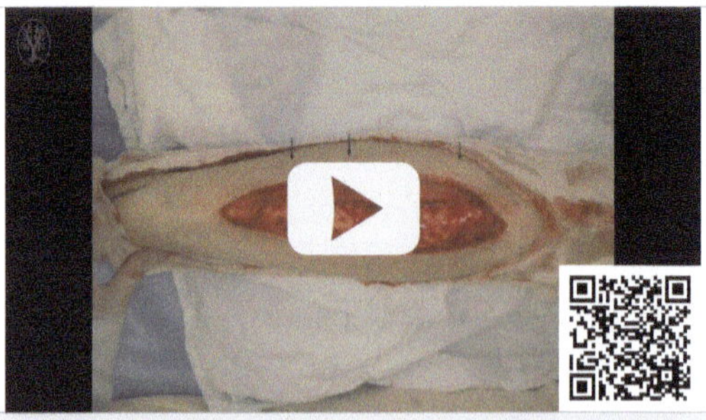

Video 17.1 Supermicrosurgery Approach. https://www.thieme.de/de/q.htm?p=opn/cs/20/7/12265281-5c759b6b

17.6 Postoperative Care Protocol

The most important part of postoperative care in this approach is maintaining the adequate flow to the lower extremity and flap. When the patient is dehydrated, the flow centers toward the vital organs and the peripheral flow decreases. Thus, keeping the patients well hydrated is important. Having the patient in the sitting position after the patient regains consciousness from anesthesia also helps increase the flow to gravity-dependent extremity. Pharmacological agents can be used as well. Vasodilator can be used intravenously; 10-µg lipoprostaglandin E1 (Eglandin, Welfide, Seoul, Korea) mixed in 5% DW is infused over 4 hours and used for 5 days. Also, still under debate, some cases may benefit from using low-molecular-weight heparin (Fraxiparine, Sanofi-Aventis, Paris, France) 3,800 IU subcutaneously for 5 days.[4,5]

Monitoring of the flap can be done with subjective methods such as looking at skin refill, temperature, and skin turgor. Objective methods includes using thermoscans to compare the temperature with the surrounding skin adjacent to the flap, using duplex to monitor the pedicle flow, and in some cases looking at the characteristics after pin prick.[15,19] Early detection of arterial insufficiencies may provide a high chance for salvage, whereas venous thrombosis be more difficult as microthrombosis of the small vessels occurs early prior to detection. Nevertheless, all attempts should be made to salvage the flap once it is at risk.

17.7 Conclusion

The supermicrosurgery approach will allow an increase in the selection of recipient pedicles. By using a perforator-to-perforator anastomosis approach, less time is consumed to secure the recipient vessel and to elevate the flap by taking just a short segment of the perforator pedicle, and any risk for major vessel injury is minimized or collateral circulation can be utilized without apparent flow of major vessels while having acceptable flap survival. Further studies on physiology and anatomy will be needed to evaluate the extent of application.

References

[1] Heller L, Levin LS. Lower extremity microsurgical reconstruction. Plast Reconstr Surg. 2001; 108(4):1029–1041, quiz 1042

[2] Koshima I, Inagawa K, Yamamoto M, Moriguchi T. New microsurgical breast reconstruction using free paraumbilical perforator adiposal flaps. Plast Reconstr Surg. 2000; 106(1):61–65

[3] Koshima I, Nanba Y, Tsutsui T, Takahashi Y, Itoh S, Fujitsu M. Minimal invasive lymphaticovenular anastomosis under local anesthesia for leg lymphedema: is it effective for stage III and IV? Ann Plast Surg. 2004; 53(3):261–266

[4] Hong JP. The use of supermicrosurgery in lower extremity reconstruction: the next step in evolution. Plast Reconstr Surg. 2009; 123(1):230–235

[5] Hong JP, Koshima I. Using perforators as recipient vessels (supermicrosurgery) for free flap reconstruction of the knee region. Ann Plast Surg. 2010; 64(3):291–293

[6] Koshima I, Nanba Y, Tsutsui T, Takahashi Y. Medial plantar perforator flaps with supermicrosurgery. Clin Plast Surg. 2003; 30(3):447–455, vii

[7] Yamamoto T, Yamashita M, Furuya M, Hayashi A, Koshima I. Mono-canalization of adhered lymphatic vessels for lymphatic supermicrosurgery. J Plast Reconstr Aesthet Surg. 2014; 67(11):e291–e292

[8] Kompatscher P, Manestar M, Schuster A, Lang A, Beer GM. The thoracoacromial vessels as recipient vessels in microsurgery and supermicrosurgery: an anatomical and sonographic study. Plast Reconstr Surg. 2005; 115(1):77–83

[9] Song D, Pafitanis G, Yang P, et al. Innervated dorsoradial perforator free flap: a reliable supermicrosurgery fingertip reconstruction technique. J Plast Reconstr Aesthet Surg. 2017; 70(8):1001–1008

[10] Yoon CS, Noh HJ, Malzone G, Suh HS, Choi DH, Hong JP. Posterior interosseous artery perforator-free flap: treating intermediate-size hand and foot defects. J Plast Reconstr Aesthet Surg. 2014; 67(6):808–814

[11] Chang DW. Lymphaticovenular bypass for lymphedema management in breast cancer patients: a prospective study. Plast Reconstr Surg. 2010; 126(3): 752–758

[12] Chang DW. Lymphaticovenular bypass surgery for lymphedema management in breast cancer patients. Handchir Mikrochir Plast Chir. 2012; 44(6):343–347

[13] Althubaiti GA, Crosby MA, Chang DW. Vascularized supraclavicular lymph node transfer for lower extremity lymphedema treatment. Plast Reconstr Surg. 2013; 131(1):133e–135e

[14] Koshima I, Yamamoto T, Narushima M, Mihara M, Iida T. Perforator flaps and supermicrosurgery. Clin Plast Surg. 2010; 37(4):683–689, vii–iii

[15] Suh HS, Oh TS, Hong JP. Innovations in diabetic foot reconstruction using supermicrosurgery. Diabetes Metab Res Rev. 2016; 32 Suppl 1:275–280

[16] Khouri RK, Shaw WW. Reconstruction of the lower extremity with microvascular free flaps: a 10-year experience with 304 consecutive cases. J Trauma. 1989; 29(8):1086–1094

[17] Parrett BM, Matros E, Pribaz JJ, Orgill DP. Lower extremity trauma: trends in the management of soft-tissue reconstruction of open tibia-fibula fractures. Plast Reconstr Surg. 2006; 117(4):1315–1322, discussion 1323–1324

[18] Hong JP, Shin HW, Kim JJ, Wei FC, Chung YK. The use of anterolateral thigh perforator flaps in chronic osteomyelitis of the lower extremity. Plast Reconstr Surg. 2005; 115(1):142–147

[19] Taylor GI. The angiosomes of the body and their supply to perforator flaps. Clin Plast Surg. 2003; 30(3):331–342, v

[20] Taylor GI, Chubb DP, Ashton MW. True and "choke" anastomoses between perforator angiosomes: Part I. Anatomical location. Plast Reconstr Surg. 2013; 132(6):1447–1456

[21] Chubb DP, Taylor GI, Ashton MW. True and "choke" anastomoses between perforator angiosomes: Part II. Dynamic thermographic identification. Plast Reconstr Surg. 2013; 132(6):1457–1464

[22] Chang CC, Shen JH, Chan KK, Wei FC. Selection of ideal perforators and the use of a free-style free flap during dissection of an anterolateral thigh flap for reconstruction in the head and neck. Br J Oral Maxillofac Surg. 2016; 54(7): 830–832

[23] Chang CC, Wong CH, Wei FC. Free-style free flap. Injury. 2008; 39 Suppl 3: S57–S61

[24] Wallace CG, Kao HK, Jeng SF, Wei FC. Free-style flaps: a further step forward for perforator flap surgery. Plast Reconstr Surg. 2009; 124(6) Suppl:e419–e426

[25] Hong JP, Sun SH, Ben-Nakhi M. Modified superficial circumflex iliac artery perforator flap and supermicrosurgery technique for lower extremity reconstruction: a new approach for moderate-sized defects. Ann Plast Surg. 2013; 71(4):380–383

[26] Hong JP, Yim JH, Malzone G, Lee KJ, Dashti T, Suh HS. The thin gluteal artery perforator free flap to resurface the posterior aspect of the leg and foot. Plast Reconstr Surg. 2014; 133(5):1184–1191

[27] Eom JS, Sun SH, Hong JP. Use of the upper medial thigh perforator flap (gracilis perforator flap) for lower extremity reconstruction. Plast Reconstr Surg. 2011; 127(2):731–737

[28] Suh HS, Oh TS, Lee HS, et al. A new approach for reconstruction of diabetic foot wounds using the angiosome and supermicrosurgery concept. Plast Reconstr Surg. 2016; 138(4):702e–709e

[29] Suh HP, Kim Y, Suh Y, Hong J. Multidetector computed tomography (CT) analysis of 168 cases in diabetic patients with total superficial femoral artery occlusion: is it safe to use an anterolateral thigh flap without CT angiography in diabetic patients? J Reconstr Microsurg. 2018; 34(1):65–70

[30] Morris SF, Tang M, Almutari K, Geddes C, Yang D. The anatomic basis of perforator flaps. Clin Plast Surg. 2010; 37(4):553–570, xi

[31] Schaverien M, Saint-Cyr M. Perforators of the lower leg: analysis of perforator locations and clinical application for pedicled perforator flaps. Plast Reconstr Surg. 2008; 122(1):161–170

18 Diabetic Foot Reconstruction

Joon Pio Hong

Summary

The treatment of diabetic foot ulceration is complex with multiple considerations and unfortunately often leads to amputation. A multidisciplinary approach along with an algorithm to manage and salvage diabetic foot ulcers from amputation is now a highly doable approach. Knowing the spectrum of care and reconstructive principles can prevent diabetic foot ulcers from amputation. Further understanding of supermicrosurgery and angiosome principles can extend the possibility for reconstruction in patients with severe ischemic diabetic foot.

Keywords: diabetic foot, supermicrosurgery, angiosomes, diabetic foot reconstruction

18.1 Introduction

According to the statistics given, approximately 3 to 4% of individuals with diabetes currently have foot ulcers or deep infections and 25% will develop foot ulcers sometime during their lifetime.[1,2] The risk of lower leg amputation increases by a factor of 8 once an ulcer develops. It is estimated that the age-adjusted rate of lower extremity amputation in diabetic patients is 15-fold that of nondiabetic patients.[3] Intractable diabetic foot ulcers can not only cause decreased physical, emotional, and social functions but also be a huge economic impact to the patient.[4,5,6] Furthermore, the 5-year mortality after major amputations may range from 39% to as high as 80%.[1,7,8] These are the reasons why salvage for diabetic foot ulcers remains important as it will reduce economic burden and improve the quality of life.[8]

Limb salvage from diabetic foot using the microsurgical approach showed similar success comparable to nondiabetic patients.[9,10,11,12,13,14] Meta-analysis of a systematic review of free tissue transfer in 528 diabetes patients in 18 studies showed flap survival of 92% and limb salvage rate of 83.4% over a 28-month average follow-up period. This study indicates that free tissue transfer in the management of nontraumatic lower extremity wounds in patients with diabetes may avoid amputations.[13] Free flaps and microsurgery technique now play an important role to salvage the limb from chronic ulcerations. A previous study showed that using microsurgery can achieve an overall limb salvage rate of 84.9% and 5-year survival of 86.8%.[8] There is no doubt that a well-vascularized free flap will enhance healing, quality of life, and survival chances.

In this chapter, we will focus on the clinical aspect of reconstruction and show a step-by-step approach on how to achieve reconstructive goals.

18.2 Attributes and Detriments

18.2.1 Attributes

- Limb salvage using reconstruction is an alternative to amputation.
- A multidisciplinary approach is essential in managing diabetic foot ulcers as diabetic patients have high comorbidity.
- Once good vascular supply is secured, microsurgical or local reconstruction can be performed with reliable outcome.
- The key is the status of the recipient artery and supermicrosurgery approach using small vessels can be considered.
- Limb salvage not only leads to better quality of life but may also increase 5-year survival.

18.2.2 Detriments

- A multidisciplinary approach is needed to adequately obtain good systemic condition and vascularity for reconstruction and may not be readily available.
- Learning curve is needed to understand the algorithm of reconstruction and care.

18.3 Considerations

18.3.1 Multidisciplinary Approach and Spectrum of Care

The spectrum of diabetic foot disease may vary from asymptomatic to critically ischemic limb with unavoidable amputation. The spectrum of care for diabetic foot patients ranges from managing blood glucose, education on prevention, and managing small ulcers with good standard of care to using multiple new techniques and approaching with surgery (▶ Fig. 18.1).[15] The wide manifestation of symptoms is due to multifactor pathophysiology. The principal pathogenesis involves ischemia, neuropathy, and infection. The addition of external trauma, peripheral edema, and foot deformity may further increase the risk for diabetic foot ulceration.[16] They may act alone or synergistically to result in Charcot's deformities, Achilles tendon contractures, ulcerations, necrosis, and gangrene. One must consider these pathologies and manage them in sequence in order to provide an efficient care for the foot. Treatment must begin with strict blood sugar control and nutritional support while aggressively managing the wound and infection to achieve closure of the defect.[17] In the cases with ischemic limb, vascular bypass or angioplasty may play a vital role to enhance circulation allowing further reconstruction of soft tissue and bone.[15]

The nurse specialist or coordinator helps use the team recourses efficiently. After gathering general information about the patient and initial screening of the systemic and foot condition, the specialist would refer to an endocrinologist, nutritionist, and proper departments for further treatment and evaluation. There are four categories for initial foot evaluation: vascular, neuropathic, orthopaedic, and infectious wounds.[15] Multiple departments may be involved simultaneously to improve the patient's foot condition. In the cases of emergent wound, a dedicated team needs to be notified immediately for emergency debridement and further clinical decision. This is the first and a major step to limit the spread of acute infection that may be critical in salvaging the diabetic foot.[18] ▶ Fig. 18.2

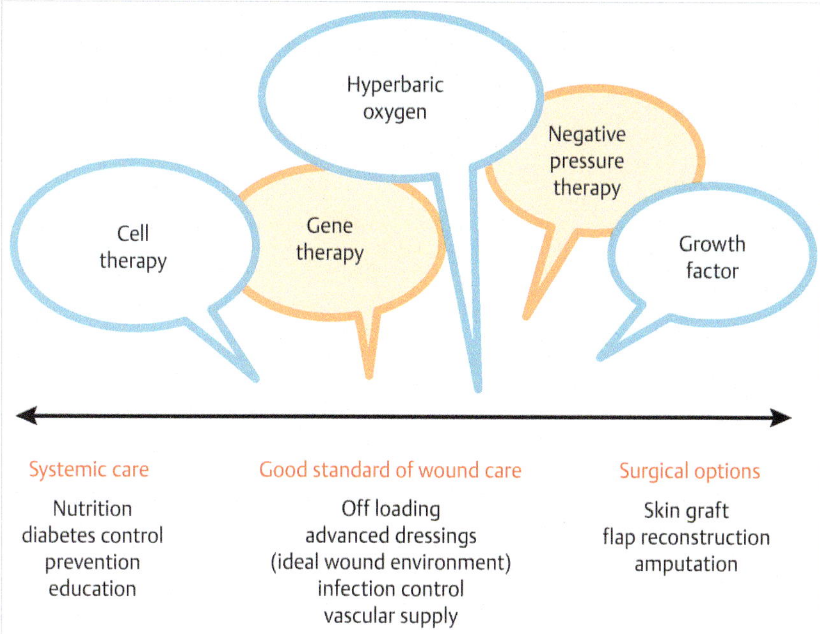

Fig. 18.1 Treating diabetic foot requires a multidisciplinary care as the spectrum of care is very wide from managing blood glucose, education on prevention, and managing small ulcers with good standard of care to using multiple new techniques and approaching with surgery.

shows the multidisciplinary algorithm for primary screening and initial treatment for wounds.[15]

With the introduction of the multidisciplinary approach, the trend of management has shifted from major amputation to limb salvage.[19] Addressing the issues of perfusion, infection, wound treatment, off-loading, and bone surgery, we are able to increase the salvage rate. Similar with other reports, the major amputation rate for diabetic foot in our center has reduced significantly after a multidisciplinary approach and recently maintains to be about 3 to 4%.[20,21] Although the indications for major amputation still exist and are often caused by multiple factors such as systemic sepsis, major tissue loss, significant comorbid factors, poor patient compliance, and non-reconstructable peripheral vascular disease, the goal remains the same: to salvage the limb under good clinical judgment. A nonhealing ulcer itself should not be considered an indication for amputation but be explored to solve the pathology behind it.[15,22,23]

18.3.2 Role of Microsurgery

Till recently, reconstruction with microsurgical techniques has been under debate.[15] This was due to the incorrect "myth" that patients with diabetes have an increased incidence of small-vessel disease that results in foot ulcers. Particularly, it was felt that patients with diabetes have arteriolar occlusive disease, which can cause ischemic lesions. This concept was first attributed to Goldenberg et al in 1959.[24] They studied amputation specimens from patients with gangrene and concluded that diabetic patients have endothelial hypertrophy and proliferation in the smaller arteries, with complete occlusion of the lumen in several cases. But subsequent studies have failed to demonstrate increased arteriolar occlusive disease or endothelial proliferation.[25,26,27] A thickening of the capillary basement membrane has been documented, but capillary narrowing or occlusion has not been documented.[25] The same study showed that diabetics often have atherosclerotic occlusion of the tibial arteries, but the occlusive disease occurs mainly in the leg so that the arterial system in the foot is less involved. Also as the patient undergoes obstruction of major vessels, new collateral sprouts to maintain a relatively stable vascularity to the foot.[28] Based on these studies, limb salvage from diabetic foot using microsurgical approach showed similar success in nondiabetic patients.[9,10,11,12,13,14] Meta-analysis of a systematic review of free tissue transfer in 528 diabetes patients in 18 studies showed flap survival of 92% and limb salvage rate of 83.4% over a 28-month average follow-up period. This study indicates that free tissue transfer in the management of nontraumatic lower extremity wounds in patients with diabetes may avoid amputations.[13] Free flaps and microsurgery technique now play an important role to salvage the limb from chronic ulcerations.[8,10,15,29,30]

18.4 Surgical Algorithm

While the medical care for the patient with diabetic foot ulceration begins with stabilization of the patient's systemic condition including blood glucose, the surgical care begins with debridement and control of infection. After the patient and the wound stabilized, further evaluation of the wound is made. Unless indicated for major amputation, the reconstructive algorithm is followed as shown in ▶ Fig. 18.3.[15] If it is a simple wound with minimal or no vital structures exposed, conservative care with various treatments can be considered. If well granulating after wound preparation, skin graft or a small local flap can be performed.[31] Well-granulating wounds can be an indication for good vascularity. However, if healing is stalling, then further evaluation using transcutaneous oxygen pressure measurement ($TcPO_2$) or angiograms are warranted to evaluate the arterial flow and prepare for vascular intervention. The same evaluation and approach to ensure vascularity are needed for complex wounds waiting reconstructive procedure.

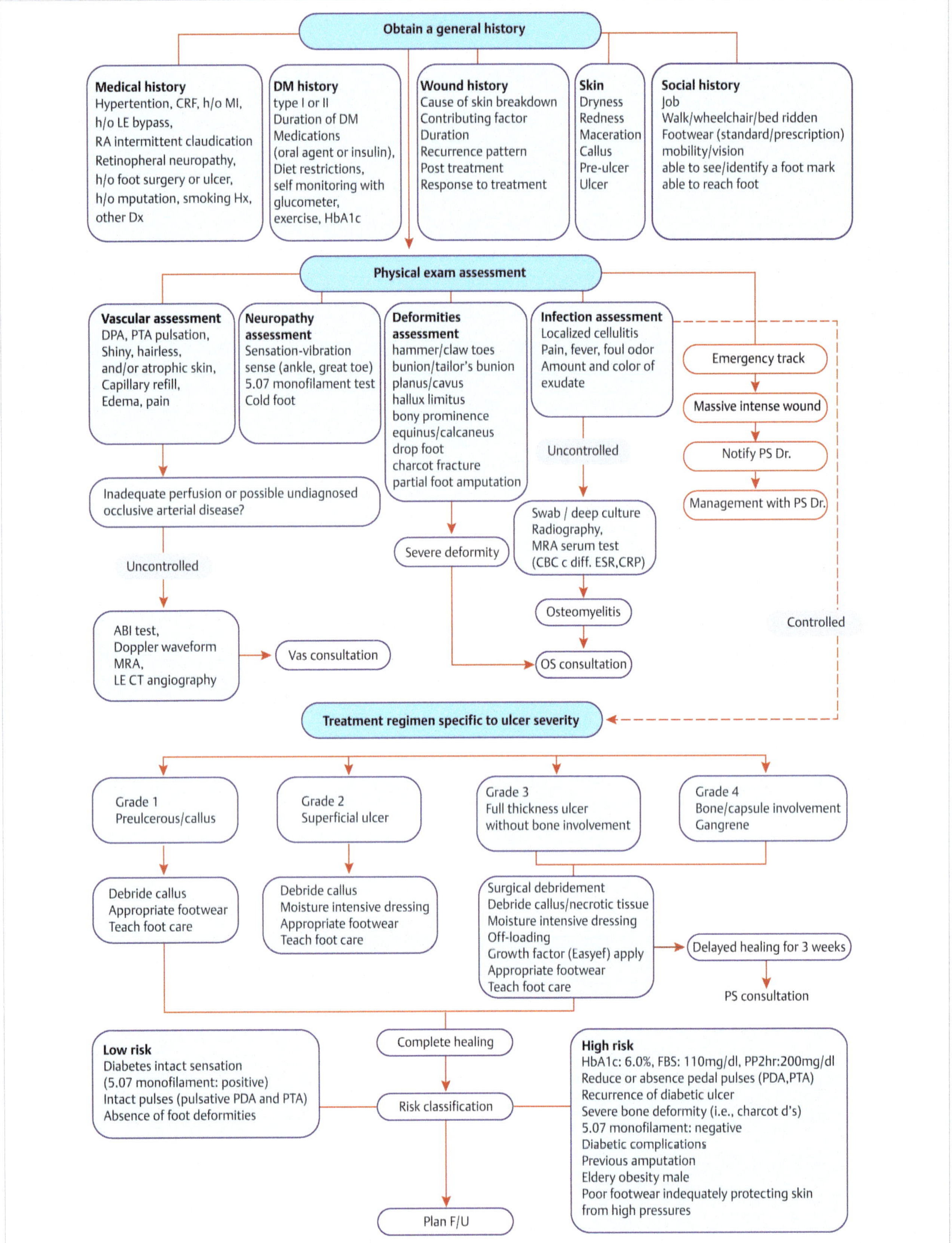

Fig. 18.2 The multidisciplinary algorithm for primary screening and initial treatment for wounds is shown. Note the emergency track that requires immediate surgical attention. Once the problem resolved, routine follow-up is important to prevent further recurrence.

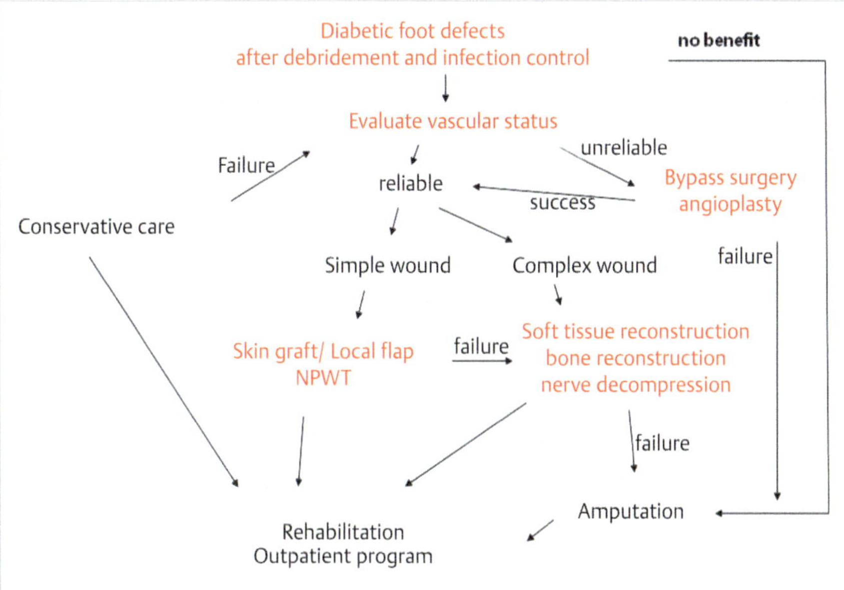

Fig. 18.3 Reconstructive algorithm is shown. Depending on the defect and the available vascularity, reconstructive planning can be done accordingly.

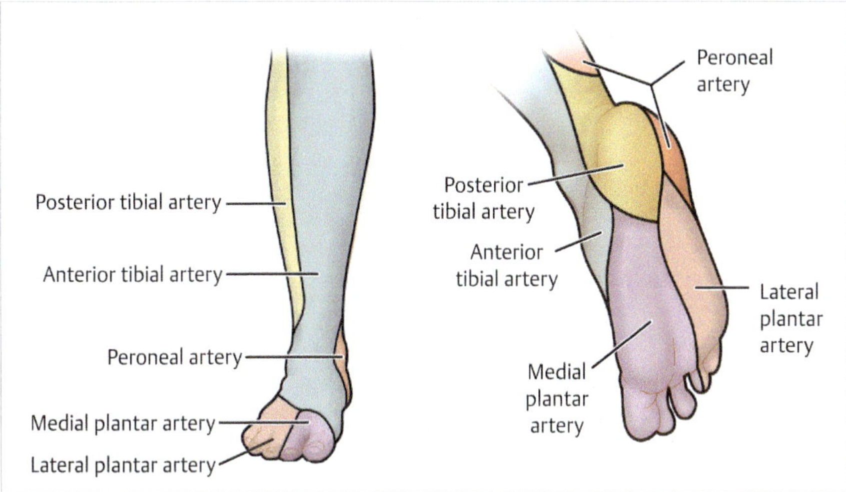

Fig. 18.4 The angiosome of the foot is shown. The six angiosomes of the foot and ankle are fed by the three main arteries. The anterior tibial artery becomes the dorsalis pedis artery supplying the dorsum of the foot. The posterior tibial artery (PTA) supplies the toes, the sole, and heel of the foot. The three main branches of the PTA supply distinct portions of the sole: the calcaneal branch to the heel, the medial plantar artery to the instep, and the lateral plantar artery to the lateral midfoot and the forefoot. The peroneal artery supplies the lateral border of the ankle and heel.

18.4.1 Debridement

The first step of treatment for a diabetic foot wound is to evaluate, debride, and treat the infection.[32] Missing timely management will lead to amputations and longer hospital stays.[33] If symptoms and sign of infection are clinically suspected, proper treatment must be provided without delay. If superficial infection is suspected without systemic infection, antibiotics treatment along with non-weight bearing of the foot should be ensued. Optimal management of a diabetic foot infection can potentially reduce incidence of major limb amputations and other related morbidities. All non-viable and infected soft tissue and bone should be excised during debridement. Milking along the proximal tendon can be helpful to identify and limit ascending infection. Tissue culture should be sent. Sufficient irrigation should follow after debridement to reduce bacterial count.[34] Recent advance in technology introduced the hydrosurgery system and negative-pressure wound therapy allows achievement of cleaner and better granulation.[35,36]

Understanding of vascular distribution of the foot angiosome is crucial in planning not only reconstruction but also debridement (▶ Fig. 18.4).[37] When planning for reconstruction, one should avoid violating the angiosome territory even when designing a local flap that may lead to flap breakdown in patients with low vascular perfusion.[38] Performing debridement according to the angiosome territory will enhance flap survival as the marginal vascularization from healthy surrounding angiosome territory occurs.[39] Repetitive debridement should be performed as part of wound preparation for reconstruction while monitoring C-reactive protein (CRP) for possible hidden infections and using it as an index for possible infection after reconstruction.[15]

18.5 Soft-Tissue Reconstruction

Once an adequate debridement and reasonable vascular perfusion are achieved, in extensive and complex diabetic foot defects, reconstruction should be considered. It is crucial that one improve the vascularity of the leg thorough endovascular procedures or bypass graft depending on the patient's status. Local flaps are useful when the patient has a good vascular status on the leg and foot. However, when the foot has compromised flow, the utilization of local flaps may breach the distal flow of the small collateral vessels especially the subdermal flow.[15] One must consider the vascular status as well as future flow where small collateral vessels may play an important role for distal circulation. Thus, the microsurgical approach may be considered for the following conditions: (1) lower limb defect that has not displayed any signs of granulation or healing despite adequate debridement or necrotic tissue and conservative treatment; (2) no significant systemic illness likely to be exacerbated by multiple operations and prolong rehabilitation; (3) previously ambulatory with the aim to restore a functional limb; (4) likely to engage with the significant physical therapy required for return to normal living; and (5) peak flow velocity of greater than 15 cm/s in the recipient artery.[8,29,39,40,41] The following can be high risk for patients who may undergo reconstructive microsurgery: (1) patients who have had multiple angioplasties; (2) patients with severe peripheral artery disease; and (3) patients after kidney transplantation who are using immunesuppression.[8,29,39] Among these considerations, the most significant one will be perfusion of the recipient vessel. If any small vessel is seen with good pulsatile flow, it would be indicated for microsurgery. Thus, an absolute contraindication would be no flow to the foot without any sign of perfusion from any distal small vessels. This supermicrosurgery and free style reconstruction approach, however, will require a refined skill along with a paradigm shift for reconstruction.[15,29,39]

18.5.1 Step-by-Step Approach for Reconstructive Microsurgery

1. Evaluate the general systemic condition of the patient.
2. Evaluate the vascular status and consider vascular intervention if needed to maximize flow to the foot. Identify potential vascular recipient site as well as flap donor site. ▶ Fig. 18.5 shows that the anterior tibial artery is calcified and nonviable; thus, the choice to use the posterior tibial artery has to be made. ▶ Fig. 18.6 shows that the major collateral vessel distally is the descending branch of the lateral circumflex femoral artery and one must avoid using the anterolateral thigh (ALT) as this would diminish the flow to the entire lower leg.
3. Debride the wound using angiosome concept and confirm the bleeding from the margins of the skin.
4. Identify the recipient vessels, visualize adequate pulse, and evaluate the relationship with the defect to determine the pedicle length.
   The biggest challenge in reconstructive microsurgery for a diabetic foot is finding the recipient vessel. Even with an adequate flow to the foot, atherosclerosis of the artery may make anastomosis very difficult. If a named artery will be used as recipient, one must try to find a small segment spared from calcification.[10] End to side on the major artery, end to end on a branch form the major vessels, or a T-anastomosis can be considered to minimize the flow deprivation after anastomosis. Small perforators can be used as recipients as well. During debridement, pulsatile arteries are marked. If there is no pulsating small arteries in the lesion, search for an adequate small recipient artery can be extended to the adjacent healthy angiosome territory. Once a pulsatile perforator or a small artery is found, it is dissected and preserved. For the recipient veins, there is no preference over superficial or deep veins. Easily available veins during debridement are mostly used.[29,39]
5. Elevation of flap with adequate pedicle length.
   The flap for reconstruction of a diabetic foot should provide a

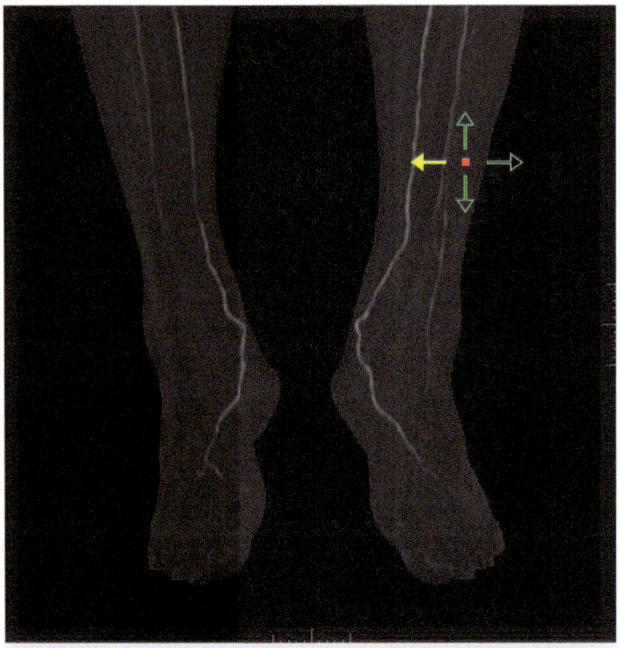

Fig. 18.5 CT angiography plays an important role in evaluating the overall flow of the leg. In addition, it provides information on potential recipient vessels. This examination shows that the anterior tibial artery is calcified and nonviable; thus, the choice to use the posterior tibial artery has to be made.

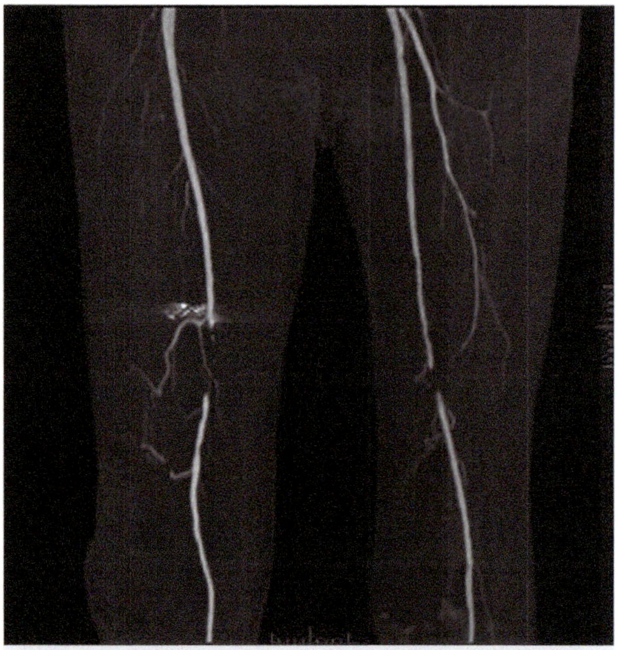

Fig. 18.6 CT angiography plays an important role in evaluating the overall flow of the leg. In addition, it also provides information in selecting potential flap donor sites. This examination shows that the major collateral vessel distally is the descending branch of the lateral circumflex femoral artery and one must avoid using the anterolateral thigh as this would diminish the flow to the entire lower leg.

well-vascularized tissue to control infection, adequate contour for footwear, durability, and solid anchorage to resist shearing forces. Controversy still remains as to which flap, whether muscle flaps with skin grafts, fasciocutaneous flaps, and recently added perforator flaps, offers the optimal solution to reconstruct the foot, especially the weight-bearing surface. But as long as the large defect is covered with any well-vascularized tissue, it will provide an independent and well-nourished vascular supply to eradicate infection, increase local oxygen tension, enhancing antibiotics activity, and neovascularization to the adjacent ischemic tissue.[42,43]
In our clinical experience, we are shifting toward using perforator flaps such as ALT perforator, gluteal artery perforator flap, and superficial circumflex iliac perforator flap as it provides a thin flap to minimize shearing, can take only the superficial fat to imitate the fibrous septa of the sole to adhere tightly, enhance neovascularization of the subdermal plexus with adjacent tissue, and provide adequate blood supply to fight infection.[10]

6. Check the recipient vessel again prior to cutting the flap pedicle.
7. Cut the pedicle and anastomosis of the vessels. If the pulse or the pulsatile flow of the recipient artery looks poor, consider elevating the systemic blood pressure.
An end-to-side anastomosis is highly recommended to preserve the flow to the feet. If vessels are calcified, one should look for a calcification spared segment or use a small branch from the major vessel as recipient. It is relatively rare to see branches from posterior tibial and dorsalis pedis arteries to be calcified and by using this branch one can easily anastomose to a supple and soft artery without diminishing distal flow. An alternative anastomosis may be the T-style anastomosis where bypassing artery segment with a branch to the flap is interanastomosed between the proximal and distal recipient artery. All efforts should be made to preserve the distal flow to the foot.
8. Insetting of the flap.

18.6 Postoperative Care

Postoperative care with splinting, maintenance of adequate hydration, patient in sitting position, and use of vasodilators such as prostaglandin E1 are routine. Along with subjective findings of the flap, duplex scan was used to evaluate the actual velocity of the blood flow into the flap. The patient can begin wheelchair ambulation on day 4 or 5 and compression garment applied on day 7. One should remember that the diabetic patients are prone to infection and should follow up with the CRP level closely until discharge. The patient can be discharged or transferred within 10 days.

18.7 Conclusion

The treatment of diabetic foot ulceration is complex with multiple considerations often leading to limb amputation. The multidisciplinary approach along with an algorithm to manage and salvage diabetic foot ulcers from amputation is a doable approach. Knowing the spectrum of care and reconstructive principles can prevent diabetic foot ulcers from amputation. Further understanding of supermicrosurgery and angiosome principles can extend the possibility for reconstruction in patients with severe ischemic diabetic foot.

References

[1] Reiber GE. The epidemiology of diabetic foot problems. Diabet Med. 1996; 13 Suppl 1:S6–S11

[2] Singh N, Armstrong DG, Lipsky BA. Preventing foot ulcers in patients with diabetes. JAMA. 2005; 293(2):217–228

[3] Most RS, Sinnock P. The epidemiology of lower extremity amputations in diabetic individuals. Diabetes Care. 1983; 6(1):87–91

[4] Saar WE, Lee TH, Berlet GC. The economic burden of diabetic foot and ankle disorders. Foot Ankle Int. 2005; 26(1):27–31

[5] Apelqvist J, Ragnarson-Tennvall G, Larsson J, Persson U. Long-term costs for foot ulcers in diabetic patients in a multidisciplinary setting. Foot Ankle Int. 1995; 16(7):388–394

[6] Reiber GE, Lipsky BA, Gibbons GW. The burden of diabetic foot ulcers. Am J Surg. 1998; 176(2A) Suppl:5S–10S

[7] Moulik PK, Mtonga R, Gill GV. Amputation and mortality in new-onset diabetic foot ulcers stratified by etiology. Diabetes Care. 2003; 26(2): 491–494

[8] Oh TS, Lee HS, Hong JP. Diabetic foot reconstruction using free flaps increases 5-year-survival rate. J Plast Reconstr Aesthet Surg. 2013; 66(2):243–250

[9] Colen LB. Limb salvage in the patient with severe peripheral vascular disease: the role of microsurgical free-tissue transfer. Plast Reconstr Surg. 1987; 79(3):389–395

[10] Hong JP. Reconstruction of the diabetic foot using the anterolateral thigh perforator flap. Plast Reconstr Surg. 2006; 117(5):1599–1608

[11] Searles JM, Jr, Colen LB. Foot reconstruction in diabetes mellitus and peripheral vascular insufficiency. Clin Plast Surg. 1991; 18(3):467–483

[12] Shenaq SM, Dinh TA. Foot salvage in arteriolosclerotic and diabetic patients by free flaps after vascular bypass: report of two cases. Microsurgery. 1989; 10(4):310–314

[13] Fitzgerald O'Connor EJ, Vesely M, Holt PJ, Jones KG, Thompson MM, Hinchliffe RJ. A systematic review of free tissue transfer in the management of non-traumatic lower extremity wounds in patients with diabetes. Eur J Vasc Endovasc Surg. 2011; 41(3):391–399

[14] Oishi SN, Levin LS, Pederson WC. Microsurgical management of extremity wounds in diabetics with peripheral vascular disease. Plast Reconstr Surg. 1993; 92(3):485–492

[15] Hong JP, Oh TS. An algorithm for limb salvage for diabetic foot ulcers. Clin Plast Surg. 2012; 39(3):341–352

[16] Boulton AJ. The diabetic foot: from art to science. The 18th Camillo Golgi lecture. Diabetologia. 2004; 47(8):1343–1353

[17] Endara M, Masden D, Goldstein J, Gondek S, Steinberg J, Attinger C. The role of chronic and perioperative glucose management in high-risk surgical closures: a case for tighter glycemic control. Plast Reconstr Surg. 2013; 132(4): 996–1004

[18] Childers BJ, Potyondy LD, Nachreiner R, et al. Necrotizing fasciitis: a fourteen-year retrospective study of 163 consecutive patients. Am Surg. 2002; 68(2): 109–116

[19] Wraight PR, Lawrence SM, Campbell DA, Colman PG. Creation of a multidisciplinary, evidence based, clinical guideline for the assessment, investigation and management of acute diabetes related foot complications. Diabet Med. 2005; 22(2):127–136

[20] Krishnan N, Becker DF. Characterization of a bifunctional PutA homologue from Bradyrhizobium japonicum and identification of an active site residue that modulates proline reduction of the flavin adenine dinucleotide cofactor. Biochemistry. 2005; 44(25):9130–9139

[21] Holstein P, Ellitsgaard N, Olsen BB, Ellitsgaard V. Decreasing incidence of major amputations in people with diabetes. Diabetologia. 2000; 43(7):844–847

[22] Apelqvist J. Wound healing in diabetes. Outcome and costs. Clin Podiatr Med Surg. 1998; 15(1):21–39

[23] Cavanagh PR, Ulbrecht JS, Caputo GM. The non-healing diabetic foot wound: fact or fiction? Ostomy Wound Manage. 1998; 44(3A) Suppl:6S–12S, discussion 13S

[24] Goldenberg S, Alex M, Joshi RA, Blumenthal HT. Nonatheromatous peripheral vascular disease of the lower extremity in diabetes mellitus. Diabetes. 1959; 8(4):261–273

[25] Strandness DE, Jr, Priest RE, Gibbons GE. Combined clinical and pathologic study of diabetic and nondiabetic peripheral arterial disease. Diabetes. 1964; 13:366–372

[26] Conrad MC. Large and small artery occlusion in diabetics and nondiabetics with severe vascular disease. Circulation. 1967; 36(1):83–91

[27] LoGerfo FW, Coffman JD. Current concepts. Vascular and microvascular disease of the foot in diabetes. Implications for foot care. N Engl J Med. 1984; 311(25):1615–1619

[28] Suh HP, Kim Y, Suh Y, Hong J. Multidetector computed tomography (CT) analysis of 168 cases in diabetic patients with total superficial femoral artery occlusion: is it safe to use an anterolateral thigh flap without CT angiography in diabetic patients? J Reconstr Microsurg. 2018; 34(1):65–70

[29] Suh HS, Oh TS, Hong JP. Innovations in diabetic foot reconstruction using supermicrosurgery. Diabetes Metab Res Rev. 2016; 32 Suppl 1:275–280

[30] Moran SL, Illig KA, Green RM, Serletti JM. Free-tissue transfer in patients with peripheral vascular disease: a 10-year experience. Plast Reconstr Surg. 2002; 109(3):999–1006

[31] Knox KR, Datiashvili RO, Granick MS. Surgical wound bed preparation of chronic and acute wounds. Clin Plast Surg. 2007; 34(4):633–641

[32] Attinger CE, Bulan EJ. Débridement. The key initial first step in wound healing. Foot Ankle Clin. 2001; 6(4):627–660

[33] Reiber GE, Vileikyte L, Boyko EJ, et al. Causal pathways for incident lower-extremity ulcers in patients with diabetes from two settings. Diabetes Care. 1999; 22(1):157–162

[34] Badia JM, Torres JM, Tur C, Sitges-Serra A. Saline wound irrigation reduces the postoperative infection rate in guinea pigs. J Surg Res. 1996; 63(2):457–459

[35] Granick M, Boykin J, Gamelli R, Schultz G, Tenenhaus M. Toward a common language: surgical wound bed preparation and debridement. Wound Repair Regen. 2006; 14 Suppl 1:S1–S10

[36] Granick MS, Posnett J, Jacoby M, Noruthun S, Ganchi PA, Datiashvili RO. Efficacy and cost-effectiveness of a high-powered parallel waterjet for wound debridement. Wound Repair Regen. 2006; 14(4):394–397

[37] Clemens MW, Attinger CE. Angiosomes and wound care in the diabetic foot. Foot Ankle Clin. 2010; 15(3):439–464

[38] Attinger C, Cooper P, Blume P, Bulan E. The safest surgical incisions and amputations applying the angiosome principles and using the Doppler to assess the arterial-arterial connections of the foot and ankle. Foot Ankle Clin. 2001; 6(4):745–799

[39] Suh HS, Oh TS, Lee HS, et al. A new approach for reconstruction of diabetic foot wounds using the angiosome and supermicrosurgery concept. Plast Reconstr Surg. 2016; 138(4):702e–709e

[40] Yue DK, McLennan S, Marsh M, et al. Effects of experimental diabetes, uremia, and malnutrition on wound healing. Diabetes. 1987; 36(3):295–299

[41] Berman SJ. Infections in patients with end-stage renal disease. An overview. Infect Dis Clin North Am. 2001; 15(3):709–720, vii

[42] Shestak KC, Hendricks DL, Webster MW. Indirect revascularization of the lower extremity by means of microvascular free-muscle flap: a preliminary report. J Vasc Surg. 1990; 12(5):581–585

[43] Chang N, Mathes SJ. Comparison of the effect of bacterial inoculation in musculocutaneous and random-pattern flaps. Plast Reconstr Surg. 1982; 70(1): 1–10

19 Rationale for Lower Limb Sensate Flaps

Joon Pio Hong

Summary

The ideal reconstruction of sole should lead to optimal functional and aesthetic results, achieving durable coverage for weight bearing, adequate contour for footwear, protective sensation, and solid anchorage to deep tissue to resist shearing. Thin flaps accommodating the defect can be the best chance for prolong stability. A sensate flap with thin skin component may be ideal in providing plantar surface reconstruction. However, if a sensate flap cannot be used, a thin flap without including deep fat and deep fascia may regain some protective sensation within a 12-month period.

Keywords: sensate flaps, plantar reconstruction, microsurgery, nerve flap, thin skin flap

19.1 Introduction

Sensate flaps are flaps that provide sensation on the recipient site and innervated flaps are flaps that have direct nerve coaptation. It has been known that skin flaps and muscle flaps do have the ability to regain sensation to a certain level with or without direct nerve reinnervation.[1,2,3,4] Thus, theoretically any flap can be potentially sensate flaps, but the nomenclature of sensate flap is frequently used synonymously with innervated flaps. In this chapter, the same traditional definition will be used. The weight-bearing plantar foot remains the most important recipient site for sensate flaps. The importance of sensation during gait cannot be overemphasized. This section will elaborate the approach in using sensate flap mostly in regard to plantar reconstruction.

In flaps with skin components, specific sensory nerves are identified above the deep fascia. When a cutaneous nerve is identified, flaps using the skin component can be designed to incorporate the sensory nerve. The recipient cutaneous nerve is located around the defect and is used as a recipient nerve.

Muscle flaps are frequently needed to cover large defects of the extremity and foot. Free muscle flaps with skin grafts have been traditionally popular, considered to be easier in tailoring into the soft-tissue defects, providing good cushioning and solid anchorage to the deep structure and thus can best replace the complex subcutaneous architectural structure of the plantar surface.[3,5,6] But questions have been raised with regard to their durability against long-standing pressure.[7,8] In muscle flaps that were used to reconstruct the foot without reinnervation, gait and stance analysis with nonsensory innervated muscle flaps revealed the ability to bear weight, but with decreased pressure and duration.[1,2,3] Other reports speculate that functional reconstruction outcome may be more related to underlying bony deformities.[9] Nevertheless, muscle flaps with skin graft to reconstruct the foot may be bulky and require frequent secondary debulking proceudres.[3] Furthermore, frequent ulceration has been reported with muscle flaps with skin grafts that may need high maintenance (▶ Fig. 19.1).[3] This is most likely due to the lack of normal skin anatomy and sensory recovery. Although there have been multiple reports that muscle flaps regain deep pressure sensation even without cutaneous innervation, they will never regain complete sensory recovery.[1,2,3,10] Muscle flaps with intact motor nerves or with reanastomosis of the motor nerve to suitable motor or sensory nerves at the recipient site may have higher chance to retain protective sensibility.[1,2,3] Nevertheless, with good maintenance involving visual inspection, proper footwear, and daily management, muscle flaps do provide a good solution especially for extensive defects of the foot.

Second choice for plantar reconstruction will be fasciocutaneous flaps. The first lesson in plastic surgery starts with the concept of "like-with-like" reconstruction. Reconstruction of the weight-bearing sole remains difficult and challenging due to the specialized dermal–epidermal histology, and fibrous septa of the subcutaneous layer provide a unique property to withstand pressure and absorb shock of the gait.[11,12,13,14] The only skin that is identical to the plantar skin is the palmer skin, which is limited in source. Conventional local flaps from the plantar regions can be used to achieve ideal reconstruction but is limited to small defects. For larger and extensive defects, microvascular flap reconstruction is often required. But whatever flap is chosen, it is nearly impossible to replace the unique property of the weight-bearing sole. The ideal reconstruction of the sole should lead to optimal functional and aesthetic results, performing successful function in everyday life and occupation, wearing usual footwear with minimal donor site morbidity. To achieve these goals, characteristics such as durable coverage for weight bearing, adequate contour, protective sensation, and solid anchoring to deep tissue to resist shearing should be provided. The fasciocutaneous flaps may be able to provide some of the characteristics of an ideal flap for plantar reconstruction. However, the problem of sliding phenomenon has made it a controversial option.[8,15] The anatomical structure of multiple fat layers in addition to the superficial fascia between the deep

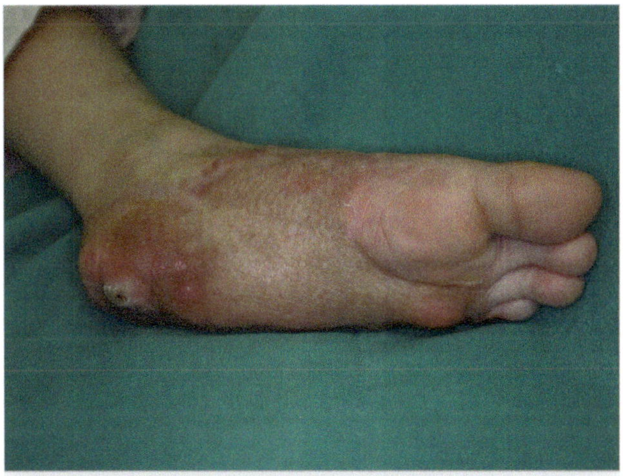

Fig. 19.1 Minor ulceration after muscle free flap with skin graft is noted during follow-up. Although the overall contour looks fine, minor complications continues to occur.

fascia and the skin makes the skin surface slide resilient to external environment, but this property of the fasciocutaneous flap increases the gliding of the skin and makes it less ideal to resist shearing. The thicker the flap and the more the fat structure, the greater the gliding of the flap. Rautio et al reported that the optimal thickness of the flap should be less than 6 mm for adequate tightening and to resist shearing.[10,16] The third choice for reconstruction can be the perforator flap. Perforator flaps can be elevated as a fasciocutaneous flap, but when raised above the deep fascia it becomes a skin flap with subcutaneous fat. When using the perforator flaps such as the anterolateral thigh flap, which is one of the most frequently used perforator flaps, with the fat component present despite elevating it suprafascially, it can still be very bulky making it a less ideal choice for foot reconstruction. Since the introduction of thin perforator flaps elevating it above the superficial fascia and including only superficial fat and the skin, it may become thin enough to mimic the ideal thickness of the flap for plantar reconstruction.[17,18] Further report in using perforator flaps after thinning removing the deep fat and the deep fascia show that it may reduce the shearing in plantar surface reconstruction.[4] Another interesting finding from this study showed that perforator flaps with adequate subcutaneous fat after removing the deep fat may provide a cushioning effect over the plantar surface unlike that seen with forearm free flap.[4] Within the superficial fat layer, multiple small lobules surrounded by fibrous network may attach firmly to the surface of the defect and limit the sliding of the skin surface. One must ask, due to the anatomical position of the sensory nerves in the skin lying just above the deep fascia, whether it is better to include the nerve as a sensate flap despite the flap being thick. Although there is no clear study to answer this question, our experience shows that there is a difference in sensory recovery between sensory perforator flaps and insensate perforator flaps. The difference was statistically significant only at the third month, suggesting that earlier sensory recovery is expected by sensory nerve coaptation.[4] However in nonsensate flaps, it ultimately regained protective sensation in 83.3% at 1 year without sensory nerve coaptation. This result is similar with the reports in which forearm fasciocutaneous flaps were used. Santanelli et al presented that flaps gained protective sensibility in 12 months regardless of surgical nerve repair.[16] It is most likely, as seen in the case of forearm and anterolateral thigh perforator flap, that thinness of the flap may play an important role in reestablishing sensibility. Thus, in this chapter we will talk about the application of thin flaps for plantar surface reconstruction. The thinning technique of perforator flaps will be covered in another chapter.

Maintenance of protective sensation is essential especially for the feet and other weight-bearing areas. Without protective sensation, one can be at risk of ulcers and injuries from shoes and objects stepped on without shoes. Thus, the controversy on which flap can best accommodate the sensation after reconstruction has been under continuous debate. The ideal reconstruction of the foot, especially the weight-bearing areas of the plantar surface, should result in adequate contour for normal footwear, thick durable skin, protective sensation, and solid anchorage to the deep structures to resist shearing forces.[19] Studies have shown benefits of protective sensation for ankle and heel reconstruction both with rotational flaps and by microvascular tissue transfer.[16,20,21] Sensory reinnervation for free flaps showed faster sensory recovery and flaps without sensory reinnervation did recover protective sensation to a certain degree.[4,16]

19.1.1 Nerve Flaps

The sensory nerves are supplied by an extrinsic and intrinsic blood supply. The extrinsic blood supply to the peripheral nerves consists of arteriae nervorum that rises directly from the perforating vessels. These perforating vessels may originate from various deeper vessels as seen from Nakajima et al's perforator classification.[22] These small arteriae nervorum enters the nerve and terminates intraneurally. The intrinsic blood supplies are the longitudinally oriented arterioles located on the epineurium, perineurium, and endoneurium. The intrinsic vessels communicate and receive vascular supply from the extrinsic arteries (vasa nervosum) and the end branches.[23,24] Thus, the nerve flap can be harvested from superficially located sensory nerves based on perforating vessels originating from a proximal source vessel. Based on this clear distinction of tissue being supplied by a vascular source, the term "vascularized nerve graft" would be a misnomer and "nerve flap" should be used as the right term to minimize confusion. There has not been an extensive report in using nerve flaps for nerve defects. However, sporadic reports are showing that the regeneration of nerve may be faster and thus functionally beneficial.

Well-known examples of nerve flaps would be superficial radial nerve flap based on the radial artery and accompanying veins, saphenous nerve flap proximally based on the branches from femoral artery and distally based on the saphenous artery, and sural nerve flap based on the superficial sural artery or medial sural artery.[25,26,27,28,29]

In the cases where perforators are not found leading to the superficial nerve, one can use the accompanying vein along the superficial nerve in an arterialized fashion. Typical example would be the sural nerve flap where an arterial supply such as superficial sural artery and medial or lateral sural artery would be missing and the lesser saphenous vein would be arterialized[30,31,32]

19.2 Attributes and Detriments

19.2.1 Attributes

- Sensate flaps may benefit plantar reconstruction.
- Sensate flaps will regain faster sensory recovery.
- Muscle flaps and nonsensate skin flaps will regain some form of sensation when the flap is thin enough.

19.2.2 Detriments

- Sensate flaps may be too thick as the sensory nerve is located just above the deep fascia.
- One must decide the benefits of sensate flaps versus thin flaps.

19.3 Anatomical Considerations

There are several anatomical considerations. Foremost, the thickness of the flap should be considered. Despite what flap

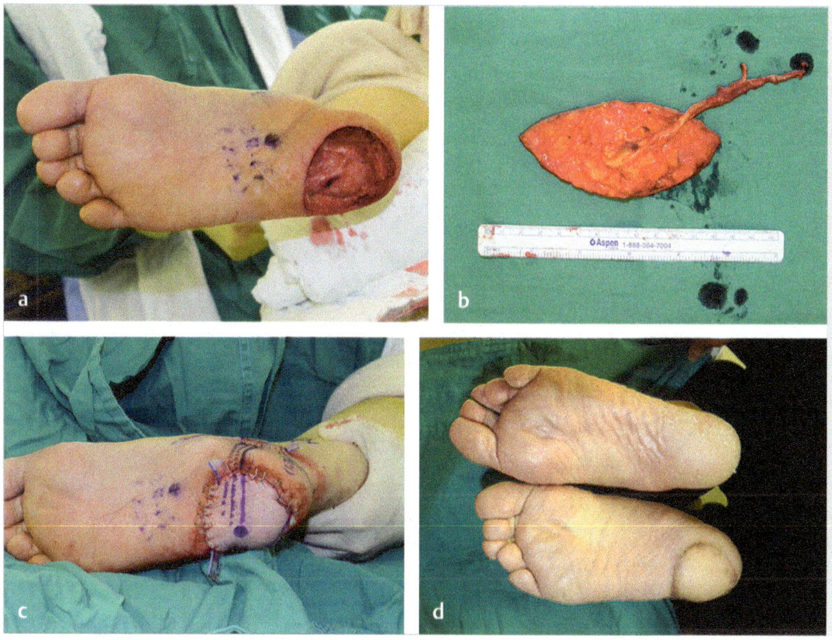

Fig. 19.2 **(a)** A patient after cancer resection is shown with heal defect. **(b)** A naturally thin anterolateral thigh flap is elevated above the deep fascia including the superficial femoral nerve. **(c)** Notice the good contour immediately after reconstruction with nerve anastomosis. **(d)** Long-term follow-up shows good contour without further complications.

you use, muscle, fasciocutaneous, or perforator, thin flaps mimicking and providing the missing depth of the defect would be ideal to minimize shearing. When including the sensory nerve in skin component, one must decide whether thickness will accommodate the defect. If the flap is thin enough even when including the nerve, it can be the ideal flap as it will regain sensation early as well as provide better sensation (▶ Fig. 19.2). When not including the nerve, one should achieve the ideal thickness. Next is to minimize gliding by removing the deep fascia and deep fat of the perforator flaps. Using fasciocutaneous flaps will be less ideal as the gliding will not be prevented by having the deep fascia intact.

19.4 Anatomical Variants and Potential Pitfalls

See perforator flap thinning in Chapter 22.

19.5 Flap Design and Harvest

See perforator flap thinning in Chapter 22 and Chapter 26.

19.6 Postoperative Care Protocols

As in the case of any plantar surface reconstruction, patient education and patient compliance are vital in achieving long-term success after reconstruction. One of the keys to maintaining prolong durable reconstruction is minimizing shearing of the flap that may lead to secondary breakdowns. To allow early weight bearing of the reconstructed foot, pressure stocking plays an important role in maintaining the integrity of the flap. The pressure of the stocking allows the premature flap to bear weight without shearing and it also reduces the edema, leading to early molding.

The compression pressure of 30 to 35 mm Hg is safe based on the fact that regular compressions stocking to minimize and prevent orthostatic swelling uses compression pressure of 20 to 30 mm Hg. We further determined the safety of compression by looking at the survival of the flap as well as the effect on the pedicle flow velocity and volume. Our results at 30 to 35 mm Hg compression on flaps show no difference prior to (29.21 cm/s) and post (29.42 cm/s) compression. The same can be seen for flow prior to (7.13 cm^3/s) and post (6.56 cm^3/s) compression. Another interesting finding we made was that the type of anastomosis was not affected by compression either. We usually start compression at day 5 after reconstruction. The reason for starting at day 5 was to allow the flap to inosculate to the surrounding structure without stress and to monitor the flap for complications. Our protocol specifying the pressure and timing showed safe results as the flaps had no major complication during the follow-up. To standardize the pressure application, we decided to use the custom-designed garments as mirroring the uninjured contralateral leg would be able to deliver an even compression throughout the reconstruction area mimicking the normal contour of the leg. This garment is frequently used in burn patients to minimize burn scar and thus is easily obtainable. It has a zipper and can be easily and safely applied by the patient without any aid from a caregiver while providing constant even pressure. Thus, we showed that the use of compression garment at 30 to 35 mm Hg is safe and easy to apply beginning from day 5 (▶ Fig. 19.3).

Unless using a local flap or a plantar skin free flap, the anatomy of the plantar surface will never be identical. All other flaps will be suboptimal. The only way to overcome this gap is good postoperative follow-up and education. Regular visual inspection, palpation, and temperature monitoring will be essential to detect early complication. In our institute, the patient is required to go through early rehabilitation program, vigorous education, and serial follow-ups.

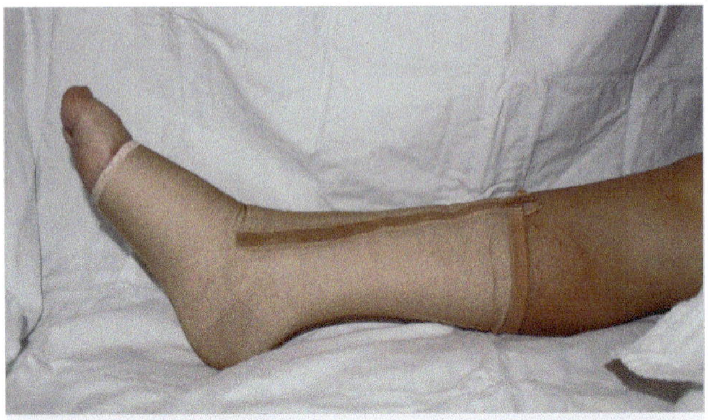

Fig. 19.3 Using compression garment with 30 to 35 mm Hg allows the flap to tightly adhere to the plantar base minimizing any shearing during gait.

19.7 Conclusion

The ideal reconstruction of the sole should lead to optimal functional and aesthetic results, performing successful function in everyday life and occupation, wearing usual footwear with minimal donor site morbidity. To achieve these goals, characteristics such as durable coverage for weight bearing, adequate contour, protective sensation, and solid anchoring to deep tissue to resist shearing should be provided. Flaps with thin thickness accommodating the defect can be the best chance for prolong stability. A sensate flap with thin skin component may be ideal in providing plantar surface reconstruction. If a sensate flap cannot be used, a thin flap without including deep fat and deep fascia may regain some protective sensation within a 12-month period.

References

[1] Ducic I, Hung V, Dellon AL. Innervated free flaps for foot reconstruction: a review. J Reconstr Microsurg. 2006; 22(6):433–442

[2] Yücel A, Senyuva C, Aydin Y, Cinar C, Güzel Z. Soft-tissue reconstruction of sole and heel defects with free tissue transfers. Ann Plast Surg. 2000; 44(3): 259–268, discussion 268–269

[3] May JW, Jr, Halls MJ, Simon SR. Free microvascular muscle flaps with skin graft reconstruction of extensive defects of the foot: a clinical and gait analysis study. Plast Reconstr Surg. 1985; 75(5):627–641

[4] Hong JP, Kim EK. Sole reconstruction using anterolateral thigh perforator free flaps. Plast Reconstr Surg. 2007; 119(1):186–193

[5] May JW, Jr, Gallico GG, III, Jupiter J, Savage RC. Free latissimus dorsi muscle flap with skin graft for treatment of traumatic chronic bony wounds. Plast Reconstr Surg. 1984; 73(4):641–651

[6] Ferreira MC, Besteiro JM, Monteiro Júnior AA, Zumiotti A. Reconstruction of the foot with microvascular free flaps. Microsurgery. 1994; 15(1):33–36

[7] Ohjimi H, Taniguchi Y, Kawano K, Kinoshita K, Manabe T. A comparison of thinning and conventional free-flap transfers to the lower extremity. Plast Reconstr Surg. 2000; 105(2):558–566

[8] Sönmez A, Bayramiçli M, Sönmez B, Numanoğlu A. Reconstruction of the weight-bearing surface of the foot with nonneurosensory free flaps. Plast Reconstr Surg. 2003; 111(7):2230–2236

[9] Potparić Z, Rajacić N. Long-term results of weight-bearing foot reconstruction with non-innervated and reinnervated free flaps. Br J Plast Surg. 1997; 50(3): 176–181

[10] Rautio J. Patterns of recovery of sensibility in free flaps transferred to the foot: a prospective study. J Reconstr Microsurg. 1990; 6(1):37–41

[11] Gidumal R, Carl A, Evanski P, Shaw W, Waugh TR. Functional evaluation of nonsensate free flaps to the sole of the foot. Foot Ankle. 1986; 7(2):118–123

[12] Masquelet AC, Romana MC. The medialis pedis flap: a new fasciocutaneous flap. Plast Reconstr Surg. 1990; 85(5):765–772

[13] Morrison WA, Crabb DM, O'Brien BM, Jenkins A. The instep of the foot as a fasciocutaneous island and as a free flap for heel defects. Plast Reconstr Surg. 1983; 72(1):56–65

[14] Shaw WW, Hidalgo DA. Anatomic basis of plantar flap design: clinical applications. Plast Reconstr Surg. 1986; 78(5):637–649

[15] Weinzweig N, Davies BW. Foot and ankle reconstruction using the radial forearm flap: a review of 25 cases. Plast Reconstr Surg. 1998; 102(6):1999–2005

[16] Santanelli F, Tenna S, Pace A, Scuderi N. Free flap reconstruction of the sole of the foot with or without sensory nerve coaptation. Plast Reconstr Surg. 2002; 109(7):2314–2322, discussion 2323–2324

[17] Hong JP, Choi DH, Suh H, et al. A new plane of elevation: the superficial fascial plane for perforator flap elevation. J Reconstr Microsurg. 2014; 30(7):491–496

[18] Hong JP, Chung IW. The superficial fascia as a new plane of elevation for anterolateral thigh flaps. Ann Plast Surg. 2013; 70(2):192–195

[19] Harris PG, Letrosne E, Caouette-Laberge L, Egerszegi EP. Long-term follow-up of coverage of weight bearing surface of the foot with free muscular flap in a pediatric population. Microsurgery. 1994; 15(6):424–429

[20] Chen SL, Chen TM, Chou TD, Chen SG, Wang HJ. The distally based lesser saphenous venofasciocutaneous flap for ankle and heel reconstruction. Plast Reconstr Surg. 2002; 110(7):1664–1672

[21] Matthews RN, Fatah F, Davies DM, Eyre J, Hodge RA, Walsh-Waring GP. Experience with the radial forearm flap in 14 cases. Scand J Plast Reconstr Surg. 1984; 18(3):303–310

[22] Nakajima H, Fujino T, Adachi S. A new concept of vascular supply to the skin and classification of skin flaps according to their vascularization. Ann Plast Surg. 1986; 16(1):1–19

[23] Breidenbach WC, Terzis JK. The blood supply of vascularized nerve grafts. J Reconstr Microsurg. 1986; 3(1):43–58

[24] Breidenbach W, Terzis JK. The anatomy of free vascularized nerve grafts. Clin Plast Surg. 1984; 11(1):65–71

[25] Taylor GI, Ham FJ. The free vascularized nerve graft. A further experimental and clinical application of microvascular techniques. Plast Reconstr Surg. 1976; 57(4):413–426

[26] Daniel RK, Terzis J, Schwarz G. Neurovascular free flaps. A preliminary report. Plast Reconstr Surg. 1975; 56(1):13–20

[27] Acland RD, Schusterman M, Godina M, Eder E, Taylor GI, Carlisle I. The saphenous neurovascular free flap. Plast Reconstr Surg. 1981; 67(6):763–774

[28] Gilbert A. Vascularized sural nerve graft. Clin Plast Surg. 1984; 11(1):73–77

[29] Doi K, Kuwata N, Kawakami F, Tamaru K, Kawai S. The free vascularized sural nerve graft. Microsurgery. 1984; 5(4):175–184

[30] Terzis JK, Kostopoulos VK. Vascularized nerve grafts for lower extremity nerve reconstruction. Ann Plast Surg. 2010; 64(2):169–176

[31] Terzis JK, Kostopoulos VK. Vascularized ulnar nerve graft: 151 reconstructions for posttraumatic brachial plexus palsy. Plast Reconstr Surg. 2009; 123(4):1276–1291

[32] Terzis JK, Skoulis TG, Soucacos PN. Vascularized nerve grafts. A review. International Angiology. 1995; 14:264

20 A New Concept in Drop Foot Treatment: Ninković's Technique—the Neuromusculotendinous Gastrocnemius Transfer

Milomir Ninković, Marina Ninković, and Alexander de Heinrich

Summary

A "drop foot" deformity may be due to peroneal nerve injury or muscle damage of the anterior and/or lateral compartments. When not treated, in addition to ambulatory impediment, a secondary equinovarus deformity with Achilles tendon shortening develops due to the uncompensated activity of the posterior muscle compartments innervated by the tibial nerve. Whereas previously transfer of any of the latter functionally antagonistic plantar-flexing muscles to restore dorsiflexion would simultaneously contract with all other remaining posterior compartment muscles, this generated a tenodesis effect to keep the foot in a neutral position without voluntary range of motion of the ankle joint. A more physiological approach would be the transfer of usually the lateral head of the gastrocnemius muscle still attached to the superficial portion of the Achilles tendon. In the first stage, a viable proximal portion of the deep peroneal nerve as well as the tibial nerve to the chosen gastrocnemius muscle is dissected. Tenorrhaphy of the Achilles tendon is next completed with the anterior compartment tendons. Finally, a tension-free microscopic neurorrhaphy of the deep peroneal and sural nerves is performed. Nerve regeneration and concomitant rehabilitation can be a prolonged period even up to 18 months before full muscle strength can be expected. This, however, when usually successful, will best restore a more normal, fully automatic walking pattern, with stability of the foot without being dependent on any successful muscle reeducation.

Keywords: drop foot, neuromusculotendinous gastrocnemius transfer, dynamic muscle transfer

20.1 Introduction

Innervated by the common peroneal nerve, the muscles of the anterior and lateral compartments of the lower leg control eversion, inversion, and dorsiflexion of the foot and toes. Thus, injury to the peroneal nerve or muscle damage of the anterior and/or lateral compartment causes muscular imbalance and drop foot. If the condition is not treated, secondary equinovarus deformities and Achilles tendon shortening develop because of the uncompensated activity of the posterior muscle compartments innervated by the tibial nerve. The most common surgical treatment for drop foot deformity is a tendon transfer of the tibial posterior muscle, sometimes combined with transfer of additional muscles of the posterior compartment.

The muscles of the anterior compartment of the leg are innervated by the deep peroneal nerve, and are mainly responsible for dorsiflexion of the foot at the ankle joint as well as extension of the toes, which implies that any reconstructive options for them, if needed, be adjusted to suit these specific anatomical features. The deep peroneal nerve provides muscular branches to the extensor muscles including the tibialis anterior (TA), extensor hallucis longus (EHL), extensor digitorum longus (EDL), as well as the fibularis (peroneus) tertius (PT). These muscles are collectively accountable for dorsiflexion of the foot at the ankle joint, extension of the toes, and a normal walking pattern. Moreover, the deep peroneal nerve innervates some of the intrinsic muscles of the foot along with the extensor digitorum brevis and the extensor hallucis brevis. Any kind of trauma to the deep peroneal nerve or the anterior compartment muscles may consequently lead to a material deterioration of dorsiflexion of the foot, which clinically is defined as "drop foot syndrome." This is exemplified by a characteristic steppage gait with patients dragging their foot and having a compensatory excessive raising of their knee while walking. The common treatment of the drop foot syndrome includes the surgical single and split dynamic tendon transposition of the tibialis posterior (TP) tendon along with the "bridle manner," in which the tendon is inserted into the affected muscle tissues of the anterior and lateral muscle compartments.

In 1933, Ober[1] was the first to describe a surgical technique for the treatment of drop foot, which used transfer of the TP tendon around the medial border of the tibia to the dorsum of the foot. Watkins et al[2] improved this approach by transferring the TP tendon through the interosseous membrane between the tibia and the fibula. Further improvements were the dual insertion of the TP tendon to balance the foot by Anderson,[3] who split the TP tendon into two tails and inserted them into the tendons of the EHL and the EDL in the so-called tendon-to-tendon technique. Using existing tendons as distal attachment points helped avoid foot deformities resulting from direct insertion into bone.[4] The most frequently used "bridle" transfer described by McCall et al[5] works by transfer of the TP tendon through the interosseous membrane, then dual insertion into the tendons of the TA and the rerouted peroneus longus muscle.

All of these previously published procedures use transfer of functionally antagonistic plantar-flexing muscles of the posterior muscle compartments in order to restore dorsiflexion and replace missing function of the muscles of the anterior compartment. The muscles themselves used for transfer remain innervated by the tibial nerve, and thus simultaneously contract with all the remaining muscles of the posterior compartment, generating a tenodesis effect to keep the foot at a neutral position without voluntary range of motion (ROM) of the ankle joint. Improvement of function is only attainable with intensive reeducation and training to increase strength and achieve voluntary contraction.

A functional gastrocnemius muscular transfer technique, which effectively overcomes the limitations of TP muscle transfer, was first described in 1994 by Ninković et al[6] and followed up with a second study in 2013. This physiological approach restores a normal, fully automatic walking pattern, and results in stability of the foot without being dependent on successful muscle reeducation. Over time, this "Ninković procedure" has become a more common and favorable method of treatment for drop foot,[7] a new philosophy that relies on careful patient selection and precise surgical technique to obtain the satisfactory result.

20.2 Indications

The use of the antagonistic muscle mass of the posterior compartment as the most widely applied method for rehabilitation of impaired dorsiflexion of the foot is a functional discrepancy in itself, and has an inherent fundamental downside that leads to the need for pervasive patient retraining and reeducation in order to accomplish voluntary contraction.

Disposing of the aforementioned requirement for muscle reeducation, the neuromusculotendinous transfer of the gastrocnemius muscle, as first defined by Ninković and Ninković[8] was intended to overcome these barriers to permit a total intuitive approach to the natural and functional reestablishment of foot dorsiflexion. By providing suitable force and ROM, the gastrocnemius muscle offers adequate size, strength, topography, and neurovascular anatomy for achieving these goals.

Patients must meet specific prerequisites in order to be regarded as appropriate candidates for a gastrocnemius neuromusculotendinous transfer:

- Lack of muscle function within the anterior or both anterior and lateral compartments of the lower leg due to irreversible posttraumatic paralysis of the peroneal nerve or massive muscle damage following trauma, compartment syndrome, or tumor resection (▸ Fig. 20.1). Posttraumatic paralysis is defined as irreversible when no signs of functional improvement are found and lack of reinnervation potentials seen in electromyographic studies after a minimum of 18 months subsequent to the initial injury or most recent surgery. However, patients with lesions at the myoneural junction or muscle loss (e.g., after severe compartment syndrome and muscles necrosis) may be operated on earlier because they stand no chance of spontaneous nerve recovery.
- Lesions of the peroneal nerve must be detected distal to its branching from the tibial nerve, and therefore an intact proximal portion of the deep or common peroneal nerve must be identified either clinically via Tinel test or by ultrasound, magnetic resonance imaging, or intraoperative exploration.
- Adequate passive dorsal foot flexion at the ankle joint to at least 0 degrees.
- Presence of viable muscles innervated by the tibial nerve.
- Adequate soft-tissue coverage in the anterior distal third of the lower leg that will be within the operative field.

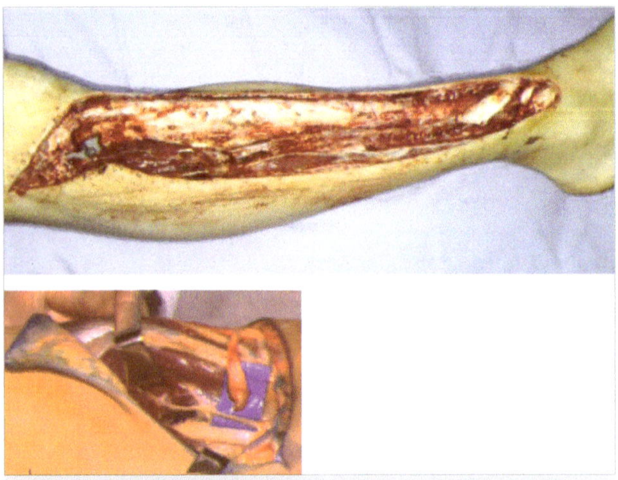

Fig. 20.1 S/P severe compartment syndrome with debridement of all necrotic muscle, but peroneal nerve (on microgrid) still intact.

20.3 Operative Technique

The neuromusculotendinous gastrocnemius transfer is performed in three stages (▸ Video 20.1). At the first stage, the viable proximal portion of the deep peroneal nerve has to be identified and isolated (▸ Fig. 20.2). After lower limb exsanguination and mid-thigh tourniquet elevation so as to obtain a clear bloodless field, a skin incision is made in the lateral popliteal region to expose the common peroneal nerve and, in due course, the proximal part of the deep peroneal nerve that proceeds to innervate the extensors of the foot. Should the proximal stump of the peroneal nerve prove viable by surgical view under the microscope and by histopathology, the operation as

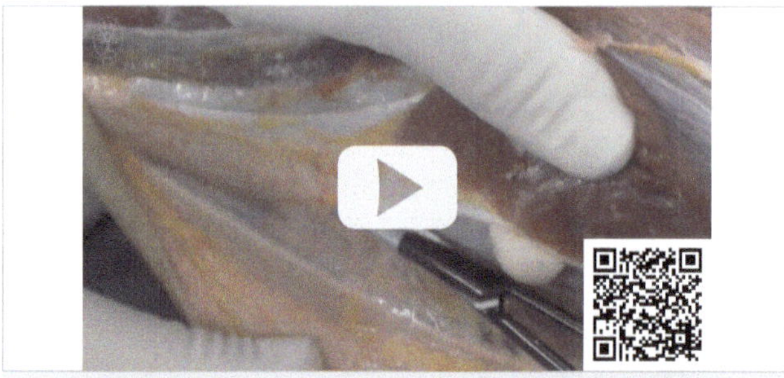

Video 20.1 How to Dissect a Musculocutaneous Perforator. https://www.thieme.de/de/q.htm?p=opn/cs/20/7/12265282-f4ef4966

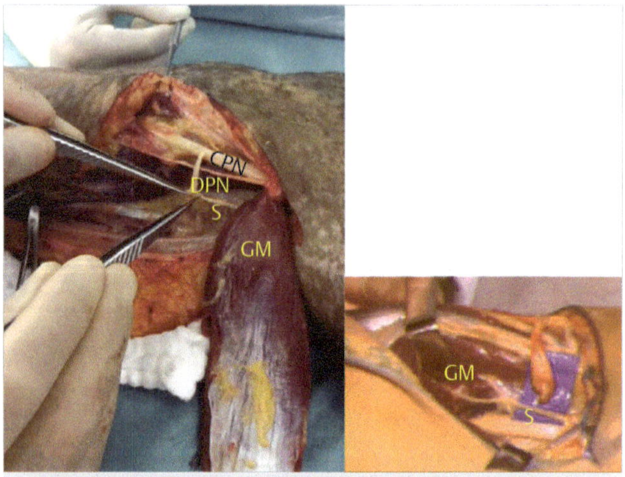

Fig. 20.2 Principles of the operative technique. Left: Identification of a viable proximal portion of the deep peroneal nerve and dissection of the motor branch of the gastrocnemius muscle from the tibial nerve has been accomplished. Right: Dissection of the lateral head of the gastrocnemius muscle with its neurovascular pedicle has been prepared for transfer to the anterior compartment. CPN, common peroneal nerve; DPN, deep peroneal nerve; GM, gastrocnemius muscle with motor nerve branch (S = sural) from the tibial nerve.

planned can proceed. Under the microscope, the deep motor branch is separated from the common peroneal nerve and its accompanying vessels, and dissected free until an adequate length of intact nerve fibers for a tension-free nerve coaptation is obtained (▶ Fig. 20.2).

Stage two starts with a perpendicular stocking seam skin incision beginning in the calf to expose the gastrocnemius muscle, followed distally to disconnect the more superficial Achilles tendon from the soleus muscle lying underneath, while remaining still attached to the gastrocnemius muscle (▶ Fig. 20.3). This dissection continues proximally, releasing and isolating the gastrocnemius muscle up to its origin and neurovascular pedicle, so as to permit it to be pivoted to the anterior lower extremity. Alternatively, the primary incision can be extended distally in a lazy-S manner for even fuller exposure of the gastrocnemius muscle and Achilles tendon (▶ Fig. 20.3). This approach can always be applied in patients who have had a compartment syndrome. They usually have scarring in this region due to previous surgery and removal of necrotic tissue. It is crucial to gain ample length and thickness of the Achilles tendon to be able to suture this tendon sufficiently to the tendons of the anterior compartment.

Now, moving to the anterior aspect of the lower limb, the TA, EDL, and EHL tendons are exposed through separate anterior incisions (▶ Fig. 20.4). Consequently, the dissected gastrocnemius muscle is now pulled through the subcutaneous tunnel to the anterior aspect of the lower leg and sutured to the tendons of the anterior compartment/lateral compartment proximal to the extensor retinaculum under maximal dorsiflexion in the ankle joint.

Whether the medial or lateral head of the gastrocnemius is transferred for restoring the anterior compartment function, the surgical procedure remains the same.[9] Careful attention must be paid to equilibrate the tendon attachments in order to keep the foot in anatomical balance. Utilization of both gastrocnemius muscles to rebuild the lateral compartment represents an exception to the rule, and requires a modification of the method of tendon attachment. This variation is indicated for severe cases of anterior and lateral compartment syndrome or after loss of all muscle tissue in those regions, as well as for patients who have suffered a prolonged complete nerve palsy of the deep and superficial peroneal nerve. In these cases, the lateral gastrocnemius muscle will remain innervated by the tibial nerve and will be attached to the peroneus brevis tendon along the lateral border of the fibula to avoid foot inversion and to achieve a fully stabilized foot. This will oppose tension by the medial gastrocnemius muscle that will be reinnervated by the deep peroneal nerve, so as to insure equilibration, active dorsal extension, and stabilization of the foot. To obtain anatomical balance when using only one gastrocnemius head, maximum tension on the EDL tendon must be applied in order to avoid inversion of the foot.

The third and last, but the most essential stage to perform correctly, is the microscopic epineural coaptation of the motor branch of the tibial nerve innervating the gastrocnemius muscle to the deep branch of the peroneal nerve using 10–0 nylon sutures without tension.[10] It is key for rapid reinnervation of the muscle to keep the tibial motor branch as short as possible while avoiding any tension on the end-to-end nerve coaptation (▶ Fig. 20.5).

After thorough cleansing and hemostasis of the surgical wound area, a final check must be performed of maximum possible dorsiflexion and anatomical balance of the foot. While still in the operation room, the ankle joint must be stabilized in a padded long leg cast held in maximal dorsiflexion (▶ Fig. 20.6).

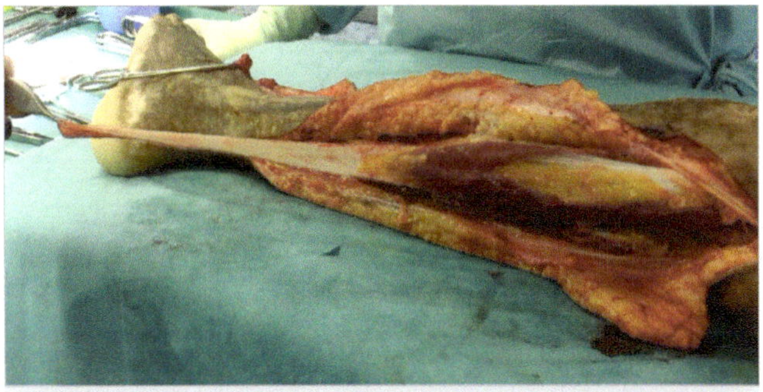

Fig. 20.3 Dissected superficial Achilles tendon kept together with the lateral gastrocnemius head, after disconnection from the underlying soleus muscle.

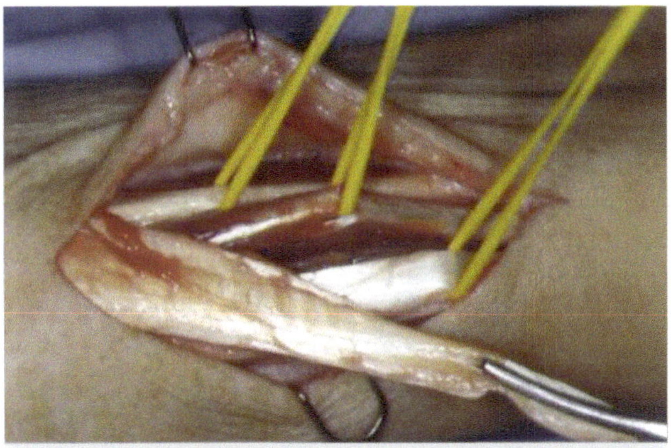

Fig. 20.4 Transposed gastrocnemius muscle and dissected tibialis anterior, extensor hallucis longus, and extensor digitorum longus, prior to tenorrhaphy.

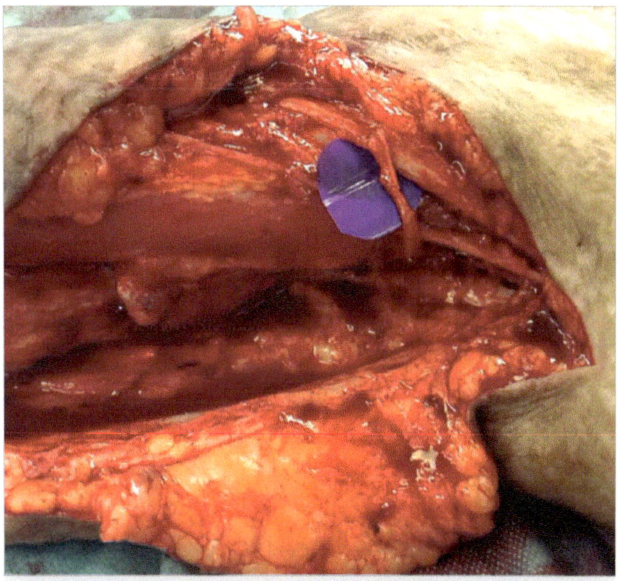

Fig. 20.5 The deep peroneal nerve and motor branch of the gastrocnemius muscle are prepared for microsurgical coaptation.

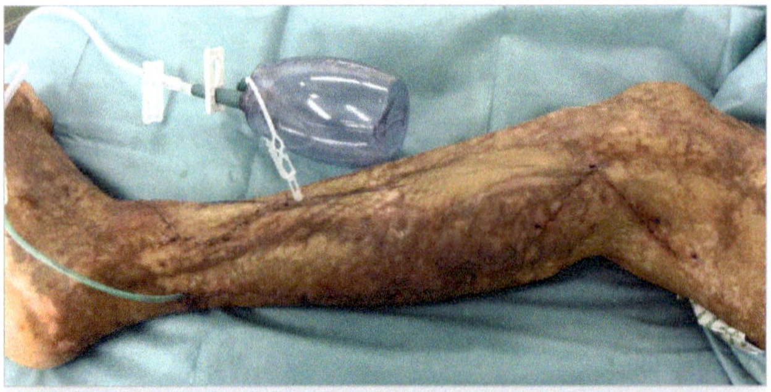

Fig. 20.6 Maximum dorsiflexion of the foot after wound closure is maintained, with a surgical drain of the anterior compartment.

20.4 Postoperative Considerations

After an immobilization period of 6 weeks in a vacuum-assisted stabilizing system, the patient will need to continue wearing an ankle–foot orthosis for several months in a neutral position to prevent extension of the denervated gastrocnemius muscle throughout the reinnervation period. Simultaneously, adjuvant physical therapy is begun. The therapy combines ROM practice and electrostimulation of the transplanted muscle. Supportive stimulation treatment is pursued until a spontaneous muscle contraction grade 3 according to the Medical Research Council Scale for Muscle Strength is accomplished. Only when achieving this level of reinnervation is the ankle–foot orthosis no longer necessary.

20.5 Complications

In order to reach a functional outcome in patients treated with this unique approach, their selection must meet stringent criteria as previously outlined. A successful result primarily requires preoperative viable neural and musculotendinous structures, but the microsurgical expertise of the surgeon and ideal circumstances as well as timing of the procedure and social infrastructure are also concerns. Potential postoperative complications unique to this procedure include inadequate reinnervation of the transferred muscle, tendon adhesions encouraged by the necessary postsurgical immobility, and foot imbalance, if there is insufficient distal tendon connection to the anterior compartment extensor tendons, with either over-supination or over-pronation of the ankle joint. Although postoperative wound healing disturbances, bleeding and hematomas, and wound infections occur as with any surgery, the worst complication theoretically would be a compartment syndrome.

20.6 Outcomes

In most patients, excellent enhancement of gait will be obtained as demonstrated by a rehabilitated walking pattern without use of an ankle–foot orthosis. After a mean hospitalization of 8 days (range: 4–28 days), no donor site morbidity is usually observed. At the 6-month follow-up, all patients should be able to voluntarily contract the transferred gastrocnemius muscle while finally reaching full active ROM within 18 months postoperatively. In the Ninković experience,[8,11,12] 56% of the patients achieved excellent results with normal gait and a

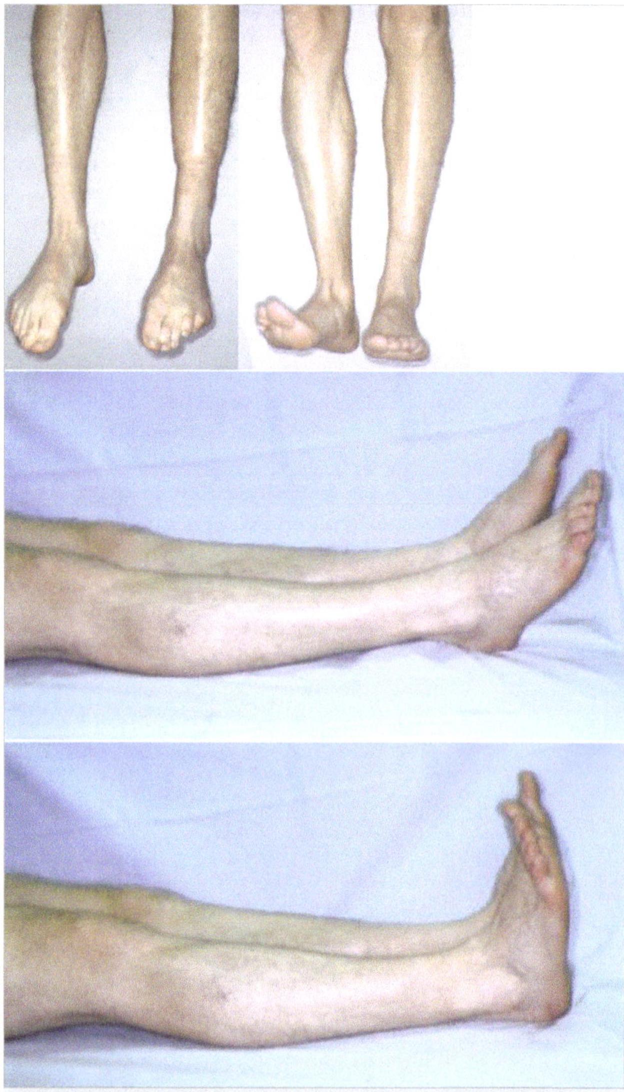

Fig. 20.7 Postoperative view 1 year after surgery with (above) full range of voluntary plantar flexion at the ankle joint and (below) full range of voluntary foot dorsiflexion with a good functional outcome.

balanced ankle joint with an active ROM of ≥ 40 degrees and normal electromyographic (EMG) results (▶ Fig. 20.7). Good results were found in 22% of the patients who had an adequate walking pattern, minimal foot imbalance, and active ROM ≥ 30 degrees. Fair outcomes were seen in another 22% of patients who had satisfactory function on EMG, yet a normal walking pattern with only sporadic dropping of the foot and active ROM ≥ 20 degrees. Only 5% showed moderate gait improvement with a still noticeable drop foot and active ROM ≤ 20 degrees.

20.7 Conclusion

Our surgical approach to the drop foot deformity uses the gastrocnemius muscle instead of the standard tibial posterior muscle for a dynamic transfer for several reasons. The gastrocnemius muscle has a well-suited size, topography, and neurovascular anatomy, in addition to adequate strength and range of excursion, to substitute for the nonfunctioning muscle mass of the anterior and/or lateral compartment. A single motor branch of the tibial nerve innervates each head of the gastrocnemius muscle. The close anatomical relationship between this motor branch and the location of the proximal part of the deep peroneal nerve (▶ Fig. 20.2) makes a tension-free neurorrhaphy close to the muscle possible to minimize muscle denervation time. The patient can use the transferred muscle voluntarily right after reinnervation is successful. Only postoperative physical therapy is needed to build up muscle strength. It must be emphasized that nerve regeneration takes time as does a prolonged rehabilitation period before full muscle strength can be expected, often even up to 18 months later. Another major advantage is that this surgical approach does not require a tenodesis effect to be effective. Because of the orthotopic reinnervation, the transferred muscle acts independently during movement. By transferring the gastrocnemius muscle, the anterior and lateral compartments are strengthened, as opposed to just maintaining muscle balance, and power is restored. The straight and superficial route chosen for the transfer of the muscle–tendon unit allows a normal gliding pattern and prevents adhesions.

Diagrams of dynamic ankle motion (▶ Fig. 20.8) and dynamic EMG (▶ Fig. 20.9) show the physiological balance between a transposed gastrocnemius muscle and remaining muscle innervated by the tibial nerve, as well as a normal walking pattern that is to be expected. Finally, this transfer does not cause any considerable functional or aesthetic defects. Note that transfer of the TP muscle in the long term changes the normal tension of the plantar aponeurosis, producing drooping of the instep region where normally inset and causing a flat foot. Transfer of the gastrocnemius muscle, as well known, is a standard procedure for soft-tissue coverage of the proximal third of the lower leg with virtually no donor site morbidity[13] as the soleus muscle will take over most of the function of the missing gastrocnemius muscle. Furthermore, transfer of one or both gastrocnemius muscles reduces the total strength of the posterior muscle group leading to a more physiological balance between the transferred gastrocnemius and remaining muscles of the posterior compartment.

The neuromusculotendinous transfer of the gastrocnemius and the subsequent reinnervation by the peroneal nerve for treatment of the drop foot is a simple yet extremely effective

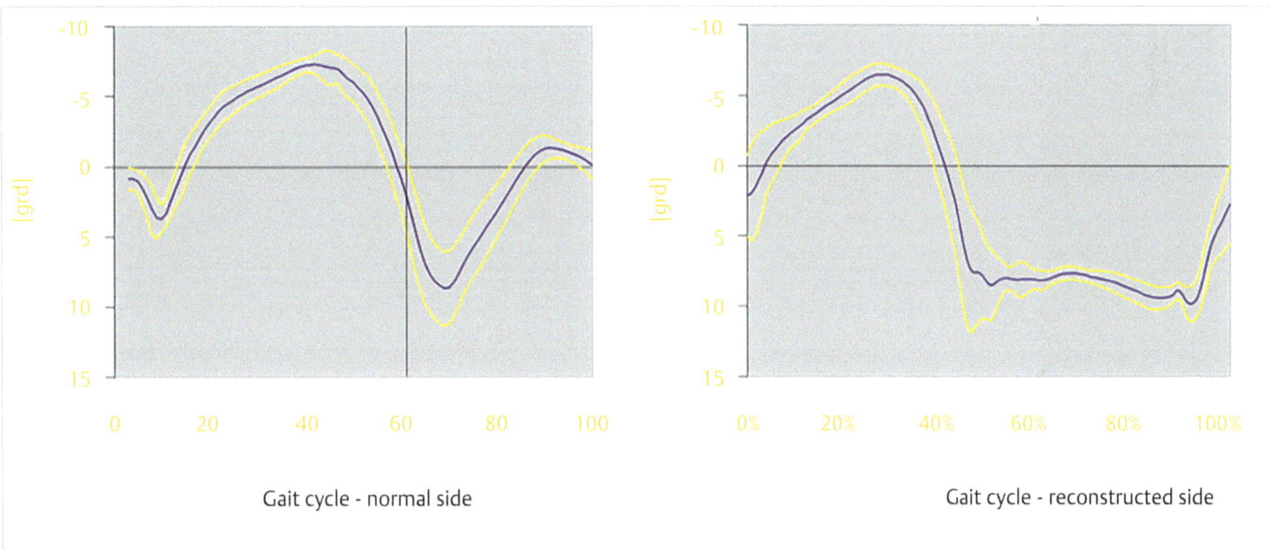

Fig. 20.8 Dynamic ankle motion of normal and reconstructed side showing a very similar graph of dynamic ankle motion.

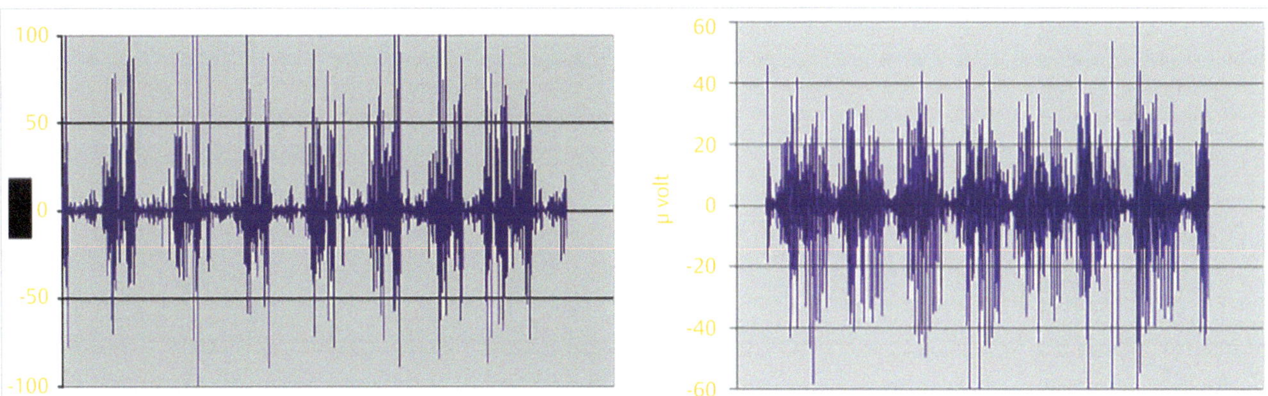

Fig. 20.9 Dynamic electromyography during seven steps for the healthy side (left) and for the transferred head of the gastrocnemius muscle (right).

procedure for functional rehabilitation. It grants restoration of voluntary dorsiflexion without influencing regular plantar flexion, and permits a normal gait. It is a straightforward operation making use of antagonistic plantar-flexing muscles for reconstruction of defective dorsal extension, yet **necessitating no supplementary** patient reeducation in restoring physiologic conditions. The Ninković technique is exceptionally effective in the cases with muscle necrosis after compartment syndrome or after muscle resection, since no peroneal nerve injury has occurred. In well-selected patients with a permanent peroneal palsy, those who have a healthy proximal part of the deep peroneal nerve, excellent results can also be obtained.

References

[1] Ober FR. Tendon transplantation in the lower extremity. N Engl J Med. 1933; 209:52–59

[2] Watkins MB, Jones JB, Ryder CT, Jr, Brown TH, Jr. Transplantation of the posterior tibial tendon. J Bone Joint Surg Am. 1954; 36-A(6):1181–1189

[3] Anderson JG. Foot drop in leprosy and its surgical correction. Acta Orthop Scand. 1963; 33(1–4):151–171

[4] Carayon A, Bourrel P, Bourges M, Touzé M. Dual transfer of the posterior tibial and flexor digitorum longus tendons for drop foot. Report of thirty-one cases. J Bone Joint Surg Am. 1967; 49(1):144–148

[5] McCall RE, Frederick HA, McCluskey GM, Riordan DC. The Bridle procedure: a new treatment for equinus and equinovarus deformities in children. J Pediatr Orthop. 1991; 11(1):83–89

[6] Ninković M, Sućur D, Starović B, Marković S. A new approach to persistent traumatic peroneal nerve palsy. Br J Plast Surg. 1994; 47(3):185–189

[7] Giuffre JL, Bishop AT, Spinner RJ, Levy BA, Shin AY. Partial tibial nerve transfer to the tibialis anterior motor branch to treat peroneal nerve injury after knee trauma. Clin Orthop Relat Res. 2012; 470(3):779–790

[8] Ninković M, Ninković M. Neuromusculotendinous transfer: an original surgical concept for the treatment of drop foot with long-term follow-up. Plast Reconstr Surg. 2013; 132(3):438e–445e

[9] Leclère FM, Badur N, Mathys L, Vögelin E. Neurotized lateral gastrocnemius muscle transfer for persistent traumatic peroneal nerve palsy: Surgical technique. Neurochirurgie. 2015; 61(4):292–297

[10] Flores LP, Martins RS, Siqueira MG. Clinical results of transferring a motor branch of the tibial nerve to the deep peroneal nerve for treatment of foot drop. Neurosurgery. 2013; 73(4):609–615, discussion 615–616

[11] Leclère FM, Badur N, Mathys L, Vögelin E. Nerve transfers for persistent traumatic peroneal nerve palsy: the Inselspital Bern experience. Neurosurgery. 2015; 77(4):572–579, discussion 579–580

[12] Nath RK, Somasundaram C. Gait improvements after peroneal or tibial nerve transfer in patients with foot drop: a retrospective study. Eplasty. 2017; 17: e31

[13] Barfod B, Pers M. Gastrocnemius-plasty for primary closure of compound injuries of the knee. J Bone Joint Sug Br. 1970; 52:124

21 Modern Concepts of Prosthetic Rehabilitation in Amputation of the Lower Extremity

Stefan Salminger, Clemens Gstoettner, Agnes Sturma, and Oskar C. Aszmann

Summary

Targeted muscle reinnervation offers a proven method for the treatment of amputation-related pain in lower limb amputees. It is recommended for any patient suffering from painful terminal neuromas and/or phantom limb pain and has also shown good effects in preventing these conditions, when performed during the amputation procedure. Targeted sensory reinnervation may provide a similar approach for purely sensory nerves with the additional benefit of improved sensory feedback at the stump.

Keywords: neuromas, phantom pain, amputation-related pain, targeted muscle reinnervation

21.1 Introduction to Targeted Muscle and Sensory Reinnervation

The majority of lower limb amputees suffer from some type of amputation-related pain.[1,2] Generally, these painful sensations may include neuroma and/or phantom limb pain, which are both related to loss of continuity of the affected extremity nerves.[3] After a peripheral nerve loses its physiological target through trauma or surgery, its axons regrow at the nerve stump. If they do not find a target to innervate, they sprout in an unguided manner, leading to the formation of a terminal neuroma.[1,4] When sensory fibers are included, these neuromas are generally painful upon external stimuli such as increased pressure. Located at an area of weight bearing, stump neuromas frequently inflict pain upon loading and thereby prevent the use of a prosthetic device. Phantom limb pain, in contrast, is not directly associated with mechanical stimuli at the stump. It affects up to 80% of amputees and entails painful sensation of the missing parts of the limb. It usually appears as intermittent background pain, with intervals that range from 1 day to several weeks and some additional short exacerbations.[5] The underlying pathomechanisms of phantom limb pain are not well understood. While there are different theories about its origin, there is an agreement that various peripheral and central factors along the neuraxis are at play.[6] Furthermore, external factors such as emotional stress or psychiatric disorders might also contribute to an increase in pain.[7,8,9]

Both stump neuromas and phantom limb pain do not respond well to standard pain medication. While as first-line medication the use of paracetamol and nonsteroidal anti-inflammatory drugs (NSAIDs) is recommended before other pharmacologic agents, there is still limited evidence on the effect of these.[10,11] Regarding stump neuromas, over 150 surgical treatment methods[4] have been described and traditionally the best, although still limited, results have been achieved by shortening of the nerve and transposition into muscle tissue. Phantom limb pain treatment has generally been conducted in a multimodal manner, including pharmacological interventions, behavioral approaches, physical and occupational therapy, surgical approaches such as sympathectomy, aimed at lesioning certain neural pathways, and neurostimulation. Several studies have shown that most of these treatments are ineffective, often not exceeding the placebo effect.[6,12] Other studies showing positive effects of treatment approaches lack the methodological rigor and robust reporting needed to confirm effectiveness.[13]

Targeted muscle reinnervation (TMR) was first introduced in 2004 by Kuiken et al as a technique for improved prosthesis control in upper limb amputees.[14] The main concept is the transferal of blindly ending nerves onto the motor nerves of remaining muscles in the stump, thereby creating novel neuromuscular units. While the primary emphasis of this technique was to create an increased number of intuitive myosignals for upper limb amputees in order to facilitate improved prosthetic control, it has also shown to be effective in the treatment of amputation-related pain. It also prevents neuroma formation by offering the nerves new terminal receptors. While it may be argued that muscles only provide a target for motor fibers, experience has shown that sensory fibers also regrow into the skin overlying the reinnervated muscles after TMR.[15] This "reafferentiation" of a peripheral target to the central nervous system, that is, the recreation of a complete and functional neuraxis, is believed to be a driving factor behind the positive effects of TMR on phantom limb pain.

In the first randomized clinical trial on surgical treatment of amputation-related pain, TMR has shown better outcomes for phantom limb pain and neuroma-related residual limb pain compared with conventional neurectomy, that is, shortening of the nerve.[16] More recently, it has also been explored as a preventive treatment performed during amputation, showing similarly encouraging results.[17,18]

Targeted sensory reinnervation (TSR) applies the same concept to the reinnervation of sensory nerves. While theoretically providing the same benefits as TMR with regard to pain management, it offers the additional benefit of creating specialized sensation at the stump of lower limb amputees. For example, after transfer of the sensory tibial nerve onto the sural/saphenous nerve, a transtibial amputee will feel their planta pedis at the stump.[19] This can be employed with the idea in mind to create more natural gait feedback for the amputee.[20] It is hypothesized that such an approach to create meaningful and intuitive feedback can help improve postural stability and embodiment of the device, while reducing falls.[19] However, not much work has been done on this topic and its feasibility is yet to be investigated.

21.1.1 Indications and Contraindications

TMR should be considered for any patient with lower extremity amputation, suffering from either phantom limb or neuroma pain. In light of recent research, it is recommended to perform TMR already during the amputation procedure, thereby effectively preventing neuroma formation and acting against phantom limb pain after successful muscle reinnervation.[17,18] There are no specific contraindications for this procedure. In the cases where there is no viable musculature left at the stump or soft-tissue coverage at the weight-bearing area is insufficient, which may happen in certain avulsion traumas, a free muscle transfer may be used as target for nerve transfers.

21.1.2 Preoperative Management

In the case of terminal neuromas at the stump, these can in most cases be located in clinical examination by elicitation of a Tinel–Hoffmann sign. In addition, high-resolution ultrasound can be helpful to determine the exact location and type of neuroma, and ultrasound-guided nerve block may be used to secure the diagnosis. Phantom limb pain, on the other hand, is a purely clinical diagnosis, associated with painful sensations at missing parts of the limb. The availability of sufficient stump muscles for TMR may be assessed clinically. In the cases where there is doubt about the condition of stump musculature, high-resolution ultrasound and MRI may prove helpful and surface or needle electromyogram (EMG) is recommended to test muscular activity.[21]

21.1.3 Technique

The patient is placed in a prone or lateral position. In above-knee amputees, the main nerves of the thigh are exposed via a longitudinal dorsal incision. In below-knee amputees, the incision crosses the knee joint in a Z-fashion, continuing laterally along the course of the peroneal nerve.

As an example, we report the case of a 17-year-old adolescent boy who lost his lower limb at the below-knee level in a traumatic accident with a boats' propeller. Prosthetic fitting was not successful, as the patient developed chronic ulcerations at the scarred distal stump end as well as painful neuromas. To save the below-knee level of amputation and improve the soft-tissue quality, a free musculocutaneous latissimus dorsi flap was performed. In this case, the deep peroneal nerve was coapted to the thoracodorsal nerve of the latissimus flap, and the distal tibial nerve was coapted to the nerve branches of the gastrocnemius heads. With this complex procedure, painless weight bearing at the distal stump end and therefore excellent prosthetic use could be achieved (▶ Fig. 21.1, ▶ Fig. 21.2, ▶ Fig. 21.3).

The nerve transfers used in the treatment of neuroma and phantom limb pain should be chosen based on clinical examination (location of neuromas) and available anatomy. The donor nerves have to be neurotomized at least to a level of palpable healthy fascicles. Nerve transfers can be performed under loupe magnification in an end-to-end fashion using 8–0 or 9–0 nylon sutures and fibrin glue.

21.1.4 Postoperative Management

Depending on the exact site of nerve coaptation, successful reinnervation of the target muscles may take 3 to 6 months. If there is neuropathic pain during this period, this can be managed with specific analgesics such as pregabalin. Neuropathic

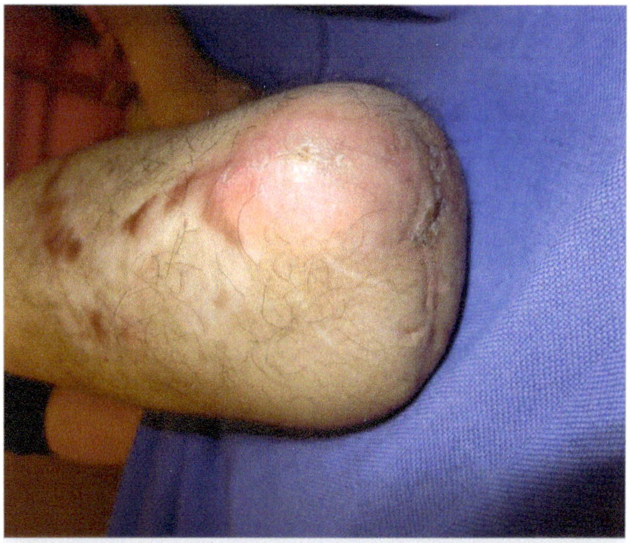

Fig. 21.1 Chronic ulcerations at the scarred stump end.

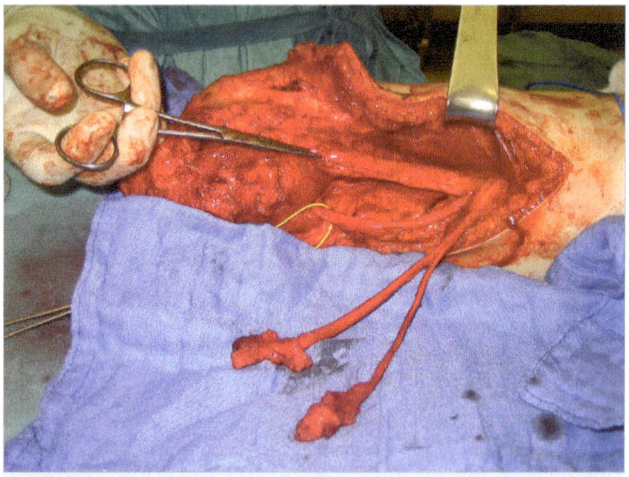

Fig. 21.2 Dissected neuromas.

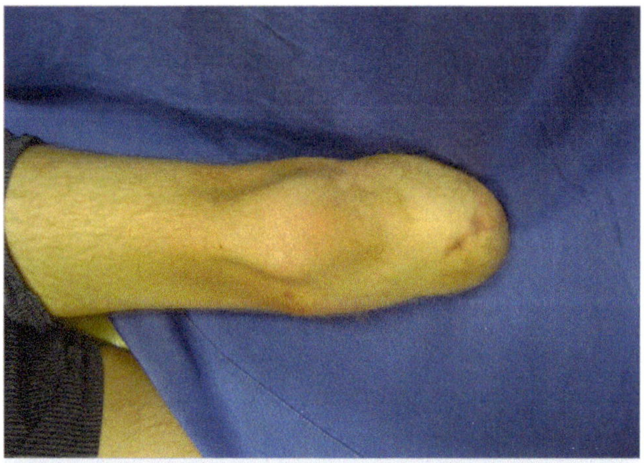

Fig. 21.3 Stump 6 months after soft-tissue correction with free latissimus dorsi flap.

and phantom limb pain should subside once the nerves have reached the targets. After reinnervation, selective activation and training of the newly innervated stump muscles can be helpful if phantom limb pain persists. This is done with the aim to effectively strengthen the cortical representation of the lost limb and may be guided by surface EMG biofeedback or approaches for sensory training.[21,22]

21.1.5 Conclusion

TMR offers a proven method for the treatment of amputation-related pain in lower limb amputees. It is recommended for any patient suffering from painful terminal neuromas and/or phantom limb pain and has also shown good effects in preventing these conditions, when performed during the amputation procedure.

TSR may provide a similar approach for purely sensory nerves with the additional benefit of improved sensory feedback at the stump.

21.2 Introduction to Osseointegration at Below- and Above-Knee Level of Amputation

The quality of the interface between the residual limb and the fabricated socket is of utmost importance for the success and functional outcome of any prosthesis, regardless of whether the amputation is below or above the knee. However, the residual limb is a dynamic organ with surrounding soft tissue resulting in relative movements and stump volume changes. Additionally, the tibial and femoral bones only have a limited transsectional surface and the overlying skin is not designed for full weight bearing. Therefore, the most commonly faced issues with conventional sockets reported are skin irritations, sweating within the socket, and pain during activity[23] with skin problems alone affecting 24 to 74% of lower-limb amputees.[24,25] These issues can result in a significantly reduced walking distance or even prosthetic abandonment.[26]

These problems led to the development of osseointegration. Adapted from early concepts of dental implants, the first osseointegration with a titanium implant in a lower limb amputee was performed in the 1990s by Rickard Brånemark.[27] The concept of osseointegration allows a direct prosthetic bone anchorage without interfering with skin and soft tissue. Thus, it avoids the inherent problems with conventional socket suspension. Additionally, studies have shown that patients using osseointegrated limbs receive some sensory feedback through this new interface, a phenomenon that was termed osseoperception.[28] Still, as osseointegration necessitates a percutaneous interface of the metal implant, there is the risk of superficial and deep infections.[29]

21.2.1 Indications and Contraindications

Osseointegration is indicated if patients report about problems with conventional socket prostheses, for example, discomfort, pain, poor suspension, or inability to use conventional socket prostheses at all. However, it is important to rule out that these issues are due to a poorly fitted socket or inadequate training. In order to assess these indications, it is recommended to see the patient in a multidisciplinary team including a surgeon, a physical or occupational therapist, and a prosthetist. If there is any doubt on the patient's psychological state allowing to fully follow clinical instructions, the consultation of a psychologist/psychiatrist is necessary. Furthermore, patients should have reached full skeletal maturity, have normal skeletal anatomy, and agree to comply with a strict treatment and follow-up program. Contraindications are severe peripheral vascular disease, diabetes, smoking, limb exposure to radiation, osteoporosis or current chemotherapy, as well as corticosteroid use.[23]

21.2.2 Preoperative Management

For preoperative planning, a CT scan of the stump is performed to evaluate bone quality and determine the size and length of the implant.

21.2.3 Technique

Depending on the implant used, the surgical procedure can be done in a single stage or in two stages. Most of the currently available implants use the press-fit technique. The percutaneous interface is of great importance in regard to the risk of infection. Therefore, the skin surrounding the implant is thinned to a minimum and subcutaneous tissue is removed in this area. This enables a stable interface with minimum soft-tissue movement around the implant, minimizing fluid secretion and risk of infection (▶ Fig. 21.4, ▶ Fig. 21.5).

21.2.4 Postoperative Management

The postoperative phase is divided into a healing period and a loading period. Depending on the surgical technique, single- or two-staged approach, the amount of time in the healing phase varies. During load training process, the patient is fitted with a

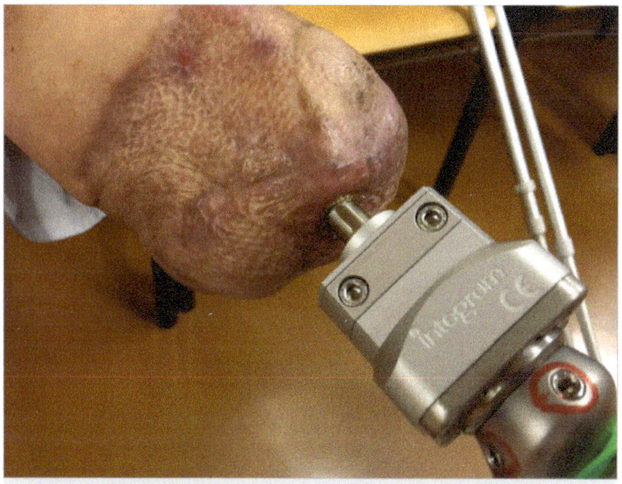

Fig. 21.4 Percutaneous interface in a patient with below-knee osseointegration.

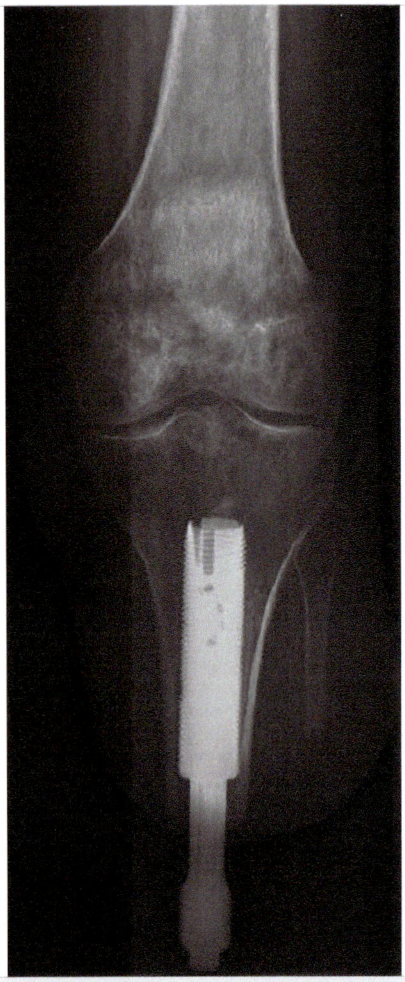

Fig. 21.5 X-ray of below-knee osseointegration.

short training prosthesis to stand on a bathroom scale. Weight bearing usually begins with 10 kg on the prosthesis and is increased every week by additional 10 kg until full body weight can be loaded painlessly. This process normally takes 6 to 8 weeks and varies depending on the used system and bone healing. If the loading training is successful, gait training is initiated at about 12 weeks postoperatively. In the beginning, the patient is asked to use two crutches and limit prosthesis use to no more than 2 hours per day. The wearing time, prosthetic activity, and weight bearing are then gradually increased over the following weeks. After radiologic control and successful gait training, about 6 months postoperatively, the patient can stop using walking aids. During the entire loading process, pain is an important indicator for implant loosening or overloading.

21.2.5 Conclusion

Osseointegration in below- and above-knee amputation has become an established treatment option in patients not tolerating or not applicable for conventional socket fittings. It has been shown that osseointegration is able to improve patients' quality of life, functional prosthetic outcome, body image, range of motion of the hip joint, comfort especially in the sitting position, as well as easing donning and doffing of the prosthetic device. Additionally, osseoperception provides sensory feedback that improves the ability to walking and secureness, especially on rough surfaces. Nonetheless, patients have to be aware of the potential risks and complications. Additionally, some restrictions in the use of the system apply as for most current systems running or cycling is not recommended.

21.3 Introduction to Femoral Shortening Osteotomy in Through-Knee Amputees

In patients in whom a below-knee amputation is not feasible, the through-knee level should be the primary goal.[30,31,32] Compared to above-knee amputation, the through-knee level has several advantages.[33] It represents a relatively simple operative technique with decreased surgical blood loss, preserves all thigh muscles, especially the adductors, leading to a better prosthetic control, and, most importantly, delivers a fully weight-bearing distal bulbous stump end.[33,34] Thus, the prosthetic socket does not need ischial weight bearing, and donning and doffing can be performed much easier.[35] By maintaining the cartilage barrier, through-knee amputations tend to have a higher resistance to infections and although the distal growth plate is preserved, there is no risk of bony overgrowth or exostosis especially in young patients.[31] Additionally, the metabolic costs of walking strongly depend on the amputation level, showing substantially less effort for through-knee compared to above-knee amputees.[30,34] This results in relatively slower walking velocities, both self-selected and maximum walking speed, in patients with above-knee amputation compared to through-knee amputation.[34] Despite these advantages, through-knee amputation is only performed in approximately 5% of all amputations proximal to the transtibial level.[31]

However, prosthetic fitting in above-knee amputees results in excess length of the thigh together with the prosthetic knee joint. Thus, in earlier days, through-knee amputations were fitted with prostheses lacking knee-control mechanisms.[36] This specially designed prosthetic knee joints or anchors have been developed to overcome the burden of excess length in through-knee amputees, however, all compromising stability or swing-phase control compared to normal microprocessor controlled prosthetic knee joints.[35]

Using modern prosthetic knee joints, the artificial joint is positioned distally onto the socket resulting in lengthening of the thigh. This difference in length compared to the sound side leads to difficulties, for example, when sitting in narrow spaces like in the car.[35] The excess length of the thigh, together with the prosthetic knee joint ultimately, necessitates a shortening of the shank. Thus, pivot points of the knee joints differ between both legs. Obviously, this has a negative influence on the gait cycle; however, it also leads to a poor cosmetic outcome especially in the sitting position.[35] Due to the shortening of the shank, the foot is lifted off the floor in the sitting position, which is reported as uncomfortable by the patients.[37] The prosthetic socket with both the inner lining and rigid outer sockets, together with the anchor of the knee joint and the prosthetic knee, itself adds, depending on the type of knee joint, between 5 and 10 cm of length to the through-knee amputation stump.[35]

To overcome the difficulties in prosthetic fitting due to the excess length together with the artificial knee joint, a femoral shortening osteotomy can be performed, preserving the weight-bearing distal stump end.

21.3.1 Indication and Contraindications

Patients with through-knee amputations are eligible for this procedure if they have reached full skeletal maturity, are successfully fitted with a prosthesis, report dissatisfaction or functional limitations due to the excess in length, and show good skin quality at the distal weight-bearing stump end. In the cases with poor skin quality or even initial soft-tissue deficits at the distal stump end, additional soft-tissue surgery can be necessary. Contraindications are severe peripheral vascular disease, diabetes, smoking, osteoporosis, or current chemotherapy as well as corticosteroid use.

21.3.2 Technique

In the supine position, the femur is prepared through about a 20-cm-long lateral incision at the mid-diaphysial level. The femur is freed at a length of 15 cm. The distal osteotomy is performed about 12 cm proximal to the stump end to avoid pressure on the plate after prosthetic fitting within the condylar region. An 8.5- to 10-cm-long femur segment is then resected and osteosynthesis is performed with an eight-hole locking plate. The patients receive intra- and postoperative antibiotic prophylaxis with amoxicillin. The femoral shortening osteotomy can be combined with other procedures to improve the stump–socket interface or patients' comfort while wearing the prosthesis. In our experience, these have been soft-tissue alignments, for example, thigh lift, different free flaps for distal soft-tissue coverage, or neuroma resection/nerve transfers.

21.3.3 Postoperative Management

No weight bearing or prosthetic use is allowed until bony union is confirmed with conventional X-ray. The first X-ray control is performed 3 months postoperatively. In the majority of cases, bony union is achieved at this point and prosthetic fitting can be started. Implant removal is only performed if patients report pain within the socket at the region of the plate.

21.3.4 Conclusion

The femoral shortening osteotomy with preservation of the distal weight-bearing stump end allows a prosthetic fitting with the knee joint at an anatomical level, resulting in increased functional outcome, aesthetic appearance, and thus patient satisfaction. As there is no need for ischial weight bearing resulting from distal loading of the stump, the range of motion of the hip joint is not impaired and thus permits a more natural and less energy-consuming gait compared to above-knee amputees.[33] Additionally, it has been shown that the favorable prosthetic suspension permitted by the femoral condyles leads to less pain when using the prosthesis compared to above-knee amputees.[30] However, due to the risk of bony nonunion, femoral shortening osteotomy should be performed in patients after traumatic amputations with normal vascular status.

Femoral shortening osteotomy can also be performed at the stage of the initial amputation if there is a substantial tissue loss. In these cases, the femoral segment resection may allow primary wound closure or, as proposed by Wendt et al, in a secondary procedure to remove split skin graft at the distal stump end.[38,39]

References

[1] Ephraim PL, Wegener ST, MacKenzie EJ, Dillingham TR, Pezzin LE. Phantom pain, residual limb pain, and back pain in amputees: results of a national survey. Arch Phys Med Rehabil. 2005; 86(10):1910–1919

[2] Penn-Barwell JG. Outcomes in lower limb amputation following trauma: a systematic review and meta-analysis. Injury. 2011; 42(12):1474–1479

[3] Ehde DM, Czerniecki JM, Smith DG, et al. Chronic phantom sensations, phantom pain, residual limb pain, and other regional pain after lower limb amputation. Arch Phys Med Rehabil. 2000; 81(8):1039–1044

[4] Vernadakis AJ, Koch H, Mackinnon SE. Management of neuromas. Clin Plast Surg. 2003; 30:247–68, vii

[5] Wolff A, Vanduynhoven E, van Kleef M, Huygen F, Pope JE, Mekhail N. 21. Phantom pain. Pain Pract. 2011; 11(4):403–413

[6] Flor H. Phantom-limb pain: characteristics, causes, and treatment. Lancet Neurol. 2002; 1(3):182–189

[7] Flor H. Maladaptive plasticity, memory for pain and phantom limb pain: review and suggestions for new therapies. Expert Rev Neurother. 2008; 8(5): 809–818

[8] Vase L, Nikolajsen L, Christensen B, et al. Cognitive-emotional sensitization contributes to wind-up-like pain in phantom limb pain patients. Pain. 2011; 152(1):157–162

[9] Kern U, Busch V, Müller R, Kohl M, Birklein F. Phantom limb pain in daily practice: still a lot of work to do! Pain Med. 2012; 13(12):1611–1626

[10] Moore RA, Chi C-C, Wiffen PJ, Derry S, Rice ASC. Oral nonsteroidal anti-inflammatory drugs for neuropathic pain. Cochrane Database Syst Rev. 2015(10):CD010902

[11] Moore RA, Straube S, Wiffen PJ, Derry S, McQuay HJ. Pregabalin for acute and chronic pain in adults. Cochrane Database Syst Rev. 2009(3):CD007076

[12] Subedi B, Grossberg GT. Phantom limb pain: mechanisms and treatment approaches. Pain Res Treat. 2011; 2011:864605

[13] Ferraro F, Jacopetti M, Spallone V, et al. Italian Consensus Conference on Pain in Neurorehabilitation (ICCPN). Diagnosis and treatment of pain in plexopathy, radiculopathy, peripheral neuropathy and phantom limb pain. Evidence and recommendations from the Italian Consensus Conference on Pain on Neurorehabilitation. Eur J Phys Rehabil Med. 2016; 52(6):855–866

[14] Kuiken TA, Dumanian GA, Lipschutz RD, Miller LA, Stubblefield KA. The use of targeted muscle reinnervation for improved myoelectric prosthesis control in a bilateral shoulder disarticulation amputee. Prosthet Orthot Int. 2004; 28(3): 245–253

[15] Kuiken TA, Miller LA, Lipschutz RD, et al. Targeted reinnervation for enhanced prosthetic arm function in a woman with a proximal amputation: a case study. Lancet. 2007; 369(9559):371–380

[16] Dumanian GA, Potter BK, Mioton LM, et al. Targeted muscle reinnervation treats neuroma and phantom pain in major limb amputees: a randomized clinical trial. Ann Surg. 2019; 270(2):238–246

[17] Bowen JB, Ruter D, Wee C, West J, Valerio IL. Targeted muscle reinnervation technique in below-knee amputation. Plast Reconstr Surg. 2019; 143(1):309–312

[18] Valerio IL, Dumanian GA, Jordan SW, et al. Preemptive treatment of phantom and residual limb pain with targeted muscle reinnervation at the time of major limb amputation. J Am Coll Surg. 2019; 228(3):217–226

[19] Baur EM, Bauer T, Egger H, Salzmann S, Haslwanter T. Ein neuer Ansatz für einer sensitiven Beinprothese. Orthopädietechnik. 2016; 7:62–66

[20] Plauche A, Villarreal D, Gregg RD. A haptic feedback system for phase-based sensory restoration in above-knee prosthetic leg users. IEEE Trans Haptics. 2016; 9(3):421–426

[21] Sturma A, Hruby LA, Prahm C, Mayer JA, Aszmann OC. Rehabilitation of upper extremity nerve injuries using surface EMG biofeedback: protocols for clinical application. Front Neurosci. 2018; 12:906

[22] Wakolbinger R, Diers M, Hruby LA, Sturma A, Aszmann OC. Home-based tactile discrimination training reduces phantom limb pain. Pain Pract. 2018; 18(6):709–715

[23] Hebert JS, Rehani M, Stiegelmar R. Osseointegration for lower-limb amputation: a systematic review of clinical outcomes. JBJS Rev. 2017; 5(10):e10

[24] Dillingham TR, Pezzin LE, MacKenzie EJ, Burgess AR. Use and satisfaction with prosthetic devices among persons with trauma-related amputations: a long-term outcome study. Am J Phys Med Rehabil. 2001; 80(8):563–571

[25] Koc E, Tunca M, Akar A, Erbil AH, Demiralp B, Arca E. Skin problems in amputees: a descriptive study. Int J Dermatol. 2008; 47(5):463–466

[26] Meulenbelt HEJ, Geertzen JHB, Jonkman MF, Dijkstra PU. Skin problems of the stump in lower limb amputees: 1. A clinical study. Acta Derm Venereol. 2011; 91(2):173–177

[27] Brånemark R, Brånemark PI, Rydevik B, Myers RR. Osseointegration in skeletal reconstruction and rehabilitation: a review. J Rehabil Res Dev. 2001; 38(2):175–181

[28] Häggström E, Hagberg K, Rydevik B, Brånemark R. Vibrotactile evaluation: osseointegrated versus socket-suspended transfemoral prostheses. J Rehabil Res Dev. 2013; 50(10):1423–1434

[29] Tillander J, Hagberg K, Hagberg L, Brånemark R. Osseointegrated titanium implants for limb prostheses attachments: infectious complications. Clin Orthop Relat Res. 2010; 468(10):2781–2788

[30] Hagberg E, Berlin OK, Renström P. Function after through-knee compared with below-knee and above-knee amputation. Prosthet Orthot Int. 1992; 16(3):168–173

[31] Baumgartner R. Knee disarticulation and through-knee amputation [in German]. Oper Orthop Traumatol. 2011; 23(4):289–295

[32] Green PW, Hawkins BS, Irvine WT, Jamieson CW. An assessment of above- and through-knee amputations. Br J Surg. 1972; 59(11):873–875

[33] Baumgartner RF. Knee disarticulation versus above-knee amputation. Prosthet Orthot Int. 1979; 3(1):15–19

[34] Pinzur MS. Gait analysis in peripheral vascular insufficiency through-knee amputation. J Rehabil Res Dev. 1993; 30(4):388–392

[35] de Laat FA, van der Pluijm MJ, van Kuijk AA, Geertzen JH, Roorda LD. Cosmetic effect of knee joint in a knee disarticulation prosthesis. J Rehabil Res Dev. 2014; 51(10):1545–1554

[36] Early PF. Rehabilitation of patients with through-knee amputation. BMJ. 1968; 4(5628):418–421

[37] Oberg K. Knee mechanisms for through-knee prostheses. Prosthet Orthot Int. 1983; 7(2):107–112

[38] Wendt KW, Zimmerman KW. Shortening osteotomy of the femur after knee joint exarticulation [in German]. Unfallchirurg. 1994; 97(12):652–654

[39] de Kruijff LGM, Bemelman M, Holtslag HR. Salvage of a through-knee amputation by performing a femoral shortening osteotomy: a case report. JBJS Case Connect. 2014; 4(3):e72–e5

22 Procurement of Thin Flaps as Indicated in the Lower Extremity

Joon Pio Hong

Summary

Elevation on the superficial fascia (super-thin) is a new approach for elevating flaps. It has advantages such as providing a thin flap allowing increased versatility to achieve better contour of flap, minimizing the need for secondary debulking, and being hemodynamically reliable.

Keywords: super-thin flap, superficial fascia elevation, flap elevation

22.1 Introduction

The goals of microsurgery reconstruction are functional outcome and aesthetic result. To achieve these goals, we often need a thin flap that is pliable and viable. Perforator flaps have been extensively used for these purposes from head and neck reconstruction, trunk reconstruction, and extremity reconstruction. But often when reconstructing for coverage, the bulk of the perforator flaps makes it difficult to achieve good contour at a single stage especially in obese patients.[1]

The current method of elevation of the perforator flap is either subfascial where the flap is elevated with the deep muscle fascia or suprafascial where the elevation is made just above the deep fascial plane.[2] In either case, the flap frequently remains too bulky to resurface the defect. Immediate debulking procedures can follow but may result in partial loss of the flap.[3] Microdissection can be applied with better success to achieve a thin flap but may be to tedious and time consuming.[4] Thus, secondary debulking procedures are chosen to minimize flap loss, and procedures such as liposuction or surgical resection are followed to achieve better contour of the reconstruction site. But if possible, one should aim to have the ideal reconstruction at a given single stage like the concept of the reconstructive elevator.[5]

In this chapter, we will focus on how to thin the flap based on a new plane, the superficial fascial plane, which may provide a constant safe and reliable plane.[6] Since the anterolateral thigh (ALT) flap and the thoracodorsal artery perforator (TDAP) flap have been discussed in detail in the previous chapters, only the superficial circumflex iliac artery perforator (SCIP) flap and the gluteal artery perforator (GAP) flap will be exemplified in this chapter.[7,8,9,10]

22.1.1 Attributes

- There are three distinctive layers for elevation: subfascial, suprafascial, and superficial fascia.
- The superficial fascia is a distinct white film-like layer between the deep and superficial fat that is easily identifiable.
- The linking vessels may be connected in the superficial fat that stabilizes vascular reliability of the flap when elevating on this plane.
- The indirect linking vessels allow the flap to capture multiple perforasomes.
- The superficial fascia is a relatively avascular plane that allows easy dissection.
- The elevation on this plane allows for a thin skin flap harvest.

22.1.2 Detriments

- Elevation on the superficial fascia will be thick in very obese patients and may need further debulking secondarily, but far thinner than taking the whole thickness.
- When near the pedicle, one should be careful and take note of the small perforators and the branches.
- It cannot be used as a sensate flap as the nerve is usually located just above the deep fascia.
- A steep learning curve may be needed.

22.2 Anatomical Considerations

Using the superficial fascial plane in flap elevation is a different approach from the classical subfascial or suprafascial approach. The subfascial approach is made by incising the deep fascia, and then elevating beneath this fascia, which makes it easier to identify the perforators before it penetrates the fascia. It is the easiest and, maybe, fastest way to elevate the flap.[2,11,12] The disadvantage, however, is that this approach leaves the thickest flap with possibility of muscle hernia. The suprafascial approach elevates the flap above the fascia until the perforator is reached and then opening the hiatus of the deep fascia and dissecting the perforator proximally toward the source vessel. Although it reduces the risk of muscle hernia by keeping the deep fascia intact, the risk of skin graft loss and depression of scar remains a problem if the donor site is not closed primarily. Finally, despite being thinner than the subfascial approach, it may still be too thick and not adequate for resurfacing defects with thin surrounding skin.[6]

The critical anatomy when elevating the thin flap is the identification of layers: deep fascia, deep fat, superficial fat, and the superficial fascia that lies between the two fat layers (▶ Fig. 22.1).[3,13,14] According to the perforasome concept by Saint-Cyr et al, viability of the flap with the superficial fascia plane will be derived from perfusion of the perforator and the ability of indirect linking vessels connecting to each other.[15,16] Based on this knowledge, a large thin flap will survive even without direct linking vessels.[17,18] Therefore, despite the debulking of the deep fat where the direct linking vessels might be found, the thin flap harvested on the superficial plane will still have adequate blood supply.[6]

The superficial fascia acts to maintain the skin integrity. Once removed, the skin can expand mimicking the full-thickness skin graft. Thus, the ability to stretch allows the flap to have thinner appearance while maintaining adequate circulation to the flap.

Another critical component of elevation on a superficial fascia plane is to identify perforators. When elevating on the

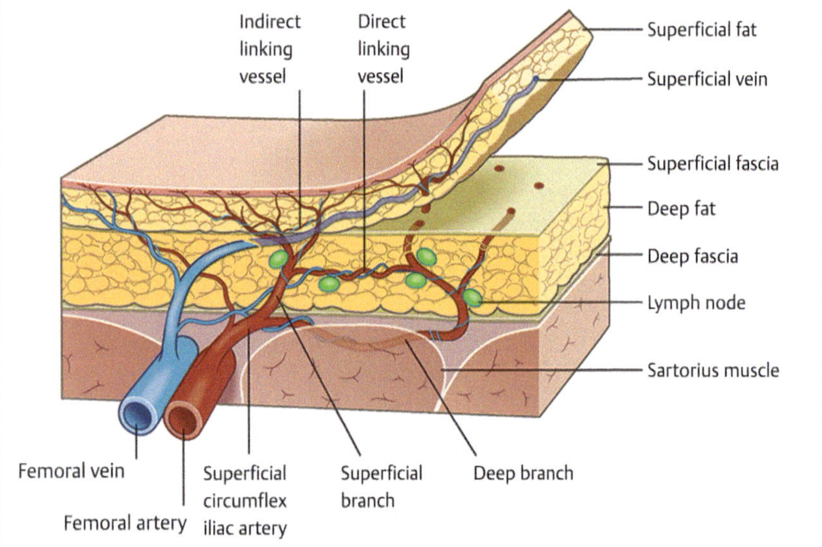

Fig. 22.1 The critical anatomy when elevating the thin flap is the identification of layers: deep fascia, deep fat, superficial fat, and the superficial fascia that lies between the two fat layers. This illustration depicts the elevation on the superficial fascial plane.

superficial fascia plane, one can come across multiple perforators heading upward toward the skin. If multiple ones are identified, the perforator with the largest diameter is usually preferred. Once the perforator of choice is determined, dissection has to head toward the source vessel until an adequate length of the perforator is achieved; this is known as the freestyle approach. The final critical component of elevating on the superficial fascia can be the superficial veins. The importance of the superficial veins is known especially when elevating flaps having a potentially dominant superficial venous system. Among the commonly used flaps in the extremity, DIEP (deep inferior epigastric perforator) and SCIP flaps can be such examples. In these flaps, it is wise to include the superficial vein even when accompanying veins of the perforator allow adequate drainage.

The skin of the flap itself can vary in thickness. The only part of the skin that has a large epidermal component other than the hand and foot is the buttock skin. While the back (TDAP flap, parascapular flap) and the buttock (GAP flap) have a similar or a lightly thicker skin thickness (epidermis and dermis) compared to the plantar surface, the back skin has only half the epidermal component compared to the buttock.[19] On the contrary, the skin thickness of the anterior body may be thinner. Furthermore, the SCIP flap has one of the thinnest fat deposits as the skin is relatively tightly adhered to the deep fascia compared to other sites such as the abdomen and thigh. Thus, one can consider the skin thickness when reconstructing a defect.

22.3 Anatomical Variants and Potential Pitfalls

When elevating the flap on the superficial fascia, the identification of this layer can be tricky especially in thin patients. In a thin patient, there might be lack of deep fat as well as superficial fat, making the distinction difficult. Nevertheless, adequate tension can show the superficial fascia. Adequate tension and countertension during elevation of the perforator flap is critical to identify the superficial fascia. This maneuver allows identifying the avascular thin white film-like structure with better clarity.

The elevation in freestyle allows coping with any variant of perforator location. However, pre-elevation Doppler marking will guide you to expect where and when meticulous approach is needed. The concept of hot and cold zones of the flap may come in handy when elevating any perforator flap. Rapid elevation can occur during the elevation of the cold zone where there are no meaningful perforators and meticulous dissection is required as you come close to the vicinity of the marked perforators (hot zones).

There can be multiple perforator variants derived from the ALT, TDAP, GAP, and SCIP flaps. The perforators may not originate from the commonly known named sources. However, the freestyle approach lets you overcome these variations by quickly identifying another perforator in the adjacent region and change the flap design accordingly.

The SCIP flap can be raised as a fasciocutaneous flap known as the groin flap.[20] When raised on the suprafascial plane, it is Dr. Koshima's original description of the SCIP flap.[21] On this plane, one can take the SCIP flap as a chimeric flap to include lymph nodes to address patients with lymphedema or extend the dissection to the iliac bone to reconstruct small bone defects.[22] The dissection to include the bone may become very tedious as the small branches from the perforator can be difficult to identify. The donor site may have prolonged leakage of the lymphatic fluid if the lymphatic vessels and nodes are not adequately coagulated.

The GAP flap can be based on either the superior or the inferior gluteal artery.[23] When elevating with the full fat layers, it can be used to reconstruct the breast.[24] When elevating above the superficial fascia, it can be used to resurface the lower extremity or a weight-bearing foot. There can be many designs available from each GAP.[25,26] It can be designed in multiple axes directing to the trochanter or toward the flank. The design variation depends on the donor site appearance or the position of the defect if it is used as a local flap to cover the defect usually originating from a pressure sore.

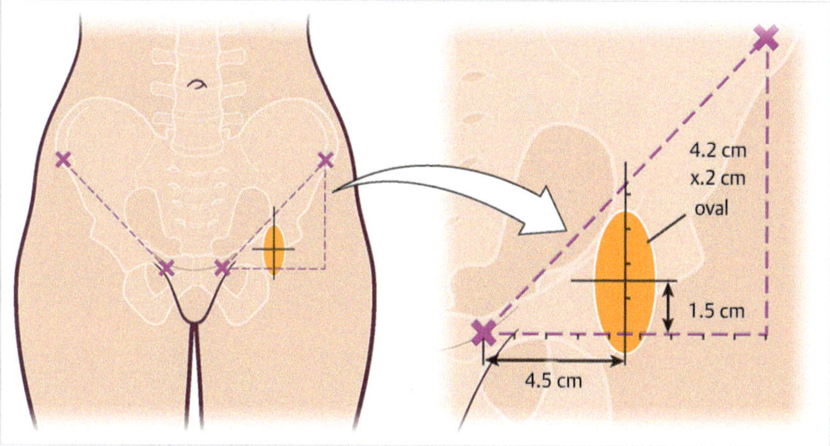

Fig. 22.2 The medial (superficial) branch is a direct cutaneous branch and in 95% of cases it penetrates the deep fascia within an oval of 4.2 × 2 cm (vertical × horizontal) with the center of the oval point located 4.5 cm lateral and 1.5 cm superior from the superolateral corner of the pelvic tubercle.

22.4 Flap Design

The flap design for the ALT and TDAP has been covered in the previous chapters and will not be covered in duplication.

Preoperative multidetector row computed tomography (MDCT) angiograms or conventional angiograms when hardware was used were obtained in the patients to evaluate the vascular status of the extremity. It can help identify the perforators rising from the thigh, buttock, and groin region. Preoperative markings of perforators are made based on the anatomical landmarks as described in previous chapters with the exception of the SCIP and GAP flaps. Additionally, a handheld Doppler was used to locate the actual perforator for a freestyle approach. When using a perforator as recipient, a strong visible pulse of the perforator is the main indicator for use.[27] For all flaps, especially the SCIP and the GAP flaps, a pinch test of the skin should be made to maximize the chance for primary closure of the donor site. In large defects, ALT or TDAP flaps can be designed in multiple skin paddles based on multiple perforators originating from the source vessel allowing the primary closure of the leg.[28]

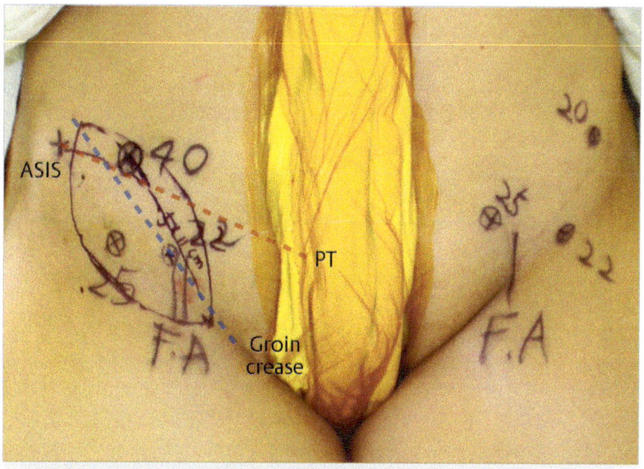

Fig. 22.3 In the groin region, there are three different systems: superficial circumflex iliac, external pudendal, and the superficial inferior epigastric systems. Multiple perforators are noted, but the medial branch of the superficial circumflex iliac artery perforator flap is relatively constant at 4.5 cm lateral and 1.5 cm superior from the superolateral corner of the pelvic tubercle.

22.4.1 Flap Design for the Superficial Circumflex Iliac Artery Perforator Flap

A line is drawn from the inguinal crease to the anterosuperior iliac spine (ASIS), marking the topographical pathway of the perforator. An acoustic Doppler is used to locate and identify the perforators from the superficial circumflex iliac artery (SCIA). Multiple perforators can be traced along this axis. There are usually two major perforators originating from the SCIA along this axis. The medial (superficial) branch is a direct cutaneous branch and in 95% of cases it penetrates the deep fascia within an oval of 4.2 × 2 cm (vertical × horizontal) with the center of the oval point located 4.5 cm lateral and 1.5 cm superior from the superolateral corner of the pelvic tubercle (▶ Fig. 22.2, ▶ Fig. 22.3).[29]

The lateral (deep) branch often travels through the sartorius muscle and then penetrates the deep fascia traveling further down to the flank region. If a large skin paddle were desired, it would be prudent to base the SCIP flap on this lateral perforator. The flap design is outlined so as to include as many perforators as possible and also to center the flap toward the medial aspect of the groin. A pinch test is done to confirm primary closure of the donor site. The maximum width of the flap that can be raised while permitting primary closure is 8 cm. The length of the flap can be extended beyond the anterior iliac spine or medially toward the buttock crease.

22.4.2 Flap Design of the Gluteal Artery Perforator Flap

To locate the SGAP perforators, a line is drawn from the posterosuperior iliac spine to the greater trochanter. Perforators are usually found adjacent to the medial two-thirds of the drawn line. A skin paddle is positioned over the most suitable perforator. In general, the more lateral the perforator, the longer the pedicle (▶ Fig. 22.4, ▶ Fig. 22.5).[26] To locate the inferior gluteal artery perforators (IGAPs), a line is drawn from the greater trochanter to the middle of the distance between the posterosuperior iliac spine and the medial border of the gluteal crease. The perforators are located on the middle third of this line in the marked areas (▶ Fig. 22.4).[26] A skin paddle is positioned over a desirable perforator and dissection proceeds as a freestyle elevation.

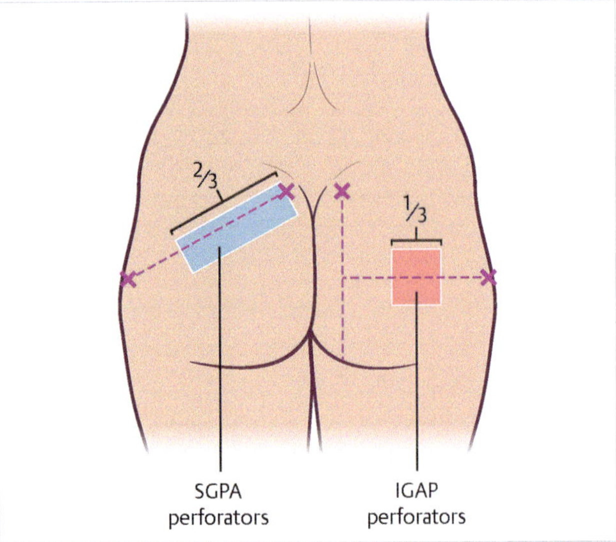

Fig. 22.4 To locate the inferior gluteal artery perforators, a line is drawn from the greater trochanter to the middle of the distance between the posterosuperior iliac spine and the medial border of the gluteal crease. The perforators are located on the middle third of this line in the marked areas.

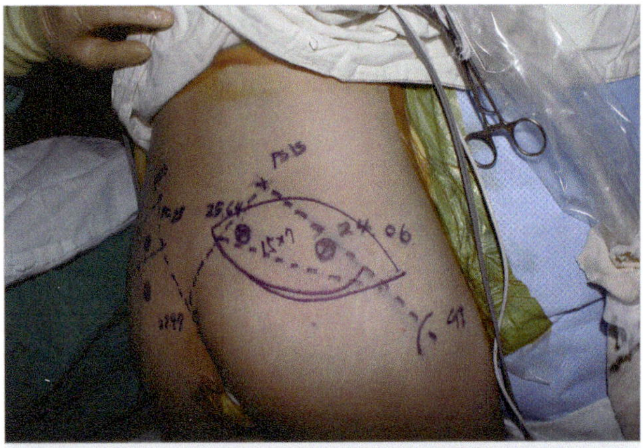

Fig. 22.5 Further use of Doppler can assist in localizing the perforator for the inferior gluteal artery perforator.

22.5 Flap Harvest

The elevation is a freestyle approach under loupe magnification and begins from either the lateral or the medial border of the flap. The incision is made deep to the superficial fascia dividing the superficial and deep fats. The superficial fascia is between the large deep fat lobules and smaller superficial fat lobules. The small lobules suddenly become larger as it passes a very thin fascia-like structure. This may be more apparent in patients with high BMI. It is easier to identify this thin white film-like fascia while retracting the skin from both sides of the incision. The elevation technique on the superficial plane can be made easy once the white film-like layer is identified under the right traction and countertraction of the skin immediately upon incision of the skin. After locating the fascia, elevation is made on this plane until the perforator marked previously on the skin is reached (hot zone). Then the same approach is made from the contralateral side. Based on the pulse and diameter of the vessels, a single perforator can be chosen and dissected into the deep fascia and muscle. The fat around the perforator can be skeletonized or maintained with a cuff of fat. We prefer to skeletonize the pedicel as it allows identifying relevant branches to the flap. After reaching adequate length, the pedicle is cut and made ready for microsurgery (see ▶ Video 22.1).

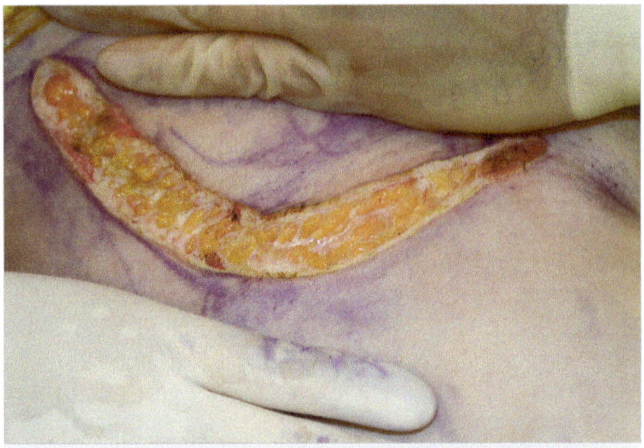

Fig. 22.6 The dissection plane, which is identified most clearly inferolaterally, lies above the Scarpa fascia (superficial fascia, super-thin plane), in between the superficial and deep fat. There is a distinct white fascial layer noted with the right amount of traction separating the smaller fat lobules from the deeper, larger fat lobules

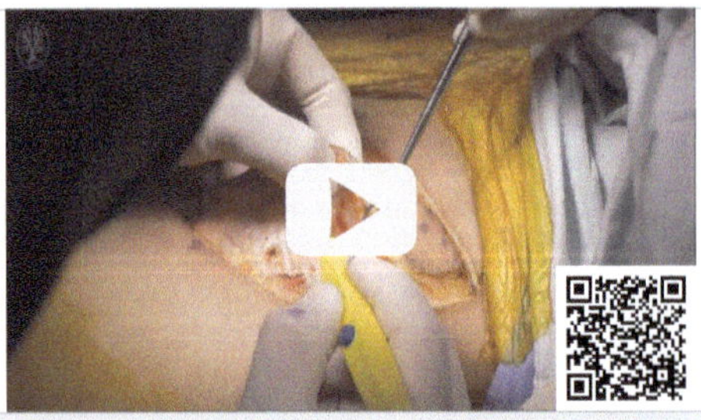

Video 22.1 Design of SCIP Flap. https://www.thieme.de/de/q.htm?p=opn/cs/20/7/12265283-c76663af

22.5.1 Elevation of Superficial Circumflex Iliac Artery Perforator flap

Required dimensions of the SCIP flap are outlined as per the defect. The flap is elevated along the inferior and lateral borders under × 4 loupe magnification. The dissection plane, which is identified most clearly inferolaterally, lies above the Scarpa fascia, in between the superficial and deep fat. There is a distinct white fascial layer noted with the right amount of traction separating the smaller fat lobules from the deeper, larger fat lobules (▶ Fig. 22.6, ▶ Fig. 22.7). Superficial lymphatics and lymph nodes are spared as they are found in the deeper adipose tissue. A bloodless field, essential so that staining of the tissue does not interfere with the identification of the perforators, is achieved through diathermy needle dissection.

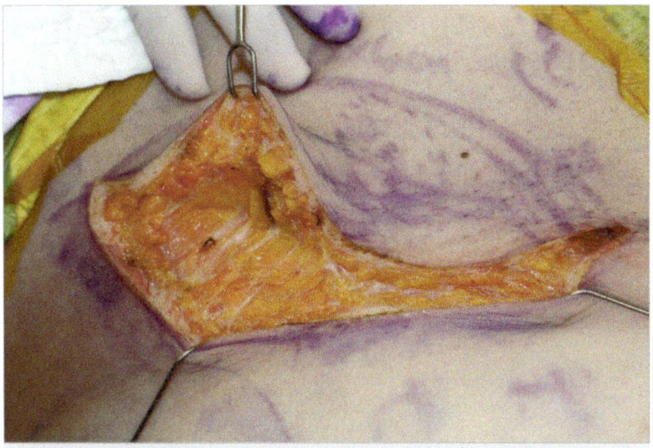

Fig. 22.7 Further elevation with the right traction will clearly show the white film-like superficial fascia. This avascular plane will allow you to visualize the perforators entering into the skin.

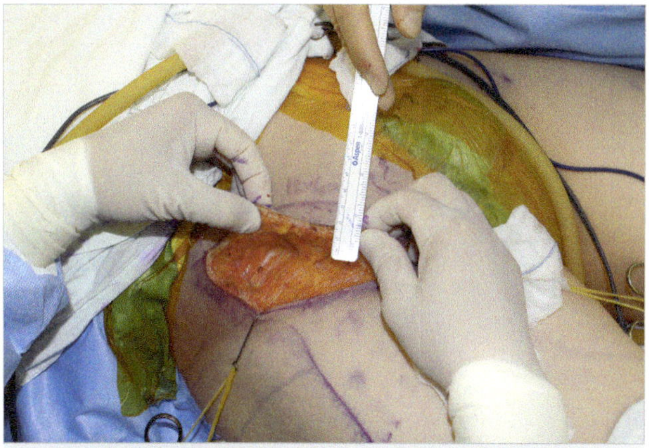

Fig. 22.8 Once the perforator(s) are seen from the inferolateral approach, the elevation progresses from lateral to medial and the lateral (deep) branch from the superficial circumflex iliac artery is identified/dissected first, followed by the medial (superficial) branch.

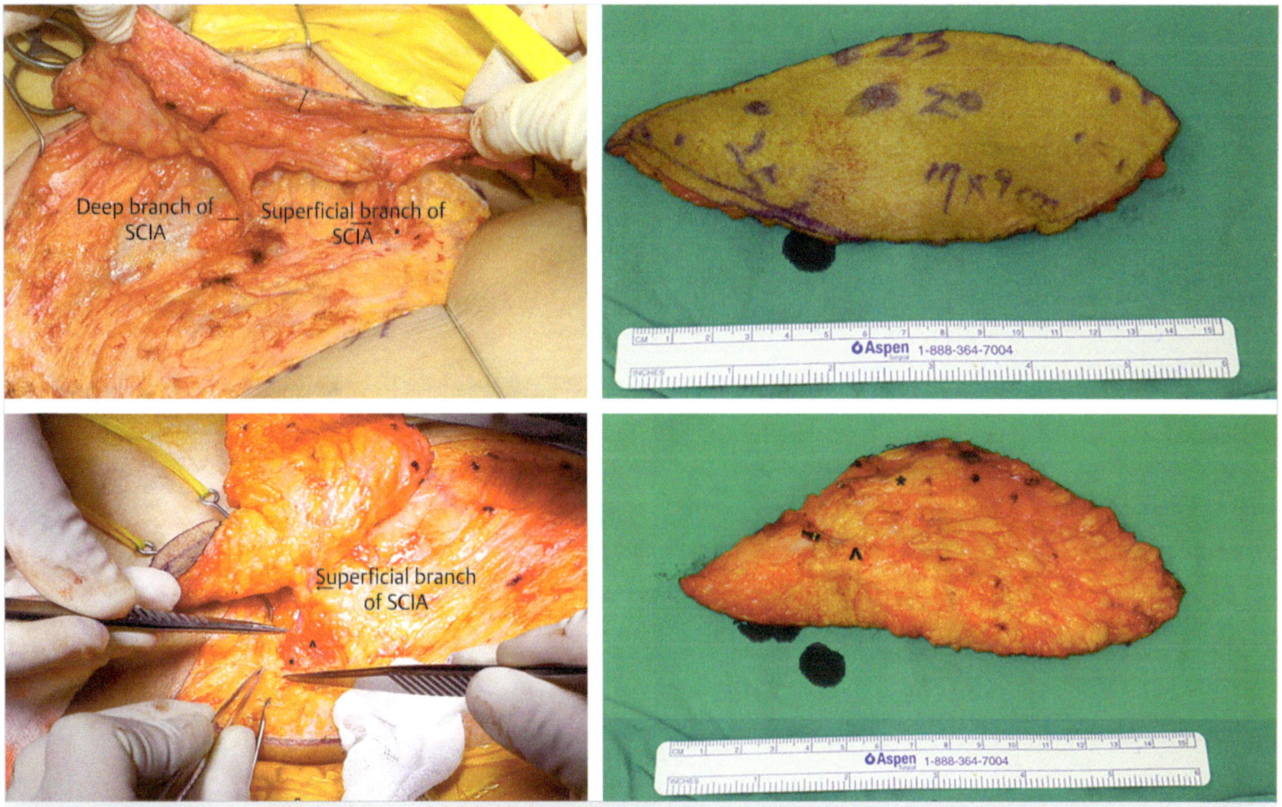

Fig. 22.9 Once both perforators are noted, or sometime just the medial one depending on the flap size, dissection of the pedicle is made toward the source vessel. The pedicle is cut once the adequate length is achieved or at the root of superficial circumflex iliac artery

Elevation progresses from lateral to medial and the lateral (deep) branch from the SCIA is identified first, followed by the medial (superficial) branch (▶ Fig. 22.8, ▶ Fig. 22.9). Perforators are skeletonized toward the deep fascia and examined for their suitability (▶ Fig. 22.10).

The deep branch is clamped to assess for sufficiency of the corresponding superficial branches. If the perfusion of the flap continues to be sufficient, the deep branch is ligated and the flap is raised on the superficial branch. Pedicle dissection is performed retrogradely toward the SCIA. The deep fascia can be incised to obtain a longer pedicle length and larger vessel diameter. A superficial vein running from the ASIS toward the pubis is normally identified and preserved. It is often that the accompanying vein drains into the superficial vein. In the cases where there is a small or absent superficial vein, the comitantes vein is usually of a larger caliber. In the cases where the donor vessels are small, dissection is done under the microscope. The average time for flap harvest is 45 minutes. ▶ Video 22.2 demonstrates the elevation of SCIP flap.

To close the donor site, the superficial fascia layer is plicated together with absorbable 2–0 sutures before the dermis and skin sutures are placed. This is important to obliterate the dead space and prevent seroma formation. Closure is done over one Jackson–Pratt drain. If the flap width exceeds 8 cm or the closure is tight, the groin is flexed to 45 degrees for 5 days to reduce tension on the wound.[7,8]

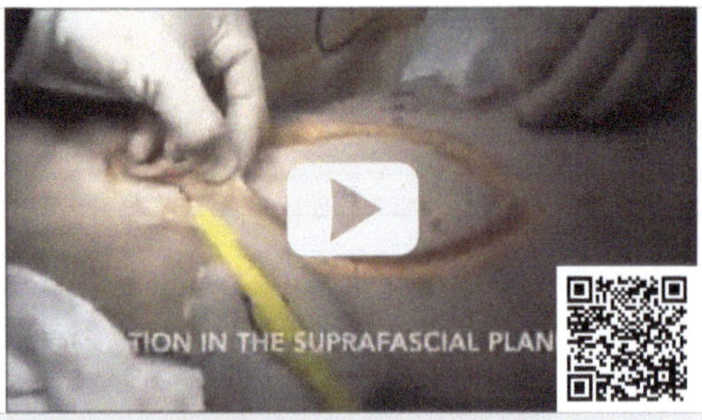

Video 22.2 Elevation of Anterolateral Thigh Flap in the Suprafascial Plane. https://www.thieme.de/de/q.htm?p=opn/cs/20/7/12265284-efd91947

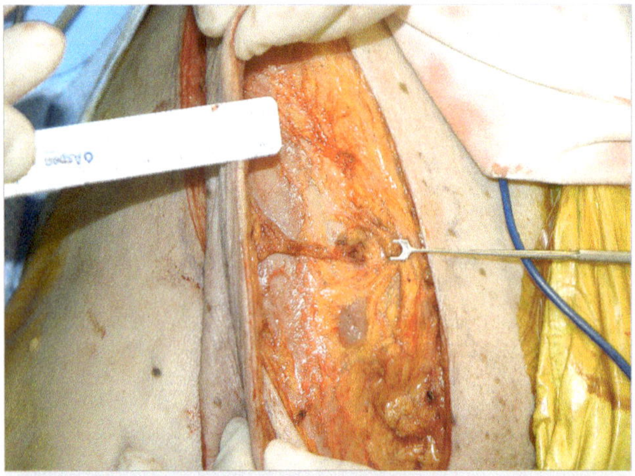

Fig. 22.10 After elevating the flap, pedicel dissection is made. Note the thin flap on the superficial fascial plane.

22.5.2 Elevation of Gluteal Artery Perforator Flap

A pinch test of the skin should be made to assure primary closure of the donor site. This flap can be used when reconstructing the posterior aspect of the body excluding the need to change patient position during the operation. A two-team approach can be used, one on the donor area to harvest the flap and one on the recipient area to prepare the recipient vessels. Using the preoperative marking of the perforator, either SGAP or IGAP, the elevation is a freestyle approach under loupe magnification and begins from the lateral border of the flap. The incision is made deep to the superficial fascia dividing the superficial and deep fats (▶ Fig. 22.11). The superficial fascia is between the large deep fat lobules and smaller superficial fat lobules and easy to identify with the right traction (▶ Fig. 22.12).

After locating the fascia, elevation is made on this plane until the perforator marked previously on the skin is reached (hot zone). Then the same approach is made from the medial side. There can be multiple perforators identified along this plane. Based on the pulse and diameter of the vessels, a single perforator is chosen and dissected into the deep fascia and muscle. The fat around the perforator can be skeletonized or maintained with a cuff of fat. We prefer to skeletonize the pedicel as it allows clear identification of relevant branches to the flap. After reaching adequate length (not longer than 8 cm), the pedicle is cut and made ready for microsurgery.[23] The video demonstrates the elevation technique for the thin GAP free flap elevation. ▶ Video 22.3 The donor site is always closed primarily. Plication of the superficial fascia is performed first followed by the subdermal and skin sutures.

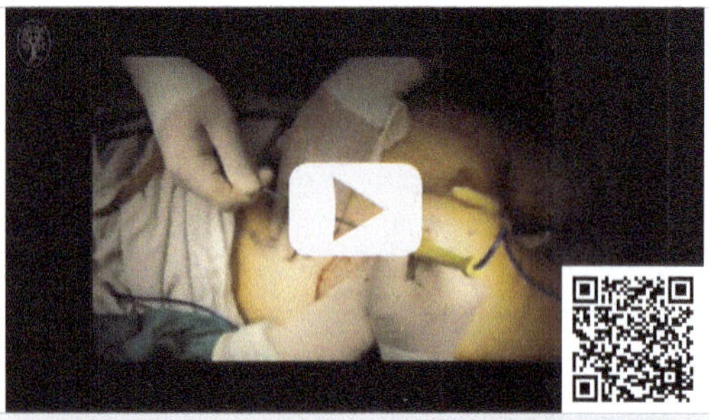

Video 22.3 GAP Free Flap Elevation. https://www.thieme.de/de/q.htm?p=opn/cs/20/9/12586549-88d9231b

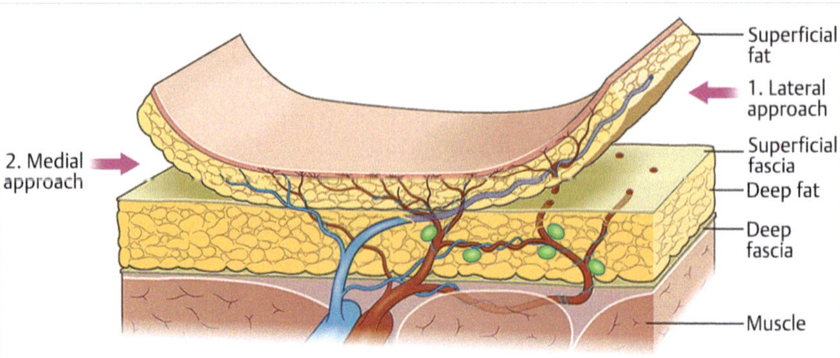

Fig. 22.11 Using the preoperative marking of the perforator, either superior gluteal artery perforator or inferior gluteal artery perforator, the elevation is a freestyle approach under loupe magnification and begins from the lateral border of the flap. The incision is made deep to the superficial fascia dividing superficial and deep fat. The superficial fascia is between the large deep fat lobules and smaller superficial fat lobules and easy to identify with the right traction

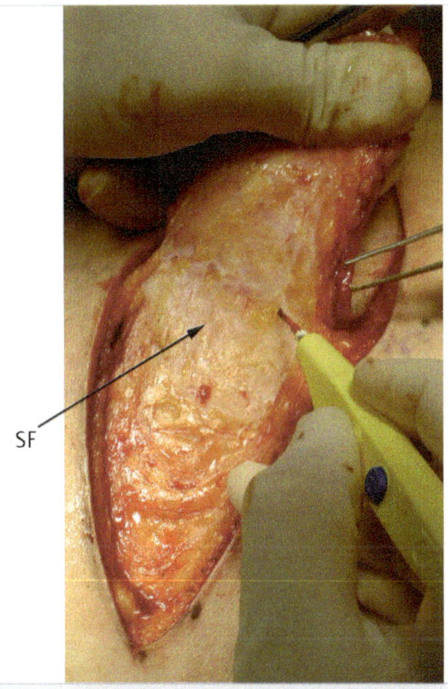

Fig. 22.12 From the preoperative markings using Doppler, a swift elevation can be made along the cold zone and transitioned into a meticulous dissection when the hot zone is reached.

22.6 Postoperative Care Protocols

Like any other flap, the importance of hydration to maximize perfusion to the flap and to the extremities cannot be overemphasized enough. Potent vessel dilators such as prostaglandins may help as well as low molecular heparin although still under debate. In our center, we like to start graduated pressure garments (30–60 mm Hg) from day 5 to 7 to reduce edema and to mold the flap. This also enables early ambulation by day 7 to 10, especially in the lower extremity reconstruction. Upper extremity cases and head and neck cases are ambulated on postoperative day 1. Patients are discharged from the hospital within 10 days unless there are other medical problems.

22.7 Conclusion

The elevation on the superficial fascia is a new approach for elevating flaps. It has advantages such as providing a thin flap allowing increased versatility to achieve better contour of flap, minimizing the need for secondary debulking, and being hemodynamically reliable.

References

[1] Pribaz JJ, Chan RK. Where do perforator flaps fit in our armamentarium? Clin Plast Surg. 2010; 37(4):571–579, xi

[2] Wei FC, Jain V, Celik N, Chen HC, Chuang DC, Lin CH. Have we found an ideal soft-tissue flap? An experience with 672 anterolateral thigh flaps. Plast Reconstr Surg. 2002; 109(7):2219–2226, discussion 2227–2230

[3] Kimura N, Satoh K. Consideration of a thin flap as an entity and clinical applications of the thin anterolateral thigh flap. Plast Reconstr Surg. 1996; 97(5): 985–992

[4] Kimura N. A microdissected thin tensor fasciae latae perforator flap. Plast Reconstr Surg. 2002; 109(1):69–77, discussion 78–80

[5] Gottlieb LJ, Krieger LM. From the reconstructive ladder to the reconstructive elevator. Plast Reconstr Surg. 1994; 93(7):1503–1504

[6] Hong JP, Choi DH, Suh H, et al. A new plane of elevation: the superficial fascial plane for perforator flap elevation. J Reconstr Microsurg. 2014; 30(7):491–496

[7] Hong JP, Sun SH, Ben-Nakhi M. Modified superficial circumflex iliac artery perforator flap and supermicrosurgery technique for lower extremity reconstruction: a new approach for moderate-sized defects. Ann Plast Surg. 2013; 71(4):380–383

[8] Goh TL, Park SW, Cho JY, Choi JW, Hong JP. The search for the ideal thin skin flap: superficial circumflex iliac artery perforator flap: a review of 210 cases. Plast Reconstr Surg. 2015; 135(2):592–601

[9] Hong JP, Chung IW. The superficial fascia as a new plane of elevation for anterolateral thigh flaps. Ann Plast Surg. 2013; 70(2):192–195

[10] Kim KN, Hong JP, Park CR, Yoon CS. Modification of the elevation plane and defatting technique to create a thin thoracodorsal artery perforator flap. J Reconstr Microsurg. 2016; 32(2):142–146

[11] Celik N, Wei FC. Technical tips in perforator flap harvest. Clin Plast Surg. 2003; 30(3):469–472

[12] Celik N, Wei FC, Lin CH, et al. Technique and strategy in anterolateral thigh perforator flap surgery, based on an analysis of 15 complete and partial failures in 439 cases. Plast Reconstr Surg. 2002; 109(7):2211–2216, discussion 2217–2218

[13] Tsai FC, Yang JY, Mardini S, Chuang SS, Wei FC. Free split-cutaneous perforator flaps procured using a three-dimensional harvest technique for the reconstruction of postburn contracture defects. Plast Reconstr Surg. 2004; 113(1): 185–193, discussion 194–195

[14] Yang WG, Chiang YC, Wei FC, Feng GM, Chen KT. Thin anterolateral thigh perforator flap using a modified perforator microdissection technique and its clinical application for foot resurfacing. Plast Reconstr Surg. 2006; 117(3): 1004–1008

[15] Saint-Cyr M, Schaverien M, Wong C, et al. The extended anterolateral thigh flap: anatomical basis and clinical experience. Plast Reconstr Surg. 2009; 123(4):1245–1255

[16] Saint-Cyr M, Wong C, Schaverien M, Mojallal A, Rohrich RJ. The perforasome theory: vascular anatomy and clinical implications. Plast Reconstr Surg. 2009; 124(5):1529–1544

[17] Ross GL, Dunn R, Kirkpatrick J, et al. To thin or not to thin: the use of the anterolateral thigh flap in the reconstruction of intraoral defects. Br J Plast Surg. 2003; 56(4):409–413

[18] Alkureishi LW, Shaw-Dunn J, Ross GL. Effects of thinning the anterolateral thigh flap on the blood supply to the skin. Br J Plast Surg. 2003; 56(4):401–408

[19] Lee Y, Hwang K. Skin thickness of Korean adults. Surg Radiol Anat. 2002; 24(3–4):183–189

[20] Hsu WM, Chao WN, Yang C, et al. Evolution of the free groin flap: the superficial circumflex iliac artery perforator flap. Plast Reconstr Surg. 2007; 119(5): 1491–1498

[21] Koshima I, Nanba Y, Tsutsui T, et al. Superficial circumflex iliac artery perforator flap for reconstruction of limb defects. Plast Reconstr Surg. 2004; 113(1): 233–240

[22] Koshima I, Nanba Y, Tsutsui T, Itoh S. Sequential vascularized iliac bone graft and a superficial circumflex iliac artery perforator flap with a single source vessel for established mandibular defects. Plast Reconstr Surg. 2004; 113(1): 101–106

[23] Hong JP, Yim JH, Malzone G, Lee KJ, Dashti T, Suh HS. The thin gluteal artery perforator free flap to resurface the posterior aspect of the leg and foot. Plast Reconstr Surg. 2014; 133(5):1184–1191

[24] LoTempio MM, Allen RJ. Breast reconstruction with SGAP and IGAP flaps. Plast Reconstr Surg. 2010; 126(2):393–401

[25] Nojima K, Brown SA, Acikel C, et al. Defining vascular supply and territory of thinned perforator flaps: part II. Superior gluteal artery perforator flap. Plast Reconstr Surg. 2006; 118(6):1338–1348

[26] Ahmadzadeh R, Bergeron L, Tang M, Morris SF. The superior and inferior gluteal artery perforator flaps. Plast Reconstr Surg. 2007; 120(6):1551–1556

[27] Hong JP, Koshima I. Using perforators as recipient vessels (supermicrosurgery) for free flap reconstruction of the knee region. Ann Plast Surg. 2010; 64(3):291–293

[28] Zhang YX, Hayakawa TJ, Levin LS, Hallock GG, Lazzeri D. The economy in autologous tissue transfer: part 1. The kiss flap technique. Plast Reconstr Surg. 2016; 137(3):1018–1030

[29] Suh HS, Jeong HH, Choi DH, Hong JP. Study of the medial superficial perforator of the superficial circumflex iliac artery perforator flap using computed tomographic angiography and surgical anatomy in 142 patients. Plast Reconstr Surg. 2017; 139(3):738–748

23 Bone Flaps and Bone Transport for Lower Limb Reconstruction

Matthew Iorio, Stephen Andrew Sems, and Steven L. Moran

Summary

Bone defects of greater than 5 cm are best managed with vascularized bone flaps. The vascularized fibula bone flap is the most commonly used and versatile flap for managing acute bone loss, late nonunions and allograft failure. For extensive soft-tissue loss, vascularized rib grafts used in conjunction with the serratus and latissimus muscle flap can provide soft-tissue coverage and bone reconstruction in one setting. For small recalcitrant defects, the medial femoral condylar flap provides vascularized cortical cancellous graft with vascularized skin.

Keywords: bone defect, bone reconstruction, vascularized bone graft, bone flap, fibula flap, vascularized rib bone, medial femoral condylar flap

23.1 Introduction

Functional restoration of the lower extremity following trauma, infection, or tumor extirpation can be challenging for the reconstructive surgeon; this is particularly true in the cases involving segmental bony loss of the tibia or the femur. For these defects, restoration of function requires bone reconstruction for stable weight bearing and ambulation. In addition, adequate soft tissue must be present to provide coverage of bone and hardware. Amputation of severely traumatized limbs is always an option, but amputation can be associated with morbidity in the form of increased cardiopulmonary and metabolic demands during prosthetic-based ambulation, increase in overall sedentary activity, and a resultant 5-year mortality rate of up to 68%.[1]

Efforts at limb salvage in the cases of trauma and tumor extirpation have led to the development of several strategies for the reconstruction of segmental bony defects. For defects less than 5 cm, a variety of allograft, synthetic, and nonvascularized autograft options are available. For bone defects that are greater than 5 cm in length and for smaller recalcitrant defects in areas of infection or radiation, vascularized autologous bone flaps and bone transport are reliable means of bony reconstruction. This chapter will review the major bone flaps used for reconstruction in the lower extremity and the principles of bone transport.

23.2 General Principles for Reconstruction of Bone Defects

Small bone defects, up to 5 cm, can often be repaired with shortening or nonvascularized bone grafting, provided there is an adequate soft-tissue envelope and the wound is free of infection.[2] Nonvascularized bone grafts are incorporated into defects through the process of creeping substitution and vascular ingrowth. Creeping substitution refers to a process of vascular ingrowth into the bone graft with subsequent resorption and replacement of the donor necrotic bone. Multiple donor sites exist for the harvest of nonvascularized cortical or cancellous autogenous bone; donor sites include the iliac crest, proximal ulna, and distal radius. Cancellous graft is usually preferred, unless there is the need for structural stability, as it is replaced more quickly than cortical bone by the process of creeping substitution. Nonautologous bone and bone substitutes can also be used for small bone defects; nonautologous options include cancellous and cortical allograft, calcium phosphate, and calcium sulfate. Nonautologous bone grafts are replaced more slowly than autologous bone, and often produce an immune response that inhibits complete replacement of the donor bone. A complete discussion of benefits and downsides associated with nonvascularized bone grafts is beyond the scope of this chapter; however, for small defects, it is our preference to use autologous bone if possible.

In contrast to bone graft, vascularized bone flaps allow for primary bone healing instead of depending on creeping substitution initiated by the recipient bone. The process of creeping substitution and bone remodeling may be compromised (or even absent) if the surrounding bone has been affected by radiation and infection or suffers from avascular necrosis.[3,4,5] In these situations, vascularized bone grafts have been shown to provide more rapid healing, reduce the risk of subsequent fracture, and have the ability to remodel under physiologic load allowing for early weight bearing and bone hypertrophy.[6,7]

Keys for successful reconstruction for any bone defect include thorough debridement of nonviable tissue, stable skeletal fixation, and adequate soft-tissue coverage. If these three components are not achieved, then even reconstruction with a vascularized bone flap will fail. For lower extremity reconstruction, it is best to work as a team with the orthopaedic trauma surgeons. The trauma surgeons can assist with bone debridement and fixation, while the microsurgeon provides soft-tissue coverage and bone flap reconstruction.

For most bone infections and subacute traumas, we perform debridement back to bleeding bone. In the cases of established osteomyelitis, we will place antibiotic impregnated polymethyl methacrylate cement into the defect in the form of a block spacer or as antibiotic beads for 6 to 8 weeks prior to reconstruction.[8] Bone stabilization in these cases is initially achieved with an external fixator. An eternal fixator allows for bony stability, yet places hardware away from the infected site (▶ Fig. 23.1). The polymethyl methacrylate is removed following the 6 to 8 weeks and the defect is filled with vascularized bone. The external fixator can be left in place until bony healing is achieved.

In the cases of acute open trauma, it is our preference to use internal fixation whenever possible for the definitive fixation, as this minimizes the need for external wires or fixators, which can compromise soft-tissue reconstruction and hamper rehabilitation (▸ Fig. 23.2). The concept of definitive fixation and flap coverage in a single setting is ideal to minimize the chances of hardware contamination and has been shown to produce union rates of better than 95%.[9] At the time of presentation and following the initial debridement, these patients can be managed with temporary external fixation until definitive soft-tissue and bony debridement is completed. Once the wound is free of nonviable and contaminated tissue, definitive bony fixation is achieved with intramedullary rods or plates and screws, following which the leg is covered with a free or pedicled flap. Regardless of the type of fixation used, stable bone fixation is imperative and is the cornerstone upon which successful limb salvage is based.

Similar principles are followed in the cases of tumor surgery. A multidisciplinary team is used where the oncologic surgeon can guarantee clean margins and assist in bony reconstruction. For intercalary bone reconstruction, there are many options for limb salvage, including tumor prosthesis, total prosthetic joint replacement, and massive cadaveric allograft reconstruction. While these options have all been shown to produce acceptable early limb salvage rates, they can suffer from long-term risks of fracture, nonunion, and infection.[10,11] We feel that vascularized bone flaps with or without massive cadaveric allograft reconstruction provide the most reliable means of long-term limb salvage. The one caveat in these cases is that additional nonvascularized

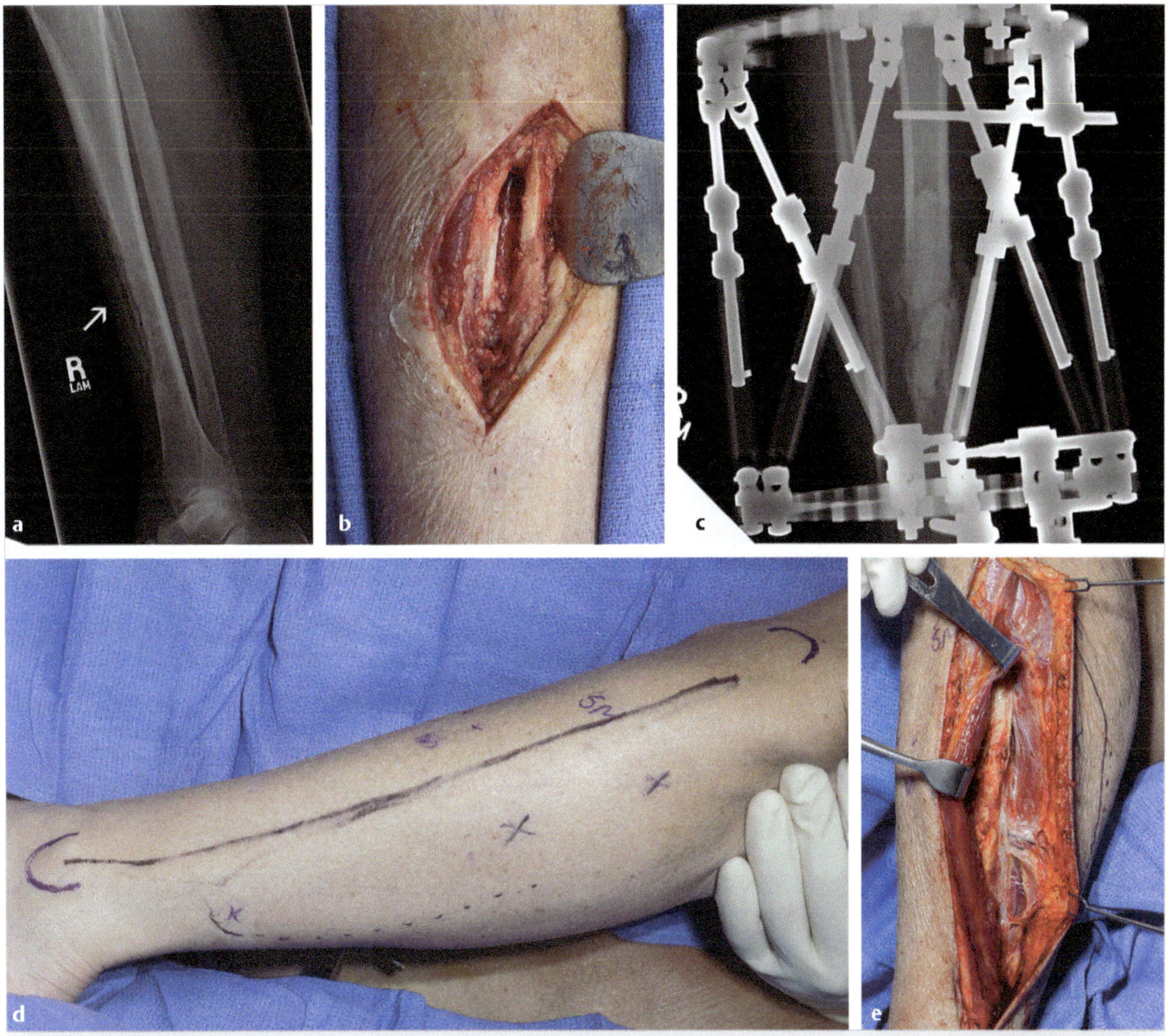

Fig. 23.1 (a) Anteroposterior radiograph of a 59-year-old woman with chronic osteomyelitis (*arrow*) of her right tibia as a result of an open fracture treated over 10 years ago. **(b)** Initial management consists of bone debridement, antibiotic bead placement for 6 weeks, and **(c)** external fixator placement for stability during treatment process. **(d)** A free fibula flap with a skin paddle is chosen for definitive treatment of the bone defect. Flap design begins by identifying Doppler signals in the skin (*marked with X*) just posterior to the fibula border, which correspond to cutaneous perforators for designing the skin island. **(e)** Dissection begins by elevating the anterior aspect of the incision until one identifies the interval between the peroneus muscles and the soleus. The fascia covering the peroneus muscle is elevated to reveal the perforators passing posterior to the fibula in the posterior crural septum.

(Continued)

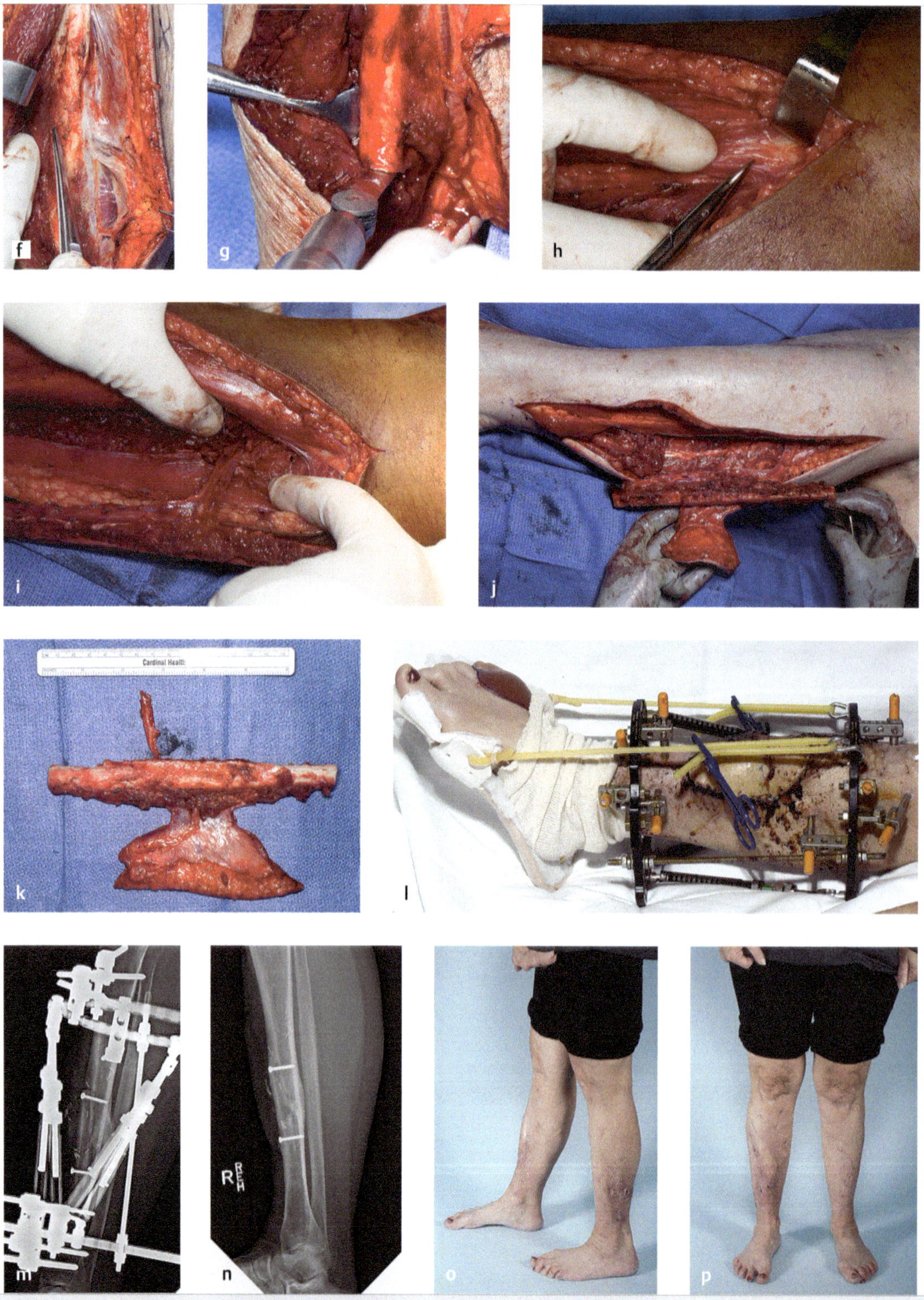

Fig. 23.1 (*Continued*) **(f)** Once the perforators are clearly identified the posterior margin of the skin island can be dissected. The major cutaneous perforator can be seen in this image along with the anterior and lateral dissection over the fibula. **(g)** The distal osteotomy is made with the aid of a Chandler retractor placed beneath the fibula to protect the peroneal vessels. **(h)** The common peroneal nerve (shown at the tip of the scissors) is identified at the superior margin of the incision prior to completing the proximal dissection and proximal osteotomy. **(i)** Once the proximal osteotomy is performed, the peroneal vessels are dissected back to the tibial peroneal trunk. **(j)** The fibula is now entirely isolated on its vascular pedicle. (*Continued*) **(k)** An image of the flap prior to insetting. **(l)** The leg is maintained in external fixator until definitive bony union. An elastic band attached to the fixator is used to prevent Achilles contracture. **(m)** Lateral radiograph showing insetting of the fibula using two compression screws. **(n)** Lateral radiograph of healed bone. **(o, p)** Clinical appearance of the salvaged limb and resultant donor site scar on the left leg at 2 years postoperatively.

autologous bone graft should be used to augment the osteosynthesis sites (either the two cut ends of the fibula or the surface beneath the vascularized bone graft). Additional autologous graft has been shown to limit cases of delayed union. The use of vascularized fibular flaps in the setting of malignant tumors has shown union rates of better than 90%.[12] In the following sections, we will discuss our workhorse flaps for segmental bone loss in the lower extremity.

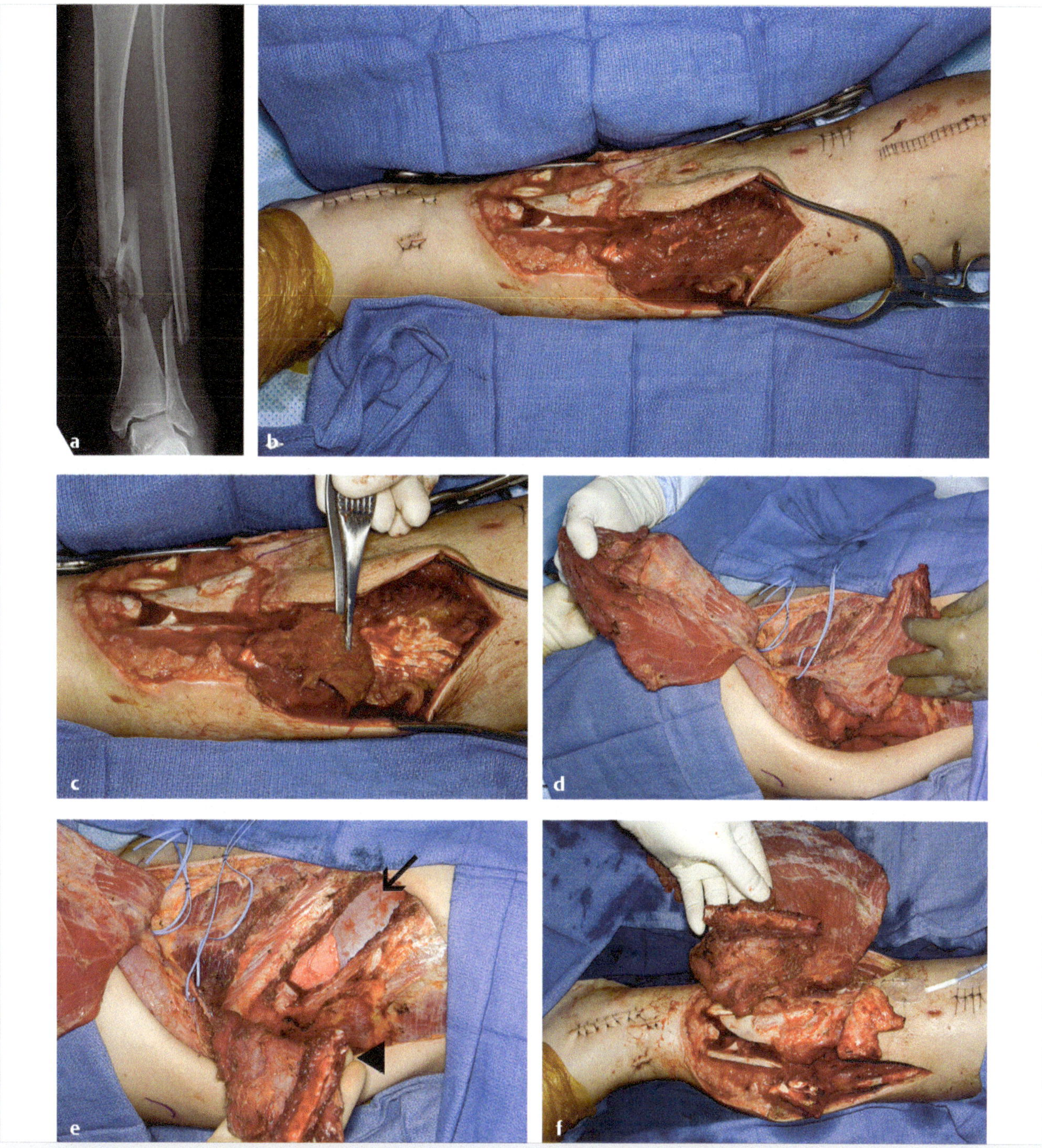

Fig. 23.2 **(a)** Anteroposterior radiograph of a 28-year-old man who suffered an open compound fracture of his tibia and fibula. **(b)** Reconstruction is started with debridement of the bone defect and **(c)** extensive debridement of the surrounding dead muscle and soft tissue. **(d)** A single rib is harvested with the serratus and latissimus for soft-tissue coverage and bony reconstruction. **(e)** This intraoperative image shows the vessel loops surrounding branches of thoracodorsal vessels. The *arrowhead* points to the rib and the *arrow* points to the pleura. The chest defect can be covered with synthetic mesh or acellular dermal matrix. **(f)** The chimeric flap is transferred to the leg where an end-to-side anastomosis is performed between the thoracodorsal artery and the posterior tibial artery. The long pedicle length allows for easy insetting of the rib.

(*Continued*)

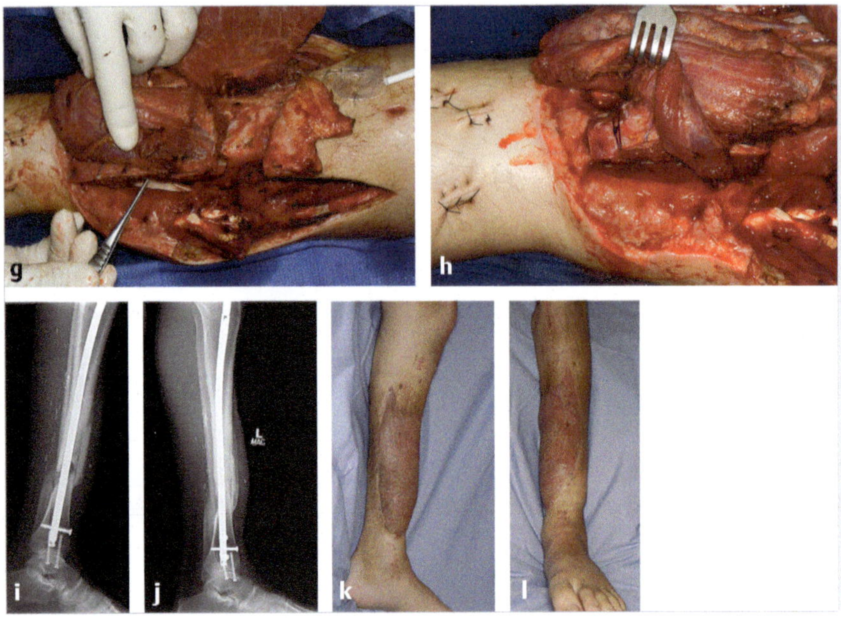

Fig. 23.2 *(Continued)* **(g)** The rib is secured to the tibia with sutures placed **(h)** through bone tunnels. The fracture is also stabilized with an intramedullary rod. **(i)** Postoperative radiograph at 5 months showing early consolidation and at 2 years **(j)** showing bony union with hypertrophy of rib graft. **(k, l)** Clinical appearance of the leg at 5 months postoperatively.

23.3 Fibula Flap

23.3.1 Introduction

The fibula flap was originally described by Taylor et al in 1975 as a vascularized bone flap for augmented osteoinduction in a large tibial defect.[13] The flap was then modified by Chen and Yan in 1983 to include a skin paddle. The fibula osteocutaneous flap has remained a workhorse flap for segmental and intercalary bony defects in combination with soft-tissue reconstruction.[14] The ubiquitous use of this flap for long bone reconstruction is due to the length of bone one can obtain (over 25 cm) and the ability to reliably carry a cutaneous paddle with the flap. Multiple reports have demonstrated excellent rates of union, with up to 80% primary union rates and as high as 97% following supplemental bone grafting.[12]

23.3.2 Attributes

- Bicortical bone for increased mechanical strength and potential weight bearing.
- Longest available piece of vascularized bone for reconstruction (~25–30 cm).
- It can be osteotomized to fit recipient defect.
- Multiple configurations include longitudinal strut, double-barreled, onlay, and as a hybrid used in conjunction with massive cadaveric allograft.
- Large diameter vascular pedicle based on peroneal artery and comitantes.

23.3.3 Detriments

- It sacrifices a major blood vessel to the lower leg.
- Proximal and distal osteotomies must be carefully placed to avoid injury to the common peroneal nerve (CPN) or ankle mortise.
- Skin paddle design inclusion frequently results in the need for skin grafting at the donor site.
- Dissection through the flexor hallucis can result in a stiff or contracted toe.
- It can result in chronic ankle instability.

23.3.4 Anatomic Considerations

The fibula receives its blood supply from the peroneal, anterior interosseous, and lateral geniculate arteries[15]; however, the majority of flaps are designed to utilize the peroneal artery as the flaps' major blood supply. All of the vessels supplying the fibula originate from the popliteal artery. After passing beneath the popliteus muscle, the popliteal artery divides into two major terminal branches: the anterior tibial artery and the tibioperoneal trunk. The anterior tibial artery branches proximal to the tibioperoneal trunk and perforates the interosseous membrane to travel within the anterior compartment of the leg. After passing through the interosseous membrane, the anterior tibial artery gives off several branches that supply the fibular head and fibular physis in children. These branches include the circumflex fibular artery as well as the first and second recurrent epiphyseal arteries.[15] Distal to the anterior tibial artery's branch point, the popliteal artery terminates in the tibioperoneal trunk, which divides into the posterior tibial artery (coursing medial) and peroneal artery passing laterally to run along the posterior medial surface of the fibula.

After branching to the fibula, the peroneal artery runs in close proximity to the medial surface of the fibula between the tibialis posterior muscle and the flexor hallucis muscle. The peroneal artery provides both a nutrient vessel for endosteal blood flow and multiple periosteal perforating branches. The nutrient artery to the fibula diaphysis enters in the middle third of the bone and should be preserved during dissection. Additionally, the peroneal artery gives off several perforators to the lateral leg skin. These perforators pass along the posterior margin of the fibula, within the septum of the deep posterior compartment, also referred to as the posterior crural septum. A pooled analysis of 1,710 peroneal perforators was performed to evaluate the location and frequency of these cutaneous perforators along the axis of the fibula. The authors found that if the total length of the fibula is marked off into tenths from proximal to distal, the area with the highest density of perforators was localized in the sixth interval from the fibular head, with 19% of all perforators being found in this region. There was a 79% positive predictive probability of finding a skin perforator in this region. More proximal along the fibula, perforators are more likely to travel through the muscle belly of the soleus prior to irrigating the skin, whereas distal perforators are more likely to be septocutaneous due to the Achilles musculotendinous interface.[16]

Finally, the surgeon should be aware of the course of the CPN, as it runs close to the proximal limits of the fibula dissection (▶ Fig. 23.1). The nerve originates from the apex of the popliteal fossa after splitting from the sciatic nerve, which continues distally as the tibial nerve. The CPN then travels between the head of the lateral gastrocnemius and the medial margin of the biceps femoris. At the fibular head, the CPN will often be encountered in the plane of dissection of the fibular flap as it moves from the popliteal fossa to the lateral compartment. At the level of the peroneus longus, the nerve divides into the superficial branch and deep peroneal branch. To protect the nerve and its branches, the proximal osteotomy is typically made 5 to 7 cm distal to the fibular head; however, if necessary, the head of the fibula may be taken for added length or for cases that require a growth plate transfer. In such cases, the nerve should be identified and protected during flap elevation.

23.3.5 Anatomic Variations and Potential Pitfalls

The complications seen with the fibular flap are often related to lower leg anatomic variation and fibula donor site morbidity. Due to the limited skin laxity, intramuscular dissection, and ankle mortise changes, removal of the fibula can be associated with several donor site complications. Momoh et al[17] evaluated 157 consecutive patients who underwent a free fibula flap for head and neck reconstruction, in order to determine the risk factors for acute and long-term morbidity following use of the flap. They found a 31.2% incidence of perioperative complications, most commonly due to local wound disruptions, including skin graft loss at the closure site (15%), cellulitis (10%), and dehiscence (8%). Additionally, long-term complications were identified in 17% of patients, and were commonly related to gait disturbances, with decreased ankle mobility (12%), hallux contracture (9%), leg weakness (8%), and ankle instability (4%). Despite these complications, the authors reported that 96% of patients returned to their preoperative level of ambulatory activity.

From a vascular standpoint, in patients with normal three-vessel runoff the harvest of the peroneal artery appears to have minimal impact to the overall vascularity and viability of the distal leg and foot. To demonstrate this, near-infrared spectroscopy has been utilized pre- and postoperatively following the removal of the fibula flap and the corresponding peroneal artery. The study found that the distal oxygen saturation decreased less than 5% in the first 8 hours postoperatively; however, the oxygen saturation subsequently recovered to the baseline after 8 hours.[18]

In rare instances, the posterior tibial or anterior tibial arteries can be hypoplastic or injured, and the peroneal artery subsequently becomes a dominant arterial supply to the lower leg and foot. In rarer instances, both the posterior tibial and the anterior tibial are aplastic, creating a hypertrophied peroneal artery, referred to as a *peronea arteria magna*. To determine the incidence of these rare variations, a systematic review was conducted among 26 studies, which examined a total of 5,790 limbs.[19] The study found that abnormal branching patterns with at least one hypoplastic artery have been reported in 5% of patients. The most frequent variation reported was a hypoplastic posterior tibial artery, whereas the incidence of the peronea arteria magna was only found in 0.4% of limbs.

While the incidence of anatomic variation is low, we still recommend preoperative evaluation of the lower extremity prior to flap elevation. In the cases of lower extremity trauma, this may be even more important for the recipient limb, where single vessel traumatic occlusion can be seen in greater than 25% of patients requiring free tissue transfer.[20] A CT angiogram can provide detailed anatomic arterial information of both lower limbs and can be obtained with little risk to the patient. Finally, during flap elevation, the surgeon should carefully verify that the peroneal artery is the selected vessel, as retractors or dissection within the posterior compartment can place the posterior tibial artery in close proximity to the fibula, potentially resulting in injury to the posterior tibial artery or common tibioperoneal trunk.

23.3.6 Flap Design

The fibula can be either oriented as a single longitudinal flap or osteotomized to create a "double-barreled" paired configuration (▶ Fig. 23.3). The paired endosteal, or "internal," and periosteal ("external") circulations allow the segments to remain well vascularized if the intervening periosteal sleeve is left intact without injury. The double barrel may be especially useful when reconstructing large metaphyseal defects or areas subjected to high axial strain and weight bearing. However, in order to have sufficient bone for reconstruction, the double-barrel configuration should be limited to defects less than 13 cm in length, based on the average available length of the fibula.

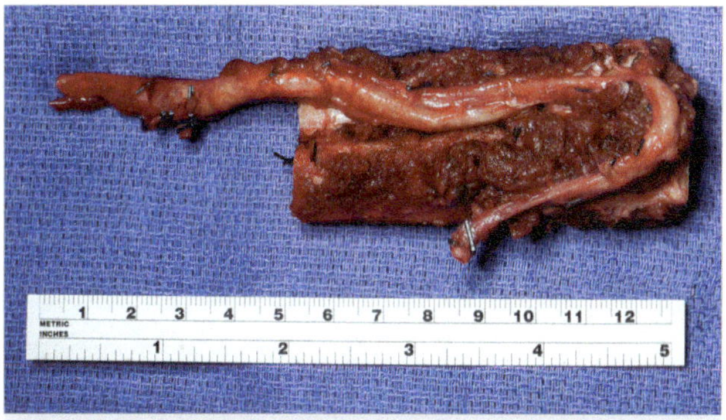

Fig. 23.3 Intraoperative image of a double-barreled fibula flap construct. The peroneal artery is carefully left in continuity as a portion of the fibula is excised or osteotomized to allow for folding of the fibula. This configuration allows for easier reconstruction of metaphyseal defects.

Some authors have advocated for the use of the longitudinal vascularized fibular strut with a combination of rigid plating, as the fibular flap will eventually hypertrophy following repetitive load. Sainsbury reported on 18 patients with fibula flap interposition following resection for sarcoma. In this group, the mean time to union was 24 months (range, 9–72 months), and the authors found that the fibula underwent significant hypertrophy following axial loading, with resultant diameters of 71% of the recipient bone.[21]

Alternatively, in the cases of chronic nonunion, the fibula can be utilized to augment primary bone healing in combination with autograft or allograft. The "onlay" technique describes a technique where the fibula is used to span the site of nonunion to increase osteogenesis and primary bone healing; this technique is especially useful in the cases of chronic infection, failed massive allograft, or irradiated avascular bone.[22] Friedrich et al evaluated the outcomes of 25 patients who received an onlay fibular flap, and found fracture union in 21 patients at an average of 11 months postoperatively, 22 of these patients having received prior bone irradiation. The authors noted that 21 of the fractures were pathologic secondary to irradiation and avascular necrosis. Prior to fibular flap treatment, 10 patients had failed operative fixation of the fracture with a nonunion for an average of 14 months, and the remaining 15 had trialed and failed cast immobilization.[23]

In oncologic cases where the intercalary bone defect exceeds the length requirements of a double-barreled design, or in those that may require more rigid osteosynthesis, the fibula flap can be placed within the center of an allograft. This hybrid technique was originally described by Capanna in 1993 for reconstruction of large oncologic intercalary bone defects of the tibia, and utilizes an allograft that has been cored or hallowed to allow the passage of the fibula flap internally (▶ Fig. 23.4). The fibula can be slotted into the intramedullary canal of the allograft. A channel is then created within the allograft with a rotary burr to allow access and passage of the vascular pedicle (▶ Fig. 23.4). The Capanna technique allows for immediate rigid fixation as large plates, or double plating can be applied to the allograft, while the fibula remains protected from injury during hardware fixation. In the long term, the fibula allows for accelerated healing at the osteosynthesis sites. In addition, the fibula helps revascularize the allograft leading to lower rates of infection and late fracture.[11]

Studies evaluating the outcome of the Capanna technique have demonstrated improved time to bone healing and subsequent weight bearing. Houdek et al evaluated their outcomes

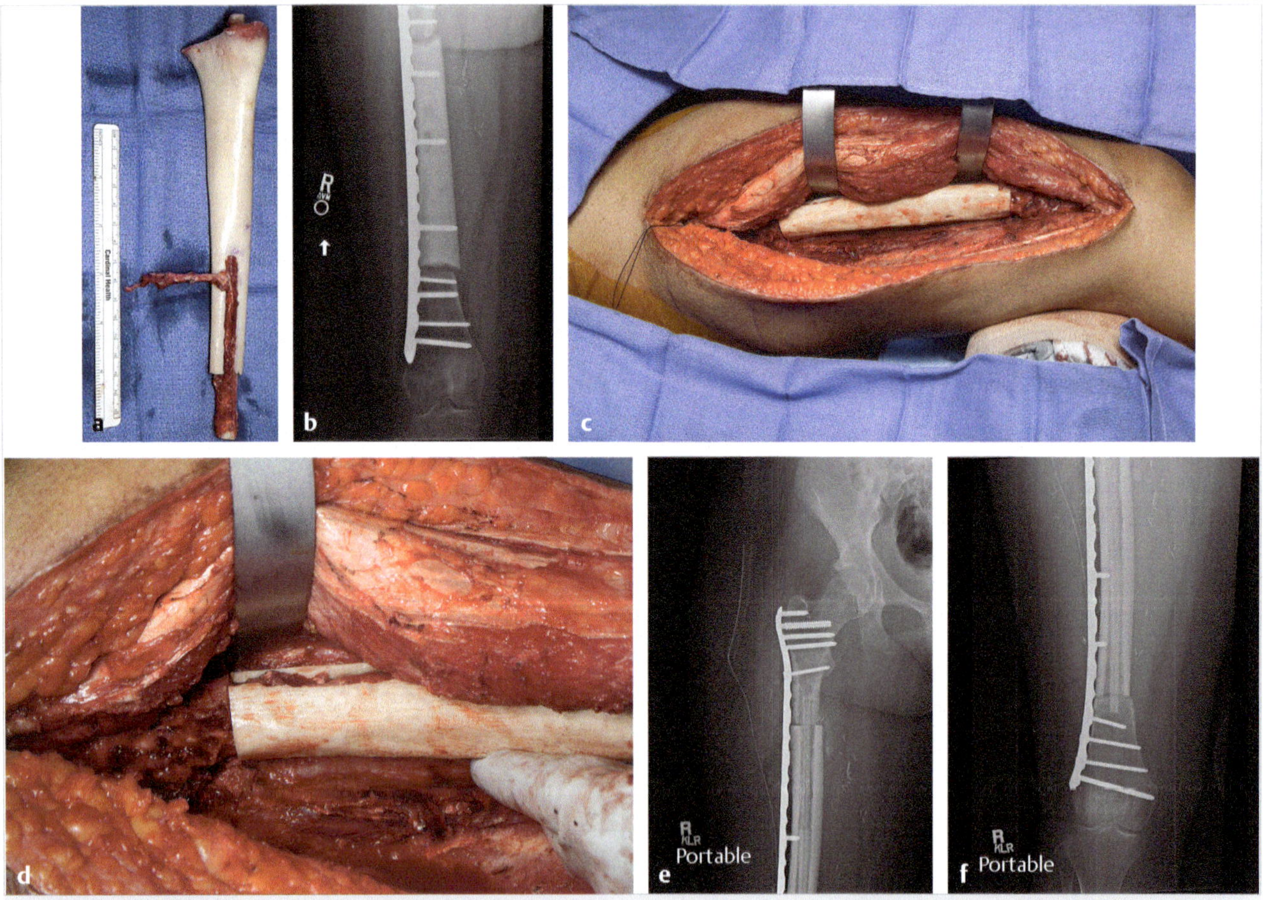

Fig. 23.4 An example of the Capanna technique. **(a)** The fibula flap is placed within a large cadaveric allograft. The vessels are protected by creating a slot into the allograft. **(b)** Anteroposterior radiograph of a failed allograft reconstruction of an intercalated bone defect in a 14-year-old adolescent girl following resection of Ewing sarcoma of bone. **(c, d)** Intraoperative image of a Capanna construct in place. **(d)** Vessels exiting the slot within the allograft. **(e, f)** The postoperative clinical radiographs showing fibula spanning the ends of the allograft, allowing for accelerated bony union.

with the technique in 18 pediatric patients who underwent limb salvage following oncologic tibial resections. In this group, the overall limb salvage rate was 94% and despite 6 patients requiring a secondary procedure for a symptomatic nonunion, 17 of these patients had good or excellent outcome as indicated by their Mankin score.[24,25] Similar findings were demonstrated by Schwarz et al. In their retrospective review of 13 patients, 8 required secondary bone grafting for nonunion, but the median time to union was 10 months (range, 3–40 months) and of the surviving patients, 91% achieved full weight bearing by 2 years and were able to participate in sports.[26]

Finally, the fibula flap design can be modified to include the proximal fibular head for either a vascularized physeal transfer or an osteochondral flap. Dissection is modified in these cases to harvest the fibular head on the anterior tibial artery and subsequent nutrient branches to the fibular head and physis.[15] In these cases, the fibula is approached through the interval between the tibialis anterior and extensor digitorum longus. The motor branches from the deep peroneal nerve must be carefully preserved to the anterior compartment, while including a strip of muscle and interosseous membrane with the recurrent epiphyseal branch of the anterior tibial artery.

23.3.7 Flap Harvest

The total length of the fibula should be marked out to identify a safe interval for the proximal and distal osteotomies. Typically, 6 cm is left proximally to prevent iatrogenic injury to the CPN proximally and 6 cm is left distally to avoid the development of ankle instability distally (▶ Fig. 23.1).

If a skin paddle is to be included, the perforators are identified with a handheld Doppler along the posterior border of the fibula, whereas any skin perforators on the anterior margin are most likely from the anterior tibial artery and should not be included. The paddle should be marked out, with the anticipation that skin paddles in excess of 4 cm may require a skin graft for donor site closure.[17] Under tourniquet control, the anterior skin margin can be incised, and the surgeon should consider a suprafascial dissection to maintain a potential surface for skin grafting in larger skin paddles. Additionally, this may help identify and avoid injury to the superficial peroneal nerve.

The division between the anterior and lateral compartments can be identified by a longitudinal fibrofatty strip, and based on the Doppler, dissection proceeds to the posterior margin of the peroneus longus and brevis muscles to the marked perforators. We find it helpful to separate the soleus insertion from the fibula. This allows one to create a window into the posterior compartment to visualize the peroneal vessels proximally. At this point, we will often also identify the peroneal nerve and mark it with a vessel loop to prevent any retraction injury.

Once the peroneal artery has been visualized, dissection begins to elevate the peroneus muscles and the extensor digitorum muscles medially. The skin perforators can be isolated on their perforator passing through the posterior crural septum. Proximally, skin perforators can be dissected through the soleus without a muscular cuff by following the course of the perforator and associated fascial envelope. At this point, the skin flap can be tacked to the bone with several temporary stitches to prevent avulsion during the remainder of the harvest. If there is no skin paddle, the elevation of the fibula flap can proceed directly without identification of perforators or posterior dissection of the soleus.

The peroneal and anterior compartment muscles are then reflected sharply to keep a minimal (1–2 mm) cuff of muscle intact to prevent injury to the periosteum. Following this, the interosseous membrane is identified and carefully incised near the fibula. At the site of the bone cuts, a periosteal elevator is used to carefully create space between the peroneal artery and the fibula, and a curved retractor is placed to protect the vessels. Distally, in the instance of heavy atherosclerosis or if there is potential difficulty controlling the pedicle, a 1-cm paired osteotomy can be performed to remove a small block of bone and allow direct visualization and control of the pedicle. Following the proximal and distal osteotomies, the flap is elevated from distal to proximal, freeing the pedicle from the flexor hallucis muscle and preserving the skin perforators, if included. The proximal peroneal artery and venae comitantes are identified at the tibioperoneal trunk, and if possible, the tourniquet is deflated prior to ligation to ensure adequate perfusion to both the flap and the foot.

Following harvest, the flexor hallucis muscle can be suspended to the interosseous membrane with the hallux in extension to prevent postoperative toe contractures. Additionally, the operative leg should be immobilized for 5 to 7 days in a well-padded posterior splint with the ankle in neutral.

23.4 Vascularized Rib

23.4.1 Introduction

Free rib flaps were first described in 1977 for reconstruction of lower extremity injuries.[27] The rib is composed of membranous bone that possesses a dual blood supply, from the posterior intercostal artery and an abundant periosteal blood supply from the serratus anterior muscle. The periosteal blood supply is derived from the thoracodorsal artery providing a long reliable pedicle to be used in vascularized bone grafting. Typically, this graft is used to reconstruct lower extremity defects when the contralateral fibula is damaged or absent.[28]

One advantage of this flap is the combination of a large serratus muscle soft-tissue envelope with or without the latissimus.[29] This allows for bone reconstruction and extensive soft-tissue coverage with the use of a single pedicle. Double-rib transfers are also possible without the need for excessive chest wall reconstruction. Double-rib transfers have been shown to be biomechanically superior to single-rib transfer for some nonunions.[30]

23.4.2 Attributes

- Cortical cancellous vascularized bone of up to 10 to 15 cm can be easily harvested.
- Can be harvested in combination with the serratus, latissimus, or scapular flap.
- Minimal functional donor site morbidity.
- Can be osteotomized to ease insetting.

23.4.3 Detriments

- Risk of pneumothorax.
- Potential risk to long thoracic nerve injury, which could lead to winged scapula.
- Proximal serratus resection can lead to scapular dysfunction.
- Bone does not provide sufficient biomechanical strength for unrestricted weight bearing alone, and is best used to augment existing structural bone.

23.4.4 Anatomic Considerations

The rib receives its blood supply from the intercostal vessels, which provide endosteal and periosteal perforators. The thoracodorsal arterial contribution to the serratus muscle anastomoses with the intercostal system, allowing the rib to be harvested on the serratus muscle. Additionally, the serratus muscle supplies intramuscular perforators directly to the rib periosteum.

As the ribs are curved, we find it best to osteotomize the pleural cortex with an oscillating saw prior to placing them within the leg. This allows one to straighten the rib against the tibia or the femur.[31] We also prefer to fix the ribs with 3.5 compression screws or with heavy suture in a cerclage fashion. While the rib lacks the structural strength of the fibula, the high cancellous content may accelerate bony consolidation.[32]

23.4.5 Anatomic Variations and Potential Pitfalls

When harvesting the rib with the serratus anterior as part of a combination "chimeric" flap with the latissimus dorsi or scapular flap, the pedicle must be dissected all the way to the axillary artery in order to rule out any vascular anomalies and to ensure that the latissimus dorsi and the other components are nourished by a single thoracodorsal pedicle. Once the pedicle has been adequately visualized, the serratus anterior digitations between the 5th and 10th ribs can be harvested in conjunction with the latissimus dorsi. Most surgeons prefer to take the digitations between the 5th and 8th ribs as the 9th and 10th rib digitations are not always reliable. Harvesting only between the sixth and eighth digitations has been shown to be helpful in minimizing functional morbidity created by sacrificing the serratus muscle. Preservation of the most cephalad portion of the serratus and its attachment to the scapula prevents the possibility of postoperative scapular winging.

23.4.6 Flap Design

Skin incision is the same as one would use for a serratus muscle harvest. We prefer to make an incision in the anterior axillary line and carry it into the inframammary fold in a woman and anteriorly into the fifth to sixth intercostal space in men. This allows for a broad exposure of the serratus in addition to allowing rib harvest to the anterior thorax if necessary.

23.4.7 Flap Elevation

▶ Fig. 23.2 depicts the elevation. Elevation of the flap begins by raising skin flaps anteriorly and posteriorly to identify the latissimus muscle. The anterior border of the latissimus is elevated so that one can see the serratus anterior and the long thoracic nerve. The thoracodorsal vessels are then identified and traced distally until they give off the branch to the serratus. This arterial branch to the serratus runs on the anterior surface of the muscle, unlike the branch to the latissimus, which runs on the deep posterior surface of the latissimus muscle.

One to two ribs can be safely included with the serratus muscle flap for reconstruction of composite bone and soft-tissue defects. Perfusion to the ribs is provided by the periosteal blood supply and small anastomoses between the muscular branches of the serratus muscle and the intercostal system. Harvest of the fifth to eighth ribs is preferred because these ribs can be centered beneath the serratus flap. The selected rib is taken with the intercostal bundle, which runs inferior to it. We prefer to take sequential ribs; however, Lin et al have recommended taking alternating ribs to avoid chest wall reconstruction.[28]

Rib with serratus muscle harvest is started by separating the inferior digitations from the rest of the serratus muscle. Then to raise the flap, the lower anterior border of the planned flap is opened with a cautery. By placing a finger in the plane between the flap and the ribs, blunt dissection can be carried out away from the bone to be harvested. The latissimus dorsi is retracted as far as possible dorsally to expose the origins of the lower digitations on the inferior scapular angle. After the planned flap has been separated, sharp dissection can be performed to detach the flap from its insertions on the scapula.

After the serratus muscle has been isolated from the superior slips of the proximal muscle, an electrocautery is used to dissect beneath the serratus toward the rib, which is to be included within the flap. It is important to leave all the small perforating branches from the serratus to the underlying rib periosteum, as well as a generous piece of intercostal muscle above and below the rib segment. The intercostal muscles attaching to the ribs are dissected toward the rib. At the anterior border of the flap, dissection is carried out over the surface of the rib. This allows the surgeon to carefully dissect below the rib to create a plane between the rib and the pleura. Once the pleura has been identified, the rib can be divided anteriorly and posteriorly with rib cutters or a large bone biter. At this point, the rib is elevated from its pleural surface with a periosteal elevator. The pleural surface of the rib should be carefully dissected to avoid injury to the underlying pleura; in some cases, subperiosteal dissection may be required if there are dense adhesions to the pleura. The intercostal vessels must be ligated anteriorly and posteriorly to fully mobilize the flap. Finally, unicortical osteotomies can be made on the pleural surface of the rib to allow them to straighten for reconstruction of forearm or metacarpal defects.

The resultant donor site in the chest wall can be closed with acellular dermis or some other form of bioprosthetic mesh. If an injury to the pleura occurs, one may place a chest tube attached to water seal for 24 to 48 hours or one can evacuate the air from the chest cavity with a suction device and then repair the pleural tear with absorbable suture. A postoperative chest radiograph should always be obtained at the completion of the case to verify there is no residual or expanding pneumothorax.

Combined Latissimus Dorsi and Serratus Anterior with Rib Flap

The latissimus and serratus muscles can be elevated together on a single pedicle for reconstruction of large defects in the lower extremity (▸ Fig. 23.2). After exposing the anterior border of the latissimus dorsi, the thoracodorsal artery and its branches to the serratus anterior muscle digitations are identified. The main trunk of the thoracodorsal neurovascular bundle can be easily located by dorsally retracting the anterior segment of the latissimus dorsi. The trunk lies superficially to the serratus anterior muscle. One or two branches supply the serratus anterior digitations and usually arise 3 to 6 cm inferior to the vessels point of entry into the latissimus dorsi. It is important to identify and preserve the long thoracic nerve branches to minimize functional morbidity and winging of the scapula. The long thoracic nerve usually lies on the surface of the muscle and joins the vascular bundle at the level of the sixth rib. The serratus anterior muscle can be mobilized by meticulously dividing its attachments on the corresponding ribs. Extreme care should be taken to preserve the innervations at the upper and lower borders to avoid scapular winging.

23.5 Medial Femoral Condyle Flap

23.5.1 Introduction

The medial femoral condyle (MFC) flap is a versatile piece of the cortical cancellous bone harvested from the distal femur (▸ Fig. 23.5). Originally described as a thin corticoperiosteal flap, the osteogenic ability of the vascularized flap has been utilized in nonunion sites throughout the upper and lower extremities, with excellent results.[33,34,35] A systematic review of 248 cases of the MFC flap used for both upper and lower extremities was performed by Kazmers et al. The review found that the union rate averaged 98.7% (range, 66–100%). Within this review, the majority of MFC flaps were used to treat previously operated recalcitrant nonunions. In addition to excellent outcomes, the donor site morbidity of the MFC, including iatrogenic fracture and knee dysfunction, is quite low at 0.8 and 0.4%, respectively, making this flap a good choice for recalcitrant nonunions of the lower extremity.[36]

23.5.2 Attributes

- Thick corticocancellous block of vascularized bone.
- Can be harvested in combination with a skin paddle.
- Minimal functional donor site morbidity.
- Can be harvested with portions of the adductor tendon, vastus medialis for composite defects around the Achilles tendon.
- Inclusion of the trochlea allows for a vascularized osteochondral flap.

23.5.3 Detriments

- Risk of iatrogenic femur fracture.
- Risk of knee instability if the medial collateral ligament (MCL) complex is injured.
- A unicortical bone flap may not provide sufficient biomechanical strength for unrestricted weight bearing and is best used

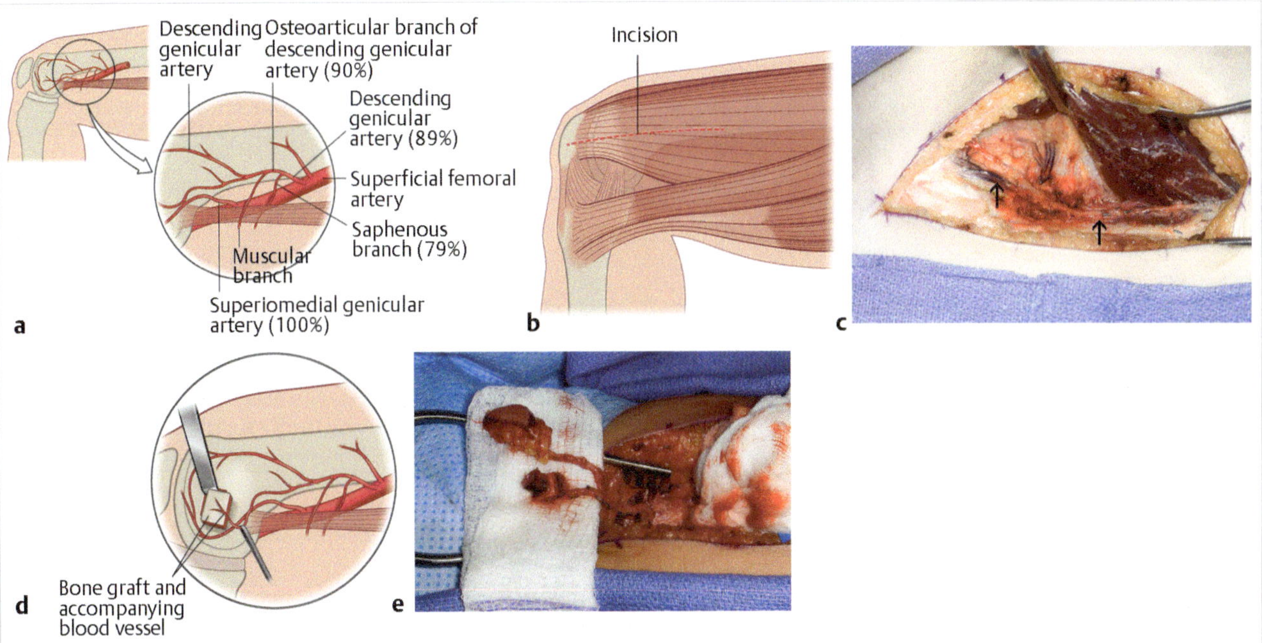

Fig. 23.5 (a) Artist's rendition of descending genicular artery and superomedial geniculate artery. The percentages represent the percentage of specimens containing the respective arteries based on the study of Yamamoto.[37] **(b)** Representation of the line of initial incision for elevation of the medial femoral condyle flap. **(c)** After elevation of the vastus medialis muscle, the descending geniculate artery (*arrows*) can be seen running on top the medial femoral condyle. **(d)** Artist's rendition of vessel isolation and use of osteotome to harvest bone graft. **(e)** Clinical image of a graft with associated skin paddle prior to pedicle division. (Reproduced with permission from Mayo Clinic.)

in combination with rigid fixation in the cases of recalcitrant nonunion.[33]

23.5.4 Anatomic Considerations

The MFC is irrigated by nutrient vessels from the deep femoral artery, which creates an endosteal circulation and centrifugal flow pattern from the cancellous to cortical bone. However, the overlying periosteum has multiple perforating branches from the superficial femoral artery (SFA) that communicates with this deep system to provide perfusion when elevating a corticocancellous bone flap. Specifically, the MFC is perfused primarily from the descending genicular arterial (DGA) system and the superior geniculate artery (SGA). Iorio et al evaluated the periosteal circulation over the MFC through subtraction angiography and demonstrated that up to 29% of the distal femoral length (13.7 ± 1.3 cm from the knee joint line) is irrigated through the distal periosteal circulation of the DGA.[38] Subsequent authors have also found rich periosteal connections with the DGA circulation, and the greatest density of cortical perforating branches appears to be in the posterodistal quadrant of the MFC.[37]

As the DGA branch enters the MFC periosteum, a dense filigree emerges with two main trunks: the longitudinal branch and the transverse branch. The longitudinal branch passes parallel to the long axis of the femur to provide irrigation to the level of the joint line. In comparison, the transverse branch courses perpendicular to the long axis toward the superior pole of the condyle and the articular surface at the trochlea. As such, the transverse branch can be elevated from the periosteum and utilized to create an osteochondral flap, or the medial femoral trochlea (MFT) flap. The average cartilage thickness at the edge of the trochlea is near 1.65 mm, creating an excellent source of cartilage for resurfacing chondral defects.

23.5.5 Anatomic Variations and Potential Pitfalls

When considering the inclusion of a skin paddle, either for resurfacing or for flap monitoring, skin perforators can be included as direct cutaneous branches from the distal DGA, or the saphenous artery branch (SAB) more proximally. In a study evaluating the region of skin perfusion, the SAB perfused an average area of 361 cm^2, extending to the posterior thigh and distal to the knee joint along the medial column. In comparison, the DGA cutaneous branch originates from the DGA just at the level of the condylar flare, passes perpendicular to the sartorius tendon, and had an average 70 cm^2 of skin irrigation. The DGA zone is directly over the MFC, but has some overlap with the saphenous artery distribution at the posterior margin.[39]

Typically, the DGA arises directly from the SFA, though there can be some variability in combination with the saphenous artery branch. In a cadaveric evaluation of branching patterns, three separate patterns were noted with the saphenous artery branch originating directly from the DGA in a majority of cases (64%). Minor variations also include the potential for a common origin from the SFA (27%) and an independent origin from the SFA (9%).[39] In addition, Yamamoto found that 10% of anatomic specimens lacked the DGA and the MFC is perfused solely by the SGA. In these cases, the MFC flap would need to be elevated on the SGA pedicle[37]

Dissection around the knee should proceed carefully to limit the potential injury to the knee joint and retaining ligaments. Most at risk is the MCL complex, as it originates on the distal inferior portion of the MFC. The MCL acts as the primary restraint against valgus laxity at neutral and in 30-degree knee flexion. The ligament is part of the capsuloligamentous complex of the medial knee, and coalesces with part of the medial patellofemoral ligament. The fibers originate on the posterior aspect of the MFC and attach distally to the tibia 5 to 7 cm below the joint line.[40]

23.5.6 Flap Design

The bone flap should be designed along the medial column of the femur, again taking care to avoid injury to the far cortex, or encroachment within the anterior or posterior femoral columns (▶ Fig. 23.5, ▶ Fig. 23.6).

Biomechanical studies have been performed in cadaveric specimens to determine the threshold for a safe bone flap size. In a report of 16 cadaveric limbs, bone defects measuring 3, 5, or 7 cm were created and compared to a control group without osteotomies. The risk of fracture increased with larger osteotomies, with bone failure rates of 12.5, 12.5, 28.6, and 55.6% for control, 3-, 5-, and 7-cm defect groups, respectively. Failure torque was seen at 45.5, 29.35, 27.4, and 30.83 Nm for the control, 3-, 5-, and 7-cm groups, respectively. Additionally, any osteotomy within the medial column will demonstrate some decreased resistance to torsion, and may create a risk of fracture if not properly monitored.[41]

If a skin paddle is to be included, or for exposure of the MFT, a curvilinear line between the patella and the MFC is marked following identification of the skin perforator on Doppler ultrasound. If a bone-only flap is intended, the incision can be a straight line parallel to the long axis of the femur on the posteromedial margin. When accessing the articular surface of the knee, care should be taken to avoid injury to the medial patellofemoral and meniscal ligaments, attaching from the lower margin of the articular patella to the femur and the anteromedial meniscus. Injury to these structures can result in lateral patellar instability and chronic knee pain.[42]

23.5.7 Flap Harvest

A skin incision is made down to the level of the muscular fascia over the vastus medialis. The inferior margin of the muscle interdigitates with the fascia of the sartorius tendon and this interval is carefully reflected in a superior direction to allow exposure of the MFC. On average, there are two muscle branches from the DGA pedicle to the vastus medialis that occur on average 12.5 ± 2.0 and 9.8 ± 1.9 cm from the joint line. Carefully ligate these branches to prevent inadvertent injury to the main pedicle.

Once the periosteum is exposed, dissection can proceed in either a retrograde or an antegrade fashion in reference to the pedicle origin and arborization, based on the surgeon's preference. When starting distally, the thin fibrofatty envelope overlying and superficial to the periosteum is reflected while

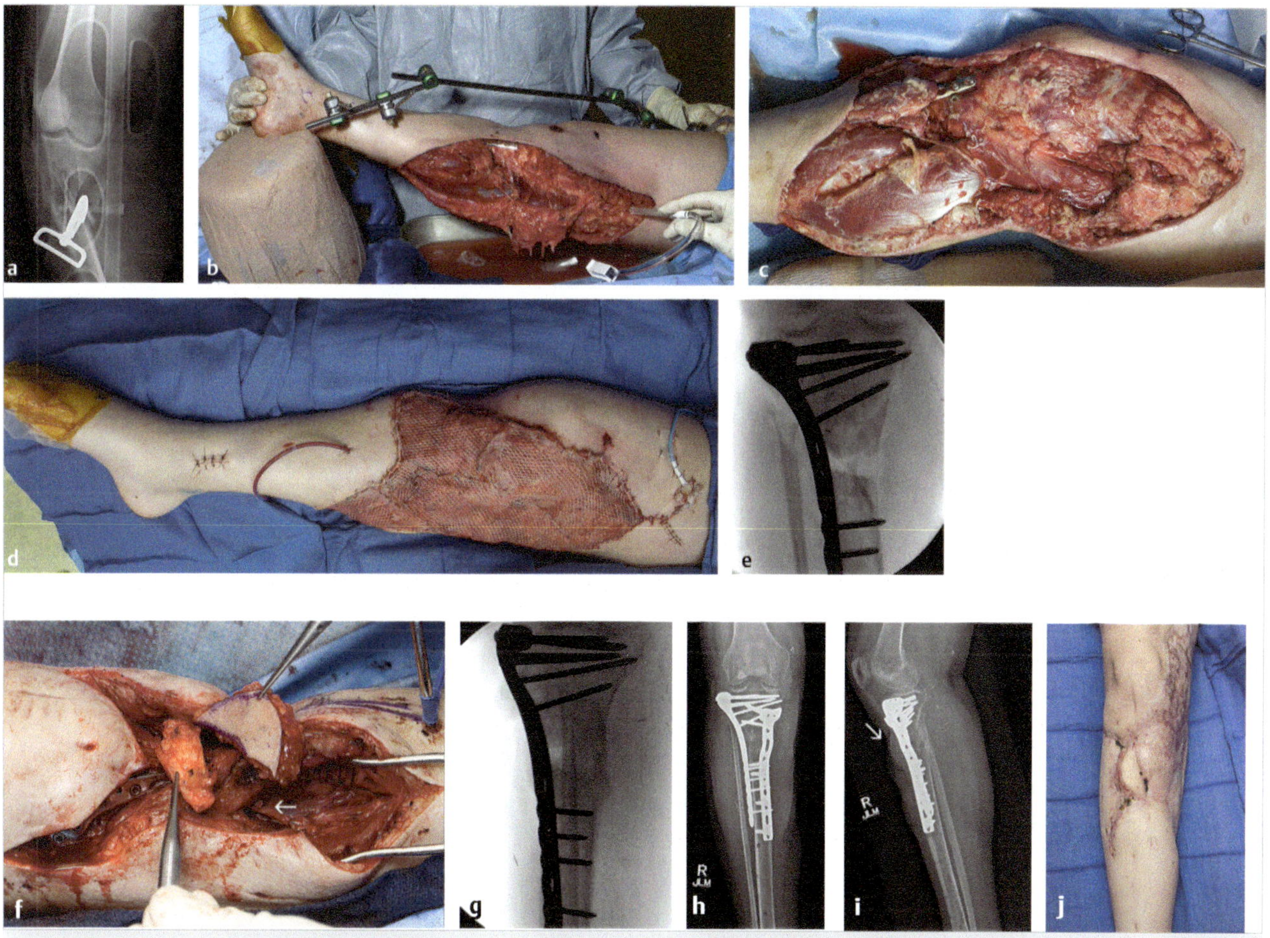

Fig. 23.6 Clinical case of the medial femoral condylar (MFC) flap for treatment of a tibial nonunion. **(a)** Initial anteroposterior (AP) radiograph of a 31-year-old woman with Gustilo IIIc injury to the right leg. The popliteal artery was transected at the time of injury and repaired at the time of initial debridement. **(b)** Preliminary fixation was obtained with external fixator until completion of debridement surgeries. **(c,d)** Soft-tissue coverage was obtained with a free latissimus flap anastomosed into the distal femoral artery while plate fixation was performed for the tibia fracture. At 6 months, the patient presents with a persistent nonunion of proximal tibia, seen in the AP radiograph in **(e)**. An MFC bone flap with skin paddle was used to treat the nonunion. **(f)** Skin paddle to the right and bone flap to the left. The vascular pedicle (*arrow*) was passed beneath the anterior tibialis muscle to anastomose to the anterior tibial artery. **(g)** Intraoperative inset. **(h, i)** incorporation of graft over 2 months (*arrow* points to graft location). **(j)** Appearance of the leg at 4 weeks post-op, with viable skin paddle.

keeping the densely adherent periosteum intact. The DGA pedicle and comitantes can then be dissected free from the adductor tendon to the point of origination from the SFA just distal to the adductor hiatus.

As the pedicle is dissected and the recipient bone defect templated onto the MFC, the surrounding margin of the periosteum is incised with a monopolar cautery. The periosteum directly over the intended bone flap should not be elevated, and the osteogenic cambium layer between the vascular and cortical tissue is left intact. A small sagittal saw or curved and straight osteotomes are utilized to elevate the flap. To avoid creating a stress riser during flap elevation, one can predrill the margins of the flap with a small Kirschner wire. Once the straight osteotomies have made a uniform bone cut around the flap, curved osteotomes are used to carefully elevate the posterior margin on the flap and prevent corticocancellous delamination.

Rao et al evaluated the MFC donor site in 15 patients with postoperative CT and found that there is minimal reparative bone regrowth at the femoral margin, even at an average follow-up of 18 months. As such, whenever possible the donor site should be packed with cancellous allograft to encourage restoration of the medial column of the femur.[43] The design, harvest and application is show on ▶ Video 23.1.

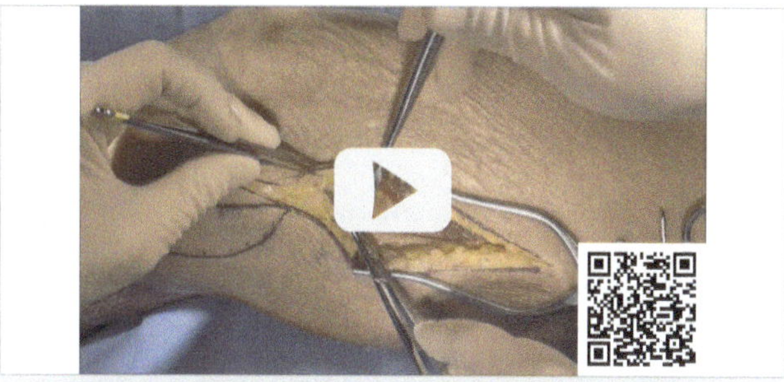

Video 23.1 Medial Femoral Condyle Flap with Skin Paddle. https://www.thieme.de/de/q.htm?p=opn/cs/20/7/12265285-ab78d7fa

23.6 Bone Transport and Distraction Osteogenesis

23.6.1 Introduction

Bone transport is a technique used to treat intercalary bony defects with the process of distraction osteogenesis. The technique involves cutting a segment of the surrounding healthy bone and gradually moving the osteotomized segment into the defect. Distraction osteogenesis generates new bone in the space created by the distraction through a mechanical process of callus distraction. Distraction osteogenesis results in the formation of immature regenerate bone mainly through intramembranous ossification.[44] This regenerate bone subsequently matures and solidifies over time, creating a mechanically stable limb. This technique is dependent on slow distraction occurring at a rate of 0.75 to 1 mm per day. Thus, bone transport can be a lengthy process and because of this, complications can occur. Common complications include hardware failure, hardware infection, nonunion, and knee and ankle stiffness.[45]

The choice to use distraction osteogenesis over a vascularized bone flap is multifactorial; however, regenerate bone avoids a flap donor site, avoids microsurgery, and a lengthy, operative procedure. In many cases, patients are able to avoid retained hardware and large segmental allografts (▶ Fig. 23.7). Limb length discrepancies and rotational deformities can be corrected with the distraction process. Obviously, the downsides are related to the time necessary for the process to occur.

23.6.2 Attributes

- Can be used to restore bone in the setting of massive bone loss.
- May avoid the need for autograft harvest. Thus, there is no donor site morbidity.
- Does not rely on internal fixation, which may be desirable in the setting of previous infection.
- Allows adjustments for corrections of deformities as bone position can be modified throughout the transport process.

23.6.3 Detriments

- A time-consuming process that requires many postoperative clinic visits.
- High rate of complications, including pin site infections, regenerate fractures, and docking site nonunions.
- Requires the patient to wear an external fixator.
- Depends on patient compliance and understanding of process to adjust external fixator daily.

23.6.4 Anatomical Considerations

Bone transport may be considered in the setting of bone loss from traumatic, iatrogenic, or congenital conditions (▶ Fig. 23.7). It requires a soft-tissue envelope capable of accommodating external fixation pins and these wires will then be pulled through the skin. Additionally, the transported segment and distraction site need a level of perfusion and viability to permit osteogenesis to occur. The bone ends that will dock together must be inspected for perfusion. To do this, a burr or rasp can be used to debride the ends back to punctate bleeding bone. The ends should be contoured to allow maximal surface area upon docking.

The external fixator generally requires three rings to perform bone transport. The proximal and distal rings are affixed to the bone, aligning the segments in their anatomic position. In the setting of preexisting deformity, gradual correction can be accomplished during the transport process. If there are no preexisting angular deformities, the proximal and distal rings remain static in relationship to each other throughout the

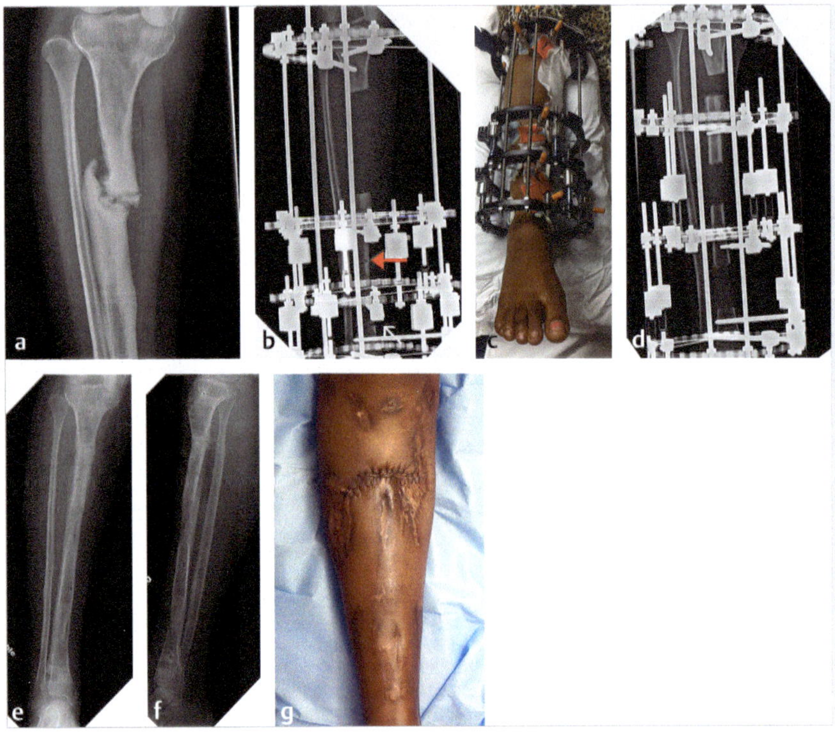

Fig. 23.7 **(a)** Anteroposterior radiograph of long-standing nonunion due to osteomyelitis. Bone is resected and distraction osteogenesis is initiated by placing a ring fixator and creating two distal corticotomies (*red and white arrow*) in **(b)**. **(c)** Appearance of the leg in the ring fixator. Because two osteotomies were used, the distraction process can proceed more rapidly along for each fragment to be mobilized 1 mm a day. **(d)** Early consolidation and **(e)** late consolidation at the time of fixator removal **(f)**. **(g)** Final appearance of the leg at the time of fixator removal.

process. The middle ring is attached to the segment to be transported. Half pin and smooth wire placement in the transport segment should be carefully considered to prevent the transport ring from impinging on the docking site ring before the bone ends abut. Once the rings are secured to the bone, a low-energy cortical osteotomy is completed to create a transport segment. This can be accomplished by making several drill holes in the bone at the desired level, followed by closed manipulation or completion with an osteotome.

A latency period of 7 to 10 days follows, in which the osteotomized segment is held stable and not distracted. After this period, the transport begins at a rate of 0.75 to 1.0 mm per day. This rate is adjusted based on the quality of regenerate bone that forms, as well as the compliance of the soft tissues around the area. In the cases in which hypertrophic regenerate bone forms (evidenced by bone forming outside the margins of the cortex), or in the subperiosteal region along the cortex, the rate of transport may temporarily be increased to prevent premature consolidation. In the instances where the regenerate bone does not form robustly, the rate is decreased to allow bone formation.

The bone is transported until it docks with the native cortex. The final weeks of transport require close observation and radiographs to ensure that the cortices align and that the skin and soft tissue do not invaginate into the defect, potentially necrosing as the bone docks. If the skin does become pinched in the docking site, it must be surgically elevated from the site to allow docking. Bone grafting may be necessary to promote healing at the docking site, and this can be done a week or two before the docking would occur. Once the bone ends are docked, the docking site should be periodically compressed to encourage healing. Compressing the site can be accomplished by turning the struts or lengtheners to move the rings a few millimeters closer to each other. Once the docking site has united and the regenerate has matured and formed well-defined cortices, the external fixator may be removed.

23.6.5 Anatomical Variations and Potential Pitfalls

Large bony defects treated with bone transport will frequently experience complications. Pin site infections are common and can typically be treated with oral antibiotics. In the instances when this is not successful or there is a more severe infection, removal of the pin may be necessary. The surgeon should be sure to maintain adequate stability to the construct when pins or wires are removed. Adding pins or wires to the construct when one pin or wire is removed due to a pin site infection is periodically required.

As the transport segment is dragged through the defect, the pins or wires securing it must also be pulled through the skin and soft tissues. Free flaps can accommodate bone transport without concern for microvascular compromise of the flap.[46,47] However, performing transport through a flap may result in pin tracts that are not cosmetically appealing. These pin sites may experience more drainage and irritation than the pins or wires attached to the proximal or distal rings.

Formation of hypertrophic regenerate may result in premature consolidation. It is recommended to obtain serial radiographs during the transport process to evaluate for this condition. Increasing the rate of distraction temporarily may prevent the consolidation from occurring. Should the bone consolidate, a surgical procedure to either free the consolidation or to make a new corticotomy is necessary to release the transport segment so it can move. In distinction, in the cases where the bone transport segment has been compromised by previous surgery, trauma, or other vascular insult, the regenerate bone may form more slowly. In this instance, the rate may be decreased to allow regenerate bone to form at a slower rate.

Joint contractions may occur during the transport process. The soft tissues adherent to the transport segment that cross the adjacent joint may not accommodate movement of the joint. Patients undergoing transport should continually work on the range of motion of the joints around bone being transported. Physical therapy is helpful to maintain range of motion during this process. Patients should be started with the therapy immediately after surgery, before a joint contracture has developed. Full weight bearing is usually permitted and often encouraged during the bone transport process. This may also minimize the risk of joint contracture.

Finally, docking site nonunions are a frequent problem with bone transport. The docking site may be bone grafted to encourage healing. Sequential compression may also promote docking site union. Once the docking site has been closed and the bone ends opposed, further compression is generated by adjusting the fixator to shorten by 3 to 5 mm. This compression is left in place for 2 to 3 weeks, and then compression is applied by shortening the site weekly in very small increments, to maintain continuous compression on the site. In the instances where the docking site or the regenerate bone formation has not consolidated adequately, adjunctive fixation with plates or intramedullary rods may provide the necessary stability to permit healing.[48,49]

23.7 Summary

Bone defects of greater than 5 cm are best managed with vascularized bone flaps. A variety of bone flaps are available, but the fibula has remained the most versatile for managing acute bone defects in addition to allograft failure and late nonunions. For cases of extensive soft-tissue loss, we have preferred the use of vascularized rib grafts used in conjunction with the serratus and latissimus muscle flap to provide soft-tissue coverage and bone reconstruction in one setting. Finally, for small recalcitrant defects, the medial femoral condylar flap provides vascularized cortical cancellous graft with vascularized skin. Studies evaluating all of these flaps have shown better than 90% union rates for the appropriately selected patient.

For those situations where there is adequate soft-tissue coverage and the patient is willing to tolerate an external fixator, bone transport also offers the option of regenerating large segments of missing bone. The bone created can match the diameter of the native femur or tibia and avoid the need for hypertrophy as well as avoiding the need for internal hardware. Despite the method or flap chosen, successful bone reconstruction is predicated on adequate debridement, adequate soft-tissue coverage, and stable fixation.

References

[1] Iorio ML, Goldstein J, Adams M, Steinberg J, Attinger C. Functional limb salvage in the diabetic patient: the use of a collagen bilayer matrix and risk factors for amputation. Plast Reconstr Surg. 2011; 127(1):260–267
[2] Bieber EJ, Wood MB. Bone reconstruction. Clin Plast Surg. 1986; 13(4):645–655
[3] Arata MA, Wood MB, Cooney WP, III. Revascularized segmental diaphyseal bone transfers in the canine. An analysis of viability. J Reconstr Microsurg. 1984; 1(1):11–19
[4] de Boer HH, Wood MB. Bone changes in the vascularised fibular graft. J Bone Joint Surg Br. 1989; 71(3):374–378
[5] Friedrich JB, Moran SL, Bishop AT, Shin AY. Free vascularized fibula grafts for salvage of failed oncologic long bone reconstruction and pathologic fractures. Microsurgery. 2009; 29(5):385–392
[6] Fujimaki A, Suda H. Experimental study and clinical observations on hypertrophy of vascularized bone grafts. Microsurgery. 1994; 15(10):726–732
[7] Han CS, Wood MB, Bishop AT, Cooney WP, III. Vascularized bone transfer. J Bone Joint Surg Am. 1992; 74(10):1441–1449
[8] Zalavras CG, Patzakis MJ, Holtom P. Local antibiotic therapy in the treatment of open fractures and osteomyelitis. Clin Orthop Relat Res. 2004(427):86–93
[9] Yazar S, Lin CH, Wei FC. One-stage reconstruction of composite bone and soft-tissue defects in traumatic lower extremities. Plast Reconstr Surg. 2004; 114(6):1457–1466
[10] Friedrich JB, Moran SL, Bishop AT, Wood CM, Shin AY. Free vascularized fibular graft salvage of complications of long-bone allograft after tumor reconstruction. J Bone Joint Surg Am. 2008; 90(1):93–100
[11] Moran SL, Shin AY, Bishop AT. The use of massive bone allograft with intramedullary free fibular flap for limb salvage in a pediatric and adolescent population. Plast Reconstr Surg. 2006; 118(2):413–419
[12] Houdek MT, Wagner ER, Wyles CC, Nanos GP, III, Moran SL. New options for vascularized bone reconstruction in the upper extremity. Semin Plast Surg. 2015; 29(1):20–29
[13] Taylor GI, Miller GD, Ham FJ. The free vascularized bone graft. A clinical extension of microvascular techniques. Plast Reconstr Surg. 1975; 55(5):533–544
[14] Chen ZW, Yan W. The study and clinical application of the osteocutaneous flap of fibula. Microsurgery. 1983; 4(1):11–16
[15] Morsy M, Moran SL. Vascularity of the proximal fibula and its implications in vascularized epiphyseal transfer: an anatomic and high-resolution computed tomographic angiography study. Plast Reconstr Surg. 2019; 143(1):172e–183e
[16] Iorio ML, Cheerharan M, Olding M. A systematic review and pooled analysis of peroneal artery perforators for fibula osteocutaneous and perforator flaps. Plast Reconstr Surg. 2012; 130(3):600–607
[17] Momoh AO, Yu P, Skoracki RJ, Liu S, Feng L, Hanasono MM. A prospective cohort study of fibula free flap donor-site morbidity in 157 consecutive patients. Plast Reconstr Surg. 2011; 128(3):714–720
[18] Shan XF, Ouyang SY, Cai ZG, Zhang J. Evaluation of foot perfusion after fibula flap surgery. J Craniofac Surg. 2014; 25(4):1346–1347
[19] Abou-Foul AK, Borumandi F. Anatomical variants of lower limb vasculature and implications for free fibula flap: systematic review and critical analysis. Microsurgery. 2016; 36(2):165–172
[20] Duymaz A, Karabekmez FE, Vrtiska TJ, Mardini S, Moran SL. Free tissue transfer for lower extremity reconstruction: a study of the role of computed angiography in the planning of free tissue transfer in the posttraumatic setting. Plast Reconstr Surg. 2009; 124(2):523–529
[21] Sainsbury DC, Liu EH, Alvarez-Veronesi MC, et al. Long-term outcomes following lower extremity sarcoma resection and reconstruction with vascularized fibula flaps in children. Plast Reconstr Surg. 2014; 134(4):808–820
[22] Chang DW, Weber KL. Use of a vascularized fibula bone flap and intercalary allograft for diaphyseal reconstruction after resection of primary extremity bone sarcomas. Plast Reconstr Surg. 2005; 116(7):1918–1925
[23] Friedrich JB, Moran SL, Bishop AT, Wood CM, Shin AY. Vascularized fibula flap onlay for salvage of pathologic fracture of the long bones. Plast Reconstr Surg. 2008; 121(6):2001–2009
[24] Houdek MT, Wagner ER, Stans AA, et al. What is the outcome of allograft and intramedullary free fibula (Capanna technique) in pediatric and adolescent patients with bone tumors? Clin Orthop Relat Res. 2016; 474(3):660–668
[25] Houdek MT, Wagner ER, Bishop AT, et al. Complications and long-term outcomes of free fibula reconstruction following resection of a malignant tumor in the extremities. Plast Reconstr Surg. 2017; 139(2):510e–519e
[26] Schwarz GS, Disa JJ, Mehrara BJ, Healey JH, Cordeiro PG. Reconstruction of oncologic tibial defects in children using vascularized fibula flaps. Plast Reconstr Surg. 2012; 129(1):195–206
[27] Buncke HJ, Furnas DW, Gordon L, Achauer BM. Free osteocutaneous flap from a rib to the tibia. Plast Reconstr Surg. 1977; 59(6):799–804
[28] Lin CH, Wei FC, Levin LS, et al. Free composite serratus anterior and rib flaps for tibial composite bone and soft-tissue defect. Plast Reconstr Surg. 1997; 99(6):1656–1665
[29] Onishi K, Maruyama Y. Compound rib-latissimus dorsi osteomusculocutaneous flap in reconstruction of the upper arm. Ann Plast Surg. 1996; 37(2): 191–194
[30] Ueng WN, Chuang CC, Shih CH. Double-rib composite free transfer to reconstruct a single-spared lower extremity defect. J Trauma. 1995; 38(2):210–212
[31] Wilden JA, Moran SL, Dekutoski MB, Bishop AT, Shin AY. Results of vascularized rib grafts in complex spinal reconstruction. Surgical technique. J Bone Joint Surg Am. 2007; 89 Suppl 2, Pt 1:128–141
[32] Houdek MT, Wagner ER, Watts CD, Sems SA, Moran SL. Free composite serratus anterior-latissimus-rib flaps for acute one-stage reconstruction of Gustilo IIIB tibia fractures. Am J Orthop. 2018; 47(6)
[33] Choudry UH, Bakri K, Moran SL, Karacor Z, Shin AY. The vascularized medial femoral condyle periosteal bone flap for the treatment of recalcitrant bony nonunions. Ann Plast Surg. 2008; 60(2):174–180
[34] Hayashi A, Maruyama Y. The medial genicular artery flap. Ann Plast Surg. 1990; 25(3):174–180
[35] Kakar S, Duymaz A, Steinmann S, Shin AY, Moran SL. Vascularized medial femoral condyle corticoperiosteal flaps for the treatment of recalcitrant humeral nonunions. Microsurgery. 2011; 31(2):85–92
[36] Kazmers NH, Thibaudeau S, Steinberger Z, Levin LS. Upper and lower extremity reconstructive applications utilizing free flaps from the medial genicular arterial system: a systematic review. Microsurgery. 2018; 38(3):328–343
[37] Yamamoto H, Jones DB, Jr, Moran SL, Bishop AT, Shin AY. The arterial anatomy of the medial femoral condyle and its clinical implications. J Hand Surg Eur Vol. 2010; 35(7):569–574
[38] Iorio ML, Masden DL, Higgins JP. The limits of medial femoral condyle corticoperiosteal flaps. J Hand Surg Am. 2011; 36(10):1592–1596
[39] Iorio ML, Masden DL, Higgins JP. Cutaneous angiosome territory of the medial femoral condyle osteocutaneous flap. J Hand Surg Am. 2012; 37(5):1033–1041
[40] Andrews K, Lu A, Mckean L, Ebraheim N. Review: medial collateral ligament injuries. J Orthop. 2017; 14(4):550–554
[41] Endara MR, Brown BJ, Shuck J, Bachabi M, Parks BG, Higgins JP. Torsional stability of the femur after harvest of the medial femoral condyle corticocancellous flap. J Reconstr Microsurg. 2015; 31(5):364–368
[42] Hinckel BB, Gobbi RG, Kaleka CC, Camanho GL, Arendt EA. Medial patellotibial ligament and medial patellomeniscal ligament: anatomy, imaging, biomechanics, and clinical review. Knee Surg Sports Traumatol Arthrosc. 2018; 26(3):685–696
[43] Rao SS, Sexton CC, Higgins JP. Medial femoral condyle flap donor-site morbidity: a radiographic assessment. Plast Reconstr Surg. 2013; 131(3):357e–362e
[44] López-Pliego EM, Giráldez-Sánchez MÁ, Mora-Macías J, Reina-Romo E, Domínguez J. Histological evolution of the regenerate during bone transport: an experimental study in sheep. Injury. 2016; 47 Suppl 3:S7–S14
[45] Papakostidis C, Bhandari M, Giannoudis PV. Distraction osteogenesis in the treatment of long bone defects of the lower limbs: effectiveness, complications and clinical results; a systematic review and meta-analysis. Bone Joint J. 2013; 95-B(12):1673–1680
[46] Lowenberg DW, Buntic RF, Buncke GM, Parrett BM. Long-term results and costs of muscle flap coverage with Ilizarov bone transport in lower limb salvage. J Orthop Trauma. 2013; 27(10):576–581
[47] Repo JP, Barner-Rasmussen I, Roine RP, Sintonen H, Tukiainen EJ. Treatment of compound tibia fracture with microvascular latissimus dorsi flap and the Ilizarov technique: a cross-sectional study of long-term outcomes. J Plast Reconstr Aesthet Surg. 2016; 69(4):524–532
[48] Aktuglu K, Günay H, Alakbarov J. Monofocal bone transport technique for bone defects greater than 5 cm in tibia: our experience in a case series of 24 patients. Injury. 2016; 47 Suppl 6:S40–S46
[49] Napora JK, Weinberg DS, Eagle BA, Kaufman BR, Sontich JK. Hexapod frame stacked transport for tibial infected nonunions with bone loss: analysis of use of adjunctive stability. J Orthop Trauma. 2017; 31(7):393–399

24 Surgical Treatment for Lower Extremity Lymphedema

Isao Koshima, Hirofumi Imai, Shuhei Yoshida, Shogo Nagamatsu, Kazunori Yokota, Mitsunobu Harima, Shuji Yamashita, and Haruki Mizuta

Summary

Physiologic surgical treatment for lymphedema includes lymphovenous anastomosis, lymph node transfers, and lymph vessel transplantation. With these physiologic approaches, lymphedema can be treated by reestablishing the drainage of lymphatics of the extremity.

Keywords: lymphedema, lymphovenous anastomosis, lymph vessel transplantations

24.1 Introduction

24.1.1 History of Lymphatic Channel and LVA

The description of the lymph duct began with the coinage of the word "white blood" by Hippocrates in the 5th century BC. The nature of lymphatic vessels was first revealed by Gasparo Asellius (1581–1626) of the University of Pavia, Pavia, Italy. Asellius, while dissecting a dog immediately after it had been fed, observed a series of vessels filled with a white milky fluid in the peritoneum and intestines. He misunderstood this as a blood vessel leading to the liver and named it the "chilo-duct." From the 1600s, the anatomy of lymphatic vessels using mercury began and its detailed distribution became clear. In Japan, Genpaku Sugita et al listed lymphatic vessels for the first time in 1774 in the new anatomical book "Kaitai Schinsyo" translated from Dutch to Japanese. Professor Buntaro Adachi, Kyoto University's first anatomy professor, was passionate about the study of lymphatic vessels, and his successor Professor Shogo Funaoka performed lymphangiography in rabbits for the first time in the world and published it as a German paper in 1929. Furthermore, in 1969 Dr. Yamada of Nagoya University performed a lymphaticovenular anastomosis (LVA) in a dog and patients with lymphedema using a microscope. Efforts of the pioneers in Japan have led to the current treatment of lymphedema.

About 1988, Professor O'Brien (Melbourne) was the only person who performed lymph bypass surgery for the treatment of lymphedema.[1] This method had already been tried by many surgeons, but found to be ineffective. In his last speech on lymphedema for us, O'Brien expressed unhappiness at the fact that there were no followers of surgical treatment of lymphedema. This has been the motivation for Dr. Koshima to continue the use of surgery for the treatment of lymphedema since 1990.[2,3] Around 1980, the authors developed supermicrosurgical techniques that have made possible the anastomosis of more precise vessels of 0.3- to 0.8-mm caliber size. This technique allows the use of 12–0 nylon with a 50- to 30-μm needle in vascular anastomosis of vessels less than 0.8 mm in diameter. Even in legs with lymphedema of long duration, we found that there remain a sizable number of precise lymphatics and subdermal venules (0.5 mm). With the supermicrosurgical techniques, anastomosis of precise lymphatics and the subdermal venular system with a higher patency rate is possible. The application of these techniques to the drainage of lymphatic fluid into the subdermal precise venular system (LVA) has been achieved with improved results. Since 1990, the authors have performed LVA in 2,000 patients including primary edema of the legs (300 upper arms and 1,700 legs) under local anesthesia. As a result, complete recovery and/or remarkable improvement was obtained in mild and moderate cases with primary edema,[2,3] and now new strategies combining LVA with functional lymph channel transfers are established for severe cases with primary edema.

24.2 Definition of Lymphedema

Lymphedema is a disorder of the lymphatic transport caused by congenital abnormality and acquired injury of the lymphatic system, resulting in pathological excessive accumulation of lymph fluid in the interstitial space. If this condition persists, fibrous tissue and adipose tissue will proliferate secondarily. Lymphedema is distinguished from physiological "swelling" caused by retention of lymph fluid after standing for a long period of time.

24.3 Classification

From the cause of its onset, it is classified as (1) primary (idiopathic) lymphedema and (2) secondary lymphedema.

24.3.1 Primary (idiopathic) Lymphedema

- Congenital edemas are those already developed at birth. Sometimes, there is an example showing unilateral seminal edema including the face. There are cases in which edema of the limb is combined with neonatal thoracic fluid and ascites, often complicating protein leaky gastroenteropathy. Although it was considered a congenital edema up to now, the authors believe this is the secondary because it is caused by stenosis or obstruction of the thoracic duct. Hereditary lymphedema (Milroy disease) is congenital edema of both lower limbs and is a rare disorder with autosomal dominant inheritance without other anomalies. Recent developments in molecular biological techniques have revealed vascular endothelial growth factor receptor 3 (VEGFR3), which is responsible for establishing the causative gene and expression of vascular endothelium. This makes it possible to perform genetic diagnosis and it is said to recognize Ala → Thr mutation in exon 18 constituting the kinase domain of VEGFR3.

- Premature edemas are those developed at adolescents without incentives or at younger than 35 years.
- *Delayed edemas*: As for these idiopathic edemas, lymphatic vessels always exist when they are confirmed by surgery. The existence of congenital missing or obstruction (hypoplasia) of thoracic duct is also conceivable, but the details are unknown at this time.

24.3.2 Secondary Lymphedema

Depending on the cause of the condition, it is subdivided as follows:

- *After treatments for malignant disease:* onset after lymph node dissection and radiotherapy and/or chemotherapy.
- *Those accompanying progression and recurrence of malignant tumor:* so-called malignant lymphedema.
- *Trauma:* damage of lymphatic vessel, or extensive scarring.
- *Infections:* filariasis, etc.

Secondary edema is lymphedema of the limbs after the surgery for breast or uterine cancers, and most cases in the upper limb are secondary. In the lower limb, 87% of the cases are secondary after uterine cancer surgery, but there are male cases, such as after testicular tumor resection. In the lower extremity cases, 29% of cases are bilateral and tend to progress from one side to both sides.

24.4 Stage of Lymphedema

Recently, advanced stage classification of edema for surgical treatment is beginning to be used frequently.

- Stage I: reversible edema in the initial state.
- Stage II: irreversible persistent edema.
- Stage III: sustained progressive edema (often accompanied by acute lymphangitis or cellulitis).
- Stage IV: elephantiasis.
- Stage V: critical edema (septic shock).

Normally, it is considered that after the second phase, it is an indication for compression therapy, and stages II to IV are indication for lymphaticovenous anastomosis. The authors believe all stages are indicated.[2,3]

24.5 Symptoms and Complications

Redness of the affected limb is a common symptom in the majority of cases. It is mild when getting up; swelling increases when the patients work in the standing position or in the evening. For this reason, many refractory cases are males who cannot get enough resting time. Patients have a fever about once a month to once a year (especially in the summer), and the occurrence of inflammatory symptoms like cellulitis or erysipelas is the most serious complication. The longer the repetition of this, the stronger the fibrosis of the subcutaneous tissue. In the cases where no treatment was given for a long period of time, some become typical elephantiasis. Other frequent complications are tinea and/or ingrown toe nail, requiring treatment with phenol or antifungal topical medication. Frequent complications are lichen planus of the lower leg and edema of the genital region. In the edema of the genital region, some refractory pudendal skin lymph fistula is followed. In the cases of edema of the lower limb after treatment of uterine cancer, treatment including mental care is necessary because there are significant quality of life disorders such as sexual dysfunction due to vaginal stenosis resulting from irradiation failure and pudendal edema. Protein-losing gastroenteropathy associated with obstruction of thoracic duct complicates hypoproteinemia and may have growth disorders in the cases with congenital lymphedema.

24.6 Diagnosis

Although the definite diagnosis method is a classical "lymphangiogram," it has now become unpopular because it involves incision of the skin of the affected limb and injecting the contrast medium directly into the lymphatic channel. "Lymphoscintigraphy" using isotopes cannot confirm the state of fine lymphatic vessels. Ultrasound, CT, and MRI examination are useful for easily diagnosing the state of edema. Since lymphatic vessels are not confirmed directly, we do not know the site of lymphatic obstruction or condition of lymphatic damage, but we can sufficiently confirm the distribution of moisture in the subcutaneous tissue and the degree of increase in fibrosis and adipose tissue. Moreover, if the Doppler method is used, the presence or absence of merger of venous disease (especially deep venous thrombosis) can also be confirmed. The photodynamic eye method is currently being used clinically and is expected to be promising. Since indocyanine green (ICG) emits fluorescence when it is injected intradermally and then infrared rays are applied, the remaining drainage function can be confirmed with the distribution of ICG incorporated in the lymphatic vessel.[4]

24.6.1 Differential Diagnosis

It is important to distinguish it from other systemic diseases that cause edema (heart failure, renal failure, hepatic disorder, etc.). Other diseases include the following:

- *Deep vein thrombosis*: The onset is rapid, unilateral, painful, and often complicates varicose veins, congestive dermatitis, pigmentation, and ulcer.
- *Lymphatic malformation (lymphangioma)*: There is no difference in the degree of edema in the morning and evening and no acupressure trace on the lesion.
- *Transient swelling*: Swelling at the distal side of the lower leg appears especially in the evening due to prolonged standing and sitting, and the swelling disappears in the morning.
- *Lipodystrophy (fat hyperplasia due to abnormal fat metabolism)*: It is usually symmetrical and does not cause infection without skin hardening.
- *Lymphangiosarcoma (Stewart–Treves syndrome)*: In long-term lymphedema cases (about 10 years), injured lymphatic

endothelial cells develop to highly malignant lymphangiosarcoma. Superficial erythema progressively expands, but this noninflammatory legion resists the treatment by antibiotic and therapeutic agents for skin diseases.[5] Lymphovenous bypass surgery has now become absolute indication to cure sarcoma (surgical anticancer immune therapy).

24.7 Treatments

- *Compression by elastic stocking*: It is used to increase tissue pressure by applying external pressure and to prevent exacerbation of edema. Patients must wear it especially when they need to stand for a long period of time in the daytime. Because it is washed frequently, it loosens up in a short period of time; so, it needs to be changed frequently, and stockings must be made to suit individual's needs with attached chucks, rubber, etc. There is a special order item for those larger than the standard size.
- *Skin resection/skin grafting (Charles method, Sistrunk method, Thompson method)*[6]: It is a method of extensive resection of diseased tissue. Although it is effective immediately after surgery, it is said that there are many cosmetic problems such as hypertrophic scars in the long term and recurrence of edema in the resected area.
- *Liposuction*: It is a method of aspirating fat of the edema part with a liposuction device. Improvement is seen immediately after surgery, but the effect tends to decrease within a few months. Based on the authors' experience, liposuction shows good results only for the effective cases with lymph bypass surgery.
- *Lymphovenous anastomosis (LVA; lymph bypass surgery)*: Operative treatment was applied to all patients with mild and severe edema with or without preoperative conservative treatment including compression. Under local anesthesia for adult patients (general anesthesia for children), after making short incisions on the medial aspects (totally two or more incisions, each 3 cm in length), the lymphatics and subdermal venules (each 0.5 mm in diameter) are explored using a loupe or operating microscope. The affected lymphatics are often dilated or sclerotic. Dye staining is not always a good indicator for finding lymphatics. When no suitable lymphatics are found in one site, incisions are made in other portions of the leg and foot dorsum. The subdermal venules, which exist anywhere beneath the dermis, can be usually detected adjacent to the lymphatics. Regarding the selection of these channels, lymphatics with strong drainage function, which are easily detected after transecting them under an operating microscope, should be selected to establish powerful lymphovenous shunting. Small subdermal venules of 0.5 mm caliber size are most suitable for joining with the lymphatics, because larger cutaneous veins may have higher intravascular pressure than that of the lymphatics. Larger dilated lymphatics greater than 0.5 mm, which are sometimes detected in either the superficial or the deep adipose layer, are anastomosed to the small branches of the main cutaneous vein. Without a vascular clamp, end-to-end lymphaticovenular anastomoses of the same size are carried out using 50-µm needle sutures (with 12–0 nylon) with a fine needle holder under high magnification (× 20–30 magnifications; ▶ Fig. 24.1, ▶ Fig. 24.2). Although this operation can be completed within 3 hours, some patients with an irradiated bladder need catheter urination. Postoperatively, a low-pressure bandage and a vascular dilating drug (prostaglandin E1) are applied and the patients are allowed to walk freely. Use of elastic stockings is started 2 weeks later for at least half a year.[2,3]
- *Combined surgical treatment including lymph vessel transplantation*: Since 2004, for severe limb lymphedema against LVA, we have been performing combined surgery including lymphatic vessel with functioning smooth muscle cells from the normal donors, multiple LVA, and liposuction, simultaneously or consequently.[7] In the lymphatic transplantation method, lymphatic vessels having drainage functions of the lateral chest and the first web space are collected with nutrient blood vessels. It is divided into multiple pieces, transferred into the affected portions and limbs, and anastomosed with a fain recipient vessel (muscle penetrating branch), which nourishes the skin of the affected limb. If possible, LVA both inside and outside of the flap is established. Loss of drainage function of lymphatic vessel can be reconstructed with this method. This method has been followed in about 200 cases resisted to multiple LVA up to now; 10% did not required compression therapy (functional recovery) and 50% showed improvement. As we are currently popularizing this combined technique overseas, it will be a mainstream in the future (▶ Video 24.1).

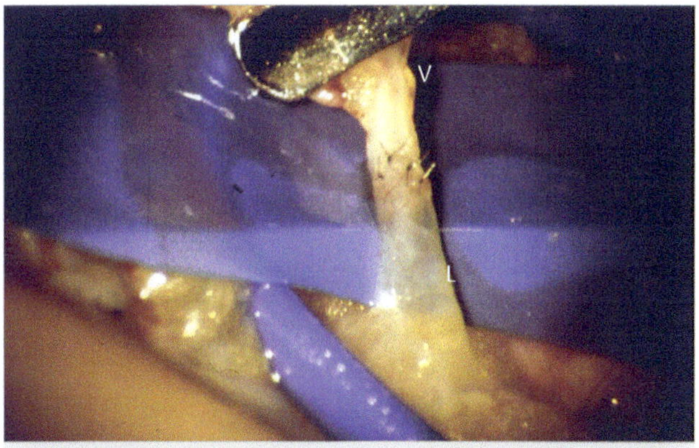

Fig. 24.1 Microscopic lymph venous anastomosis. Lymphaticovenous anastomosis with six stiches using a 50-µm needle under magnification about 30 times.

From now on, prophylactic anastomoses are being considered early after resection of breast or uterine cancer with lymph node dissection. In addition, multidisciplinary therapy with a team approach that is combined with plastic surgery, breast surgery, obstetrics and gynecology, urology, etc., is beginning to be adopted more frequently.

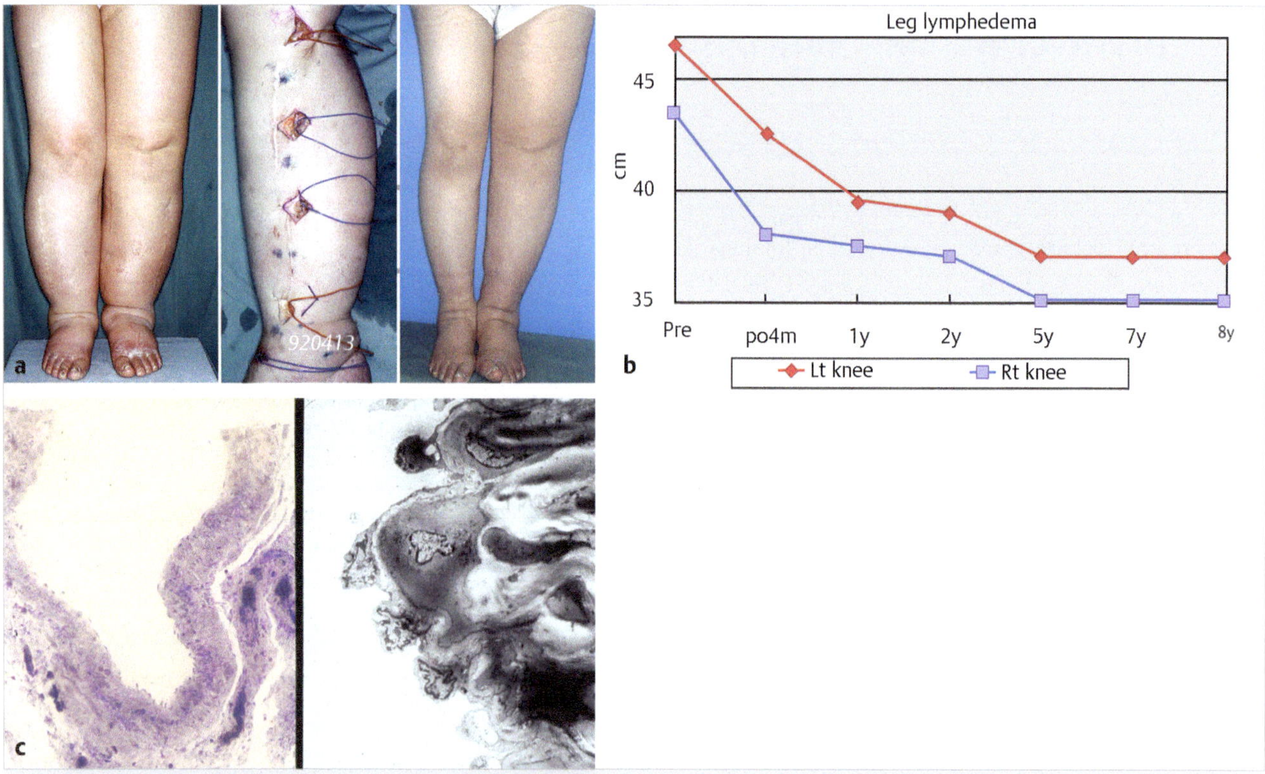

Fig. 24.2 (a) Primary edema of a 42-year-old woman. Left: A leg edema of 24 years' duration. Compression did not stop the progression of edema and phlegmon. Center: Five LVA for the right leg and island groin dermal fat flap for the left leg. Right: 9 years after the operation. Dramatic improvement and no infection with the same compression as before the surgery. **(b)** Postoperative change on circumferential length of bilateral lower legs. They show periodical decrease until 9 years after surgery. **(c)** Left: biopsied lymph channel shows dilatation (× 40, toluidine blue stain). Right: Regenerated smooth muscle cells and proliferated collagen fibrils (electron microscopic study).[4]

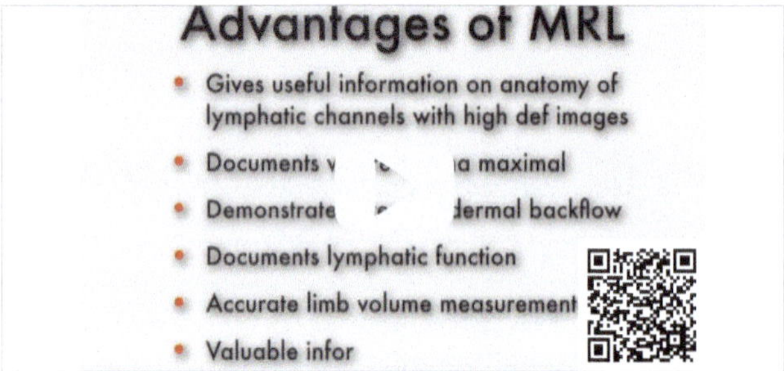

Video 24.1 Surgical Treatment for Lower Extremity Lymphedema.
https://www.thieme.de/de/q.htm?p=opn/cs/20/7/12265286-fe49921e

References

[1] O'Brien BM, Sykes P, Threlfall GN, Browning FS. Microlymphaticovenous anastomoses for obstructive lymphedema. Plast Reconstr Surg. 1977; 60(2): 197–211

[2] Koshima I, Kawada S, Moriguchi T, Kajiwara Y. Ultrastructural observations of lymphatic vessels in lymphedema in human extremities. Plast Reconstr Surg. 1996; 97(2):397–405, discussion 406–407

[3] Koshima I, Nanba Y, Tsutsui T, Takahashi Y, Itoh S, Fujitsu M. Minimal invasive lymphaticovenular anastomosis under local anesthesia for leg lymphedema: is it effective for stage III and IV? Ann Plast Surg. 2004; 53(3):261–266

[4] Ogata F, Azuma R, Kikuchi M, Koshima I, Morimoto Y. Novel lymphography using indocyanine green dye for near-infrared fluorescence labeling. Ann Plast Surg. 2007; 58(6):652–655

[5] Stewart FW, Treves N. Lymphangiosarcoma in postmastectomy lymphedema; a report of six cases in elephantiasis chirurgica. Cancer. 1948; 1(1):64–81

[6] Thompson N. Buried dermal flap operation for chronic lymphedema of the extremities. Ten-year survey of results in 79 cases. Plast Reconstr Surg. 1970; 45(6):541–548

[7] Koshima I, Narushima M, Mihara M, et al. Lymphadiposal flaps and lymphaticovenular anastomoses for severe leg edema: functional reconstruction for lymph drainage system. J Reconstr Microsurg. 2016; 32(1):50–55

25 Lower Limb Vascularized Composite Allotransplantation

Pedro C. Cavadas

Summary

Lower limb vascularized composite allotransplantation (VCA) is not immunologically different from solid organ transplantation; so any recipients will require lifelong immune suppression (IS) to prevent rejection, and expect the risks of significant metabolic and renal toxicity, opportunistic infections, and an increased peril of malignancy. As such, lower limb VCA would be justifiable only if the expected improvement of the quality of life of the patient would be enormous. Prior knee joint VCA has been reported with overall negative results. Presented here is the first case of lower limb VCA in a wheelchair-dependent bilateral traumatic above-knee amputee. Active range of motion even of the feet was subsequently possible, but complications at postoperative month 15 required reamputation of both legs. Lower limb VCA therefore remains very controversial and is a subject of continuing debate as for any clear indications. The limiting factor as shown is not the surgical technique, but rather the necessary IS treatment that must first be mastered.

Keywords: vascularized composite allotransplantation, lower limb allotransplantation, immune suppression

25.1 Introduction

Solid organ transplantation (SOT) is now considered a standard of care for various end-stage organ failures. Based on the wealth of knowledge generated by SOT during the past five decades, nonvital organ transplantation (mainly visible segments of the musculoskeletal system) has been introduced relatively recently. These "organs," the so-called vascularized composite allotransplantations (VCAs), are a markedly heterogeneous group of structures (limbs, abdominal wall, face, uterus, larynx, penis) grouped together because of their composite-tissue nature and/or the need for nerve regeneration to achieve function. VCAs are not immunologically different from SOT; so recipients of VCA require lifelong immune suppression (IS) to prevent rejection, at the expense of significant metabolic and renal toxicity, opportunistic infections (such as cytomegalovirus [CMV] infections), and an increased risk of malignancy. Given these risks, VCAs are indicated only if the expected improvement of the quality of life of the patient is enormous.

The world's experience in VCA approaches 150 cases, mainly including the upper limb (hand, forearm, and arm), abdominal wall, and facial segments.[1,2] The short- and mid-term results obtained in upper limb transplantation have been remarkably good with functional results comparable to same-level replantations.[2]

Lower limb allotransplantation enthusiasm has not paralleled that of the upper limb. There are several reasonable explanations. Below-knee (BK) amputees are generally able to walk quite well with prostheses. Above-knee (AK) amputees, especially if bilateral, are much more difficult to rehabilitate.[3,4] Osseointegrated AK prostheses have been described, although the complication rate is high.[5] Lower limb replantation itself has historically been discouraged, in sharp contrast to upper limb replantation. Results have been stated to be poor, and prostheses traditionally considered the better treatment of choice.[6,7,8] Most surgeons are thus not familiar with systematic lower limb replantation. However, encouraging results of leg replantation have been published recently.[9,10]

Compared to the upper limb, the lower limb performs a much more basic function in most people. For a fundamental gait, hip extensor–abductors (glutei medii muscles), knee extensors (quadriceps), and a plantigrade support are the minimum requisites. Plantar protective sensation is also desirable for long-term plantar integrity. Achieving all these basic functions with a lower limb VCA seemed to be a realistic goal in a bilateral AK amputee, and for this reason, Cavadas et al performed the first lower limb allotransplantation in July 2011.[11,12] There were no precedents in the medical literature, but planning was based on solid clinical grounds.

A case usually cited as the first lower limb allotransplantation was the excellent clinical report by Zuker et al in 2006 in which one leg was transferred between conjoined twins.[13,14] Although technically brilliant, this was autologous tissue, without IS therapy, and thus cannot be considered an allotransplantation. Experience with knee joint VCA has been reported by Diefenbeck et al[15] and Hoffmann and Kirschner[16] in a heterogeneous group of patients, some without a skin island monitor to detect acute rejection (AR), with overall negative results. This is in striking contrast with the relatively benign behavior of allogenic joints in upper limb transplants.

25.2 Clinical Example of Lower Limb Vascularized Composite Allotransplantation

The recipient was a 22-year-old man, who was a wheelchair-dependent bilateral traumatic AK amputee. The right side level was mid-shaft femur, and left side was the distal third (▶ Fig. 25.1). CMV immunoglobulin G (IgG) was negative and Epstein–Barr virus (EBV) IgG was positive. The donor was a 26-year-old woman ABO-compatible multiorgan donor. CMV and EBV IgG were negative, and there was total HLA mismatch—and a complete human leukocyte antigen (HLA) mismatch. Transplantation was performed on July 11, 2011, by a single surgeon with three assistants. Relevant structures were dissected and tagged bilaterally in the stumps of the recipient. The external iliac vessels were used as the recipient vascular sites. The procurement of the legs was performed in an adjacent operating room after cardiac and liver retrieval. The infrarenal aorta was not cross-clamped, allowing simultaneous in situ perfusion of the lower extremities with cold UW (University of Wisconsin) solution.

The right leg was transplanted first (▶ Fig. 25.2). The sequence of repairs was the same on both sides. Bone fixation was

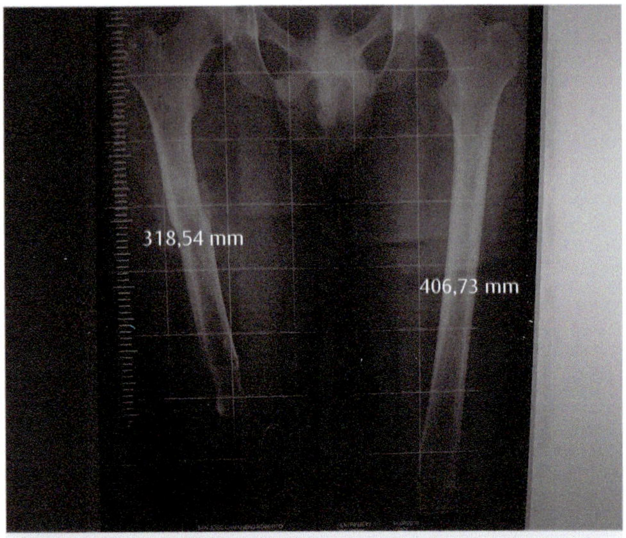

Fig. 25.1 Preoperative X-ray of the recipient with bilateral transfemoral amputation.

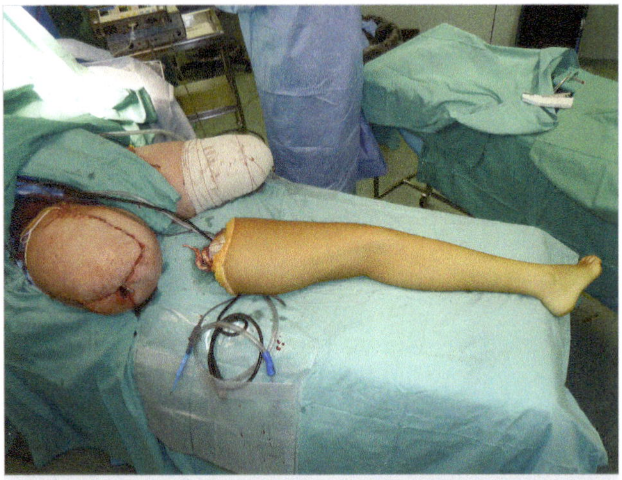

Fig. 25.2 Intraoperative view of the donor right limb as transplantation is about to start.

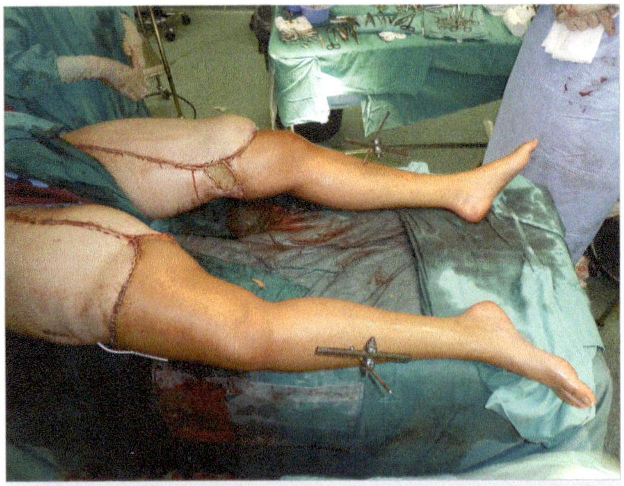

Fig. 25.3 Intraoperative view after both limbs have been transplanted. The external fixators of the tibiae were for suspending the transplanted limbs during the early postoperative period to avoid pressure on the dorsal aspect of the legs.

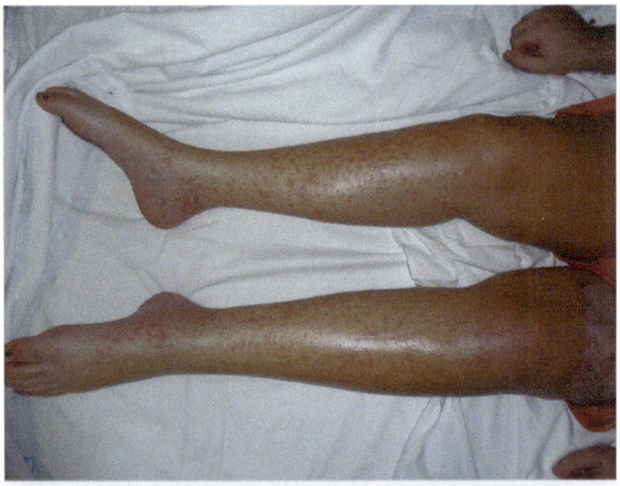

Fig. 25.4 Acute rejection at postoperative month (POM) 3 manifested by cutaneous maculae with a histopathological diagnosis of lymphocyte infiltration of the dermis BANFF grade 1.

performed initially with lateral 4.5-mm locking plates without X-ray control for expediency. Hamstring muscles were next repaired en bloc with moderate tension. The knee was extended and the sciatic nerve repaired. The quadriceps muscle was sutured under maximal tension. In order to minimize the hemodynamic and hypothermic insult, the following sequence of limb rewarming, vascular refilling, and clamp management was performed. The iliac artery of the VCA was flushed with warm (35 °C) Ringer's solution. The vascular bed of the leg was filled with warm Ringer's solution and the artery and vein clamped. End-to-side anastomoses were performed to the recipient's external iliac vessels. The vein clamp was released first, and then the arterial clamps, allowing revascularization. The left leg was kept cooled during the right side reattachment, and the same sequence of surgical maneuvers was followed on the left side (▶ Fig. 25.3). Total ischemia time was 3.5 hours on the right side and 5.5 hours on the left side. No fasciotomies were performed. No adverse intraoperative hemodynamic events occurred.

IS treatment consisted of induction with anti-CD52 alemtuzumab 30 mg IV, and maintenance with mycophenolate mofetil (MMF) 1 g/12 h, tacrolimus (Tac) titrated for trough levels of 10 to 17 ng/mL during the first month and 7 to 12 ng/mL thereafter, and tapering prednisone doses. No CMV prophylaxis was instituted, because of donor and recipient negative (D^-/R^-) combination. CMV replication was monitored for preemptive treatment.

No significant complications developed in the early postoperative period. At postoperative day 90, there was a steroid-resistant AR coincident with CMV primary infection and shift from Tac to rapamycin chosen (in order to reduce the long-term risk of malignancy; ▶ Fig. 25.4). The rapamycin exchange for Tac resulted in rapid clinical and histological resolution (▶ Fig. 25.5). Lymphodepleting antibodies were specifically avoided in this case to reduce the risk of posttransplant lymphoproliferative disease (PTLD). A second AR occurred on

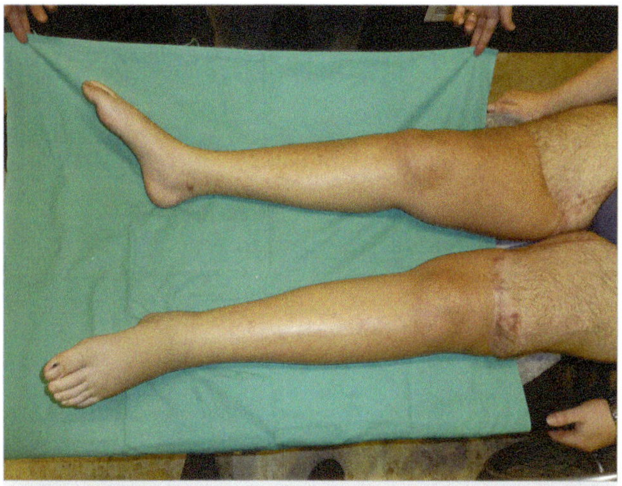

Fig. 25.5 Appearance of the successful bilateral lower limb vascularized composite allotransplantation after treatment and resolution of the first acute rejection.

postoperative month (POM) 9, related to low through levels of Tac and MMF. Dose adjustment resolved the rejection.

Active foot flexion started at POM 7 on the left side and POM 8 on the right side. Strengthening exercises were performed accordingly. Active foot extension was recovered on POM 12 on the right side. At POM 15, the patient had full passive range of motion in both knees, with active knee extension with some extension lag. There was active flexion of both knees. Foot plantar flexion was M4 (Medical Research Council (MRC) score) on the left side and M3 + on the right. Foot dorsal flexion was M2 on the right side and M1 on the left side. Tinel sign was advancing to the mid-plantar level. The patient had fully incorporated the transplanted legs into his body image and was able to walk on parallel bars. On POM 15, the patient developed diplopia and strabismus of the left eye with hypertropia. Brain MRI showed a 25-mm mass in the brainstem (▶ Fig. 25.6). EBV polymerase chain reaction was negative in the blood but positive in the cerebrospinal fluid. Stereotaxic biopsy confirmed the diagnosis of primary central nervous system (PCNS) PTLD.

After discussion with the patient and his family, the IS therapy was abruptly interrupted and the legs removed. The patient was treated with high-dose methotrexate and stereotaxic radiotherapy with complete remission. Five years after the diagnosis of PCNS PTLD, the patient is asymptomatic and continues in complete remission.

25.3 Discussion

Hand and upper extremity VCA is now a well-accepted procedure, with a favorable risk-to-benefit ratio, especially in bilateral cases.[17] Lower limb VCA is, however, very controversial. The risk-to-benefit ratio of lower limb VCA in bilateral transfemoral amputees has not yet been determined, and is a subject of continuing debate.[18,19] The limiting factor in general allotransplantation is not the surgical technique (although bilateral lower limb allotransplantation is a formidable surgery), but rather the IS treatment. With proper planning and execution, this surgery for the lower extremity can be safely performed. IS therapy is not different from other VCA (induction with antibodies and triple therapy with Tac, MMF, and prednisone), and the risk of potentially lethal complications is similar to other SOT or VCAs. Allograft longevity is a major concern in general transplantation. Recent advancements in IS treatment have achieved excellent short-term allograft survival, but has failed to improve long-term survival of the transplanted organ. Chronic allograft vasculopathy (chronic rejection) eventually occurs in the majority of SOT given enough time, and is starting to occur in VCA as the follow-up duration of the cases increases.

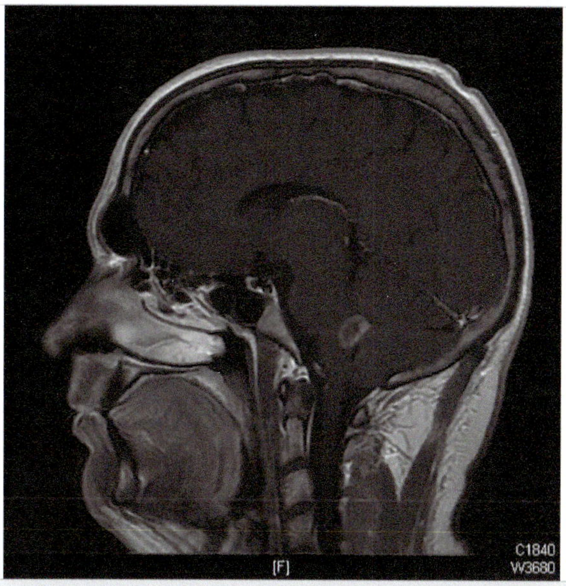

Fig. 25.6 An MRI on postoperative month (POM) 15 found a brainstem lymphoma. Immune suppression treatment was stopped and the limbs reamputated immediately.

In order to reduce the associated risks, CMV matching is important in VCA, and avoidance of high-risk D^+/R^- combinations has been recommended.[20] A primary CMV infection is exceedingly rare in D^-/R^- with preemptive therapy.[21,22] The association between CMV replication and AR is well described in the literature. IS treatment increases the risk of malignancy, and PTLD is a major problem in transplanted patients. The incidence of PTLD is highest in small intestine transplants and lowest in heart recipients.[23] In VCA, due to the relatively small number of cases, the incidence of PTLD has not yet been established. EBV mismatch (D^+/R^-), pediatric age, and use of lymphodepleting antibodies are also significant risk factors. The prognosis of PCNS PTLD is poor. Reduction or cessation of immunosuppression, with the obvious risk of allograft rejection and loss, and various combinations of chemotherapy and radiation therapy are the backbone of the treatment of PCNS PTLD.[24]

Limb transplants require a long period of rehabilitation and lengthy time for nerve regeneration before gaining useful function, despite the positive effect of calcineurin inhibitors in nerve regeneration.[25] This period is 6 to 18 months in hand transplantations, and, in a transfemoral transplantation, could exceed 2 years. This extended rehabilitation process is unique to VCA. A SOT recipient is getting benefit from the transplant from day 1, whereas VCA recipients have to go through many months of rehabilitation and toxic IS before obtaining any functional benefit.

There are other relevant questions that still remain unanswered regarding the hypothetical long-term performance of transplanted lower limbs. Apart from the "chronic rejection" issue, there are concerns unique to the lower limbs. It is well described that any proinflammatory stimulus can trigger an AR in VCA, such as remarkably minor trauma or even sunburns.[26] The cyclic mechanical microtrauma to the sole of the foot during physiologic walking could or could not be a significant proinflammatory stimulus for allogenic limbs. Similar microtraumatisms are known to have elicited AR in hand transplants. If this is the case, lower limb VCA may never be a viable treatment option. In the case report presented here, protected walking with parallel bars with increasing weight bearing was achieved daily without evidence of AR, but this limited observation time frame cannot be extrapolated to normal, long-term walking conditions. Other issues such as the possibility of developing neuropathic arthropathy are also relevant and cannot be inferred from the experience in upper limb VCA, since upper limb joints do not bear axial loads as lower limb joints do.

Apart from the unfortunate and rare complication that resulted in reamputation in this reported case, lower limb VCA remains controversial by itself. The risk-to-benefit ratio is difficult to define with current knowledge. The only possible indication may be for the transfemoral quadrimembral amputee who already has a stable bilateral upper limb transplant but is unable to use prostheses. The required IS treatment is already being administered, and although a third-party transplant can trigger an AR in a stable SOT patient, the probability is low. Simultaneous quadrimembral transplantation has been attempted and consistently resulted in fatal intraoperative complications, likely because of the massive hemodynamic insult, so probably even this does not seem to be warranted.

25.4 Conclusion

With current IS treatment, lower limb allotransplantation does not have a clear indication at this time. Future improvements in IS treatment and further research in validated animal models may help define eventually the role of this intriguing procedure for those unfortunate enough not to have any other viable alternatives.

References

[1] Shores JT, Brandacher G, Lee WP. Hand and upper extremity transplantation: an update of outcomes in the worldwide experience. Plast Reconstr Surg. 2015; 135(2):351e–360e

[2] Petruzzo P, Lanzetta M, Dubernard JM, et al. The International Registry on Hand and Composite Tissue Transplantation. Transplantation. 2010; 90(12): 1590–1594

[3] Bondurant FJ, Cotler HB, Buckle R, Miller-Crotchett P, Browner BD. The medical and economic impact of severely injured lower extremities. J Trauma. 1988; 28(8):1270–1273

[4] Crouse SF, Lessard CS, Rhodes J, Lowe RC. Oxygen consumption and cardiac response of short-leg and long-leg prosthetic ambulation in a patient with bilateral above-knee amputation: comparisons with able-bodied men. Arch Phys Med Rehabil. 1990; 71(5):313–317

[5] Hagberg K, Brånemark R. One hundred patients treated with osseointegrated transfemoral amputation prostheses: rehabilitation perspective. J Rehabil Res Dev. 2009; 46(3):331–344

[6] Hierner R, Berger AK, Frederix PR. Lower leg replantation: decision-making, treatment, and long-term results. Microsurgery. 2007; 27(5):398–410

[7] Battiston B, Tos P, Pontini I, Ferrero S. Lower limb replantations: indications and a new scoring system. Microsurgery. 2002; 22(5):187–192

[8] Kutz JE, Jupiter JB, Tsai TM. Lower limb replantation. A report of nine cases. Foot Ankle. 1983; 3(4):197–202

[9] Cavadas PC, Landín L, Ibáñez J, Roger I, Nthumba P. Infrapopliteal lower extremity replantation. Plast Reconstr Surg. 2009; 124(2):532–539

[10] Cavadas PC, Thione A. Lower limb replantation. In: Salyapongse AN, Poore S, Afifi A, Bentz M, eds. Extremity Replantation: A Comprehensive Clinical Guide. New York, NY: Springer Science + Business Media; 2015:145–159

[11] Cavadas PC, Thione A, Carballeira A, Blanes M. Bilateral transfemoral lower extremity transplantation: result at 1 year. Am J Transplant. 2013; 13(5): 1343–1349

[12] Cavadas PC, Thione A, Blanes M, Mayordomo-Aranda E. Primary central nervous system posttransplant lymphoproliferative disease in a bilateral transfemoral lower extremity transplantation recipient. Am J Transplant. 2015; 15(10):2758–2761

[13] Zuker RM, Redett R, Alman B, Coles JG, Timoney N, Ein SH. First successful lower-extremity transplantation: technique and functional result. J Reconstr Microsurg. 2006; 22(4):239–244

[14] Fattah A, Cypel T, Donner EJ, Wang F, Alman BA, Zuker RM. The first successful lower extremity transplantation: 6-year follow-up and implications for cortical plasticity. Am J Transplant. 2011; 11(12):2762–2767

[15] Diefenbeck M, Nerlich A, Schneeberger S, Wagner F, Hofmann GO. Allograft vasculopathy after allogeneic vascularized knee transplantation. Transpl Int. 2011; 24(1):e1–e5

[16] Hofmann GO, Kirschner MH. Clinical experience in allogeneic vascularized bone and joint allografting. Microsurgery. 2000; 20(8):375–383

[17] Shores JT, Imbriglia JE, Lee WP. The current state of hand transplantation. J Hand Surg Am. 2011; 36(11):1862–1867

[18] Carty MJ, Zuker R, Cavadas P, Pribaz JJ, Talbot SG, Pomahac B. The case for lower extremity allotransplantation. Plast Reconstr Surg. 2013; 131(6):1272–1277

[19] Carty MJ, Duclos A, Talbot SG, Tullius SG, Pribaz JJ, Pomahac B. Attitudes regarding lower extremity allotransplantation among lower extremity amputees. Plast Reconstr Surg. 2014; 134(6):1334–1342

[20] Schneeberger S, Lucchina S, Lanzetta M, et al. Cytomegalovirus-related complications in human hand transplantation. Transplantation. 2005; 80(4):441–447

[21] Zhang LF, Wang YT, Tian JH, Yang KH, Wang JQ. Preemptive versus prophylactic protocol to prevent cytomegalovirus infection after renal transplantation: a meta-analysis and systematic review of randomized controlled trials. Transpl Infect Dis. 2011; 13(6):622–632

[22] George B, Pati N, Gilroy N, et al. Pre-transplant cytomegalovirus (CMV) serostatus remains the most important determinant of CMV reactivation after allogeneic hematopoietic stem cell transplantation in the era of surveillance and preemptive therapy. Transpl Infect Dis. 2010; 12(4):322–329

[23] Jagadeesh D, Woda BA, Draper J, Evens AM. Post transplant lymphoproliferative disorders: risk, classification, and therapeutic recommendations. Curr Treat Options Oncol. 2012; 13(1):122–136

[24] Cavaliere R, Petroni G, Lopes MB, Schiff D, International Primary Central Nervous System Lymphoma Collaborative Group. Primary central nervous system post-transplantation lymphoproliferative disorder: an International Primary Central Nervous System Lymphoma Collaborative Group Report. Cancer. 2010; 116(4):863–870

[25] Glaus SW, Johnson PJ, Mackinnon SE. Clinical strategies to enhance nerve regeneration in composite tissue allotransplantation. Hand Clin. 2011; 27(4):495–509, ix

[26] Cavadas PC, Ibañez J, Thione A. Secondary surgery for functional improvement after hand transplantation. Ann Plast Surg. 2011; 67(4):421–422

26 Perioperative Care and Rehabilitation Specific to the Lower Limb

Manas Nigam, Michael V. Defazio, and Karen K. Evans

Summary
The lower extremity is subject to unique stresses and pathophysiologies that make reconstruction, particularly with free tissue transfer, a challenging but rewarding process. In order to ensure a successful outcome, the reconstructive surgeon should optimize the patient's comorbidities in the preoperative period and adhere to tried and true perioperative management principles. Postoperative rehabilitation is crucial for a patient to achieve her ultimate functional goal, which is typically ambulation. Important preoperative considerations include hardware/prosthesis presence, diabetic and vascular disease, oncologic resection, thrombophilia, biomechanical optimization, and malnourished states. In the perioperative period, accurate fluid intake and output management is paramount. In addition to clinical flap monitoring, there are various adjunctive measures that have shown to increase salvage rates. Though anticoagulation differs among microsurgeons, aspirin should be included in the regimen. Postoperatively, it is important to ensure the patient is still maintaining his or her cardiovascular health and prehabilitation prior to surgery can set the patient up for success. In addition to physical therapists, occupational, vocational, and mental health experts should be included in the care team. With regard to rehabilitation, it is important to consult colleagues in pedorthotics and podiatry so custom inserts and pressure-relieving footwear can be designed. Finally, the clinician should keep an eye out for pain conditions, such as neuroma pain. In the case a patient has had a partial or total amputation, chronic phantom limb pain can preclude the patient from ambulating again.

Keywords: lower extremity reconstruction, free tissue transfer, free flap, flap monitoring, lower extremity rehabilitation, perioperative management, perioperative optimization

26.1 Introduction

In many cases, free tissue transfer is required to reconstruct complex, composite defects and wounds with exposed vital structures (i.e., vessels, nerves, tendons, bones, joint space, etc.) when simpler or local options for coverage are either unavailable or inadequate to achieve structural and/or functional restoration.

In the lower extremity, reasons for transfer include large segmental bone loss, muscle and/or tendon loss resulting from low- and high-energy injuries, osteomyelitis, bony nonunions, tumor excision, exposed prostheses, irradiated wounds, burns, diabetic ulcers, and peripheral vascular disease.

Grafts, local flaps, and regional options may be inadequate due to infection, inflammation, trauma, irradiation, insufficient volume or surface area, insufficient vascular pedicle length, and/or unsuitable morbidity at the donor site.

Successful lower extremity reconstruction requires successful patient optimization as well as a multidisciplinary team, including plastic surgeon, podiatrist or pedorthotist, vascular surgeon, physical therapist, and occupational therapist. Additionally, orthopaedics, endocrinology, cardiology, hematology, rheumatology, dermatology, psychiatry, and/or pain management consultation may be needed (▶ Table 26.1).

26.2 Perioperative Optimization

26.2.1 Managing Comorbidities Preoperatively

Pertinent comorbid diseases include cardiac disease, renal disease, infection, vasculopathy, diabetes, neuropathy, venous hypertension, lymphedema, immunodeficiency, hypercoagulability, connective tissue disease, malnutrition, autoimmune disease, neoplasm, and psychiatric illness.

Exposed Hardware/Prostheses

Traditional methods to manage exposed hardware included irrigation, debridement, antibiotics, and removal of hardware. Prognostic factors for hardware salvage are location, duration, and type of infection, duration of exposure of hardware, and hardware loosening.[1] Orthopaedists separate prosthetic infections according to chronologic criteria: early (within 12 weeks of surgery), delayed (within 2 years), or late (after 2 years, usually via hematogenous spread).[2]

If hardware is clinically stable, time of exposure is short, and infection is controlled, there is a possibility that hardware can be salvaged. If the hardware is secure and used for fracture fixation, an attempt should be made to salvage until radiographic evidence of bony healing. However, delayed or late infections require one- or two-stage reimplantation.

Alternatives for chronically seeded/late-presenting infected hardware are external fixation (for fractures), minimally invasive plating, and antibiotic spacers (particularly for joint arthroplasties).[3,4,5] Antibiotic spacers can be in either a block form or an articulating form. Increased duration of intravenous antibiotics, positive initial wound cultures, chronic osteomyelitis on initial pathologic evaluation, and number of chronic morbidities are a predictor of failed hardware salvage in microsurgical lower extremity reconstruction.[6]

Exposed vascular prosthetic grafts are limb- and life-threatening and should be managed with early debridement and muscle flap coverage.

Diabetes and Peripheral Vascular Disease

In a retrospective study by Oh et al, 66 of 71 patients with diabetic lower extremity wounds were functionally salvaged using

Table 26.1 Members of the Multidisciplinary Care Team Specific to Rehabilitation

Team Member	Role
Plastic Surgery	Patient and wound evaluation, selection of reconstruction in light of functional goals
Podiatrist	Biomechanical and gait evaluation
Prosthetist/Pedorthotist	Biomechanical evaluation and design/planning of adjunctive footwear/devices for ambulation, activities of daily living
Vascular Surgery	Evaluation and treatment of impaired perfusion
Orthopaedic Surgery	Fracture and hardware management in addition to biomechanical evaluation
Infectious Disease	Antibiotic stewardship; culture-driven antibiotic selection; minimization of iatragenic drug injuries
Medicine	Management of patient comorbidities
Physical Therapist	Prehabilitation and rehabilitation
Occupational Therapist	Rehabilitation focused on activities of daily living
Nutrition	Improvement of patient's protein intake in light of his/her comorbidities
Endocrinology	Perioperative and postoperative management of blood glucose in setting of Diabetes Mellitus
Hematology	Management of thrombophilia
Rheumatology	Evaluation and treatment of rheumatologic disorders contributing to disease process
Dermatology	Evaluation and treatment of unusual wound etiologies
Cardiology	Optimization and clearance for surgery in the setting of coronary artery disease or congestive heart failure
Psychiatry	Evaluation and management of depression, anxiety, and other disorders perioperatively
Pain Management	Management of acute and chronic pain conditions, minimize opioid requirements

a microsurgical approach.[7] A separate meta-analysis of 528 diabetic patients with lower extremity wounds showed a limb salvage rate of 83.4% at 28 months in patients otherwise needing amputation.[8] Hong and Oh showed that microvascular transfer increased survival in the diabetic patient with lower extremity wounds.[7,9,10]

Diabetic patients with poor glycemic control (blood glucose > 200 mg/dL or hemoglobin A1c > 6.5%) have been noted to have an increase in dehiscence rates of closed wounds,[11] although the effect of tight glycemic control on free flap outcomes has not been studied.

In patients with peripheral vascular disease, free tissue transfer provides increased venous drainage from, supplements blood flow to, and augments angiogenesis of hypoxic areas.[12] The vascular status must be evaluated to ensure success.[13] Vascular assessment and treatment has been discussed earlier in this textbook.

In patients with severe vessel disease and soft-tissue defects, improved rates of limb salvage have been reported combining bypass and free tissue transfer in staged or simultaneous fashion.[14] Endovascular techniques allow for direct and indirect revascularization with angioplasty dilatation and atherectomy to recanalize stenosed or obstructed arteries in patients who are poor candidates for open vascular bypass.[15]

Usually additional concerns ranging from chronic renal failure, nutrition, and blood sugar control are best managed by a multidisciplinary team.[16,17,18] These conditions lead to a predisposition to chronic bacterial colonization, osteomyelitis, complex wounds, bone deformity, local wound ischemia, and vascular disease.

Oncologic Reconstruction

Surgeons should have close coordination with the oncologists and must acquire adequate knowledge of tumor characteristics, behavior, and adjuvant treatment in order to plan and choose the appropriate reconstructive procedure. For patients requiring postoperative radiation or for wounds over joints and high-friction regions, skin grafts should be avoided with a preference for durable flaps.[19]

Flaps should be carefully chosen in patients with preoperative radiation therapy where local tissues would become fibrotic and ischemic around cancer, and thus may not allow local coverage. Free flap procedures will not interfere with chemotherapy nor will chemotherapy have an impact on free flap survival, though such treatment may have an impact on local wound healing. Following reconstruction, recommended delay prior to initiation of adjuvant chemotherapy and/or radiation is 3-4 weeks or until adequate wound healing has occurred per the reconstructive surgeon.[20,21]

Thrombophilia

Patients with factor V Leiden mutation, protein C deficiency, hyperhomocysteinemia, antiphospholipid antibody syndrome, prothrombin gene mutation, factor VIII elevation, anticardiolipin antibody syndrome, and essential thrombocytosis trend toward higher rates of microvascular thromboses, though patients with microvascular transfer have comparable overall success rates when compared to nonthrombophilic patients. Thrombophilic patients also trend toward delayed thrombotic complications and nonsalvageability in the setting of postoperative thrombosis.[15,22]

It is important to screen patients for a procoagulant condition, including asking about a history of deep venous thrombosis, pulmonary embolism, history of multiple miscarriages, family history, and exogenous estrogen use. It is also important to probe for patient accounts of acquired thrombophilia risk factors (i.e., venous thromboembolism, myocardial infarction [MI], cerebrovascular accident, and miscarriage) and/or known hereditary thrombophilia (i.e., people who know they have a genetic predisposition). A hematology consultation may be needed if patient is positive for thrombophilic state. This may miss patients who are thrombophilic without a discernible history, which can still affect free flap outcomes. Universal screening is still a source of controversy.[22,23,24]

Biomechanical Optimization

A sensorimotor examination is essential to ensuring the success of any reconstruction (▶ Table 26.2). Sensibility is evaluated with a 5.07 Semmes–Weinstein filament that represents 10 g of pressure. If the patient cannot feel the filament, protective sensation is absent, and the risk of breakdown and/or ulceration is significantly increased. Motor function is assessed by looking at the resting position of the foot and by testing the strength and active range of motion of the ankle, foot, and toes.

Gait analysis will provide an assessment of personal areas of high stress. High-stress areas include the plantar surface, mobile ankle, and knee (▶ Fig. 26.1). These are subject to pressure as well as shear forces. Prolonged weight-bearing on a single spot will lead to ulceration regardless of type of reconstruction.

Preoperative assessment of gait may include an F-scan analysis or pressure mapping as well as a measure of ankle dorsiflexion. F-scan analysis uses multiple pressure-sensing probes that record pressures on multiple areas of the sole of the foot during all phases of gait. One should evaluate for equinus deformity by assessing ankle motion when the knee is in complete extension and then flexion (which reduces stretch and tension on the gastrocnemius) to evaluate for gastrocnemius tightness (during knee flexion) or both gastrocnemius and soleus tightness (during both knee flexion and extension). If percutaneous release of the relevant portion of the Achilles tendon fails to improve dorsiflexion, then a posterior capsular release of the ankle joint should be performed. These will reduce pressure and lead to high ulcer resolution rates.[25]

Table 26.2 Preoperative Biomechanical Assessment

- Evaluate sensibility with a 5.07 Semmes Weinstein filament
- Evaluate motor function by evaluating both resting position and active range of motion of ankle, foot, and toes
- Evaluate location of current ulceration representing areas of increased pressure
- Gait analysis includes F-scan analysis or pressure point-mapping of the foot
- Evaluate for equinus deformity secondary to tight Achilles tendon

Prior midfoot amputations can cause ulceration from musculotendinous imbalance within the foot, which leads to abnormal posturing and weight distribution. Patients often require Achilles tendon lengthening and/or tibialis anterior tendon transfer. Metatarsal head prominences can be remedied with "floating" neck osteotomies and internal fixation. The fifth metatarsal head can be resected. However, the first metatarsal head should rarely be resected as this is the base of the medial column of the leg. Resection of the plantar flare of the first metatarsal head is preferred in this instance.

During reconstruction, it is important to reestablish bony stability and eliminate any bony prominences. Such prominences occur particularly with collapsed midfoot bones (e.g., Charcot), osteophyte formation, or abnormal biomechanical forces (hallux valgus, hammer toe). Charcot arthropathy is a neuroarthropathy that is a destructive process of the bones, joints, and soft tissues of the foot. Reconstruction is futile when residual bone spike leads to subsequent ulceration. Soles can be difficult to reconstruct because of generalized scarcity of glabrous skin. Only the instep area of the foot provides a vascularized glabrous skin donor site.

Authors have found a higher rate of flap ulceration in muscle flaps with skin grafts, so fasciocutaneous flaps are preferred.[26] Ducic et al emphasized that sensation is not essential for durability, but sensory nerve reconstruction improves surgical outcomes, quality of life, and patient satisfaction due to earlier sensory recovery in fasciocutaneous flaps. There is earlier return to normal footwear and daily activities.[27,28]

Typical postoperative rehabilitation is similar to that of diabetic patients, including custom-made insoles that facilitate load-sharing away from high-pressure areas on the heel and forefoot. Good custom therapeutic insoles relieve and distribute plantar pressure.[29,30] Casting can be utilized for pressure ulcers.

Nutritional Optimization

Markers of nutritional status include albumin, prealbumin, C-reactive protein, and hemoglobin A1c. Albumin has a half-life of

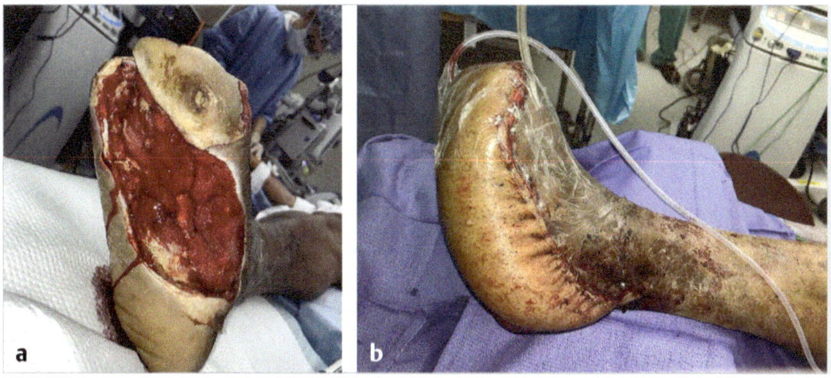

Fig. 26.1 Anterolateral thigh free tissue transfer used to construct weight-bearing portion of the foot. **(a)** Preoperative and **(b)** postoperative pictures.

Table 26.3 Nutritional Goals

- Albumin greater than 3.5 g/dL
- Prealbumin greater than 12 mg/dL
- Hemoglobin A1c less than 6.5%

21 days and prealbumin has a half-life of 48 hours, though the latter is considered an acute-phase reactant and arguably decreased in the setting of acute inflammation. Trending these markers can give critical information on host inflammatory response and if patients' health is improving. Goals should be albumin greater than 3.5, prealbumin greater than 12, and hemoglobin A1c less than 6.5 (▶ Table 26.3).

Placing surgical patients on protein-rich diets decreases levels of inflammatory cytokines postoperatively.[31] Also, a diet rich in omega-3 fatty acids has also been shown to reduce inflammatory cytokine levels. Many times, patients, even if obese, are malnourished with low protein levels required to fight infection and promote wound healing. Nutritional support decreased infectious complications and noninfectious complications, and shortened length of hospital stay—immunomodulatory nutrition diets reduced infectious complications even further.[32]

26.2.2 Perioperative Optimization

Basic perioperative principles should be regarded (▶ Table 26.4). This includes the maintenance of normothermia to reduce complications. There is debate of what may be the optimal hematocrit level, particularly in free tissue transfer; blood transfusions are associated with longer hospital stays, higher rate of vascular thrombosis, and higher rates of major surgical and medical complications. Restrictive strategies (hemoglobin level < 7 g/dL or clinically symptomatic) for blood transfusion minimize medical complications.[33] Fluid replacement is also controversial, though this is dependent on comorbidities of the patient. The surgeon can discuss with anesthesia whether a set maintenance infusion rate or replacement of calculated fluid losses is appropriate.

Postoperatively, it is important to monitor hemodynamic and pulmonary function as adequate hydration and oxygenation are critical to flap survival. Input and output of fluids should be closely monitored—distal perfusion is affected by hypotensive episodes. Fluid management can be complex for patients with end-stage renal disease who are on dialysis, which usually removes large volumes of fluid.

26.3 Immediate Postoperative Management

26.3.1 Flap Monitoring Protocols

The patient and flap should be closely monitored. Clinical examination is the gold standard; and the surgeon at the bedside can evaluate edema, turgor, color, capillary refill (too brisk can indicate venous congestion), and temperature. An experienced and knowledgeable staff is key to obtaining flap retention rates above 95%, as reported at high-volume centers.

It is important to utilize standardized flap monitoring protocols to enhance early detection of impending anastomotic complications. At the authors' institution, serial Doppler assessments are performed every 15 minutes for the first 4 hours postoperatively, then every 30 minutes for the subsequent 8 hours, and then hourly until the second postoperative day. For patients with uncomplicated recoveries, the interval between Doppler checks increases to every 2 to 4 hours until postoperative day 5.

Table 26.4 Perioperative Patient Optimization

Intraoperative
- Maintenance of normothermia (36°C to 38°C)
- Transfuse only if clinically symptomatic or hemoglobin < 7 g/dL
- Adequate discussion with anesthesia regarding goals of fluid resuscitation
- Adequate discussion with anesthesia regarding use of vasopressors

Postoperative
- Monitor hemodynamic and pulmonary function
- Strict inputs/outputs of fluids, particularly in end-stage renal disease
- Standardized flap monitoring protocols; an experienced clinical exam provides the best assessment

The threshold for surgical take-back should be very low, as microvascular compromise may be devastating. Early identification and re-exploration of a compromised flap dramatically increases salvage rate. Salvage rates are higher with arterial compromise compared with venous compromise.[34]

The first 24 hours are crucial for flap monitoring, as most thromboses will occur in this time. Up to 85% of compromised flaps can be salvaged when the first sign of vascular compromise is noted during the first 3 days.[35] Available monitoring techniques include (1) conventional clinical monitoring, (2) handheld Doppler probes, (3) implantable Doppler systems, (4) color duplex sonography, (4) near-infrared spectroscopy, (5) microdialysis, (6) laser Doppler flowmetry, and (7) glucose monitoring.

A recent review showed implantable Dopplers, near-infrared spectroscopy, and laser Doppler flowmetry were most effective.[36] The implantable Doppler uses a 20-MHz ultrasonic probe to monitor anastomosis, typically on venous segments because arterial signal will persist for hours after a venous thrombosis. The implantable Doppler around the vein can be used during the original operative flap inset to ensure the pedicle isn't kinked or compressed. Previous studies have demonstrated 100% flap salvage with a negative predictive value of 81 to 93%.[37]

Near-infrared spectroscopy detects change in oxygenated and deoxygenated hemoglobin through optical spectrometry[38] (▶ Fig. 26.2). It has the advantage of being independent of clinical experience. It detects signs of both arterial and venous compromise before experienced clinical examination, with positive and negative predictive values approaching 100%.[39,40]

The trend is the most important consideration; a gradual decrease in perioperative (over 4–16 hours) does not usually indicate flap compromise. Oxygen saturation usually returns to normal levels within 12 hours.[41] Criteria for surgical exploration are a rapid 20-point drop from baseline in 1 hour or an absolute recording less than 30%. Flaps with less than or equal to 30% tissue oxygen saturation or greater than 20% drop per hour over 30 minutes were predictive of vascular compromise.[42] Currently commercial devices are available only for

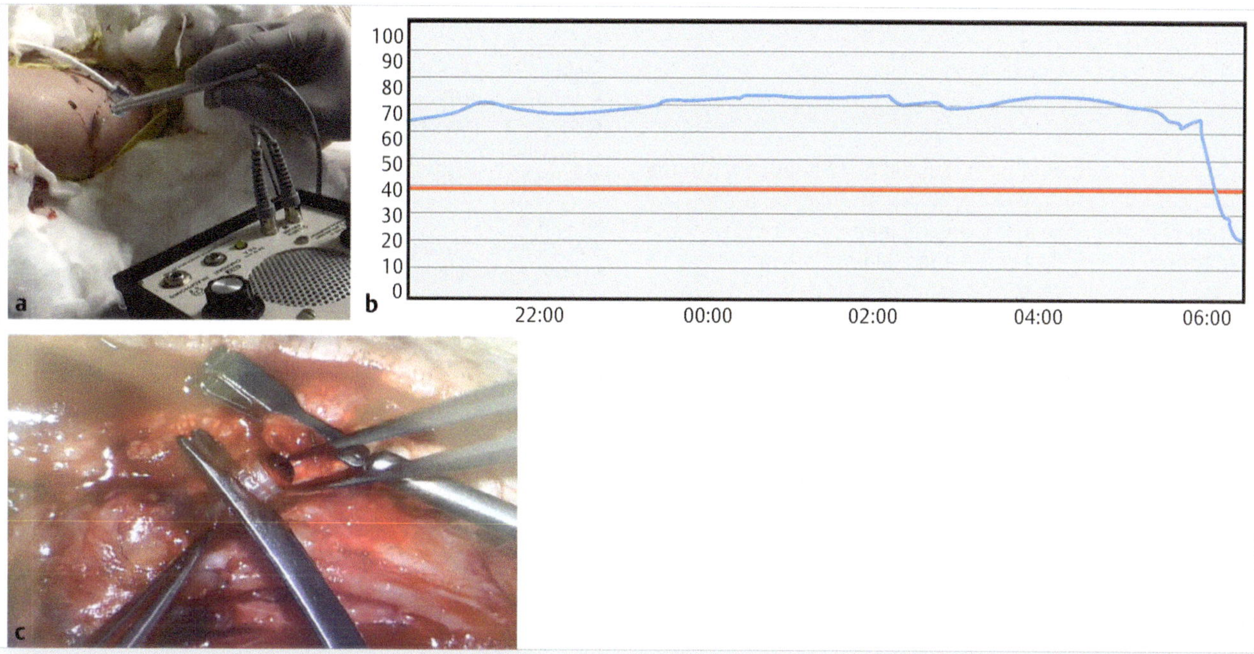

Fig. 26.2 **(a)** Both conventional handheld doppler probes and near-infrared spectroscopy visualized in photograph of anterolateral free tissue transfer to the dorsum of the foot. **(b)** Near-infrared spectroscopy over time revealed sharp drop in oxygen saturation level of the tissue. **(c)** Take-back to the operating room revealed thrombosis of one of the venae comitantes to the flap. Revision of the anastomosis resulted in successful flap salvage.

flaps with cutaneous paddles, but use has been described for buried flaps in the literature.[41]

Color Dopplers are expensive and require expertise and may be useful as a second-line tool if other monitoring suggests re-exploration. Microdialysis measures tissue content of glucose, lactate, pyruvate, and glycerol metabolite ratios to detect increases in anaerobic metabolism and arterial compromise. However, it has a steep learning curve and requires 30 minutes to analyze with wide variation in the positive predictive value.[36] Laser Doppler measures blood flow and velocity to a depth of 8 mm, but it is highly sensitive to movement and vibration of both probe and tissue, leading to inaccurate readings.[43,44]

Despite these adjunctive measures, nothing can substitute for vigilant clinical examination for flap compromise.

26.3.2 Postoperative Anticoagulation Protocols

About 96% of microsurgeons use some form of anticoagulation.[45] Anticoagulation remains controversial. Subcutaneous heparin is the only method of anticoagulation associated with decreased odds of thrombosis.[46] Other studies show increased hematoma risk with heparin, which can compromise the flap due to possible pressure on the anastomosis.

Disa et al, in a prospective randomized series, observed no effect on flap survival comparing dextran to aspirin. In the same study, dextran led to 3.9- to 7.2-fold increase in systemic complications, such as congestive heart failure, MI, pulmonary edema, pleural effusion, and pneumonia.[47]

Many reconstructive surgeons use low-dose aspirin, which has been shown to increase patency rates in lab studies, and is known to prevent microvascular thrombosis, but it is less effective than heparin.[48] More aggressive weight-based systemic heparinization/multi-agent anticoagulation protocols in thrombophilic patients have been shown to be effective at treating intraoperative thrombotic complications with low rates of recurrence and high rates of flap salvage.[49]

Leeches are a salvage measure for flaps that are not amenable to operative intervention (i.e., surgically uncorrectable venous insufficiency). Leeches can help in the cases of venous congestion by locally distributing a salivary component called hirudin, which inhibits platelet aggregation. These can be used for 5 to 7 days, but antibiotic coverage for leech-harboring *Aeromonas* must be included.

26.3.3 Offloading the Flap in Immediate Postoperative Period

The patient should be on strict bed rest in the immediate postoperative period to minimize trauma (▶ Table 26.5). Pressure on the flap and its pedicle should be minimized, particularly if the flap is in a load-bearing area of the extremity, such as the heel. It is also not uncommon for patients to develop pressure sores if the extremity is left in the same position.

Common noninvasive offloading devices include foam heel lifts, gels, air or water mattresses, and pressure-relieving ankle-foot orthoses. Compression therapy is a must postoperatively for all lower extremity flaps. Multilayer compression wraps can be useful while areas are healing. Once fully healed, these dressings can be transitioned to full compression stockings.

It may be most prudent to include orthopaedic and podiatric colleagues in order to apply a pressure-relieving external fixator device, such as a circular frame fixator. These include the Ilizarov frame and the Taylor spatial frame. A simpler, less bulky offloading device includes the "kickstand," which is constructed from bars and struts.[50]

Table 26.5 Timeline of Weightbearing of Affected Extremity

Immediate Postoperative Period
- Strict bedrest
- Compression therapy
- Noninvasive offloading: foam heel lifts, gels, air or water mattresses, ankle foot orthoses or
- Pressure relieving external fixator: Ilizarov frame, Taylor spatial frame

"Dangle Protocol" Starting at Post-operative Day 5
- Subjecting the flap to increasing time intervals of gravity
- Start as early as two days, as late as two weeks

4-6 Weeks Postoperatively
- Cleared to bear weight on affected extremity with specialized devices, e.g. Controlled ankle motion (CAM) walker and assistive devices (crutches, walker)
- Ok to remove offloading frames at this time

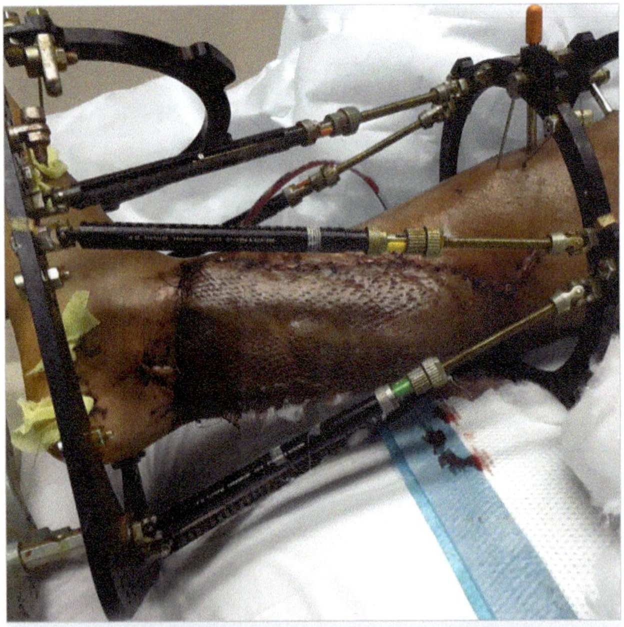

Fig. 26.3 Example of an Ilizarov frame used to offload pressure from a weight-bearing portion of the flap during the non-weight-bearing period.

The frame can be removed as patient begins to bear weight 4 to 6 weeks later. The Ilizarov frame provides superior immobilization, shortens healing times, decreases pin track infections, and promotes weight-bearing through the addition of a protective plantar foot plate (▶ Fig. 26.3).[51,52]

26.3.4 "Dangle" Protocols: Beginning to Subject the Limb to Gravity

Regarding the dangle protocol, or a protocol to subject lower extremity free tissue transfers to increasing time intervals of gravity in order for a flap to accommodate the outflow of venous blood, there is widespread controversy, and there is no general acceptance of a single method. Most are institution-specific. Some do not utilize a dangle protocol (▶ Table 26.6).

Table 26.6 Georgetown Dangle Protocol

Postoperative day	Protocol
0–5	Strict bed rest
6–9	Out of bed with leg elevated with physical therapy/ occupational therapy
10	Dangle for 15 min twice a day
11	Dangle for 15 min thrice a day
12	Dangle for 30 min once
13	Dangle for 30 min twice a day
14	Dangle for 30 min thrice a day
15	Dangle for 45 min once
16	Dangle for 45 min twice a day
17	Dangle for 45 min thrice a day

Dangle protocols are performed with extremity wrapped in compressive elastic bandage dressing

Note: Patients are allowed to begin to subject the extremity to gravity on post-op day 5/6 at increasing intervals. At post-op day 9/10, patients are cleared to leave the hospital, and perform remainder of the dangle protocol at their respective rehabilitative facilities. Oftentimes, patients are allowed to get to a chair by post-op day 3, but with strict extremity elevation and usually with the assistance of physical therapy in the hospital.

Lower extremity free flaps lack sympathetic nerves and feedback mechanisms that regulate blood flow and extremity swelling, causing venous congestion. Color-flow doppler studies have shown that arterial and venous cross-sectional areas decreased an average of 0.87 and 1.42mm^2 during dangling, but returned to baseline within 60 seconds of going to neutral.[53]

Survey data show that 43% of microsurgeons dangle at 2 to 5 days and 38% dangle at 6 to 13 days, with duration varying widely.[54] Early and aggressive start of a combined dangling/ wrapping at day 3 has not been shown to compromise flap circulation or overall outcome.[55]

The protocol can be slowed if the flap shows signs of congestion; the an experienced clinician should be on hand initially to observe for clinical signs of congestion, that is, purple discoloration, tautness of skin due to congestion, and swelling. Patients should be non–weight bearing for at least 4 to 6 weeks after surgery and at the longer end of that time frame if the flap is in a load-bearing area of the lower extremity.

26.3.5 Secondary Procedures

Any needed bone grafts are usually placed 6 weeks after soft-tissue reconstruction, after settling of tissue bed and eradication of infection.[56] Secondary tenolysis or tendon-lengthening procedures may be needed. Skin grafts increase risk for adhesions when performed over granulated tissue directly above tendons and may warrant flap coverage. Additionally, after recovery, patients frequently show scars, depression, bulky flaps, and donor site morbidities. Debulking via excision or suction-assisted lipectomy or fat grafting can be done to improve appearance. Z-plasty may be useful in scar revision.

26.4 Rehabilitation

Previous studies show that physical functioning, pain, one's belief in the ability to return to work, age, emotional score and education were all predictors of return to work, but others show that in free flap recipients, but only 62% of patients returned to work.[58,64] Rehabilitation should focus on restoring ambulation, occupational readiness, and activities of daily living in a way that does not compromise the integrity of the reconstruction.

At our institution, physical therapy should start 3-4 weeks after surgery. The initial goals of physical therapy are strength, range of motion, and gait training. The goals at this step of the process are to ambulate without bearing weight on the operated extremity so that the patient can perform his/her activities of daily living. After 4-6 weeks, if the flap is well healed, goals of physical therapy are to begin ambulating on the extremity. We use an ambulation protocol which starts at 50% weight-bearing, consisting of less than 1000 steps per day, which then progresses to full weight bearing and unlimited steps with weekly wound checks.

Once the flap edema has gone down and the foot is well healed, the patient is molded for appropriate orthotics, typically custom shoes. If there is ankle instability, ankle braces are added. For the first year after surgery, the patient should use the custom shoe. After the first year, patients can transition to regular shoes with monthly or bimonthly foot checks. Judicious foot care is essential, and patients and their family members/caretakers should inspect their operated extremity regularly and closely for signs of flap breakdown or novel ulcer formation.[70]

26.4.1 Importance of Early Motion without Use of the Extremity

The literature has elucidated across a wide variety of surgical subspecialties the importance of early mobilization on a host of patient outcomes. Though the patient may be restricted from bearing weight in the affected extremity, the patient can continue to exercise the contralateral extremity. Additionally, upper extremity workouts can be used to facilitate cardiovascular health (e.g., arm cycle machine).

Patients should wait for at least 48 hours after surgery to get out of bed, and then slowly increase activity with time, in conjunction with the preferred dangle protocol. In studies of hospitalized patients, both prehabilitation and early rehabilitation resulted in shorter length of stay, lower complications, and ability to get out of bed sooner.[64,65,66] Nutritional optimization, with protein drinks, particularly in geriatric and malnourished patients, is vital.

26.4.2 Range-of-Motion Exercises

Rehabilitation helps control edema, prevents contractures, and improves ambulation, which is the goal (▶ Table 26.7). After prolonged periods of immobilization, ambulation should begin under the guidance of physical therapy. This usually occurs with graduated weight-bearing exercises. Controlled ankle motion (CAM) walking boots equalize pressure on the plantar foot and stabilizes the ankle and should be used for the first ambulation.

Table 26.7 Important Components of Rehabilitation

- "Prehabilitation" to optimize patient's functional status prior to reconstructive surgery
- Following surgery, important to have the patient out of bed (with affected extremity elevated) by 48 hours
- Maintain/improve functional status by exercising contralateral extremity and upper extremities
- Perform range of motion of exercises even prior to weightbearing
- Psychological support is crucial
- Vocational therapy to allow patients to return to work

Prosthetists and or pedorthotist should be involved in analyzing the need for custom inserts and shoe gear. This can take up to 4 weeks for manufacturing. During this time, ambulation in the CAM boot should be continued until specialty shoe gear is ready for use.

It is important to involve physical therapy early on as maintaining range of motion is critical to a successful outcome. Contractures have a negative impact on prosthetic placement and patient function. In patients who have partial amputations or have lost function of certain muscle groups, the key is to prevent knee and ankle contractures—this occurs when dominant muscles overpower their opposing muscle groups, which results in knee flexion and ankle plantar flexion. Achilles and tibialis anterior lengthening procedures may be needed for pes equinus and pes cavus deformities, respectively.

Assistive devices include crutches and a walker. It is important to maintain and improve aerobic activity, especially in those with cardiovascular and vascular compromise.

Occupational therapy should be involved to help the patient achieve independence in activities of daily living. Self-care skills, assessment of home environment, and appropriate assistive devices should be performed.

Psychological evaluation may be needed as patients must deal with the trials of a prolonged hospital and rehabilitative course, and proper social support and necessary psychological support should be ensured.

Vocational therapy is vital as patients should be able to return to self-supporting and self-fulfilling lifestyles. As a proxy, those amputees who have returned to work have greater job satisfaction than their peers, and it is associated with younger age, higher educational level, and comfort of prostheses.[67,68] If patients can return to physically less demanding work, then they are more likely to stay working after surgery.

26.4.3 Residual Pain

It is very important to control pain, as its persistence can cause disability and delay in functional progression. Residual limb pain is local pain from the limb and prior wound site. It can come from bone, nerve, muscle, or skin. Neuromas, bone spurs, poorly fitting prostheses, intermittent claudication, or recurrence of the inciting pathology (e.g., malignancy, fracture nonunion) may be the culprits. Incisional pain tends to resolve with healing.

Phantom limb sensation is experiencing that an amputated limb or portion of a limb is still present. The input to the brain is replaced by phantom sensations. Telescoping is the sensation that an amputated limb has decreased in size. Awareness typically decreases with time, but some sensations can be felt for the rest of the patient's life.

Phantom limb pain is the sensations of pain from an amputated or partially amputated extremity. It is usually worse at night and can be exacerbated by anxiety and stress. The phenomenon does tend to decrease with time. Chronic occurrence is at 5%, with only about 14% of those feeling truly debilitated.[69] Preventive efforts at the time of the index operation have been shown to be quite effective, via targeted muscle reinnervation.

It is caused by neuron deafferentation hyperexcitability, which is loss of sensory input from elimination of sensory nerve fibers. There are then changes in the functional properties of the dorsal horn of the spinal cord that may cause the occurrence of abnormal sensations.[70]

Gabapentin—which decreases ability of nerves to depolarize —may be helpful. Efficacy rates of all the post-operative modalities have been shown to be about 30 to 70%. Additional treatments include desensitization through massage or prosthesis, and transcutaneous electrical nerve stimulation. Gabapentin—which decreases ability of nerves to depolarize. Also, other modalities such as hypnosis, biofeedback, behavioral therapy, relaxation therapy, and mirror therapy can be useful. Opioids have not been shown to be useful for treatment of phantom limb pain. Other pharmacological treatments include serotonin norepinephrine reuptake inhibitors (duloxetine, nortriptyline, amitriptyline) and anticonvulsants (pregabalin, carbamazepine). Additionally, nerve blocks, epidural blocks, and chemical sympathectomy may be used for refractory cases.

Neuromas are bundles of nerve tissue that grow after injury and can lead to pain when they are compressed. Our institution has now begun to use targeted muscle reinnervation for these postoperative neuromas with good success.[72] Targeted muscle reinnervation is rerouting of a sensory nerve into a motor nerve branch to prevent neuroma formation. Other surgical options including beurectomy, nerve implantation, capping, and coaptation may have some efficacy in improving neuroma-related pain.

References

[1] Viol A, Pradka SP, Baumeister SP, et al. Soft-tissue defects and exposed hardware: a review of indications for soft-tissue reconstruction and hardware preservation. Plast Reconstr Surg. 2009; 123(4):1256–1263

[2] Segawa H, Tsukayama DT, Kyle RF, Becker DA, Gustilo RB. Infection after total knee arthroplasty. A retrospective study of the treatment of eighty-one infections. J Bone Joint Surg Am. 1999; 81(10):1434–1445

[3] Munro JT, Garbuz DS, Masri BA, Duncan CP. Articulating antibiotic impregnated spacers in two-stage revision of infected total knee arthroplasty. J Bone Jt Surg - Br Vol. 2012; 94-B(11, Supple A):123–125

[4] Voleti PB, Baldwin KD, Lee G-C. Use of static or articulating spacers for infection following total knee arthroplasty: a systematic literature review. J Bone Joint Surg Am. 2013; 95(17):1594–1599

[5] Wyrsch B, McFerran MA, McAndrew M, et al. Operative treatment of fractures of the tibial plafond. A randomized, prospective study. J Bone Joint Surg Am. 1996; 78(11):1646–1657

[6] Patel KM, Seruya M, Franklin B, Attinger CE, Ducic I. Factors associated with failed hardware salvage in high-risk patients after microsurgical lower extremity reconstruction. Ann Plast Surg. 2012; 69(4):399–402

[7] Oh TS, Lee HS, Hong JP. Diabetic foot reconstruction using free flaps increases 5-year-survival rate. J Plast Reconstr Aesthet Surg. 2013; 66(2):243–250

[8] Fitzgerald O'Connor EJ, Vesely M, Holt PJ, Jones KG, Thompson MM, Hinchliffe RJ. A systematic review of free tissue transfer in the management of non-traumatic lower extremity wounds in patients with diabetes. Eur J Vasc Endovasc Surg. 2011; 41(3):391–399

[9] Hong JP. Reconstruction of the diabetic foot using the anterolateral thigh perforator flap. Plast Reconstr Surg. 2006; 117(5):1599–1608

[10] Hong JP, Oh TS. An algorithm for limb salvage for diabetic foot ulcers. Clin Plast Surg. 2012; 39(3):341–352

[11] Endara M, Masden D, Goldstein J, Gondek S, Steinberg J, Attinger C. The role of chronic and perioperative glucose management in high-risk surgical closures: a case for tighter glycemic control. Plast Reconstr Surg. 2013; 132 (4):996–1004

[12] Mimoun M, Hilligot P, Baux S. The nutrient flap: a new concept of the role of the flap and application to the salvage of arteriosclerotic lower limbs. Plast Reconstr Surg. 1989; 84(3):458–467

[13] Banis JC, Jr, Richardson JD, Derr JW, Jr, Acland RD. Microsurgical adjuncts in salvage of the ischemic and diabetic lower extremity. Clin Plast Surg. 1992; 19(4):881–893

[14] Shestak KC, Fitz DG, Newton ED, Swartz WM. Expanding the horizons in treatment of severe peripheral vascular disease using microsurgical techniques. Plast Reconstr Surg. 1990; 85(3):406–411

[15] DeFazio MV, Han KD, Akbari CM, Evans KK. Free tissue transfer after targeted endovascular reperfusion for complex lower extremity reconstruction: setting the stage for success in the presence of multivessel disease. Ann Vasc Surg. 2015; 29(6):1316.e7–1316.e15

[16] Lipsky BA, Berendt AR, Deery HG, et al. Infectious Diseases Society of America. Diagnosis and treatment of diabetic foot infections. Plast Reconstr Surg. 2006; 117(7) Suppl:212S–238S

[17] Caputo GM, Cavanagh PR, Ulbrecht JS, Gibbons GW, Karchmer AW. Assessment and management of foot disease in patients with diabetes. N Engl J Med. 1994; 331(13):854–860

[18] Dargis V, Pantelejeva O, Jonushaite A, Vileikyte L, Boulton AJ. Benefits of a multidisciplinary approach in the management of recurrent diabetic foot ulceration in Lithuania: a prospective study. Diabetes Care. 1999; 22 (9):1428–1431

[19] Tran NV, Evans GR, Kroll SS, et al. Postoperative adjuvant irradiation: effects on transverse rectus abdominis muscle flap breast reconstruction. Plast Reconstr Surg. 2000; 106(2):313–317–discussion 318–320

[20] Cordeiro PG, Neves RI, Hidalgo DA. The role of free tissue transfer following oncologic resection in the lower extremity. Ann Plast Surg. 1994; 33(1):9–16

[21] Evans GR, Black JJ, Robb GL, et al. Adjuvant therapy: the effects on microvascular lower extremity reconstruction. Ann Plast Surg. 1997; 39(2):141–144

[22] Wang TY, Serletti JM, Cuker A, et al. Free tissue transfer in the hypercoagulable patient: a review of 58 flaps. Plast Reconstr Surg. 2012; 129(2):443–453

[23] DeFazio MV, Hung RWY, Han KD, Bunting HA, Evans KK. Lower extremity flap salvage in thrombophilic patients: managing expectations in the setting of microvascular thrombosis. J Reconstr Microsurg. 2016; 32(6):431–444

[24] Pannucci CJ, Kovach SJ, Cuker A. Microsurgery and the hypercoagulable state: a hematologist's perspective. Plast Reconstr Surg. 2015; 136(4):545e–552e

[25] Mueller MJ, Sinacore DR, Hastings MK, Strube MJ, Johnson JE. Effect of Achilles tendon lengthening on neuropathic plantar ulcers. A randomized clinical trial. J Bone Joint Surg Am. 2003; 85(8):1436–1445

[26] Sönmez A, Bayramiçli M, Sönmez B, Numanoğlu A. Reconstruction of the weight-bearing surface of the foot with nonneurosensory free flaps. Plast Reconstr Surg. 2003; 111(7):2230–2236

[27] Ducic I, Hung V, Dellon AL. Innervated free flaps for foot reconstruction: a review. J Reconstr Microsurg. 2006; 22(6):433–442

[28] Kuran I, Turgut G, Bas L, Ozkan T, Bayri O, Gulgonen A. Comparison between sensitive and nonsensitive free flaps in reconstruction of the heel and plantar area. Plast Reconstr Surg. 2000; 105(2):574–580

[29] Owings TM, Woerner JL, Frampton JD, Cavanagh PR, Botek G. Custom therapeutic insoles based on both foot shape and plantar pressure measurement provide enhanced pressure relief. Diabetes Care. 2008; 31(5):839–844

[30] Tsung BYS, Zhang M, Mak AFT, Wong MWN. Effectiveness of insoles on plantar pressure redistribution. J Rehabil Res Dev.; 41(6A):767–774

[31] Nakamura K, Moriyama Y, Kariyazono H, et al. Influence of preoperative nutritional state on inflammatory response after surgery. Nutrition. 1999; 15 (11–12):834–841

[32] Zhong JX, Kang K, Shu XL. Effect of nutritional support on clinical outcomes in perioperative malnourished patients: a meta-analysis. Asia Pac J Clin Nutr. 2015; 24(3):367–378

[33] Fischer JP, Nelson JA, Sieber B, et al. Transfusions in autologous breast reconstructions: an analysis of risk factors, complications, and cost. Ann Plast Surg. 2014; 72(5):566–571

[34] Mirzabeigi MN, Wang T, Kovach SJ, Taylor JA, Serletti JM, Wu LC. Free flap take-back following postoperative microvascular compromise: predicting salvage versus failure. Plast Reconstr Surg. 2012; 130(3):579–589

[35] Chen CM, Halvorson EG, Disa JJ, et al. Immediate postoperative complications in DIEP versus free/muscle-sparing TRAM flaps. Plast Reconstr Surg. 2007; 120(6):1477–1482

[36] Smit JM, Zeebregts CJ, Acosta R, Werker PMN. Advancements in free flap monitoring in the last decade: a critical review. Plast Reconstr Surg. 2010; 125(1):177–185

[37] Kind GM, Buntic RF, Buncke GM, Cooper TM, Siko PP, Buncke HJ. The effect of an implantable Doppler probe on the salvage of microvascular tissue transplants. Plast Reconstr Surg. 1998; 101(5):1268–73–5. Accessed November 5, 2017

[38] Irwin MS, Thorniley MS, Doré CJ, Green CJ. Near infra-red spectroscopy: a non-invasive monitor of perfusion and oxygenation within the microcirculation of limbs and flaps. Br J Plast Surg. 1995; 48(1):14–22

[39] Colwell AS, Wright L, Karanas Y. Near-infrared spectroscopy measures tissue oxygenation in free flaps for breast reconstruction. Plast Reconstr Surg. 2008; 121(5):344e–345e

[40] Repez A, Oroszy D, Arnez ZM. Continuous postoperative monitoring of cutaneous free flaps using near infrared spectroscopy. J Plast Reconstr Aesthet Surg. 2008; 61(1):71–77

[41] Cai ZG, Zhang J, Zhang JG, et al. Evaluation of near infrared spectroscopy in monitoring postoperative regional tissue oxygen saturation for fibular flaps. J Plast Reconstr Aesthet Surg. 2008; 61(3):289–296

[42] Keller A. A new diagnostic algorithm for early prediction of vascular compromise in 208 microsurgical flaps using tissue oxygen saturation measurements. Ann Plast Surg. 2009; 62(5):538–543

[43] Heller L, Levin LS, Klitzman B. Laser Doppler flowmeter monitoring of free-tissue transfers: blood flow in normal and complicated cases. Plast Reconstr Surg. 2001; 107(7):1739–1745

[44] Yuen JC, Feng Z. Monitoring free flaps using the laser Doppler flowmeter: five-year experience. Plast Reconstr Surg. 2000; 105(1):55–61

[45] Askari M, Fisher C, Weniger FG, Bidic S, Lee WPA. Anticoagulation therapy in microsurgery: a review. J Hand Surg Am. 2006; 31(5):836–846

[46] Khouri RK, Sherman R, Buncke HJ, et al. A phase II trial of intraluminal irrigation with recombinant human tissue factor pathway inhibitor to prevent thrombosis in free flap surgery. Plast Reconstr Surg. 2001; 107(2)–408–4–15; discussion 416–418

[47] Disa JJ, Polvora VP, Pusic AL, Singh B, Cordeiro PG. Dextran-related complications in head and neck microsurgery: do the benefits outweigh the risks? A prospective randomized analysis. Plast Reconstr Surg. 2003; 112(6):1534–1539

[48] Cooley BC, Gould JS. Experimental models for evaluating antithrombotic therapies in replantation microsurgery. Microsurgery. 1987; 8(4):230–233

[49] Senchenkov A, Lemaine V, Tran NV. Management of perioperative microvascular thrombotic complications: the use of multiagent anticoagulation algorithm in 395 consecutive free flaps. J Plast Reconstr Aesthet Surg. 2015; 68 (9):1293–1303

[50] Castro-Aragon OE, Rapley JH, Trevino SG. The use of a kickstand modification for the prevention of heel decubitus ulcers in trauma patients with lower extremity external fixation. J Orthop Trauma. 2009; 23(2):145–147

[51] McKee MD, Yoo D, Schemitsch EH. Health status after Ilizarov reconstruction of post-traumatic lower-limb deformity. J Bone Joint Surg Br. 1998; 80 (2):360–364

[52] Parikh PM, Hall MM, Attinger CE, Masden DL, Steinberg JS. External fixation: indications in lower extremity reconstruction and limb salvage. Plast Reconstr Surg. 2009; 123(4):160e–161e

[53] Isenberg JS, Siegal A, Sherman R. Quantitative evaluation of the effects of gravity and dependency on microvascular tissue transfer to the lower limb, with clinical applications. J Reconstr Microsurg. 1997; 13(1):25–29

[54] Xipoleas G, Levine E, Silver L, Koch RM, Taub PJ. A survey of microvascular protocols for lower extremity free tissue transfer II: postoperative care. Ann Plast Surg. 2008; 61(3):280–284

[55] Jokuszies A, Neubert N, Herold C, Vogt PM. Early start of the dangling procedure in lower extremity free flap reconstruction does not affect the clinical outcome. J Reconstr Microsurg. 2013; 29(1):27–32

[56] Ong YS, Levin LS. Lower limb salvage in trauma. Plast Reconstr Surg. 2010; 125(2):582–588

[57] MacKenzie EJ, Bosse MJ, Kellam JF, et al. Early predictors of long-term work disability after major limb trauma. J Trauma. 2006; 61(3):688–694

[58] Guerra AB, Gill PS, Trahan CG, et al. Comparison of bacterial inoculation and transcutaneous oxygen tension in the rabbit S1 perforator and latissimus dorsi musculocutaneous flaps. J Reconstr Microsurg. 2005; 21(2):137–143

[59] Salgado CJ, Mardini S, Jamali AA, Ortiz J, Gonzales R, Chen H-C. Muscle versus nonmuscle flaps in the reconstruction of chronic osteomyelitis defects. Plast Reconstr Surg. 2006; 118(6):1401–1411

[60] Hong JP, Shin HW, Kim JJ, Wei F-C, Chung YK. The use of anterolateral thigh perforator flaps in chronic osteomyelitis of the lower extremity. Plast Reconstr Surg. 2005; 115(1):142–147

[61] Pollak AN, McCarthy ML, Burgess AR, The Lower Extremity Assessment Project (LEAP) Study Group. Short-term wound complications after application of flaps for coverage of traumatic soft-tissue defects about the tibia. J Bone Joint Surg Am. 2000; 82(12):1681–1691

[62] Parrett BM, Matros E, Pribaz JJ, Orgill DP. Lower extremity trauma: trends in the management of soft-tissue reconstruction of open tibia-fibula fractures. Plast Reconstr Surg. 2006; 117(4):1315–1322, discussion 1323–1324

[63] Rodriguez ED, Bluebond-Langner R, Copeland C, Grim TN, Singh NK, Scalea T. Functional outcomes of posttraumatic lower limb salvage: a pilot study of anterolateral thigh perforator flaps versus muscle flaps. J Trauma. 2009; 66 (5):1311–1314

[64] Nielsen PR, Jørgensen LD, Dahl B, Pedersen T, Tønnesen H. Prehabilitation and early rehabilitation after spinal surgery: randomized clinical trial. Clin Rehabil. 2010; 24(2):137–148

[65] Tayrose G, Newman D, Slover J, Jaffe F, Hunter T, Bosco J, III. Rapid mobilization decreases length-of-stay in joint replacement patients. Bull Hosp Jt Dis (2013). 2013; 71(3):222–226

[66] Wang D, Teddy PJ, Henderson NJ, Shine BS, Gardner BP. Mobilization of patients after spinal surgery for acute spinal cord injury. Spine. 2001; 26 (20):2278–2282

[67] Schoppen T, Boonstra A, Groothoff JW, De Vries J, Göeken LN, Eisma WH. Job satisfaction and health experience of people with a lower-limb amputation in comparison with healthy colleagues. Arch Phys Med Rehabil. 2002; 83 (5):628–634

[68] Schoppen T, Boonstra A, Groothoff JW, van Sonderen E, Göeken LN, Eisma WH. Factors related to successful job reintegration of people with a lower limb amputation. Arch Phys Med Rehabil. 2001; 82(10):1425–1431

[69] Dumanian, G. A., Potter, B. K., Mioton, L. M., Ko, J. H., Cheesborough, J. E., Souza, J. M., ... & Kuiken, T. A. (2019). Targeted muscle reinnervation treats neuroma and phantom pain in major limb amputees: a randomized clinical trial. Annals of surgery, 270(2), 238–246

[70] Ovelmen-Levitt J. Abnormal physiology of the dorsal horn as related to the deafferentation syndrome. Appl Neurophysiol. 1988; 51(2–5):104–116

[71] MR Z, LS L. Microvascular Reconstruction of the Lower Extremity. Seminars in surgical oncology. 2000;19(3)

[72] Nigam, M., Webb, A., Harbour, P., Devulapalli, C., & Kleiber, G. (2019). Symptomatic Neuromas in Lower Extremity Amputees: Implications for Pre-emptive-targeted Muscle Reinnervation. Plastic and Reconstructive Surgery–Global Open, 7(8S-1), 80–81

Index

Note: Page numbers set **bold** or *italic* indicate headings or figures, respectively.